THE WORDSWORTH
FAMILY MEDICAL
ENCYCLOPEDIA

THE WORDSWORTH

FAMILY
MEDICAL
ENCYCLOPEDIA

*Compiled and edited by the Staff of
MedicaPress International, Inc. and MedicaPress,
AG., The National Encyclopedia, Inc.*

WORDSWORTH EDITIONS

First published in Great Britain 1999
by Wordsworth Editions Limited
Cumberland House, Crib Street, Ware, Herts SG12 9ET

This edition published 1998
by Wordsworth Editions Limited
Cumberland House, Crib Street, Ware,
Hertfordshire SG12 9ET

ISBN 1 84022 023 6

Printed and bound in Great Britain
by Mackays of Chatham plc, Chatham, Kent.

THE WORDSWORTH
FAMILY MEDICAL ENCYCLOPEDIA

The *Wordsworth Family Medical Encyclopedia* gives you the information you need to take an active part in your own health care and has been created to help you protect your family's health and well-being.

The Encyclopedia has been prepared by a committee of authors, consultants and editors and represents the committee's understanding of medical, pharmaceutical, dental, and biological knowledge expressed in non-technical terms for the benefit of readers with no medical qualification.

The Encyclopedia has been reviewed by the committee at the latest possible date before publication to ensure that the information and advice given in the book is up to date.

The Wordsworth series of encyclopedias has been designed as a clear and comprehensive library for the lay public of information about medical, psychological and dental matters and covers also the field of healthy living with encyclopedias on prescription medicines, nonprescription medicines, family first aid, fitness programs, food & nutrition, vitamins and minerals, etc.

COLLABORATING INSTITUTIONS

National Institutes of Health, USA
National Cancer Institute, USA
Department of Medicine, University of New York
Department of Pathology, University of San Francisco
Medical Library Foundation, Switzerland
Faculty of Medicine, Free University, Brussels
Faculty of Medicine, University of Utrecht

NOTE

In this *Family Health Encyclopedia*, the authors and editors have done their best to outline the symptoms and general treatment for various conditions, injuries and diseases. Also, recommendations are made regarding certain drugs, medications, and preparations, and descriptions of certain medical tests and procedures are offered.

Different people react to the same treatment, medication, preparation, test or procedure in different ways. The Wordsworth series of encyclopedias does not attempt to answer all questions about all situations that you may encounter.

Neither the editors of Family Medical Encyclopedia, nor the consultants, authors or publisher take responsibility for any possible consequences from any treatment, procedure, test, action or application of medication or preparation by any person reading or following the information in this encyclopedia. The publication of this encyclopedia does not constitute the practice of medicine, and this book does not attempt to replace your physician. The authors, editors and publisher advise the reader to check with a physician before administering any medication or undertaking any course of treatment.

THE WORDSWORTH FAMILY MEDICAL ENCYCLOPEDIA

A – Z

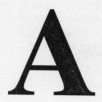

AA (Alcoholics Anonymous)

Worldwide organization numbering over 1.5 million anonymous members, in which former alcoholics aid those suffering from alcoholism. It stresses self-help, and all involved pool their experiences for mutual encouragement.

ABARTICULATION

Dislocation of a joint, for instance a pulled-out shoulder.

ABASIA

Inability to walk, generally caused by a disorder of the cerebellum.

AB BLOOD TYPE

One of the four blood groups (the others being A, B, and 0) in the AB0 blood group system, for classifying human blood based on the presence or absence of two antigens - A and B - on the surface of red blood cells; it is the least common of the four groups in our population. A person with type AB blood has both antigens and does not produce antibodies against either.

ABC LINIMENT

Liniment containing aconite, belladonna and chloroform. It is used for rubbing on painful muscles and joints but should not be used on broken skin.

ABDOMEN

The part of the body between the chest and the pelvis; the belly, including the stomach, liver, intestines, and other organs called the viscera.

ABDOMINAL BREATHING

Breathing in which the diaphragmatic muscle action is reinforced by the abdominal muscles. Such breathing occurs more in men than in women and is commonly practiced by singers.

ABDOMINAL DELIVERY

Delivery of a child through an incision in the abdomen.

ABDOMINALGIA

Pain arising within the abdomen.

ABDOMINAL HERNIA

Hernia in which a portion of an organ protrudes through the muscular walls of the abdomen, forming a swelling.

ABDOMINAL MIGRAINE

Sudden stomach aches, headaches and nausea in children, which occur every few days, weeks or months. Generally the pain lasts a few hours.

When asked to locate the ache, the child usually points to the navel. Only a small proportion of children with recurrent abdominal aches have an underlying physical problem.

ABDOMINAL PREGNANCY

Pregnancy in which the conceptus develops in the abdominal cavity, not in the uterus; occurs in about 2 percent of ectopic pregnancies and usually results in fetal death.

ABDOMINOCENTESIS

Operation of draining the peritoneal cavity abdomen of fluid which may be due to liver disease or a growth.

ABDOMINOPELVIC

Pertaining to the abdomen and pelvis.

ABDOMINOSCOPY

Examination of the interior of the abdomen by means of an instrument inserted through its wall.

ABDOMINOVAGINAL
Pertaining to the abdomen and vagina.

ABDUCENS
(abducens nerve) Sixth cranial nerve. It supplies the external rectus muscle of the eye, and paralysis of this nerve and muscle produces a squint.

ABDUCT
To draw away from the middle line of the body. If the arm is moved sideways from the body it is said to have been abducted. The reverse movement is called adduction.

ABDUCTION
The act of kidnapping, of forcibly taking away. Abduction also means the movement of a part of the body away from the midline.

ABDUCTOR
Muscle producing the movement of abduction.

ABERRANT
Departure from normal. Usually refers to a mental disorder or to an error of refraction in a lens.

ABERRATION, EMOTIONAL
Any emotional response other than that which might ordinarily be expected; an emotional illness, especially one in which the manifestation and symptoms are in themselves directly emotional.

ABIENCE
Type of behavior that moves the organism away from exposure to a stimulus.

ABILITY
Power to perform an act, physical or mental, either before or after training. The term "general ability" is used of a wide range of mental capacities or, specifically, of a general factor affecting all mental operations.

ABILITY TEST
Test to demonstrate a particular level of knowledge or skill. An individual general ability test consists of eight small subtests:
- information test;
- analogies test;
- vocabulary;
- letter memory;
- number series;
- spatial relations;
- clock test;
- sign language test.

ABIOGENESIS
Also called spontaneous generation. The doctrine that living matter may be produced by nonliving matter.

ABIOTROPHY
An early loss of function or vitality of cells or tissues.

ABLATION
The act of removal of a bodily part by surgery.

A BLOOD TYPE
One of four blood groups (the others being AB, B, and 0) in the AB0 blood group system for classifying human blood based on the presence or absence of antigen A and/or B on the surface of red blood cells. A person with type A blood produces antibodies against B antigens that cause the blood cells to agglutinate, or clump together.

ABLUTION
A form of hydrotherapy given for insomnia that usually brings quiet, restful sleep.

ABLUTOMANIA
A preoccupation with thoughts about washing that frequently accompanies an obsessive-compulsive neurosis.

ABNORMALITY
Deviation from the norm; sickness, defect, but also disturbed, disorganized, maladjustive behavior.

AB0 BLOOD GROUP SYSTEM

The most important of several systems for classifying human blood, used in blood transfusion therapy. Based on the presence or absence of two antigens - A and B -on the surface of red blood cells, the system classifies four groups, type A, B, AB, and 0.

ABOCCLUSION

Condition in which the upper and lower jaws do not meet when closed.

ABOIEMENT

The uncontrollable and involuntary production of abnormal or unusual sounds.

For example, some severely regressive schizophrenic patients make many animalistic noises.

ABORTIFACIENT

Something that produces an abortion.

ABORTION

Termination of pregnancy; expulsion or removal of the embryo or fetus before it reaches full development and can normally be expected to be capable of independent life. Abortion may be spontaneous or induced.

ABORTIONIST

One who induces abortions, especially illegal or unauthorized abortions.

ABORTUS

A dead or nonviable fetus (weighing less than 500 g (17.5 oz) at birth).

ABOULIA

Inability, usually pathological, to make or to act on decisions.

ABRACHIA

Developmental anomaly characterized by complete absence of the arms.

ABRASION

Rubbing off of the surface of the skin or of the mucous membrane due to some mechanical injury. It can be intentional or unintentional, for example a sore produced by chafing.

Small superficial abrasions can be simply treated with soap and water, but interior abrasions must be treated by a doctor.

In dentistry, abrasion means the mechanical or chemical wearing down or grinding off of the enamel and dentine (the hard bone-like part of the teeth); this is called abrasio dentinum.

ABRASIO UTERI

Term used for scraping off the lining of the uterus.

ABREACTION

Treatment used by psychiatrists to obtain a patient's emotional release. By administering various drugs, especially carbon dioxide inhalations, the patient is made to relive the incident causing his fear or worry.

As a sequel to his emotional discharge, which somewhat resembles an hysterical attack, the patient experiences a sensation of relief from his previous tensed-up and worried condition.

ABREACTION, MOTOR

Living through an unconscious emotion or experience by muscular or motor expression.

ABRIN

A potent toxin which is derived from the seeds of the jequirity plant and which causes red cells to stick together (a lectin).

ABRUPTIO PLACENTAE

Premature separation of a normally implanted placenta from the uterus. All degrees from a few mm coming apart to complete detachment may occur. The cause is unknown.

ABSCESS
A localized accumulation of pus, usually representing one response of the body to infection by bacteria and other micro-organisms.

Important terms - abscess

Acute abscess
A lesion, of recent occurrence, produced by staphylococci, streptococci or other pus-producing organisms.

Apical abscess
An abscess in the apex of a lung, or one in the alveolus in the extremity of the root of a tooth.

Appendicular abscess
An abscess in the region of the vermiform appendix.

Bone abscess
Suppuration (osteomyelitis) within the central cavity of a bone or beneath the periosteum which covers it.

Brodie's abscess
Chronic inflammation, sometimes tuberculous, of the head of a bone, especially of the tibia.

Dental abscess
A walled-off or circumscribed area of inflammation, usually within the apex of a tooth, resulting from extensive dental caries.

Douglas's abscess
Suppuration in Douglas's pouch, a pocket formed by a fold of the peritoneum from the rectum to the uterus.

Follicular abscess
One in a hair follicle.

Glandular abscess
An abscess, within any gland, but especially in or around a lymph node.

Metastatic abscess
A secondary abscess formed, at a distance from the first one, as a result of the transportation of the pus germs by the lymph system or bloodstream.

Peritonsillar abscess
Quinsy; the formation of an abscess behind the tonsils, usually as a result of acute tonsillitis.

Residual abscess
An abscess, recurring at the site of a former abscess resulting from the persistence of microbes and pus.

Retropharyngeal abscess
An abscess usually arising in retropharyngeal lymph nodes, in the back of the throat.

Subphrenic abscess
A collection of pus between the peritoneum covering the surface of the diaphragm and the peritoneum covering the surface of the liver or that of the spleen and stomach.

ABSENCE
Brief generalized seizures (epileptic attacks) manifested by a 10- to 30-second loss of consciousness, with eye or muscle flutterings at a rate of three per second, and with or without loss of muscle tone. Patients suddenly stop any activity in which they are engaged and resume it after the attack.

ABSENCE, ATONIC
A complex absence characterized by a loss of control of the postural muscles sufficient to cause the subject to slump to the ground.

ABSENCE, AUTOMATIC
A complex absence characterized by usually simple epileptic automatisms, for example, involuntary movements of the lips or tongue, or behavior such as rubbing the hands together or adjusting the clothes.

ABSENCE, ENURETIC
A complex absence characterized by urinary incontinence. Such absences must be differentiated from partial seizures of temporal lobe origin, which may be accompanied by urinary incontinence or, more frequently, by automatisms of urination.

ABSENCE, HYPERTONIC
A complex absence characterized by a tensing of the postural muscles causing the head to be pulled backwards, the eyes to roll up into the head and, sometimes, the arching of the back; the latter may force subjects to walk backwards in order to keep their balance.

ABSENTMINDEDNESS
Being so absorbed in thought so as to be largely unaware of surrounding conditions.

ABSINTHEISM
The damaging effects on tissues and organs caused by excessive amounts of absinthe, a formerly popular French liqueur or cordial consisting of brandy flavored with wormwood.

ABSOLUTE THRESHOLD
The intensity or frequency at which a stimulus becomes effective, as measured under experimental conditions. It takes a certain minimum of sense-organ stimulation to evoke any sensory experience at all. This minimum is called the absolute threshold.

Thus a spot of light coming on in a dark room must reach some measurable intensity before it can be distinguished from darkness, and a sound coming on in a soundproof room must reach a certain intensity before it can be heard.

ABSORBENT
The ability of something to absorb; a substance applied to a wound to staunch or arrest the flow of blood.

ABSORPTION
In medicine term used in two different senses.
(1) Focusing attention on one object, thereby excluding other objects.
(2) Excluding reality because the focus of one's attention is on autistic thoughts.

ABSTEMIOUSNESS
A way of life characterized by refraining from a free use of food and strong drinks.

ABSTRACTION
The mental process of forming abstract ideas. An "abstraction experiment" is the name given to a type of experiment in which the subject is required to respond verbally, or in action, to common features in objects or situations presented serially.

ABSTRUSENESS
The quality of being remote from ordinary minds or notions. It also means difficulty in being comprehended or understood.

ABSURDITIES TEST
A type of mental test in which the subject is asked to point out what is absurd about a statement, story or picture.

ABUNDANCE MOTIVE
Desire to experience enjoyment, to obtain gratification, to seek novelty, to discover and understand, to attempt to achieve and create. This motive includes the goals of satisfaction and stimulation.

ACANTHOCYTE
An abnormal red blood cell with irregular projections of protoplasm, giving it a spiny or thorny appearance.

ACANTHOCYTOSIS
Breakdown of the thorny-cell layer of the epidermis (for instance, in the skin disorder pemphigus vulgaris).

ACANTHOMA
A tumor of the outer-skin cells.

ACANTHOSIS
Overdevelopment and thickening of the prickle-cell layer of the outer skin, as in psoriasis.

ACAPNIA
Diminished carbon dioxide content of the blood; can be produced by hyperventilation.

ACARIASIS
A skin disease caused by mites.

ACCESSION
The attack or commencement of a disease or disorder.

ACCIDENT
An unexpected happening, especially one that results in injury.

ACCIDENT PREVENTION
Measures to be taken to prevent accidents in the house, on the road, in the factory or laboratory, during sports activities, etc. Both fatal and non-fatal household accidents hold a prominent place in accident statistics. Most of the fatalities - some 75 percent - occur among the aged: people over 70 years of age.

ACCIDENT-PRONE
Having a greater-than-average incidence of accidents.

ACCIDENT PRONENESS
High incidence of accidents in certain individuals.

ACCLIMATIZATION
The process of adjustment that allows an individual organism to survive under changed conditions. In a hot, sunny climate, man acclimatizes by eating less, drinking more and wearing lighter clothes; furthermore, his skin may darken. At higher altitudes, he can adjust to the diminished oxygen by increased production of red blood corpuscles.

ACCOMMODATION
(1) The adjustment of the eye lens whereby it is able to focus a clear image on to the retina.
(2) The continuing process of adjusting to one's environment.

ACCOUCHEUR
A man who acts as a midwife, attending women in childbirth.

ACCRETION
The growing together of parts naturally separated, such as the fingers or toes.

ACCUPRO
A brand name for quinapril, an ACE inhibitor with hydrochlorothiazide, a diuretic.

ACE INHIBITORS
A family of drugs used to treat hypertension and congestive heart disease. Inhibitors decrease the rate of conversion of angiotensin I into angiotensin II, which is the normal process for the angiotensin-converting enzyme.
These drugs include benazepril, captopril, enalapril, fosinopril, lisinopril, ramipril.

ACENESTHESIA
Absence or lack of the feeling or perception of one's own body.

ACEPHALY
The state of possessing no head.

ACETABULOPLASTY
Surgical repair of the cup-like socket of the haunch bone, into which the head of the femur fits to form the hip joint.

ACETABULUM
The cavity in the pelvis that receives the head of the thigh bone.

ACETAL
An organic compound formed by a combination of an aldehyde with an alcohol.

ACETATE
Any salt of acetic acid.

ACETIC ACID
Acid prepared by the oxidation of alcohol. Used as a liniment, in concentrated form to treat warts and corns, and in cough mixtures.

ACETONE
A ketone body in blood or urine produced by metabolic disease or disturbance.

ACETONEMIA
An excess of ketone bodies in the blood.

ACETONURIA
An excess of ketone bodies in the urine.

ACETYLCHOLINE (ACh)
A substance playing an important role in the transmission of nerve impulses within the nervous system. On release from the end of one nerve fiber, it stimulates the adjoining one before being rapidly broken down by the enzyme cholinesterase to choline and acetic acid, of which it is the ester.

Acetylcholine also plays an important role in the transmission of impulses from the nervous system to muscles.

ACETYLCYSTEINE
A compound with mucolytic (dissolvement of mucus) properties, used as an aid in various bronchial disorders, and is invaluable in mucoviscidosis. Also given intravenously in cases of paracetamol poisoning.

ACETYLSALICYLIC ACID
Another name for aspirin.

ACHALASIA
A spasm of the cardiac sphincter at the lower end of the esophagus. The cause of this is unknown, and it results in the impairment of esopha-geal peristalsis (involuntary swallowing). The condition may be due to a disturbed function of the myenteric plexus of the esophagus that results in denervation of esophageal muscle.

Vomiting of undigested food at night occurs in about one-third of the patients, and this may be breathed into the lungs causing lung abscesses, bronchiectasis or pneumonia.

ACHE
Pain, or continuous pain, as opposed to sudden twinges (spasmodic pain); a continuous gnawing pain as in toothache or earache.

ACHIEVEMENT
Performance in a standardized series of tests, usually educational.

ACHIEVEMENT AGE
The chronological age corresponding to any particular level on a scale of achievement tests.

ACHIEVEMENT MOTIVE
The social motive to accomplish something of value or importance, to meet standards of excellence in what one does. A great deal of human effort can be understood in relation to the motive to accomplish something of value and importance. This motive is familiar to us, since we have been reared in a culture which considers enterprise and success as marks of esteem.

ACHIEVEMENT QUOTIENT
The ratio of achievement age to the chronological age of the individual tested, expressed as a percentage.

ACHILLES HEEL
The point of weakness that is most vulnerable or susceptible. In the Achilles myth, it was the warrior's only vulnerable part.

ACHILLES TENDON
The tendon from the calf muscles to

the heel bone, important in standing, walking and running.

Achilles tendon disorders may be caused by mistakes in athletic training. The force in the Achilles tendon when the foot is flexed during running is estimated to be in the region of 600 kilograms (1320 lb), and this is repeated 1000 to 1200 times per mile. Sudden increases in training intensity and overuse through excessive mileage can produce slight damage or make existing problems worse. Uphill running demands increased flexibility and force, and can aggravate the Achilles tendon.

ACHILLES TENDON RUPTURE

Severe injury occurring in athletes who recommence training after long periods of relative inactivity. Training causes an increase in size and an increase in blood supply in active tissues; stopping training leads to a decrease in the blood supply. Upon recommencement of hard training, the diminished blood supply cannot meet the nutritional requirements of the active tendon, triggering a localized lack of blood, degeneration and rupture. A gradual return to the original level of activity can minimize the likelihood of this happening.

ACHILLODYNIA
Pain in the Achilles tendon or its bursa.

ACHILLORAPHY
Suturing of the Achilles tendon.

ACHILLOTOMY
Subcutaneous surgical division of the Achilles tendon, sometimes performed on spastic children.

ACHLORHYDRIA
Absence of hydrochloric acid from the stomach juice, a condition found in pernicious anemia and gastric cancer.

ACHOLIA
Lack or absence of bile secretion due to compression of the bile duct or its blockage by a stone.

ACHOLURIA
Lack of bile pigments in the urine: an indication of a hemolytic anemia.

ACHONDROPLASIA
Defective development of cartilage causing dwarfism.

ACHROMATIN
That portion of the nucleus of a cell which is unstainable.

ACHROMATOPSIA
Inability to distinguish colors, arising from some defect in the eye.

ACHROMYCIN
Brand name of a tetracycline antibiotic drug.

ACHYLIA
Absence or severe deficiency of hydrochloric acid, pepsinogen, or other digestive secretions.

ACID
(1) A compound that contains hydrogen as an essential constituent and has a sour taste;
(2) the hallucinogenic drug LSD.

ACID-BASE BALANCE
A normal equilibrium between the acid and base elements of the blood and body fluids.

ACIDEMIA
Abnormal acidity of the blood, caused by poor breathing or increased lactic acid from the muscles.

ACIDITY
The quality of being acid or sour.

ACIDOPHILIC
Having the quality of being easy to stain with acid.

ACIDOSIS
Abnormally acid condition of the blood.

ACID PHOSPHATASE
An enzyme capable of catalyzing the hydrolysis of esterified phosphoric acid, with liberation of inorganic phosphate. The enzyme is secreted by the prostate gland and some other organs.

ACID REFLUX
Condition in which acid fluid from the stomach wells up into the esophagus, usually caused by a hiatus hernia of the diaphragm. The condition can be tested by specific drugs.

ACIDURIA
Abnormally acid urine, usually caused by a metabolic disorder.

ACINI
Minute sacs or alveoli, filled with secreting cells. The liver acini are the smallest functional units of the liver.

ACME
The height of a crisis of disease or mental disorder.

ACMESTHESIA
Sensing sharp points with touch without pain sensation.

ACNE
An inflammatory disease of the sebaceous glands of the skin, usually on the face and upper body, characterized by papules, pustules, comedones (blackheads) and in severe cases by cysts, and scarring.

ACNE CONGLOBATA
Severe acne vulgaris with many comedones, marked by the formation of pus, cysts and scarring.

ACNEIFORM
Resembling acne, in particular acne vulgaris.

ACNE PREPARATIONS
Creams, lotions and liquids applied to the skin to treat acne. These include alcohol and acetone; alcohol and sulfur; benzoyl peroxide; clindamycin; erythromycin; salicylic acid lotion; salicylic acid and sulfur cleansing suspension; etc.

ACNE ROSACEA
Chronic disease of the skin of the nose, forehead and cheeks, marked by flushing, red coloration due to dilatation of the capillaries, with appearance of pimples and acne-like pustules.

ACORIA
An insatiable desire for food because the individual never feels full after eating.

ACOUSTIC
Pertaining to the sense or organs of hearing, or to the science of sound.

ACOUSTIC NEURINOMA
Tumor formed from the Schwann cells of the eighth cranial nerve that links the brain with the ear. Hearing loss and tinnitus are early symptoms.

ACOUSTICS
The cause, nature and phenomena of the vibrations of elastic bodies that affect the organ of hearing. individual's lifetime.

ACQUIRED IMMUNE DEFICIENCY SYNDROME
The full name of AIDS.

ACQUIRED IMMUNITY
Any form of immunity not innate but obtained during life.

ACRID
Sharp or biting to the taste or smell.

ACRIDINE DERIVATIVES
Dyers or stains (usually yellow or orange) used for some medical tests and as antiseptic agents.

ACRIFLAVINE
A derivative of acridine, a compound found in coal tar, used chiefly in medicine as an antiseptic yellow dye.

ACRO-ARTHRITIS
Arthritic condition of the joints of the hands or feet, usually rheumatoid arthritis.

ACROCYANOSIS
Persistent, painless cyanosis (a bluish tinge) of both hands and, less commonly, both feet, caused by spasms of the smaller blood vessels of the skin. The cause is unknown.

ACRODYNIA
Also called erythredema and "pink disease." A disease of infants marked by pain and swelling in, and pink coloration of, the fingers and toes and by listlessness, irritability, failure to thrive and profuse perspiration. The disease is usually caused by mercury poisoning.

ACROMEGALY
A rare disease, associated with the overgrowing of bone, especially in the jaws, hands and feet.

ACROMIAL
Pertaining to the acromion.

ACROMION
The outward end of the scapula or shoulder blade where it forms the tip of the shoulder.

ACRONYX
Ingrowing of a nail.

ACROPHOBIA
A morbid fear of heights, sometimes associated with physical symptoms; often an isolated phobia in otherwise normal people. Severe conditions require psychotherapy.

ACROTISM
An absence or weakness of the pulse.

ACTH
Adrenocorticotrop(h)in; the hormone of the anterior pituitary gland which specifically stimulates the cortex of the adrenal glands to produce corticosteroids.

ACTIN
A protein important in the contraction of muscles.

ACTING OUT
Activity as a substitute for remembering past events. The essence of the concept is the replacement of thought by action and it implies that either the impulse being acted out has never been talked about by the person, or the impulse is too intense to be put into words, or that the person lacks the capacity for inhibition. Since psychoanalysis is a "talking cure" carried out in a state of reflection, acting out is antitherapeutic. Acting out is characteristic of psychopathy and behavior disorders and reduces the accessibility of these conditions to psychoanalysis.

ACTINISM
The chemical action in cells and tissues of the body caused by the rays of light beyond the violet end of the spectrum. Actinic means producing chemical action.

ACTINODERMATITIS
An inflammation of the skin, caused by prolonged exposure to the sun's rays.

ACTINOMYCETE
A member of the order Actinomycetales, which contains rod-shaped or filamentous bacteria.

ACTINOMYCIN
One of the yellow-red polypeptide antibiotics separated from soil bacteria, used in the treatment of cancer.

ACTINOMYCIN D
An anticancer drug known to inhibit

multiplication of cancer cells.

ACTINOMYCOSIS
Chronic infectious disease caused by the microorganism Actinomyces israeli, often (and usually harmlessly) present on the gums, tonsils and teeth. The disease is seen most often in adult males.

In the form found in the neck and face, the most common point of entry is via decayed teeth; the lung disease results from the breathing in of secretions from the mouth; and the abdominal disease occurs because of a break in the mucosa of a diverticulum (a pocket in the lining of the intestine) or the appendix.

ACTINOTHERAPY
Treatment of disease by rays of light, especially ultraviolet or infrared radiation.

ACTION POTENTIAL
An electrical impulse or wave of negativity along a conducting neuron.

Not all electrical stimuli will generate action potentials. The stimulus must be large enough to decrease the membrane potential to a certain critical level, called the threshold.

ACTION SYSTEM
All the glands, nerves and muscles involved in the production of a particular response.

ACTIVATED CHARCOAL
A general antidote used to treat some forms of acute poisoning.

ACTIVATED LYMPHOCYTE
A lymphocyte altered by passage through the thymus (T cell), that has become stimulated by contact with antigen and is therefore able to induce a cell-mediated immune reaction.

ACTIVE ANALYSIS
A technique in which the analyst in psychoanalysis takes a more dominating role in the treatment process.

ACTIVE FANTASIZING
A psychotherapeutic procedure involving the analysis of the patient's spontaneous imagination.

Through the analysis of fantasized images, the analyst can uncover the unconscious roots of the patient's conflicts and help the patient to bring them into conscious awareness.

ACTIVE IMMUNITY
A form of acquired immunity in which the body produces its own antibodies against disease-causing antigens. It can occur naturally after infection or artificially after vaccination.

ACTIVE THERAPY
A method of psychoanalytic therapy sometimes used to break down a resistance.

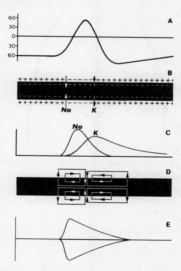

Summary of the events occurring during propagation of an impulse along a nerve.
A: action potential;
B: polarity of potential differences across the neuronal membrane;
C: changes in sodium and potassium permeabilities;
D: local circuit current flows;
E: variation in total membrane conductance.

ACUITY
Sharpness, clearness; for instance, visual acuity, the extent of how much you can see which is dependent on the clarity of the focus on the retina, how well your nerves are performing and on the interpretation of the stimuli by the brain.

ACUMEN
Quickness of perception, mental acuteness or penetration.

ACUPRESSURE
An old Japanese treatment system, comparable to acupuncture. It relies on the proper application of carefully applied pressure by the fingers or hand on specific points on the surface of the body to stimulate the natural curative abilities of the body.

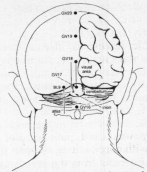

Scalp acupuncture lines superimposed on the functional zones of the brain.

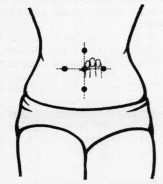

Acupressure points fort stomach and intestinal disturbances.

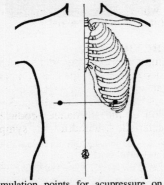

Stimulation points for acupressure on the frontal surface of the thorax.

ACUPUNCTURE
An ancient Chinese medical practice in which fine needles are inserted into the body at specific points, and is used for relieving pain and in treating a variety of conditions.

ACUTE
A term applied to a disease that is attended by more or less strong symptoms and comes speedily to a crisis.

ACUTE ABDOMEN
Acute disorder of abdominal organs, peritoneum or abdominal wall.

When no certain diagnosis can be made immediately, the best course of action may then be for the surgeon to open the abdomen and inspect the organs. This procedure is called laparotomy.

ACUTE ADRENAL FAILURE
Sudden failure of the function of the adrenal glands and their production of hormones. This can occur as a result of a condition such as Addison's disease. The symptoms are profound weakness, confusion and even collapse.

ACUTE BRAIN DISORDER
A complex collection of symptoms resulting from temporary impairment of the functions of the brain

tissue, such as disordered behavior occasionally induced by drugs.

ACUTE BRONCHITIS
Acute inflammation of the tracheo-bronchial tree of the lungs, which will generally run its course with eventual complete healing and return of function. Although usually mild, bronchitis may be serious in already weakened patients and in those with chronic lung or heart diseases. Pneumonia is a critical complication.

ACYANOSIS
Condition of the blood or blood vessels without cyanosis (a bluish tinge resulting from lack of oxygen in the blood).

ACYSTIA
Congenital absence of the bladder.

ADACTYLIA
Absence of fingers or toes or both from birth.

ADAM'S APPLE
The prominence of the thyroid cartilage at the front of the throat, predominantly in men.

ADAPTATION
The process of modification of the form or functions of a part of an organism, to make it fit for its environment and so achieve efficiency in life and reproduction. Adaptation of individual organisms is called acclimatization, and is temporary since it involves acquired characteristics; the permanent adaptation of species arises from transmitted genetic variations preserved by natural selection.

ADAPTATION SYNDROME
The syndrome comprises a series of phenomena arising in response to a trauma or lesion in man or in animals; the combined effect of the agents which cause this is called "stress.". The Canadian physician, Hans Selye, observed three stress stages:
(1) The alarm reaction: in grave stress, blood pressure falls, temperature rises, the blood thickens, etc. This stage may be fatal, but mostly it is of short duration and may go over into stage 2.
(2) The resistance phase, in which the conditions are counteracted. If the stress situation persists too long so that the compensating mechanisms cannot cope with it, the third stage may set in.
(3) The exhaustion phase, in which the symptoms of the alarm reaction recur. The adaptation syndrome is, among other things, influenced by hormones secreted by the anterior pituitary gland and the adrenal cortex.

ADAPTIVE BEHAVIOR
Behavior that brings the organism into adjustment with any variation in its environment. For an organism to survive, it must first of all maintain a favorable level of operation within its own body. Physiologists have discovered and studied a number of mechanisms that, in semi-automatic fashion, maintain the body activities at favorable levels. These mechanisms are known as homeostatic mechanisms and they are the basis of the adaptive behavior.

ADDICT
One who is addicted to a practice or a habit,especially to narcotics.

ADDICTION
A condition of strong and irresistible dependence on the use of a particular substance (for instance, cocaine, alcohol) such that abrupt deprivation of the substance produces characteristic withdrawal symptoms.

ADDICTIVE BEHAVIOR
Specific behavioral pattern of an addict.

ADDICTIVE DRUGS
Any drug that can lead to physiological dependence on the drug. These include alcohol, cocaine, marijuana, nicotine, opium, morphine, codeine, heroin (and other narcotics) and others.

ADDISON'S DISEASE
A slowly and usually progressive disease resulting from insufficient function of the cortex of the adrenal glands.
The major symptoms are:
- disturbed balance of sodium and potassium;
- lowered blood volume;
- lowered blood pressure;
- marked anemia;
- disorder of kidney function;
- low blood sugar;
- gastrointestinal upsets;
- pigmentation of the skin.

ADDITIVE
A substance added in small amounts to another for improvement, as a drug added to medicine.

ADDUCT
To draw (one's limb) toward the middle line of the body.

ADDUCTOR
The muscle that draws towards the middle line of the body.

ADENECTOMY
The surgical removal of a gland.

ADEN FEVER
An infectious, eruptive, usually epidemic fever of warm climates, characterized especially by severe pains in the joints and muscles.

ADENINE
A white, crystalline alkaloid, obtained from tea,glandular organs or uric acid.

ADENITIS
Inflammation of gland or lymph nodes.

ADENOCARCINOMA
A malignant tumor that appears in the lining tissue of glands.

ADENOFIBROMA
A benign tumor of connective tissue frequently found in the uterus.

ADENOID
A mass of lymph tissue in the nasopharynx (nasal cavity and throat).

ADENOIDECTOMY
Surgical removal of the adenoids.

ADENOID HYPERTROPHY
Enlargement of adenoidal tissue due to lymphoid hyperplasia (an abnormal increase in lymph tissue). The condition occurs in children and may have a physical cause or accompany an infection or allergy.

ADENOMA
A benign tumor in which the cells come from recognizable glandular structures or in which the cells are derived from the lining of a gland.

ADENOMATOSIS
The condition of multiple glandular enlargement.

ADENOMYOMA
The benign ingrowth of the endometrium (lining) of the uterus into its muscles. If this forms a circumscribed tumor-like nodule, it is called an adenomyoma.

ADENOPATHY
General term for a nonspecific disease of glands.

ADENOSARCOMA
A malignant growth with characteristics of adenoma and sarcoma.

ADENOSCLEROSIS
Hardening of a gland, with or without swelling, usually due to replacement by fibrous tissue or calcium salts. The condition may occur as a result of metabolic disorders.

ADENOSINE
A crystalline nucleotide which, upon undergoing hydrolysis, yields adenine and ribose.

ADENOSINE DIPHOSPHATE (ADP)
A co-enzyme, found in all living cells, important to the transfer of energy through the cell during glycolysis.

ADENOSINE TRIPHOSPHATE (ATP)
A nucleotide that occurs in all cells. It represents the reserve energy of muscle and is important in many biochemical processes that produce or require energy.

ADENOTONSILLECTOMY
Removal of both the tonsils and adenoids by a surgical procedure.

ADENOVIRUSES
A group of viruses causing a variety of acute disorders characterized by fever, inflammation of the mucous membranes in the breathing passages and around the eyes.

ADH
The abbreviation of antidiuretic hormone.

ADHESION
A growth of scar tissue resulting from an incision.

ADIPOSIS
The state of excessive obesity; an abnormally large amount of fat on the body.

ADIPOSIS DOLOROSA
Scattered areas of fat accumulation under the skin. The condition usually affects menopausal women.

ADIPOSOGENITAL DYSTROPHIA
Retarded development of the testes or ovaries and increased sugar tolerance, usually occurring in individuals during the pre- and post-adolescent period. The condition is the result of an impairment of the pituitary gland or the hypothalamus.

ADITUS
An entrance or opening. An approach to an organ.

ADIZEM-XL
A brand name for diltiazem, an anti-angina drug.

ADJUSTMENT
A change to a more satisfactory process, as in overcoming emotional problems.

ADJUSTMENT DISORDER
A maladaptive reaction to an identifiable psychosocial stressor, or stressors, that occurs within three months after onset of the stressor, and has persisted for no longer than six months. The maladaptive nature of the reaction is indicated either by impairment in occupational (including school) functioning or in unusual social activities or relationships with others or by symptoms that are in excess of a normal and expectable reaction to the stressor.

The disturbance is not merely one instance of a normal pattern of overreaction to stress or an exacerbation of one of the major mental disorders. It is assumed that the disturbance will remit soon after the stressor ceases or, if the stressor persists, when a new level of adaptation is achieved.

ADJUSTMENT REACTION
Mild or transient psychological disorders lasting longer than acute stress reactions which occur in individuals of any age without any apparent pre-existing mental disorder. Such disorders are often relatively circumscribed or situation-specific, are generally reversible and usually last only a few months. They are often closely related in time and content to stresses such as bereave-

ment, moving or separation from family. Reactions to major stress that last longer than a few days are also included here. In children such disorders are associated with no significant distortion of development.

ADJUVANT
A substance added to a prescription to aid the operation of the principal ingredient. An adjuvant is a drug that enhances the therapeutic effect of another drug, but that does not necessarily have a beneficial effect when used alone.

An example is aluminum, which is added to certain vaccines to enhance the immune response, thereby increasing the protection given by the vaccine.

ADL
Abbreviation of "Activities of Daily Living." ADL is a major program in the rehabilitation of disabled people. The ultimate goal for all disabled people is to return to gainful employment and the maximum of independence.

Although this goal is possible for many, there are others for whom minimal dependence is a triumph, those whose disability has deprived them of the ability to perform the simple, often automatic functions which are so basic that they are not appreciated until we lose them - in other words, the activities of daily living: personal hygiene, eating, dressing and other operations.

ADLER, Alfred
(1870-1939) Distinguished Austrian psychiatrist who proposed a system of psychiatric theory and therapy which he named individual psychology.

ADLER'S THEORY
An approach to psychology and psychiatry based on the hypothesis that behavior is governed by an effort to compensate for inferiority or deficiency.

ADNEXA
Adjoining parts; accessory parts equalling onestructure as, for instance, the ovaries and Fallopian tubes.

ADOLESCENCE
The period of life between childhood and the full development of the frame (between about 12 and 23 years of age).

ADOLESCENT CRISIS
The emotional changes that occur during adolescence. The adolescent ego is confronted with new challenges, achieving independence, casting off emotional ties and developing new ones. Both physiological and psychological events, during this time, present problems for the adolescent to deal with before reaching maturity.

ADOPTION
The creation of a parent-child relationship where no such natural or legal relationship exists.

ADP
Acronym for adenosine diphosphate.

ADRENAL
Pertaining to the adrenal glands or its secretions.

ADRENAL CORTICOSTEROID
Drug related to hydrocortisone, corticosterone or deoxycorticosterone used primarily for its ability to reduce inflammation. Also used to replace natural corticosteroids in deficient patients.

ADRENALECTOMY
Removal of an adrenal gland.

ADRENAL CORTEX
Center of the adrenal gland.

ADRENAL GLANDS
Small endocrine glands lying in the abdomen in the space behind the

peritoneum, closely attached to the upper part of each kidney, but not related to the function of the kidneys. The medulla produces adrenaline and noradrenaline and the cortex corticosteroids.

ADRENALINE
A hormone secreted by the adrenal glands, together with smaller quantities of noradrenaline. The nerve endings of the sympathetic nervous system also secrete both hormones (noradrenaline in greater quantities). They are similar chemically and in their effects. These constitute the 'fight or flight' response to stress situations: blood pressure is raised, smaller blood vessels are constricted, heart rate is increased, metabolism is accelerated, and levels of blood sugar and fatty acids are raised. Adrenaline is used as a heart stimulant, and to treat serious acute allergies.

ADRENAL VIRILISM
The result of adrenogenital syndrome.

ADRENERGIC
Liberated or activated by adrenaline or a similar substance.

ADRENERGIC BLOCKING AGENTS
Drugs which block the normal response of an organ or tissue to nerve impulses transmitted by the sympathetic nervous system. Blocking adrenergic nerves to the heart and blood vessels tends to decrease the heart rate and the vigor of heart contraction and to suppress the constriction of blood vessels. Adrenergic blocking agents are often used to treat angina pectoris, since by reducing heart work they reduce its need for oxygen. Some are also used to treat arrhythmias (irregular heartbeats), and to control high blood pressure, especially when is accompanied by a hyperactive heart. There are two classes of these

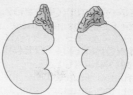

Localization of the adrenal glands on top of the kidneys.

drugs, alpha-and beta-adrenergic blocking agents. Both can be used in cardiovascular disorders, although beta-adrenergic blocking agents are used more often; of these, propranolol is the most common.

ADRENERGIC-RESPONSE RATE
Personality characteristics generally indicative of high levels of adrenaline secretion, such as high blood pressure, rapid pulse and high blood sugar level.

ADRENOCORTICOIDS
Medicines that belong to the general family of steroids. Your body naturally produces certain cortisone-like hormones which are necessary to maintain good health. If your body does not produce enough, your doctor may have prescribed this medicine to help make up the difference. Cortisone-like medicines are used also to provide relief for inflamed areas of the body. They lessen swelling, redness, itching, and allergic reactions.

They are often used as part of the treatment for a number of different diseases, such as severe allergies or skin problems, asthma, or arthritis. They may also be used for other conditions as determined by your doctor.

Possible side effects are:
- decreased or blurred vision;
- frequent urination;
- increased thirst;
- rectal bleeding;
- acne;
- stomach pain.

ADRENOCORTICOTROPHIC
Affecting the adrenal cortex.

ADRENOCORTICOTROP(H)IC HORMONE (ACTH)
A hormone secreted by the front part of the pituitary gland which stimulates the adrenal cortex.

ADRENOGENITAL SYNDROME
Any syndrome, congenital or acquired, in which excessive output of adrenal androgens causes virilization, in which male characteristics become emphasized. The effects depend on the sex and age of the patient when the disease begins, and are more marked in women than in men.

ADSORBENT
Substance which is capable of adsorbing.

ADSORPTION
Concentration of a substance on or near the surface of any solid or liquid. This is entirely different from absorption, which is the soaking up of a substance into the texture of a material.

ADULTERATION
Pollution. Usually means the fraudulent addition of a cheap substitute to foods or medicine instead of the full quantity of a more expensive article.

ADULTERY
Voluntary sexual intercourse by a married person with one who is not his or her wife or husband.

ADULTHOOD
Period of life between 24 and 45 years of age.

ADULT RUMINATION
The usually involuntary regurgitation of small amounts of food from the stomach (most often 15 to 30 minutes after eating), rechewing the material and, in most cases, again swallowing it. The reasons why this occurs are poorly understood.

ADVENTITIA
The outer of the three layers composing the walls of blood vessels.

ADVERSE REACTION
An unexpected or unpredictable reaction to a drug that is unrelated to the drug's unusual effects. The cause may sometimes be an allergic reaction or a genetic disorder, such as the lack of an enzyme that normally inactivates the drug.

AEDES
A genus of mosquitoes, including approximately 500 species; some are vectors of disease, such as Aedes aegypti, a vector of yellow fever and dengue.

AEGOPHONY
Curious noise (sometimes described as like the bleat of a goat) heard through a stethoscope when listening to the chest of someone suffering from pleurisy witheffusion (inflammation of the membranes surrounding the lungs, in which fluid accumulates between lung and chest wall).

AEREMIA
Presence of air in the blood. Usually a fatal condition and sometimes the cause of death in criminal abortion.

AEROANAEROBIC
A term applied to bacteria capable of living both in the presence and absence of oxygen.

AEROBIC ORGANISM
A microorganism that requires atmospheric oxygen in order to grow.

AEROEMBOLISM
Presence of air in the blood circulation that blocks an artery. Direct entry of air into veins may occur

through injury, cannulation (the insertion of tubes) or surgery, and a large air bubble reaching the heart may cause death.

In acute decompression (as occurs in flying to high altitude or sudden surfacing after deep diving) bubbles of air come out of solution, and these may block small blood vessels causing severe muscle pains ("bends"), tingling and choking sensations and occasionally paralysis or coma. Recompression and slow decompression is the correct treatment.

AEROGENOUS
Gas producing; said of bacteria that produce gas in their metabolism.

AEROLIN
A brand name for salbutamol, a preparation causing bronchodilation.

AEROMEDICINE
The branch of medicine concerned with disorders that result from or occur during flying.

AERONEUROSIS
Nervous disorder encountered among aircrew and pilots of aircraft. It was first noted during World War II in pilots who had undertaken so many battle missions that they were showing evidence of nervous breakdown and were overdue for a rest.

The disease was also noticed in exceptionally nervous individuals who could not take the nervous stress involved in either bombing missions or air battle. Symptoms include nausea, vomiting and headache.

AEROPAUSE
The dividing line between outer space and areas in which man and aircraft can function.

AEROPHAGIA
Swallowing of air.

AEROSOL
Atomized particles ejected into the air from apressurized can. Some medicines are distributed in the form of an aerosol.

AEROTITIS
A type of barotitis media.

AESCULAPIUS
Mythological god of healing.

AETIOLOGY
A science dealing with the causes of diseases and disorders. Also spelled etiology.

AFEBRILE
Running no temperature, without a fever.

AFFECT
A violent emotion, such as terror, fear or anger. "Affect" is derived from the Latin word affectus =diseased state of mind or body. It is no longer used in this sense and nowadays we understand affect to be an emotion or feeling attached to a mental conception or image.

The affect is a reaction of the entire personality and often expresses itself in body processes, e.g., increased heart activity or increased blood pressure.

A range of affect may be described as broad (normal), restricted (constricted), blunted, or flat. What is considered the normal range of expression of affect varies considerably, both within and among different cultures. The normal expression of affect involves variability in facial expression, pitch of voice, and hand and body movements. Restricted affect is characterized by a clear reduction in the expressive range and intensity of affects. Blunted affect is marked by a severe reduction in the intensity of affective expression. In flat affect there is virtually no affective expression; generally the voice is monotonous and the face, immobile. Affect is inappropriate when it is clearly discordant with the content of the person's speech or ideation.

Example: A patient smiled and laughed while discussing demons who were persecuting him. Affect is labile when it is characterized by repeated, rapid, and abruptshifts.

AFFECT ACT
Action made without thinking and caused by a strong affect; primitive, explosive "short-circuit" reaction.

AFFECT BLOCK
The inability to love due to a fear of love and of emotional ties. As a result of the blocking of affect, this condition involves the incapability for strong emotions and the avoidance of loving by using doubts and uncertainties.

AFFECTIVE CONTACT
Emotional relationships with others. A poor affective contact can be due to aloofness, superficialness or avoiding the emotion in an emotional atmosphere.

AFFECTIVE DEMENTIA
Mental deterioration not of the intellectual powers but of the emotional life, through which a barrier is created between the sufferer and others.

AFFECTIVE DISORDER
Psychiatric disorder in which a disturbance of affect or mood is a primary factor of the disease.

AFFECTIVE EXPERIENCE
An emotional experience, whether pleasant orunpleasant, mild or intense.

AFFECTIVE PERSONALITY DISORDER
Personality disorder characterized by lifelongpredominance of a pronounced mood which may be persistently depressive, persistently elated, or alternately one then the other. During periods of elation there is unshakable optimism and an enhanced zest for life and activity, whereas periods of depression are marked by worry, pessimism, low output of energy and a sense of futility.

AFFECTIVE PSYCHOSES
Mental disorders, usually recurrent, in which there is a severe disturbance of mood (mostly compounded of depression and anxiety but also manifested as elation and excitement) which is accompanied by one or more of the following: delusions, perplexity, disturbed attitude to self, disorder of perception and behavior.

These are all in keeping with the patient's prevailing mood (as are hallucinations when they occur). There is a strong tendency towards suicide.

AFFECTIVE REINTEGRATION
The reorganization of affects or emotions into harmony following their previous disintegration during an affective psychosis.

AFFECTIVE TRANSFORMATION
The representation in consciousness of a repressed emotion usually by its opposite.

AFFERENT
Leading towards the center. Medically, the center is frequently the brain so that nerves carrying impulses from the outside of the body towards the brain area are called afferent nerves.

AFFILIATION
The settlement of the paternity of a child on its true father.

AFFINITY
Attraction; in biochemistry, the force that impels certain atoms to

unite with certain others to form compounds.

AFFLICTION
A state of acute pain or distress of body or mind. The term is also meant in the sense of the cause of continued pain of body or mind.

AFIBROGENEMIA
Deficiency or absence of fibrinogen (a protein that aids in clotting) in the blood. The most common cause is concealed accidental hemorrhage.

AFRICAN TICK FEVER
Relapsing fever.

AFTERBIRTH
The material, primarily the placenta, expelled from the mother's body after the delivery of her child.

AFTERCARE
Further treatment of patients after discharge fromhospital or treatment center. The term aftercare is also used for the rehabilitation of offenders leaving prison.

AFTER-EFFECT
A delayed effect, an effect occurring after the first result of a drug has disappeared.

AFTER-HEARING
Hearing sounds after the stimulus causing the sound has stopped.

AFTER-IMAGE
The image or sense impression that remains after the stimulus has disappeared.

AFTER-NYSTAGMUS
Nystagmus is the coarse or fine movement of the eyeball and when this persists after the abrupt stopping of a rotation, it is called after-nystagmus.

AFTERPAIN
Pain not felt until some interval after the time when it was caused.

The term is also used for pains following childbirth associated with the contractions of the uterus.

AFTER-SENSATION
Sensation that persists after the original cause has stopped.

AFTERSOUND
Hearing of a sound after the original cause which produced it has ceased to exist.

AFTERTASTE
Taste that persists long after the food has been swallowed.

AFTER-TREATMENT
Treatment of a convalescent patient.

AGALACTIA
Non-secretion or imperfect secretion of milk after childbirth.

AGAMMAGLOBULINEMIA
An immunological deficiency state in which there is a low level of gamma globulins in the blood, resulting in heightened susceptibility to infectious diseases. People with this condition are unable to produce immunity against infections.

AGAR AGAR
Gelatinous substance derived from seaweed. It is used in bulk-forming laxative medicines, sometimes combined with liquid paraffin, and in certain preparations for the treatment of obesity.

AGENESIS
Incomplete development, sterility, sexual impotence.

AGENT
An active force or substance capable of producing an effect.

AGE RATIO
The chronological age of a child at one testing divided by the child's chronological age at a later testing. This ratio is a crude measure of a

test's predictive power.

AGEUSIA
An impairment or deficiency in the sense of taste. The cause of such a disorder may be either physiological or emotional.

AGGLUTINATION
The clumping together of bacteria or other cells because of the introduction of an antibody.

AGGLUTININS
Antibodies found in blood plasma which cause the agglutination (sticking together) of antigens such as foreign red blood cells and bacteria. Each agglutinin is produced in large quantities after a person is immunized with its particular antigen. Agglutinins which agglutinate red blood cells are called isohemagglutinins, and the blood group of an individual is determined by which of these are present in his blood.
-Group O contains isohemagglutinins anti-A and anti-B;
-group A contains anti-B;
-group B contains anti-A;
-group AB contains no isohemagglutinins.

AGGLUTINOGEN
Antigenic substance found in germs or other cells which, when injected into the bloodstream, causes the production of an antidote (agglutinin). The agglutinin then clumps together the original germs or cells, rendering them inactive and easier for the body to destroy. This process forms the basis of all the preventive inoculations against disease.

AGGRESSION
Attack on another, usually but not necessarily, as a response to opposition. Aggression is defined by psychoanalysts as a manifestation, either of the will to have power over other people, or a projection of the death impulse.

AGGRESSIVE BEHAVIOR
The acts of behavioral responses of an organism that display the quality of aggression.

AGGS
Anti-gas-gangrene serum.

AGING
The process of growing old. Generally during aging a person's height decreases, bone tissue diminishes, hair becomes gray and/or is thinned or lost, nose and ear lengthens, eye lenses become more rigid, and other physical changes occur.

AGIOLAX
A stimulant laxative containing senna as an active ingredient. The drug increases the frequency and ease of bowel movements by stimulating the bowel wall.

AGITATED DEPRESSION
Depressive disorder marked by restlessness, anxiety and increased activity intermingled with fear and tension.

AGITATED MELANCHOLIA
State of deep depression with acute anxiety and agitation.

AGITATION
A mental or physical disturbance, especially worry. Agitation is also used in the sense of a public disturbance on a large scale, or the process of creating it.

AGITATION, PSYCHOMOTOR
Excessive motor activity associated with a feeling of inner tension; the activity is usually nonproductive and repetitious. When the agitation is severe, it may be accompanied by shouting or loud complaining. The term should be used in a technical sense to refer to states of tension or restlessness that are accompanied by observable excessive motor activity.

AGITOGRAPHIA
Compulsion to write very fast with the unconscious omission of words or whole sentences. It is the manifestation of a nervous disorder.

AGITOLALIA
Excessive rapidity of speech in which words, syllables and sounds are slurred, left out or distorted.

AGLOSSIA
Congenital absence of the tongue.

AGLUTITION
Inability to swallow.

AGLYCEMIA
Absence of sugar in the blood. The more common name for this condition is now hypoglycemia.

AGNATHIA
Congenital condition in which the jaws are either absent or defectively developed.

AGNOSIA
Inability to recognize the character of objects through the senses, due to disorders of the brain or nervous system.

AGONAL
Related to agony, sometimes associated with the death agony.

AGONIST
A contracting muscle that is controlled by another opposing muscle. It is a term meaning to have a positive, stimulating effect. An agonist drug is one that binds to a receptor, thereby triggering or increasing a particular activity in that cell.

AGONY
Intense mental or physical suffering, an intense feeling.

AGORAPHOBIA
A fear of open, public places or of situations where crowds are to be found. It is the commonest of phobic disorders, comprising about 60 percent of sufferers. As a result of this fear, the person either restricts travel or needs a companion when away from home, or else endures agoraphobic situations despite intense anxiety.

Common agoraphobic situations include:
- being outside the home alone;
- being in a crowd;
- standing in a line;
- being on a bridge;
- traveling in a bus, train, or car.

Usually the person is afraid of having a limited symptom attack, that is, developing a single or small number of symptoms, such as becoming dizzy or falling, depersonalization or derealization, loss of bladder or bowel control, vomiting, or having cardiac distress. In some of these cases, such symptoms have occurred in the past, and the person may be preoccupied with fears of their recurrence. In other cases, the person has never experienced the symptoms, but nevertheless fears that the symptoms "could" develop and incapacitate him or her or be extremely embarrassing. In a small number of cases the person fears feeling incapacitated in some way, but is unable to specify what symptom he or she fears.

AGRANULOCYTE
One of the white blood cells which is devoid of granules.

AGRANULOCYTOSIS
Condition characterized by pronounced leucopenia in which there is a great reduction in the number of polymorphonuclear leukocytes (a type of white blood cell).

AGRAPHIA
Inability to write due to the disease of part of the brain.

AGROMANIA
Unhealthy desire to be left alone or in solitude. It may be the reason

why some people become hermits.

AI
Artificial insemination. A method of inducing pregnancy in which a man's semen is introduced into a woman's uterus by artificial means.

AID
Artificial insemination by donor. A method of inducing pregnancy in which semen from a donor other than the woman's partner is introduced into her uterus byartificial means.

AIDS
Acquired immunodeficiency syndrome, a disease in which the body's immune system breaks down. AIDS is caused by a virus called the human immunodeficiency virus, or HIV. A person who is infected can infect others (blood, sperm), even if no symptoms are present. People infected with HIV can develop many health problems. These can include:
- extreme weight loss;
- severe pneumonia;
- a form of cancer;
- damage to the nervous system.
There is no specific cure; some drugs can alleviate the symptoms.

AIDS DEMENTIA
Early signs of dementia in patients with AIDS. This syndrome occurs in approximately one-third of AIDS patients. The onset is usually insidious, and cognitive dysfunction predominates initially.

AIDS ENCEPHALOPATHY
Involvement of the central nervous system as a direct consequence of neurological manifestations in patients with HIV-infection, including:
- cerebral toxoplasmosis;
- lymphoma of the brain;
- herpesviral encephalitis;
- tuberculous meningitis;
- brain abscess.

AIDS-RELATED COMPLEX
A variety of chronic but nonspecific symptoms and physical findings that appear related to AIDS, which may consist of chronic generalized lymphadenopathy,recurrent fevers, weight loss, and minor infections.

AIH
Artificial insemination with sperm of the husband.

AILMENT
Disease, morbid infection of the body.

AIM INHIBITION
A state with no conscious erotic interest in the object. A relationship is said to be aim-inhibited if the subject has no conscious interest in the object. Common examples are friendships, platonic love and domestic affection between relatives. The concept assumes that, in the absence of inhibition, friendships between the same sexes would become overt homosexual relationships, platonic love would be consummated and incest would occur.

AIR EMBOLUS
Blockage of a blood vessel by an air bubble.

AIRSICKNESS
Form of motion sickness allied to seasickness, experienced by nervous individuals when flying. The cause of airsickness lies in the effect of the movement of the aircraft on the labyrinth of the inner ear where the sense of balance is located; this cause was suggested because deaf-mutes are immune to motion sickness. Changes in vertical acceleration of the aircraft is the most important factor. Susceptible persons should avoid any excess of food or drink before embarking and during the flight, sugar should be taken to avoid ketosis (poisoning by the products of the breakdown of fats).

AKATHISIA
A condition marked by restlessness, ranging from anxiety to inability to lie or sit quietly or to sleep, as seen in toxic reactions to certain drugs (phenothiazines). The person also feels a distressing inner restlessness.

AKINESIA
Marked absence of movement due to disease of the nervous system and brain.

ALA
An anatomical appendage resembling a wing.

ALACTASIA
A condition marked by malabsorption of lactose (milk sugar) due to deficiency of the digestive enzyme, lactase.

ALALIA
Inability to speak through impairment in the organs of speech.

ALARM REACTION
The release of metabolites in the affected tissues as a response to stress.

ALASTRIM
An infectious disease - variola minor -occurring especially in southern areas but also seen in Western Europe and referred to there as white pox, milk pox or kaffir pox. The skin eruptions show a strong resemblance to true smallpox - variola major - and the manner of infection is also the same, but alastrim is of a less serious nature.

ALBEE'S OPERATION
Surgical procedure for treating ankylosis of the hip joint.

ALBERS-SCHÖNBERG DISEASE
An hereditary disease marked by abnormally dense bone, and by the common occurrence of fractures of affected bone. The condition is also called marble bones.

ALBINISM
Lack of body pigment; inability to produce pigment.

ALBINO
A person of abnormally pale, milky complexion, with light hair and pink eyes, resulting from a deficiency in pigmentation.

ALBUMIN
Group of proteins soluble in water and in 50 percent saturated sulphate solution; present in animals and plants. Ovalbumin is the chief protein in egg white; serum albumin occurs in blood plasma, where it controls osmotic pressure.

ALBUMINEMIA
Abnormal amount of albumin in the blood.

ALBUMINOMETER
Apparatus for measuring the quantity of albumin in the blood or other body fluid.

ALBUMINURIA
A condition in which the urine contains albumin, often indicating kidney disease.

ALCOHOL
(1) Any class of chemical compounds derived from hydrocarbons by replacing one or more of the hydrogen atoms with an equal number of hydroxyl radicals.
(2) Term for ethyl alcohol, the alcohol of commerce and medicine.

ALCOHOL DEPENDENCE SYNDROME
A psychological state, usually also physical, resulting from taking alcohol, characterized by behavioral and other responses that always include a compulsion to take alcohol on a continuous or periodic basis in order to experience its effects, and

sometimes to avoid the discomfort of its absence; tolerance may or may not be present.

ALCOHOL HALLUCINOSIS
Hallucinosis in which vivid and persistent hallucinations develop shortly (usually within 48 hours) after cessation of or reduction in alcohol ingestion by a person who apparently has an alcohol dependence syndrome. The hallucinations may be auditory or visual. The auditory hallucinations are usually voices and, less commonly, unformed sounds such as hissing or buzzing.

In the majority of cases, the content of the hallucinations is unpleasant and disturbing. However, the hallucinatory content may be benign and leave the person undisturbed. The voices may address the person directly, but more often discuss him or her in the third person.

ALCOHOLIC JEALOUSY
Chronic paranoid psychosis characterized by delusional jealousy and associated with alcoholism.

ALCOHOLIC POISONING
Severe condition of chronic alcoholism, characterized by various conditions including nerve degeneration, mental deterioration, fatty degeneration of the liver, weight loss, personality changes, etc.

ALCOHOLIC PSYCHOSIS
Complete and ultimate mental deterioration that occurs in the chronic alcoholic. In one variety, Korsakow's psychosis (or syndrome), there is complete mental, moral and social degeneration. Sufferers steal, cheat and lie to obtain alcohol, and no longer keepthemselves clean or tidy.

ALCOHOLICS ANONYMOUS
The full name of AA.

ALCOHOL INTOXICATION
Maladaptive behavior changes due to recent ingestion of alcohol. These changes may include:
- aggressiveness;
- impaired judgment;
- impaired attention;
- irritability;
- euphoria;
- emotional lability;
- other manifestations of impaired social or occupational functioning.

Characteristic physiological signs include:
- slurred speech;
- incoordination;
- unsteady gait;
- nystagmus;
- flushed face.

The person's usual behavior may be accentuated or altered. For example, a person who tends to be somewhat suspicious may, under the influence of alcohol, become markedly paranoid. On the other hand, people who are ordinarily withdrawn and uncomfortable in social situations may become exceptionally convivial.

Alcohol intoxication is sometimes associated with an amnesia for the events that occurred during the course of the intoxication.

ALCOHOLISM
A chronic, progressive and often fatal disease of major prevalence, but one that is treatable.

ALCOHOLIZATION
The act or process of taking alcohol or the condition of being under the influence of alcohol.

ALCOHOLOPHILIA
Pathological craving for alcohol.

ALCOHOLURIA
Presence of alcohol in urine.

ALDACTIDE
A drug used for treatment of high blood pressure, water accumulation due to congestive heart failure, cirrhosis of the liver, kidney disease

and water retention of unknown cause. This preparation is a combination of two drugs which help the kidneys to pass water and salt and help reduce the symptoms of the abovementioned conditions.

ALDEHYDE
A transparent colorless liquid produced by the oxidation of pure alcohol.

ALDOSTERONE
A hormone secreted by the adrenal cortex that promotes the retention of salt and water by the kidneys.

ALDOSTERONISM
Rare illness in which an over-production of the hormone aldosterone by the adrenal cortex leads to high blood pressure.

ALEPPO BOIL
A manifestation on the skin of an infestation by Leishmania bacteria.

ALEUKEMIA
Blood disease in which white cells are either few or absent. It may occur in the course of leukemia.

ALEXIA
A disorder of language: the complete inability to comprehend the written word; word blindness.

AFLATOXIN
A toxin produced by various species of moulds, which contaminate ground nut seedlings. The toxin has been implicated as a cause of liver cancer in humans.

ALGAE
The most primitive plant variety, having no true root, stem or leaf. Algae form the food for mollusks, fish and other aquatic animals. There are many thousands of varieties such as green, brown and red algae.

In ancient times, algae were used in the treatment of goiter, skin infections and scurvy. Now algae form an important medium for the cultivation of fungi and bacteria in scientific laboratories. Further they are used as a constituent of bandages that are applied to bone fractures and as absorbent gauze for wounds.

Algae also are extensively used in the production of hair creams, hair lotions and toothpastes. In Japan women enjoy a massage with dried algae to promote smooth skin. Much research is being done at the moment on the nutritional value of algae, as they may possibly provide a solution for famine in areas with a large population growth.

ALGESIA
Pain; increased sensitivity to pain.

ALGESIC
Painful.

ALGINATES
Salts of alginic acid. Certain alginates have been used for absorbable surgical dressings. They are available in solution, as foam and in specially impregnated gauze.

ALGINURESIS
Pain on passing urine, more commonly called dysuria.

ALGOLAGNIA
A form of sexual perversion in which the infliction or the experiencing of pain increases the pleasure of the sexual act.

ALGOPHOBIA
Fear of suffering pain.

ALGOSPASM
Any painful spasm.

ALIENATION
To estrange, a mental derangement. Term also used for legal insanity.

ALIMENT
Food; nutrient.

ALIMENTARY CANAL
The canal from the mouth to the anus.

ALIMENTARY TRACT
Passage from the throat to the anus.

ALIMENTATION
The state of being nourished.

ALKALEMIA
A high alkali content in the blood.

ALKALI
Chemical which is the complete opposite in its function to an acid, and neutralizes an acid to form a salt.

ALKALINE
Substance having the reactions of an alkali.

ALKALINITY
An excess of alkali.

ALKALINURIA
Presence of alkali in the urine.

ALKALI RESERVE
Total amount of available alkali in the body which can be used to buffer against acids.

ALKALIZERS
Drugs that neutralize acidic properties of the blood and urine by making them more alkaline (or basic). Systemic alkalizers include potassium citrate and citric acid, sodium bicarbonate, sodium citrate and citric acid, and tricitrates. Urinary alkalizers include potassium citrate, potassium citrate and citric acid, potassium citrate and sodium citrate, sodium citrate and citric acid.

ALKALOIDS
Narcotic poisons found in certain plants and fungi. They have complex molecular structures and are usually heterocyclic nitrogen-containing bases. Many, such as atropine from deadly nightshade, are extremely poisonous. Others, such as morphine, nicotine and cocaine, can be highly addictive, and some, such as mescaline, are psychedelics. But in small doses alkaloids are often powerful medicines, and are used as analgesics, tranquillizers, and cardiac and respiratory stimulants. Other examples are quinine, reserpine and ephedrine. Caffeine (found in coffee and tea) is a stimulant. Although alkaloids may be found in any part of the plant, they are usually contained in the seeds, seed capsules, bark or roots. One plant, the opium poppy, contains about 30 alkaloids. Alkaloids are extracted from plants and separated by chromatography; synthetic alkaloids are seldom economically competitive.

ALKALOSIS
A condition wherein the concentration of alkali in the body is higher than normal.

ALKAPTONE BODIES
A class of substances, especially homogenistic acid, present in urine in alkaptonuria, a rare metabolic disease.

ALKAPTONURIA
Defect of the body present at birth and characterized by the excretion in the urine of a substance called homogenistic acid.

ALKA-SELTZER
Brand name of an analgesic-antacid drug containing as active ingredients: aspirin, sodium bicarbonate, and citric acid.

ALKERAN
Brand name of an anticancer drug containing melphalan as an active ingredient. The drug is used to kill or damage multiplying cells.

ALKYLATING AGENTS
Substances that disrupt the process of cell division by affecting the DNA in the nucleus, probably by

adding abnormal chemical groups to it. The chemicals are used to treat malignant diseases.

ALLANTOIC
Pertaining to the allantois.

ALLANTOIN
Generic name of a drug that has a mild antibacterial effect.

ALLANTOIS
A fetal membrane developing from the hindgut, which eventually develops into the placenta and umbilical cord.

ALLEGRON
A brand name for a drug containing as an active ingredient nortriptyline, a tricyclic antidepressant preparation.

ALLELE
Alternative forms of a gene. Each person possesses only two alleles for each gene, receiving one of each pair of alleles from each parent.

ALLER-EZE
A brand name for a drug containing as active ingredient clemastine (an antihistamine preparation).

ALLERGEN
(1) A substance, usually a protein, which, when taken into the body, makes it hypersensitive or "allergic" to it.
(2) An environmental substance that causes an allergic response in a sensitive individual.

ALLERGIC
Pertaining to or affected with allergy.

ALLERGIC BRONCHOPUL-MONARY ASPERGILLOSIS
A non-invasive form of aspergillosis (a lung disease caused by a fungi) occurring in asthmatics as pneumonia resulting from an allergic reaction to Aspergillus fumi-gatus, and characterized by a rise of eosinophils (a type of white cell) in the blood.

ALLERGIC CONJUNCTIVITIS
Atopic conjunctivitis in which the membranes around the eyes become inflamed, usually part of an allergic syndrome such as hay fever, but may also occur alone through direct contact with airborne substances such as pollen, fungus spores, various dusts or flakes of animal skin.

ALLERGIC INTERSTITIAL PNEUMONITIS
Another name for hypersensitivity pneumonitis.

ALLERGIC PURPURA
An acute or chronic bleeding from capillaries, primarily affecting skin, joints and the gastro-intestinal and urinary systems. Skin bruises vary in appearance. The disorder is often self-limited with a good prognosis.

ALLERGIC RHINITIS
A symptom complex including hay fever and perennial allergic rhinitis, characterized by seasonal or perennial sneezing, runny nose, nasal congestion, itching and often conjunctivitis (inflamed eye membranes) and pharyngitis (sore throat).

ALLERGY
(1) A hypersensitivity reaction to the presence of an agent (allergen) that is intrinsically harmless such as animal hairs, dust, pollen, or substances in certain foods.
(2) A state of sensitivity to a particular environmental substance, or allergen. An allergic reaction is the body's response, directed by the immune system, to exposure to an allergen.

ALLOCHEIRIA
Disorder of sensation where touch or pain is felt, not at the site where it occurred, but at the corresponding point on the other side of the body.

ALLOEROTISM
Erotic tendencies directed towards other people.

ALLOGENIC
Denoting tissues that are distinct as far as their antigens are concerned, but are from the same species (said of tumors and transplants).

ALLOGRAFT
Transfer of tissue or organ between members of the same species.

ALLOPATHY
The standard form of medical practice in this country; a system of therapeutics based on the production of a condition incompatible with or antagonistic to the conditions being treated. This is the opposite of homeopathy.

ALL-OR-NONE LAW
Principle relating to nerve fibers and muscles in which they either react to a complete degree or do not act at all.

ALL-OR-NONE RESPONSE
Response which is either elicited or not, and when elicited shows full intensity and no grading.

ALLOTOPIA
Displacement or malposition of an organ.

ALLOTOXIN
Any substance developed within the body which has antitoxic properties.

ALOCHIA
Absence of the lochia, the vaginal discharge that takes place for some days following childbirth.

ALOPECIA
Partial or total loss of hair from natural or abnormal causes.

ALPHA-ADRENERGIC BLOCKERS
A group of drugs used to treat hy-pertension. These drugs include prazosin, terazosin, doxazosin and labetalol (an alpha-adrenergic and beta-adrenergic combination drug).

ALPHA RHYTHM
The most common electrical brain waves of the adult cerebral cortex as observed on an electroencephalogram (EEG). During rest, the oscillations are regular and smooth, occurring at a rate of 8 to 12 per second with an amplitude of 5 to 25 microvolts.

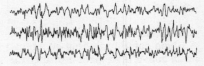

Alpha rhythm; characteristic pattern of waves in the electroencephalogram (EEG). The most prominent rhythm, noticeable when a healthy subject closes his or her eyes, shows a frequency of 8-12 cycles per second that is chiefly present at the occipital pole of the hemispheres.

ALPORT'S SYNDROME
Another name for hereditary nephritis.

ALS
Abbreviation of antilymphocyte serum. It diminishes the number of circulating lymphocytes, thus reducing the body's defense mechanisms and thereby giving a transplanted organ a better chance of survival in the recipient.

ALTER
One's conception of another human being as a distinct person like oneself.

ALTER EGO
A very intimate friend that is considered by the individual as a second or other self.

ALTERNATE GENERATION
The type of inheritance among ani-

mals by which the young do not resemble their parents, but their grandparents or some remote ancestor. This characteristic is thought also to occur in some human families.

ALTERNATIVE MEDICINE
Methods of diagnosis and treatment not regularly taught in medical schools. It is perhaps the best term among the many which have been used to describe a vast complex of treatments. In the US, such terms as "naturopathy," "nature cure," "non-orthodox medicine," "traditional medicine" and "complementary medicine" are also common.

Most of the alternative practices have been pioneered by non-registered practitioners: acupuncture from China, yoga from India, the whole-food diet, specialized diet techniques such as fasting,etc.

ALTITUDE SICKNESS
A condition of lack of oxygen in the blood and tissues due to low atmospheric pressure. Night vision is impaired, followed by breathlessness, headache and faintness. At 5000 m (16,420 ft) mental changes include indifference, euphoria and faulty judgement but complete acclimatization is possible up to this height. At very high altitudes - 6000-7000 m (19,700-22,980 ft) - cyanosis, coma and death rapidly result. Treatment is by oxygen and descent. The use of pressurized cabins in aircraft prevents the occurrence of the condition.

ALTRUISM
Consideration for the well-being of other people.

ALUMINOSIS
A chronic infection of the respiratory system due to the presence of aluminum-bearing dust in the lungs.

ALUPHOS
Brand name of an antacid containing aluminum phosphate as the active ingredient. The drug is used to relieve indigestion and heartburn by neutralizing the effects of stomach acid. Side effects are constipation and nausea.

ALVEOLAR
Pertaining to the sockets of the teeth or the alveoli in the lungs.

ALVEOLAR LOBULES
Physiologic unit of the lung consisting of a respiratory bronchiole and its branches (alveolar ducts, alveolar sacs and alveoli).

ALVEOLI (DENTAL)
The cavities or sockets in the jaws, in which the roots of the teeth are embedded.

ALVEOLI (PULMONARY)
Small air pockets that make up the alveolar sacs of the lungs, where oxygen and carbon dioxide are exchanged.

ALVEOLITIS
Inflammation of alveoli.

ALYMPHOCYTOSIS
Gross deficiency or complete absence of lymphocytes in the blood.

ALZHEIMER'S DISEASE
Presence of dementia of insidious onset and a generally progressive, deteriorating course for which all other specific causes have been excluded by the history, physical examination, and laboratory tests. The dementia involves a multifaceted loss of intellectual abilities, such as memory, judgment, abstract thought, and other higher cortical functions, and changes in personality and behavior.

The onset is insidious, and the course is generally progressive and deteriorating. In the early stages, memory impairment may be the only apparent cognitive deficit. There may also be subtle personality changes, such as the development of apathy, lack of spontaneity, and a quiet withdrawal from social interactions. People usually remain neat and well-groomed, and, aside from an occasional irritable outburst, are cooperative and behave in a socially appropriate way.

With progression to the middle stage of the disease, various cognitive disturbances become quite apparent, and behavior and personality are more obviously affected. By the late stage, the person may be completely mute and inattentive. At this point he or she is totally incapable of caring for himself or herself. This stage leads inevitably to death. With senile onset, the average duration of symptoms, from onset to death, is about five years.

AMALGAM
Soft mixture of metal and mercury used for filling teeth and may contain silver, tin, copper or various combinations of these metals.

AMASTIA
Absence of breast development.

AMATHOPHOBIA
Fear of dust or dirt.

AMAUROSIS
Blindness caused by disease in the optic nerve, without any perceptible change in the eye itself.

AMAUROTIC IDIOCY
Defective intelligence with amaurosis, and usually early death.

AMBAXIN
Brand name for a penicillin antibiotic preparation containing bacampicillin as active ingredient.

AMBIDEXTERITY
The ability to use both hands with equal ease.

AMBIGUITY
The quality of having more than one meaning or interpretation. The term is also used in the sense of an idea, statement or expression capable of being understood in more than one sense.

AMBILATERAL
Pertaining to both sides.

AMBIVALENCE
Emotional attitude towards an individual involving the alternation of the opposite feelings of love and hate. The term also means the coexistence of contradictory impulses and emotions towards the same object. Ambivalence has to be distinguished from having mixed feelings about someone. It refers to an underlying emotional attitude in which the contradictory attitudes derive from a common source and are independent, whereas mixed feelings may be based on a realistic assessment of the imperfect nature of the object. Although ambivalence is engendered by all neurotic conflict, it is mostly easily observed in obsessional neurosis, in which an attempt is made to balance the two sides of the ambivalence in the consciousness; in other neuroses, one or other side is usually repressed.

AMBIVERSION
Type of personality, balanced or oscillating between introversion and extroversion.

AMBLYOPIA
Dimness of vision or blindness for which there is no recognizable cause in the eye; it may be caused by toxins such as tobacco or alcohol.

AMBOCEPTOR
Double membrane receptor, the one combining with the blood cell, the other with complement.

AMBOSEXUAL
Having male and female characteristics, a hermaphrodite.

AMBULANCE
Vehicle fitted with suitable appliances for moving the injured and sick.

AMBULANT
Ability to walk about.

AMBULATORY
Pertaining to a disease or condition which can be dealt with while patients are able to walk about and not confined to their beds.

AMBULATORY PERITONEAL DIALYSIS
Hemodialysis (blood washing) carried out by a kidney machine at home. Patients can connect themselves up in the late evening, and sleep through the night.

AMBULATORY TRACTION
Traction exerted by a walking-splints or braces on fractured limbs while patients are up and about.

AMEBA
Also spelled amoeba; small parasite which, in the body, can cause disease.

AMEBECIDE
A drug that kills amebas (single-celled microorganisms).

AMEBIASIS
Infection with an ameba that is pathogenic. Treatment is by specific medicines.

AMEBIC DYSENTERY
A form of amebiasis characterized by ulceration of the intestinal tract, caused by the ameba.

AMEBICIDE
Drug used to treat infections caused by amebas, tiny micro-organisms commonly found in nature.

AMELIA
Congenital absence of a limb or limbs.

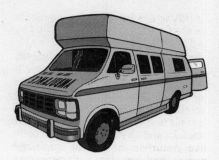

Modern ambulance equipped with apparatus to stimulate the heart in case of myocardial infarction.

AMELIORATION
Reduction of the severity of symptoms of a disease or disorder.

AMENORRHEA
Abnormal stoppage or absence of the menstrual flow.

AMENTIA
A form of passive stupor with semi-consciousness, disorientation and an inability to speak.

AMERICAN LEISHMANIASIS
Variation of leishmaniasis, a parasite infection, that may manifest itself as localized skin ulcers resembling Oriental sore (beginning as a pimple, spreading, healing slowly, leaving a scar) or as ulcers in the mucous membranes of the nose and throat. The skin ulcers usually occur on the face, when they are known as chiclero ulcers, since they primarily affect persons who enter forests to gather chicle.

AMETRIA
Congenital absence of the uterus.

AMETROPIA
An eye condition in which there is some error of refraction, in consequence of which parallel rays, with the eye at rest, are not focused on the retina.

AMIMIA
A language defect, involving the in-

ability to use significant gestures.

AMINO ACIDS

An important class of carboxylic acids containing one or more (-NH$_2$) groups. The building blocks of the proteins, found in all living matter, are composed of about 20 amino acids, and most of them are found and synthesized in cells. Amino acids are white, crystalline solids that are soluble in water; they can act as acids or bases depending on the chemical environment. An amino-acid mixture may be analyzed by chromatography. All amino acids (except glycine) contain at least one asymmetric carbon atom to which are attached the carboxyl group, the amino group, a hydrogen atom and a fourth group (R) that differs for each amino acid and determines its character. Thus amino acids can exist in two mirror-image forms. Generally only L-isomers (left-turning) occur in nature, but a few bacteria contain D-isomers (right-turning). Our bodies synthesize most of the amino acids that we need for nutrition, but we depend on protein foods for eight 'essential amino acids' that they cannot produce. Inside the body, amino acids derived from food are metabolized in various ways.

AMINO-ACIDURIA

Excessive amounts of one or more amino acids in the urine.

AMINOGLUTETHIMIDE

Generic name of a drug for advanced breast cancer and Cushing's syndrome.

AMINOGLYCOSIDES

A family of antibiotics used for serious infections. The usefulness is limited because of relative toxicity compared to some other antibiotics. These drugs include amikacin, gentamicin, kanamycin, neomycin, netilmicin, streptomycin, tobramycin.

AMINOGLYCOSIDE SERUM ASSAY

A blood test done to make sure that antibiotic drugs such as gentamicin, tobramycin and amikacin are administered in dosages that maintain therapeutic blood levels.

AMITOSIS

The direct method of cell division, characterized by the simple splitting of the nucleus, without formation of chromosomes.

AMMONIA

A substance produced by bacterial activity in the intestine. It is measured in blood to determine if the liver is functioning adequately in converting ammonia into urea, a substance excreted by the kidneys.

AMMONIA NITROGEN

A substance measured in urine to determine the body's acid/base balance and nitrogen balance.

AMMONIUM BICARBONATE

Drug used in cough mixtures as a mild expectorant.

AMMONIUM BROMIDE

Drug with sedative properties.

AMMONIUM CARBONATE

A mixture of ammonium bicarbonate and ammonium carbamate, used as a stimulant, as in smelling salts.

AMMONIUM CHLORIDE

Chemical used as a synthetic acidifier (to make a solution more acid). Ammonium chloride is also used as a drug that increases urine acidity and speeds excretion of poisons.

AMNESIA

Partial or complete loss of memory. Occurs following concussions, in dementia, hysteria and head injury.

AMNESIA, ANTEROGRADE

Loss of memory for those experiences and events following the physical or psychological trauma.

AMNESIA, CATATHYMIC
Memory loss limited and confined to a certain recollection or experience.

AMNESIA, INFANTILE
Loss of memory for the years from birth to about five years of age necessitated by the unacceptable nature of memories concerning the rise of the sexual life and the limits imposed upon the infant's power.

AMNESIA, RETROGRADE
Loss of memory for those events and experiences preceding the cause of the amnesia.

AMNESTIC SYNDROME
Impairment in short- and long-term memory that is attributed to a specific organic factor. As in dementia, the person with an amnestic syndrome has both an ongoing inability to learn new material (short-term memory deficit) and an inability to recall material that was known in the past (long-term memory deficit).

A significant degree of amnesia nearly always results in disorientation. Confabulation, the recitation of imaginary events to fill in gaps in memory, is often observed, and when present, tends to disappear with time. Most people with this syndrome lack insight into their memory deficit, and may explicitly deny it, despite evidence to the contrary. Others acknowledge a problem, but appear unconcerned. Apathy, lack of initiative, and emotional blandness are common.

AMNIOCENTESIS
A procedure whereby fluid is drawn from the liquid-filled amniotic sac surrounding the developing fetus while in the uterus. Cells shed from the fetus into the fluid can then be specially prepared within two to three weeks for chromosomal analysis to detect such conditions as spina bifida and Down's syndrome.

AMNIOGRAPHY
Method by which the amniotic fluid is made opaque by injection of radio-opaque material in order to visualize the fetal skeleton and soft tissues more clearly.

AMNION
Innermost embryonic membrane surrounding the fetus and continuing into the umbilical cord. It has no blood vessels and is smooth and transparent.

AMNION PUNCTURE
Puncture into the amnion cavity, carried out in pregnancy. This method is rapidly becoming just as important to midwifery as spinal lumbar puncture is to the neurosurgeon. Amnion puncture can be used early on in pregnancy and for the following purposes: as treatment for excess water in the amnion cavity (hydramnion), at the start of labor or for a blood transfusion to the child via the placenta and, finally, for embryonic fluid analysis (to test its composition and pressure) and also for taking blood from the embryo. Cells from the embryonic fluid may be analyzed for chromosomal and biochemical defects of the fetus.

AMNIORRHEA
Loss of the fluid surrounding the baby within the uterus shortly before birth. Popularly called 'the breaking of the waters'.

AMNIOTIC CAVITY
Fluid-filled cavity within which the unborn baby lies.

AMNIOTIC FLUID
Clear, watery fluid, secreted by the amnion, which fills the entire amniotic cavity and serves to protect the fetus. The amount of amniotic fluid increases with the duration of

the pregnancy, and in normal circumstances at the end of the pregnancy amounts to 0.5 to 1.0 liter (18-35 fl. oz). The fluid contains small fibers, skin cells and sebaceous fat from the fetus. Its functions are manifold, including:

(1) Protection of the fetus from outside pressure and violence.

(2) Making movement of the fetus possible.

(3) Making these movements less felt by the mother.

(4) Prevention of the fetus growing together with its surroundings, for example with the chorion.

(5) Moisture intake of the fetus (the fetus drinks some of the fluid).

(6) Finally, analysis of the fluid plays an important part in obstetrics. The usually colorless amniotic fluid can change to green (by mixing with excreta from the fetus, by mixing with certain medicines which act upon the intestinal system of the fetus, or in all conditions of shortage of oxygen), yellow (rhesus antagonisation), red (rupture of a blood vessel that runs through the membranes to the placenta), or brown/red (fetal death).

AMNIOTIC FLUID, CREATINE
A test done on amniotic fluid to determine the age of the fetus.

AMNIOTIC FLUID, ESTRIOL
A test done on amniotic fluid to detect fetalabnormalities, such as fetoplacental disorders, in early or late pregnancy.

AMNIOTOMY
Surgical rupture of the fetal membranes to induce labor.

AMOEBA
Also spelled ameba; small parasite which, in the body, can cause disease.

AMOEBIASIS
Infection with an ameba that is pathogenic.

AMOEBIC DYSENTERY
Also spelled amebic dysentery; a form of amebiasis characterized by ulceration of the intestinal tract, caused by the ameba.

AMOEBICIDE
Also spelled amebicide; drug used to treat infections caused by amebas, tiny microorganisms commonly found in nature.

AMOEBOID
Resembling an ameba in shape or in mode of movement, said of certain types of white blood cells.

AMOK
A furious, reckless state, comparable to a psychotic disturbance, in which the afflicted runs about frantically, attacking everyone and everything in sight.

AMPHETAMINES
A group of stimulant drugs, including Benzedrine and Methedrine, now in medical disfavor following widespread abuse and addiction. They counteract fatigue, suppress appetite, speed up performance (hence the slang word for them: 'speed') and give confidence, but pronounced depression often follows; thus psychological and then physical addiction are encouraged.

A paranoid psychosis may result from prolonged use, although it may be that amphetamine abuse is really an early symptom of the psychosis. While no longer acceptable in the treatment of obesity, they are useful in narcolepsy, a rare condition of abnormal sleepiness.

AMPHIMIXIS
The union of maternal and paternal characteristics in sexual reproduction.

AMPHORIC RESONANCE
A sound similar to that produced by blowing over the neck of an empty bottle.

AMPHORIC RESPIRATION
A hollow blowing sound heard when a stethoscope is held over cavities in the lungs, due to the echo produced from the walls of the cavity.

AMPOULE
Miniature sealed glass bottle holding one dose of a sterile solution prepared for injection into the body.

AMPULLA
Bell-like mouth of a canal such as in the tear duct of the eye and the milk ducts of the breast.

AMPUTATE
To cut off, as a limb or other member, by a surgical operation.

AMPUTATING ULCER
A penetrating ulcer encircling a part, such as a toe, leading ultimately to the complete loss of that part, such as is seen in yaws.

AMPUTATION
The surgical removal of a part of the body. Usually this is one of the limbs, sometimes a whole arm or leg, but can also be a breast or other protruding organ. A doctor may be obliged to carry out an emergency amputation in a number of dire circumstances, such as injuries in industry where a limb is caught in machinery, in those trapped in mining and railway accidents or under falling masonry during earthquakes. In most of these injuries a part of the limb, usually at its end, such as a hand or foot, is irretrievably damaged, pulped or mangled.

The simplest technique suffices and a guillotine approach is most often made with a scalpel or amputation knife cutting through all the tissues down to the bone, which is then severed or disarticulated at main joints, and the main blood vessels are caught with artery forceps and tied. If flaps have been made, these are secured with a few stitches, mainly mattress sutures left loose to be tied when the danger of bleeding or infection is over. A protective dressing of gauze, cotton wool and a bandage is applied. Elective amputation may be carried out later at the most desirable functional site; this may be done relatively close to the site of the emergency amputation.

AMPUTATION NEUROMA
Small, painful and tender growth that sometimes develops at the cut end of a nerve following amputation of a limb.

AMUSIA
A form of aphasia characterized by loss of the faculty of musical expression or of the recognition of simple musical tones.

AMYASTHENIA
Muscular weakness.

AMYELIA
Congenital malformation of the spinal cord.

AMYELINEURIA
Partial paralysis or impaired functioning of the spinal cord.

AMYGDALIN
A white glycoside powder, obtained from bitter almonds, chiefly used medically as an expectorant.

AMYLASE
An enzyme secreted by the pancreas, which becomes elevated in diseases of the pancreas or salivary glands, kidney problems, and drug ingestion.

AMYLOID
A protein complex of starchlike characteristics forming a hard substance in tissues during certain diseases.

AMYLOID DEGENERATION
Also called amyloid disease and

amyloidosis. Waxy degeneration occurring in cases of long-standing disease, such as tuberculosis, in which the tissues of the body have deposits of starch-like substances which prevent the various organs (mainly the heart, liver, kidney, spleen and intestine) from carrying out their functions, and contribute to the worsening of the patient's condition.

AMYLOID KIDNEY
State of amyloid or waxy degeneration of the kidney seen in amyloid degeneration.

AMYLOIDOSIS
Another name for amyloid degeneration.

AMYLORRHEA
Presence of excessive quantities of starch in the stools.

AMYLUM
Starch.

AMYOCARDIA
Weakness of the heart muscle.

AMYOTONIA
Extreme flaccidity and smallness of the muscles, occurring mostly in early childhood.

AMYOTONIA CONGENITA
Disease of early childhood, usually congenital and sometimes running through families, characterized by the extreme flaccidity, smallness and weakness of the muscles, which are not actually paralysed.

AMYOTROPHIC
Relating to diseases in which the wasting of muscles is a feature.

AMYOTROPHIC LATERAL SCLEROSIS
Chronic disease in which there is degeneration of the nerve cells supplying certain muscle groups resulting in a progressive muscular atrophy (wasting) of groups of muscles.

AMYTAL
Brand name of a barbiturate containing amylobarbitone sodium as the active ingredient.

ANA
"In equal quantities of each"; refers to ingredients used in prescriptions.

ANABIOSIS
A return to life from a state resembling death.

ANABOLIC STEROIDS
Group of steroids that are derivatives of the male sex hormone testosterone. They affect growth, muscle bulk and protein build-up, and have their uses in patients after major surgery or severe accidents or with debilitating disease, when there may be a breakdown of body protein. However, these drugs have been and are being abused by athletes, and for this reason, they are only prescribed by hospital doctors and are not available on normal prescriptions.

ANABOLISM
The constructive process by which living cells convert simple substances into more complex compounds, especially into living matter.

ANABOLITE
A product of an anabolic process.

ANACAL
Brand name of a preparation for the treatment of hemorrhoids containing heparinoid as the active ingredient.

ANACHLORHYDRIA
Absence of hydrochloric acid in the gastric juice.

ANACIDITY
Lack of normal acidity, especially in the gastric juice.

ANACLITIC

Term employed by psychoanalysts to describe one type of object-choice modelled after the first love object. Freud distinguished two types of object-choice: narcissistic and anaclitic.

Narcissistic object-choice occurs when people choose objects on the basis of some real or imagined similarity with themselves, while anaclitic object-choice occurs when the choice is based on the pattern of childhood dependence on those unlike themselves.

ANACLITIC DEPRESSION

Impaired development of an infant resulting from separation from its mother.

ANACROTIC PULSE

One with a "notch" in the ascending part of the pulse curve when seen on sphygmograms (graphic tracings of pulse beats), especially in aortic stenosis (narrowing of the main artery from the heart).

ANACROTISM

An abnormality of the blood circulation characterized by a secondary notch in the ascending part of a sphygmographic tracing of the pulse.

ANADIN

Pain reliever containing aspirin, salicylamide, caffeine and quinine sulphate.

ANADIPSIA

Intense thirst.

ANADONTISM

The state in which all teeth have failed to develop.

ANAEROBIC ORGANISM

Any organism whose respiration does not make use of oxygen. Many bacteria and parasites are facultative anaerobes (that is, they can survive without oxygen for short or long periods), and a few are obligate anaerobes (unable to use oxygen in respiration).

ANAEROBIOSIS

Life in the absence of air or free oxygen.

ANAGOGIC

Term employed by Carl Jung for the morally uplifting trends on the unconscious.

ANAGOGY

An elevation of mind to things celestial; the spiritual meaning or application of words.

ANAL

Related to, or situated near, the anus.

ANAL CANAL

The terminal section of the rectum.

ANAL CHARACTER

Type of character neurosis inferred to be the result of fixation at the anal stage of development. The term is usually used to refer to reaction formations against anal-erotism, in particular to compulsive obstinacy, orderliness and thrift, but can also refer to their opposites, namely untidiness and generosity.

ANALEPTIC

A drug that acts as a restorative, e.g. caffeine. Most analeptics stimulate certain parts of the brain.

ANAL EROTICISM

In psychoanalytical theory, concentration of interest on the anal region as a pregenital phase of sexual development.

ANAL FISSURE

An acute longitudinal tear or a chronic ovoid ulcer in the skin lining the anal canal.

ANAL FISTULA

Erosion of tissues caused by a

spreading abscess within the anus. The fistula itself is a tiny tube leading directly from the anal canal to a pin-hole-sized opening in the skin near the anal orifice. The treatment is a minor operation.

ANALGESIA
Loss of sensibility to pain.

ANALGESIC
Relating to, characterized by, or producing analgesia.

ANALGESICS
Drugs used for the relief of pain. They mainly impair perception of or emotional response to pain by affecting the higher brain center. Aspirin and paracetamol are mild but effective. Phenylbutazone, indomethacin and ibuprofen are, like aspirin, useful in treating rheumatoid arthritis by reducing inflammation as well as relieving pain. In principle, analgesics are agents that reduce pain without reducing consciousness.

Narcotic analgesics derived from opium alkaloids range from the milder codeine and dextropropoxyphene, suitable for general use, to the highly effective, euphoriant and addictive morphine and heroin. These last two are reserved for severe acute pain and terminal disease, where addiction is either unlikely or unimportant.

ANALGESICS, OTIC
Drugs used for the relief of pain of middle ear infections (otitis media). The preparations do not treat the infection itself. Brand names include: Aurafair, Auralgan, Aurodex, Auromid, Oto. The drug functions as a topical anesthetic/analgesic on the eardrum.

Possible adverse reactions or side effects include itching or burning in the ear (probably represents an allergic reaction). If these reactions occur, discontinue the treatment and call a doctor right away.

ANALITY
An anal psychological state, stage, or quality.

ANALOGOUS
Having similar function but a different structure and origin.

ANALOGUE
In medicine, term used in three different senses.
(1) Something that is analogous or similar to something else;
(2) an organ similar in function to an organ of another animal or plant but different in structure and origin:
(3) a chemical compound structurally similar to another but differing often by a single element of the same valence and group of the periodic table as the element it replaces.

ANALOGY
Functional similarity between anatomical parts without similarity of structure and origin.

ANAL SADISM
Refers to sadistic fantasies that originate in the anal stage.

ANAL SEX
Sexual intercourse by way of the anus. The area around the anus is an important erogenous zone, stimulating to both women and men. A couple may start with frequent manual penetration of each other's anuses and decide to try anal intercourse. If a woman has never had ana;l intercourse before, it will probably be difficult for her to accommodate a man's penis at first. Using some lubricant, the man should begin to dilate the woman's anus with a finger. If the woman is not properly prepared, anal intercourse will be painful. When the woman feels excited and ready, the man can start to enter her gradually with his penis. He should not thrust or move quickly. Both his penis and her anus should be well lubricated. The woman should bear down slightly on her

anus to relax it and facilitate initial penetration.

ANAL SPHINCTER
Ring of muscle tissue at the end of the gastrointestinal tract.

Either of two sphincters, called the outer and inner sphincter.
(1) An outer sphincter of striated muscle extending from the coccyx to the central tendinous part of the perineum and surrounding the anus immediately beneath the skin; called also external anal sphincter;
(2) an inner sphincter formed by the thickening of the circular smooth muscle of the rectum; called also internal anal sphincter.

ANAL STAGE
Stage of psychosexual development of infants postulated by instinct theory, in which the anus and defecation are the major source of sensuous pleasure and form the center of the infant's self-awareness.

Anal stage is also a stage of ego development, in which mastery of the body, particularly of its sphincters, are the infant's major preoccupation.

ANAL VERGE
The distal margin of the anal canal comprising the muscular rim of the anus.

ANALYSAND
A person who is being analyzed. The word owes what little currency it has to the fact that it makes it possible to avoid calling students 'patients'.

ANALYSIS
In its general psychological sense, the determining of the constituents of any total or complex experience or mental process; frequently used in a special sense of psychoanalysis, and kindred procedures and theories, and even as synonymous with psychoanalysis.

ANALYST
A person who analyzes or who is skilled in analysis.

ANALYTIC PSYCHOLOGY
A modification of psychoanalysis due to Carl Jung that adds to the concept of the personal unconscious a racial or collective unconscious, that objects to a narrowly sexual interpretation of libido, and that advocates that psychotherapy be conducted in terms of the patient's present-day conflicts and maladjustments rather that in terms of his early psychosexual development.

ANAMNESIS
Recalling to mind; employed also in the medical sense of the history of an illness up to the present.

ANAMNESTIC
(1) Of or relating to an anamnesis;
(2) of or relating to a second rapid increased production of antibodies in response to an immunogenic substance after serum antibodies from a first response can no longer be detected in the blood.

ANAMORPHOSIS
A gradually ascending progression or change of form from one type to another in the evolution of a group of animals or plants.

ANANCASM
Stereotyped, repetitious behavior which produces anxiety if not performed.

ANANCASTIC PERSONALITY DISORDER
Personality disorder characterized by:
- feelings of personal insecurity;
- doubt;
- incompleteness leading to excessive conscientiousness;
- checking;
- stubbornness;
- caution.
There may be insistent and unwel-

come thoughts or impulses which do not attain the severity of an obsessional neurosis. There is imperfectionism and meticulous accuracy and a need to check repeatedly in an attempt to ensure this. Rigidity and excessive doubt may be conspicuous.

ANAPHASE
The stage in mitosis (cell division) in which the chromosome halves move away from each other toward the opposite ends of the cell.

ANAPHRODISIA
Diminished sexual desire or sexual impotence.

ANAPHRODISIAC
A substance capable of dulling sexual appetite.

ANAPHYLACTIC REACTION
Severe allergic response to a substance, e.g., a drug of vaccine.
The major symptoms are:
- wheezing;
- itching;
- hives;
- nasal congestion;
- intense burning of hands and feet;
- collapse;
- loss of consciousness;
- cardiac arrest.
Symptoms appear within a few seconds or minutes after exposure. An anaphylactic reaction is a severe medical emergency.

ANAPHYLACTIC SHOCK
Sudden profound collapse following the injection of a foreign protein.

ANAPHYLACTOID PURPURA
Another name of allergic purpura.

ANAPHYLAXIS
An acute, often explosive, allergic reaction of the whole body, characterized by urticaria (skin rash), breathing problems and a dramatic drop in blood pressure and occasionally by vomiting and abdominal cramps.
Anaphylaxis occurs in people when they receive for a second time an antigen to which they have already become sensitive. It is a hypersensitive state of the body to a foreign protein (e.g., horse serum) so that the injection of a second dose after ten days brings about an acute reaction which may be fatal.

ANAPLASIA
Reversion of some highly developed cells of an organ or tissue in the body to a more primitive type, accompanied by excessive tendency to multiply, such as is seen in cancer growth.

ANAPOLON
Brand name of a hormonal preparation containing oxymetholone as the active ingredient. The hormone is given to compensate for deficiency of hormones of the pituitary gland or testicles.

ANARRHEXIS
Surgical operation of rebreaking a bone in order to reset it into a better position.

ANARTHRIA
The loss of power of articulate speech.

ANASPADIAS
Birth deformity in which the urethra opens on the top surface of the penis.

ANASTOMOSE
To join up or provide a communication between two different hollow parts or hollow organs; joining up two arteries by a surgical means. This joining-up can occur naturally when one blood vessel becomes blocked; its neighbors will open and form a network to carry blood around the blocked vessel to where it is needed. Unfortunately, the arteries that end in the brain, kidney

and intestine do not have this ability, and arteries to the heart to not have enough neighbors to deal with a blockage quickly enough.

ANA TITERS
A test to evaluate the immune system and to detect antinuclear antibodies (ANAs), substances which appear in the blood of some patients with autoimmune disease.

ANATOMY
The structure and form of biological organisms and their study.

ANATRICROTIC PULSE
A pulse wave with three breaks on the ascending curve of a tracing of heartbeats.

ANCON
The upper end of the ulna or elbow.

ANCROD
An enzyme obtained from the venom of the Malayan pit viper, acting specifically on fibrinogen in the blood, and thus prevents clotting. The enzyme is used as an anticoagulant in the treatment of retinal vein occlusion and deep vein thrombosis.

ANCYLOSTOMIASIS
Hookworm disease, caused by any of certain bloodsucking nematode worms equipped with mouth hooks, which feed off the lining of the intestine of humans and animals. The disease is characterized by severe anemia.

ANDROGENS
Steroid hormones that produce secondary male characteristics such as facial and body hair and a deep voice. They also develop the male reproductive organs. The main androgen is testosterone, produced in the testes; others are produced in small quantities in the cortex of the adrenal glands. Small amounts occur in women in addition to the fe-

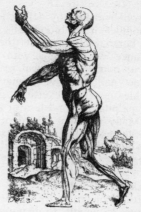

Classical anatomical drawing of the human muscular system by Andreas Vesalius, a famous anatomist of the 16th century.

male hormone, estrogen, and may produce some male characteristics.

ANDROGYNOID
A man with hermaphroditic sexual characteristics who is mistaken for a woman; a pseudohermaphrodite.

ANDROGYNY
Female pseudohermaphroditism.

ANDROID
Resembling a man in form and structure.

ANDROPHOBIA
Fear of men, or of the male sex.

ANDROSTERONE
Androgenic steroid probably manufactured by the adrenal glands and found in the urine of both men and women.

ANELECTROTONUS
The lessened irritability and conductivity of a nerve in the neighborhood of the anode (positive pole).

ANAEMIA
See Anemia.

ANAESTHESIA
See Anesthesia.

ANEMIA
A disorder caused by deficiency in the number of red blood cells or of their hemoglobin content (the red substance which binds with oxygen) or both. The clinical features include pallor, easy fatigue and breathlessness on exertion, giddiness, palpitations and less of appetite. Many different disorders may cause anemia, and it may sometimes occur as a result of drug treatment.

ANEMIA, APLASTIC
A form of anemia in which the bone marrow is unable to manufacture adequate numbers of blood cells of all types - red cells, white cells, and platelets.

ANEMIA, HEMOLYTIC
Anemia caused by a shortened lifespan of red blood cells. The body can't manufacture new cells fast enough to replace old cells.

ANEMIA, IRON-DEFICIENCY
Anemia caused by lack of iron. There are three main mechanisms by which a person becomes iron-deficient:
- nutritional insufficiency;
- intestinal malabsorption;
- blood loss.
These factors may be encountered together in the same individual.

ANEMIA, PERNICIOUS
Anemia caused by a vitamin B_{12} deficiency. Symptoms include:
- weakness;
- fatigue;
- numbness;
- vomiting;
- tingling of the hands or feet;
- degeneration of the central nervous system.

ANEMIA, SICKLE-CELL
Anemia caused by defective hemoglobin that deprives red blood cells of oxygen, making them sickle-shaped.

ANEMOPHOBIA
Morbid fear of wind and draughts.

ANENCEPHALY
Absence of the brain, or of all but the brain stem and the cerebellum.

ANERGY
Inability to react to specific antigens, either in the body fluids or in the cells themselves; usually refers to an inability to mount delayed-type skin reactions.

ANESTHESIA
Loss of sensation; absence of sensation may be of three types: general, local or pathological.

ANESTHESIA, GENERAL
A reversible state of drug-induced unconsciousness with muscle relaxation and suppression of reflexes; this facilitates many surgical procedures and avoids distress.

ANESTHESIA, INFILTRATION
Method of anesthesia by which the anesthetic is injected into the immediate area of the operation.

ANESTHESIA, LOCAL
The reversible blocking of pain impulses by the chemical action of cocaine derivatives. Large nerves are blocks for minor surgery and dentistry.

ANESTHESIA, NERVE BLOCK
Method of anesthesia by which the anesthetic is injected into the vicinity of a nerve rendering the area supplied by it insensitive.

ANESTHESIA, SPINAL
Method of anesthesia by which the anesthetic is injected into the vertebral canal outside or inside the subarachnoid space of the spinal cord.

ANESTHESIA DOLOROSA
Severe pain in part of the body which at the same time is insensible

to touch. Seen in certain diseases of the spinal cord.

ANESTHESIA, GENERAL
Gases that are used in surgery to render patients unconscious and able to withstand the pain of surgical cutting and manipulation.

ANESTHESIOLOGY
The science of administering anesthetics.

ANESTHETIC
Substance which causes the loss or reduction of sensitivity, though functional anesthesia may be produced by hypnotic suggestion or acupuncture.

ANESTHETIC, GENERAL
A drug or drug combination given to produce unconsciousness before and during surgery or potentially painful investigative procedures. General anesthesia is usually induced initially by injection of a drug such as thiopentone, and maintained by inhalation of the fumes of a volatile liquid such as halothane or a gas such as nitrous oxide mixed with oxygen.

ANESTHETIC, LOCAL
A drug applied topically or injected to numb sensation in a small area.

ANESTHETIC, TOPICAL
Medicine used to relieve pain, itching, and redness of minor skin disorders.

Topical anesthetics deaden the nerve endings in the skin. They do not cause drowsiness or unconsciousness as general anesthetics for surgery do. Benzocaine (present in many of these topical medicines) may be absorbed through the skin of young children and cause unwanted effects.

ANESTHETICS
Drugs that eliminate the sensation of pain.

ANESTHETIST
A medical doctor specializing in anesthesiology.

ANETHAINE
Brand name of a local anesthetic containing amethocaine as the active ingredient.

ANETHOPATHY
Personality disorder characterized by a lack of moral inhibitions and unethical behavior, and also including narcissistic sexual behavior and general egocentricity.

ANEUPLOIDY
An irregular number of chromosomes (e.g., 45, 47 or 48 chromosomes in humans), caused by the loss or addition of one or more chromosomes or parts of chromosomes.

ANEURINE
Vitamin B1, sometimes called thiamine. A deficiency of aneurine in the diet is the cause of beriberi.

ANEURYSM
A localized dilation of a blood vessel, usually an artery, due to local fault in the wall through defect, disease or injury,producing a pulsating swelling over which a murmur may be heard.

ANGEL'S WING
Abnormal prominence of the shoulder blades. Also called winged scapula.

ANGER
Primary emotion, provoked typically by frustration. Surprisingly, it is frequently confused with hate, despite the fact that it is a short-lasting emotion readily experienced towards those we love, whereas hate is a lasting sentiment.

ANGIITIS
Inflammation of a blood vessel or of a lymphatic.

ANGINA
Spasmodic pain associated with a sensation of choking or suffocation.

ANGINA PECTORIS
Severe but temporary attack of heart pain which may radiate to the arms, resulting from lack of oxygen to the heart muscle.

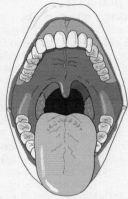

Oral cavity. The tonsils, in the back of the cavity, are the seat of angina tonsillaris.

ANGINA TONSILLARIS
Or tonsillitis, inflammatory reaction of the tonsils in the back of the mouth to an invasion of bacteria.

ANGIOCARDIOGRAM
X-ray of the heart and large blood vessels after the injection of radio-opaque substances into the bloodstream.

ANGIOCARDITIS
Inflammation of the heart and larger blood vessels attached to the heart.

ANGIOEDEMA
Local weals and a tingling redness on the skin, usually involving large fluid-filled areas.

ANGIOGRAPHY
Radiographic recording of a contrast material injected into arteries, veins or heart chambers to define anatomy, disease or direction of blood flow.

ANGIOHEMOPHILIA
Another name for Von Willebrand's disease.

ANGIOID
Pertaining to a blood vessel.

ANGIOLOGY
The branch of anatomy that deals with the blood vessels and lymphatics.

ANGIOMA
Swelling or tumor due to dilation of the blood vessels or lymphatics.

ANGIONECROSIS
Death of a blood vessel or part of a blood vessel.

ANGIONEURECTOMY
Surgical removal of blood vessels and nerves.

ANGIONEUROTIC EDEMA
Condition in which loose tissues of the body, notably the face and the scrotum in the male, swell up. It may be a manifestation of an allergy or emotional disorder.

ANGIOPLASTY
Surgical repair of blood vessels.

ANGIOSARCOMA
Malignant growth of blood vessel tissue.

ANGIOSPASM
Spasmodic contraction of the muscular coats of the smaller arteries.

ANGIOTENSIN
Hormone formed from angiotensinogen (a blood plasma constituent) by certain cells in the kidney.

When in contact with renin (also produced by the kidney), a substance is formed that raises blood pressure.

ANGSTRÖM UNIT
Unit for measuring wavelengths of ultraviolet light, X-rays or radium.

The unit is equivalent to one-hundred-millionth of a centimeter.

ANGUISH
(1) Extreme pain or distress of either body or mind.
(2) Any keen affection of the emotions or feelings.

ANHEDONIA
Absence of the capacity to experience pleasure,particularly in the sense of absence of pleasure-unpleasure feeling in situations where it is normally present.

ANHYDREMIA
Lessening or lowering of the watery constituents in the blood.

ANHYDROSIS
Abnormal decrease or absence of sweat.

ANILINE
An oily compound obtained from the dry distillation of coal and much used in the preparation of dyes. It is an important cause of serious industrial poisoning associated with malfunction of bone marrow as well as blood disorders.

ANIMA, ANIMUS
Terms of Carl Jung describing the unconscious female image in men and the unconscious male image in women.

ANIMALISM
The state of being actuated by sensual appetites only.

ANIMAL MAGNETISM
Any force or power in certain individuals said to give them the ability to induce hypnosis.

ANIMISM
The belief that anything that moves is alive.

ANIRIDIA
Absence of the iris.

ANISOCORIA
Inequality in the diameter of the pupils of the eye.

ANISOCYTOSIS
Unequal size of the red blood corpuscles and an indication of the presence of a blood disease.

ANISOMELIA
Unequal length of limbs.

ANKLE
The joint connecting the foot and the leg. Sprained ankle is a common acute injury, causing considerable discomfort and disability. Physiotherapy is the method of choice for treatment. The ankle joint may be affected in rheumatoid arthritis. Pain is often due to inflammation of the sheaths of the peroneal tendon and of the bursa. Inflammation of the bursa may be visible in an X-ray as an opacity behind the Achilles tendon. When the joint is affected, this causes local tenderness, and pain is felt especially on flexion and extension.

ANKLE CLONUS
Greatly increased ankle jerk reflex and a sign to the doctor of a disorder of the nervous system.

ANKLE JERK
Reflex jerk of the foot produced by the calf muscles when the Achilles tendon at the back of the heel is

Lateral view of the ankle joint.

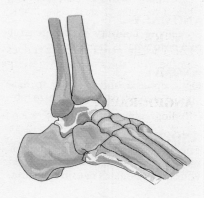

tapped with a hammer.

ANKLE TONUS REFLEX
Clonic (spasmodic) contractions of the calf muscles in response to pressure against the sole of the foot.

ANKYLOCOLPOS
Narrowing of the vagina from adhesions.

ANKYLOSE
To fuse together. This term is normally used when referring to joints in which the two surfaces are fused together by disease or are fixed together by surgical operation, the result being that the joint becomes solid and is no longer usable.

ANKYLOSING SPONDYLITIS
A chronic progressive form of arthritis distinguished by inflammation and eventual ankylosis (fusing) of a number of joints, primarily involving the spine and paraspinal structures. Characteristic are calcium deposits in the discs between the vertebrae of the spine and adjacent connective tissue, which eventually become bone-like.

ANLAGE
The initial accumulation of cells in a growing organ or part.

ANNOYANCE
The physical or mental discomfort caused by something that angers or irritates.

ANOMALY
Something contrary to the general rule or to what is expected.

ANOMIA
Optic aphasia, the inability to recognize names or to recognize objects.

ANOPHELES
The generic name of a group of mosquitoes, which, when infected with the organisms causing malaria, may transmit the disease to human beings by biting.

ANORCHUS
A male with congenital absence of testicles in the scrotum. A condition with undescended testicles may also exist.

ANORECTAL ABSCESS
Abscess resulting from bacterial invasion of the tissues surrounding the rectum, usually extending from an anal pouch or crypt.

ANORECTAL FISTULA
A tube-like tract with one opening in the anal canal and the other opening usually in the skin around the anus.

ANOREXIA
Pathological loss of appetite.

ANOREXIA NERVOSA
A disorder characterized by a disturbed sense of body image and marked anxiety about weight gain, manifested by an abnormal pattern of food handling, marked weight loss and, in women loss of periods. The disturbance in body image is manifested by the way in which the person's body weight, size, or shape is experienced.

People with this disorder say they "feel fat," or that parts of their body are "fat," when they are obviously underweight or even emaciated. They are preoccupied with their body size and usually dissatisfied with some feature of their physical appearance.

The weight loss is usually accompanied by a reduction in total food intake, often with extensive exercising. Frequently there is also self-induced vomiting or use of laxatives or diuretics.

The person usually comes to professional attention when weight loss (or failure to gain expected weight) is marked. An example is weighing less that 85% of expected

weight. By the time the person is profoundly underweight, there are other signs, such as:
- hypothermia;
- bradycardia;
- hypotension;
- edema;
- lanugo (neonatal-like hair);
- variety of metabolic changes.

In most cases amenorrhea follows weight loss, but it is not unusual for amenorrhea to appear before noticeable weight loss has occurred.

Most people with this disorder steadfastly deny or minimize the severity of their illness and are uninterested in, or resistant to, therapy. Many of the adolescents have delayed psychosexual development, and adults have a markedly decreased interest in sex.

Compulsive behavior, such as hand-washing may be present during the illness and may justify the additional diagnosis of obsessive compulsive disorder.

ANORGASMY
Absence of a climax (orgasm) in sexual relations.

ANOSMIA
Loss of the sense of smell.

ANOSPINAL
Pertaining to the spine and the anus.

ANOVESICAL
Pertaining to the anus and the urinary bladder.

ANOVULATION
Cessation of egg-cell production by the ovaries.

ANOXEMIA
Deficiency of oxygen in the blood.

ANOXIA
Lack of oxygen in blood and body tissues. Asphyxia, lung disease, paralysis of respiratory muscles and some forms of coma prevent enough oxygen reaching the blood.

Disease of the heart or circulation may also lead to tissue anoxia. Irreversible brain damage follows prolonged anoxia.

ANTACIDS
Mild alkalis or bases taken by mouth to neutralize excess stomach acidity for relief of dyspepsia, including the pain of a peptic ulcer and heartburn. Milk of magnesia, aluminum hydroxide and sodium bicarbonate are common antacids.

With larger doses than those used, magnesium oxide and milk of magnesia produce a laxative effect.

Some antacids, like aluminum carbonate and aluminum hydroxide, may be prescribed with a low-phosphate diet to treat hyperphosphatemia (too much phosphate in the blood).

ANTAGONISM
Opposition to the action of a substance on living cells or tissues.

ANTAGONIST
A term meaning to have a negative effect.
(1) A drug that counteracts the action of another drug.
(2) A muscle that counteracts another muscle.

ANTEFLEXION OF THE UTERUS
An abnormal position of the uterus, where it is sharply bent forward.

ANTEMORTEM
Before death.

ANTENATAL
Before birth. The period between conception and delivery of the child.

ANTENATAL CARE
Monitoring of the condition of a pregnant woman and of her unborn child. Advice is given about her diet, the bad effects of smoking, and other matters. One can obtain ante-

natal care from a family doctor or from a clinic.

ANTEPARTUM
Before the onset of labor.

ANTERIOR POLIOMYELITIS
A type of poliomyelitis.

ANTERIOR ROOT
Bundle of nerve fibers emerging from the front portion of the spinal cord to form a spinal nerve. Also called a motor root because it supplies the muscles with nerves.

ANTERIOR UVEITIS
Inflammation of the iris or ciliary body of the eye or, more usually, inflammation of both.

ANTEVERSION
Turning or tilting forward; displacement as in the tipping forward of an organ.

ANTHELIX
An elevated ridge of cartilage in the auricle, the external part of the ear.

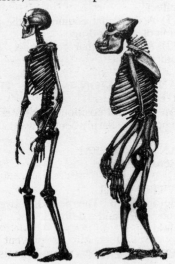

In the research on the descent of man, great value has been attached to the study of the relationship between man and anthropoid apes. Left the skeleton of man, right skeleton of an anthropoid ape.

ANTHELMINTIC
A medicine that destroys parasitic intestinal worms.

ANTHRACOSIS
Black lung; the depositing of coal dust in the lungs, occurring mainly in those who work in coal mines. It causes no ill effects.

ANTHRAX
A rare bacterial disease causing characteristic skin pustules and lung disease; it may progress to septicemia (blood poisoning) and death. Anthrax spores, which can survive for years, may be picked up from infected animals such as sheep or cattle, or from bone meal. Treatment is with penicillin, and people at risk are vaccinated; the isolation of animal cases and the disinfection of spore-bearing material is essential. It was the first disease in which bacteria were shown (by Koch) to be the cause and it had one of the earliest effective vaccines, developed by Pasteur.

ANTHROPOGRAPHY
The branch of anthropology which studies thegeographical distribution of people according to physical type, language, culture, etc.

ANTHROPOLOGY
The study of humans from biological, cultural and social viewpoints. There are two main disciplines, physical anthropology and cultural anthropology, the latter embracing social anthropology.

Physical anthropology is the study of humans as a biological species, their past evolution and their contemporary physical characteristics. In its study of prehistoric humans, it has many links with archaeology, the difference being that anthropology is concerned with the remains or fossils of humans while archaeology is concerned with the remains of their material culture. The physical anthropologist also studies the difference between races and groups, relying to a great extent on techniques of anthropometry and, more recently, genetic studies.

Cultural anthropology is divided into several classes. Ethnography is the study of the culture of a single group, either primitive or civilized.

ANTHROPOMETRY
The anthropological study of the physical characteristics of humans; originally restricted to measurements of parts of the body, it now includes blood-typing, biostatistics, etc. Anthropometry has contributed considerably to modern ideas of human evolution.

ANTHROPOMORPHISM
The attribution of human characteristics to that which is not human. It occurs in mythology, religion, literature (especially in fables where animals are credited with human feelings) and in common phrases such as "the cruel sea" and "the angry sky."

ANTHROPOPHOBIA
A pathological fear of human companionship or of society in general.

ANTHROPOSOPHY
A spiritual movement developed under Rudolf Steiner, who founded the Anthroposophical Society in 1912. It aims at higher spiritual experience and knowledge, through man's inner powers independent of the senses. Steiner claimed his "spiritual science" had practical applications, especially in education, and some schools are based on his ideas.

ANTI-ADRENALINE
Agent opposing the effects of impulses conveyed by adrenergic postganglionic fibers of the sympathetic nervous system.

ANTI-ADRENALS
Medicines or drugs that prevent the effects of the hormones liberated by the adrenal glands.

ANTI-ALLERGIC AGENT
Agent that lessens or decreases allergic reactions.

ANTI-ANGINALS
A group of drugs used to treat angina pectoris (chest pain that comes and goes, caused by coronary artery disease).

ANTI-ANTITOXIN
An antibody that inhibits or counteracts the effects of an antitoxin.

ANTI-ANXIETY DRUG
Drug used to treat symptoms of anxiety, feelings of apprehension or danger accompanied by restlessness.

ANTI-ARRHYTHMIC DRUG
Drug used to help regulate an unusual or abnormal heart rhythm.

ANTI-ASTHMATIC DRUG
Drug used to treat symptoms of asthma, including difficulty in breathing and wheezing.

ANTIBACTERIAL DRUG
Drug that is destructive to or prevents the growth of bacteria.

ANTIBACTERIAL SERUM
Blood serum that can kill bacteria or prevent their growth.

ANTIBIOSIS
A relationship between two organisms that is harmful to one, such as in parasitism.

ANTIBIOTICS
Substances produced by micro-organisms that kill or prevent the growth of other micro-organisms; their properties are made use of in the treatment of bacterial and fungal infections. Pasteur noted the effect in the 19th century, and in 1928 Alexander

Fleming first showed that the mould Penicillium notatum produced penicillin, a substance able to destroy certain bacteria. It was not until 1940 that Florey and Chain were able to manufacture sufficient amounts of penicillin for clinical use. The isolation of streptomycin by Waksman in 1944, gramicidin (from tyrothricin) by Dubois, and the cephalosporins were among early discoveries of antibiotics useful against human infection.

Numerous varieties of antibiotics now exist and the search continues for new ones. Semi-synthetic antibiotics, in which the basic molecule is chemically modified, have increased the range of naturally occurring substances.

ANTIBODY
A substance produced by body tissue or cells as a reaction to the introduction of a foreign substance (an antigen).

ANTICHOLINERGIC DRUG
A drug that antagonizes or counteracts the effects of acetylcholine, a natural substance responsible for transmitting nerve impulses from one nerve to another or from a nerve to an organ.

ANTICIPATORY REACTION
Response by a subject to a stimulus other than the proper stimulus, given by a keyed-up subject, and shown by an extremely short reaction time, in some cases even of almost zero value.

ANTICOAGULANT
Any drug that interferes with blood clotting, used to treat or to prevent thrombosis and clot embolism. The two main types are heparin, which is injected and has an immediate but short-lived effect, and the coumarins (including warfarin), which are taken by mouth and are longer-lasting. They affect different parts of the clotting mechanism, coumarins depleting certain factors made in the liver. In order for an anticoagulant to help[you without causing serious bleeding, it must be used properly and all the precautions concerning its use must be followed exactly. be sure that you have discussed the use of this medicine with your doctor.

ANTICONVULSANT DRUG
Drug used to prevent or treat any disease associated with violent involuntary contractions such as occur in epilepsy.

ANTIDEPRESSANTS
Drugs used in the treatment of depression; they are of two types: tricyclic compounds and monoamine oxidase inhibitors. Although their mode of action is obscure, they have revolutionized the treatment of depression.

ANTIDIABETIC DRUG
Drug used to treat the symptoms of diabetes mellitus.

ANTIDIABETICS, ORAL
Medicines taken by mouth to help reduce the amount of sugar present in the blood. They are used to treat certain types of diabetes mellitus (sugar diabetes). Oral antidiabetics can usually be used only by adults who develop diabetes after 30 years of age and who do not require insulin shots to control their condition. Patients who are taking oral antidiabetics may have to switch to insulin if they:
- develop diabetic coma or ketoacidosis;
- have a severe injury or burn;
- are to have major surgery;
- are pregnant.

ANTIDIARRHEAL DRUG
Drug used to treat symptoms of diarrhea.

ANTIDIURETIC
An agent that acts to reduce excretion of urine.

ANTIDIURETIC HORMONE (ADH)
Hormone produced by the posterior lobe of the pituitary gland. It acts on the kidneys and plays a large part in regulating the volume of urine.

ANTI-D IMMUNOGLOBULIN
Name of a drug used to prevent sensitization to Rhesus antigen.

ANTIDOTE
Drug used to counteract the adverse effects of a drug or chemical.

ANTIDYSKINETICS
Medicines used to treat Parkinson's disease. By improving muscle control and reducing stiffness, these medicines allow more normal movements of the body as the disease symptoms are reduced.

ANTI-EMETIC DRUG
Drug used to control vomiting.

ANTIFIBRONYLTIC DRUGS
A group of drugs used to treat fungus infections. Those listed as systemic are taken orally or given by injection. Those listed as topical are applied directly to the skin and include liquids, powders, creams, ointments and liniments. Those listed as vaginal are used topically inside the vagina and sometimes on the vaginal lips.

ANTIFLATULENT DRUG
Drug used to relieve discomfort due to excessive gas ("wind") in the stomach or intestines.

ANTIFUNGAL
Said of an agent destructive to fungi;suppressing the growth or reproduction of fungi.

ANTIGALACTIC
Agent which dries up the supply of milk in the lactating breast.

ANTIGEN
A substance capable of combining with antibody and causing a specific immune response by the body. Sometimes used to mean a substance that can combine with an antibody but cannot by itself elicit an immune response.

ANTIGENIC DETERMINANT
The specific configuration on the surface of an antigen that determines its ability to react with a corresponding configuration on an antibody.

ANTIGLAUCOMA DRUGS
Medicines used to treat glaucoma. Those listed as systemic are taken orally or given by injection. Those listed as ophthalmic are used as eye drops.

ANTIGLOBULIN
Antibody directed against an immunoglobulin molecule.

ANTIGOUT DRUGS
Drugs to treat the metabolic disease called gout. Gout causes recurrent attacks of joint pain caused by deposits of uric acid in the joint.

ANTHELMINTHIC DRUG
Drug used to treat infections caused by helminths(worms).

ANTIHEMOPHILIC FACTOR
A blood protein used to promote blood clotting in hemophilia.

ANTIHISTAMINE
Drug used for its ability to neutralize or antagonize the effects of histamine, a naturally occurring substance; used to relieve the symptoms of allergy.Some of the antihistamines are also used to prevent motion sickness, nausea, vomiting, and dizziness.

ANTIHYPERLIPIDEMIC DRUGS
Drugs used to help control high levels of fats (cholesterol, triglycerides) in the blood.

ANTIHYPERTENSIVE DRUGS

Drugs that can be used to control high blood pressure (hypertension). Those most often given are the diuretics (primarily the thiazides), which promote the natural elimination of excess fluids in the tissues and circulation. Some of the other major anti-hypertensive drugs lower blood pressure by their direct or indirect dilating effect on the arteries. Hydralazine, for example, directly relaxes the tiny muscles in the arterial walls. Other drugs block or dampen the nerves that signal the arteries to constrict. The drug propranolol slows the heartbeat, decreases the force of the heart's contractions and thus lowers the blood pressure.

ANTI-INFECTIVE

Relating to any agent used to treat an infection.

ANTI-INFLAMMATORY

Agent drug for reducing inflammation.

ANTI-INFLAMMATORY ANALGESIC

Medicine taken by mouth to relieve some symptoms caused by arthritis or rheumatism, such as inflammation, swelling, stiffness, and joint pain. The medicines do not cure arthritis and will help you only as long as you continue to take it.

Some of these medicines are also used to relieve other kinds of pain or to treat other painful conditions, such as:- gout attacks;
- bursitis;
- tendinitis;
- sprains, strains, or other injuries;
- menstrual cramps.

ANTILYMPHOCYTE SERUM

Full name of ALS.

ANTIMALARIALS

A group of drugs used to treat malaria. The choice depends on the precise type of malaria organisms and its developmental state.

ANTIMETABOLITE

An agent bearing a close structural resemblance to one required for normal functioning of the body, and exerting its effect by interfering with the utilization of the essential metabolite.

ANTIMICROBIC

Agent acting against or destroying microbes (germs).

ANTIMIGRAINE

Agent or drug against severe headache or migraine, such as methysergide.

ANTIMONIUM TARTARICUM

Homeopathic drug. Useful for respiratory diseases. The guiding symptom has been the rattling of the lungs with mucus with little coughing up. For diseases originating from exposure in damp basements and cellars.

ANTIMYASTHENICS

Medicines to treat myasthenia gravis, a muscle disorder (especially of the face and head) with increasing fatigue and weakness as muscles tire from use.

ANTIMYCOTIC

Agent acting against or destroying fungi.

ANTIMYDRIATIC

Substance which, when applied to the eye, contracts the pupil.

ANTINEOPLASTIC DRUG

Drug used to treat neoplasms (unusual growths oftissue). Cancers are neoplastic diseases.

ANTINUCLEAR ANTIBODIES

Antibody substances measured in blood to detect a wide variety of diseases, including connective tissue disease, drug-associated disease and others involving the liver, intestines and circulatory system.

ANTIPARKINSONIAN
Agent or drug effective in the treatment of Parkinson's disease.

ANTIPERIODIC
Agent or drug useful against periodic diseases such as intermittent fever.

ANTIPERISTALSIS
Peristalsis (involuntary movement of the alimentary tract) taking place in the reverse direction.

ANTIPHLOGISTIC
An agent that subdues inflammation.

ANTIPRESSAN
Brand name of a beta-blocker drug that contains atenolol as active ingredient.

ANTIPRURITIC DRUG
Drug used to relieve itching.

ANTIPSYCHOTIC DRUGS
Drugs used to treat the mental disease of psychosis, including such variants as schizophrenia, manic-depressive psychosis, anxiety states, severe behavior problems and others.

ANTIPYRETIC DRUG
Drug used to reduce fever. The most commonly used drugs are aspirin and paracetamol.

ANTIPYRINE
A white, crystalline powder used to reduce fever or relieve pain.

ANTIRHEUMATIC DRUG
Drug used to treat arthritis or other rheumatic disease.

ANTISEPTIC
Substance that kills or prevents the growth of micro-organisms (particularly bacteria and fungi). They are used to avoid sepsis (infection) from contamination of body surfaces and surgical instruments. Some antiseptics are used as disinfectants to make places or objects germ-free. Vinegar and cedar oil have been used since earlier times to treat wounds and for embalming. Commonly used antiseptics and disinfectants include iodine, chlorine, hypochlorous acid, alcohol, isopropanol, phenols (including hexachlorophene), quaternary ammonium salts, formaldehyde, hydrogen peroxide, potassium permanganate and acriflavine (an aniline dye). Heat, ultraviolet and ionizing radiations also have antiseptic effects.

ANTISEPSIS
Destruction of germs causing disease, fermentation or putrefaction.

ANTISERUM
Blood serum containing a specific type of antibody.

ANTISOCIAL
Aversion of being with people; hostility towards codes of conduct stemming from any organization of people.

ANTISOCIAL DISORDER
Personality disorder characterized by disregard for social obligations, lack of feeling for others and impetuous violence or callous unconcern. There is a gross disparity between behavior and prevailing social norms. Behavior is not readily modified by experience, including punishment. People with this personality disorder are emotionally cold and may be abnormally aggressive or irresponsible. Their tolerance to frustration is low; they blame others or offer plausible rationalizations for the behavior that brings them into conflict with society.

ANTISPASMODIC
An agent that quiets muscle spasm. The drugs reduce spasms (abnormally strong or inappropriate con-

traction) of the muscles of the gastrointestinal tract, airways, and blood vessels. Antispasmodic drugs are most commonly prescribed to relieve irritable bowel syndrome.

ANTISTREPTOLYSIN
Agent acting against streptolysis, a product of Streptococci. The quantity of antistreptolysin in the blood may be indicative of a recent infection with Streptococci.

ANTITETANUS
Agent acting against or destroying the tetanus (lockjaw) bacillus.

ANTITETANUS SERUM
The full name of ATS.

ANTITHYROID DRUGS
Drugs which decrease the amount of thyroid hormones produced by the thyroid gland.

ANTITOXINS
Antibodies produced in the body against the toxins (poisons) of some bacteria. They are also formed after inoculation with a toxoid, a chemically inactivated toxin that can still confer immunity.

ANTITUSSIVE DRUG
Drug used to relieve cough.

ANTI-ULCER DRUGS
A group of medicines used to treat peptic ulcer in the stomach, duodenum or the lower end of the esophagus.

ANTIVIRAL
Something which is effective in the treatment against a virus.

ANTIVITAMIN
A substance that makes a vitamin ineffective.

ANTIVIVISECTION
Opposition to experiments in laboratories conducted on living animals to reveal whether remedies are safe to be used on humans.

ANTRUM
A natural hollow or cavity, particularly a cavity in bone.

ANTRUM PYLORI
Part of the stomach just before the pylorus, the narrow inferior region, that communicates with the duodenum of the intestine via a sphincter.

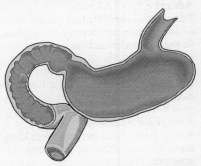

Localization of the antrum pylori just before the pylorus of the stomach.

ANURESIS
Inability to bring about the act of urination.

ANURIA
Total suppression of urine.

ANUS
Back passage, the terminal opening of the intestines.

ANVIL
The incus, one of the three small bones in the middle ear.

ANXIETY
An unpleasant and disturbing emotion. Its symptoms vary: anxious people may suffer merely an ill-defined discomfort or a profound sense of impending doom. They may be irritable, restless and agitated, or have impulses for physical activity that may be purposeless and aimless.
  Physical symptoms may include:
- increase in heart rate;

- high blood pressure;
- generalized or localized muscle tension;
- rapid and shallow breathing;
- sighing or shortness of breath;
- dizziness;
- fainting;
- dry mouth;
- sweating;
- nausea;
- vomiting;
- diarrhea;
- frequent urination.

Depending on the individual and the circumstances, the symptoms may vary in intensity from mild discomfort to attacks of severe panic. The anxiety may be acute, lasting a few minutes to a few hours, or it may become chronic, with symptoms mild to moderate in intensity but almost constantly present. The chronic state may be intermittently and unpredictably accompanied by acute increases in the severity of the symptoms.

Anxiety of some sort is one of life's most universal experiences. It is both emotional and physical, and the two aspects are closely interrelated and mutually reinforcing. The emotional aspects of anxiety are an interpretation of and a reaction to the physical changes taking place in the anxious person's body.

Anxiety is usually brought on by stress. Stress can be defined as anything perceived to be threatening to the individual's habitual state of being. The stress may be well defined and external (i.e., fear of heights, open spaces, physical injury or illness, dying, being caught in a tabooed act, being tested) or ill defined and internal (i.e., an onset of excitement, hostility, assertiveness, tenderness).

The anxiety signal sets in motion a series of voluntary and autonomic (spontaneous) responses intended to restore the individual's homeostasis. Anxiety continues to be felt as long as the person experiences movement away from his familiar steady state and doubts that efforts to reverse the direction of this movement will succeed.

It has been implied that anxiety is always undesirable and to be avoided. On the contrary, human personality development studies have demonstrated that tolerable levels of age-appropriate anxiety are largely responsible for individuals' gradual establishment of sophisticated, self-reliant behavior, attitudes and values. From these they develop their own patterns of adaptability, the ability to recognize alternatives and to explore options, and ultimately the capacity to respond appropriately to specific situations.

ANXIETY COMPLEX
Form of neurosis characterized by fear and apprehension at the outcome of any situation; a morbid attitude to personal health and a constant feeling of impending disaster.

ANXIETY DISORDER
Another name for anxiety neurosis.

ANXIETY EQUIVALENT
Intense physical response or bodily disturbance such as rapid heartbeat or breathlessness which replaces conscious anxiety or fear.

ANXIETY NEUROSIS
Condition in which apprehension is objectively out of proportion to any apparent cause.

Studies of both humans and other animals have shown that, when the intensity of age-appropriate stress evokes an anxiety exceeding the individual's capacity to adapt, restrictive, rigid and defensive behavior patterns (neurotic symptoms) result.

Such behavior was first intended to protect the individual either from apparent sources of stress or from making responses that could exaggerate movement away from his or her familiar steady state.

ANXIOLYTICS
Agents that reduce anxiety. The drugs belong to the group of benzodiazepines, such as Librium and Valium.

AORTA
The main trunk of the arterial blood circulatory system from which all arteries (except the pulmonary) branch. This large artery stems from the heart at the left ventricle.

AORTA-ARTERIOGRAPHY
X-ray studies, using a series of films, of the circulatory system of the abdomen and a portion of the lower extremities, after injecting contrast medium through a needle or catheter into an artery or vein in the lower part of the body.

AORTIC ANEURYSM
Blood-filled sac formed by localized swelling of the aorta wall.

AORTIC ARCH SYNDROME
A collection of symptoms resulting from disease that obstructs one or more of the large branches of the aortic arch, commonly the innominate, the left common carotid and

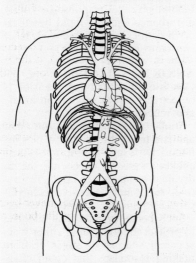

Distribution of the aorta in the abdominal cavity and thorax.

the left subclavian arteries.

AORTIC INCOMPETENCE
Incorrect closure of the aortic valve (between the aorta and the heart), whereby blood may leak back from the aorta to the left ventricle.

AORTIC STENOSIS
Narrowing of the aorta. May particularly refer to a narrowing of the aortic valve area in the heart.

AORTIC VALVE
A valve at the junction of the aorta and the left ventricle of the heart.

AORTITIS
Inflammation of the aorta, either weakening the aortic wall, leading to aneurysm formation, or obstructing the aortic lumen (the cavity inside the aorta) or of the openings of major branches, leading to symptoms and signs of ischemia (a lack of blood to the tissues).

AORTOGRAPHY
Visualization by X-rays of the aorta and its branches after the injection of a contrast medium.

APAREUNIA
Inability to have sexual intercourse.

APATHY
Lack of feeling or emotion.

APE HAND
Deformity of the hand seen in progressive muscular atrophy and in amyotrophic lateral sclerosis.

APERISTALSIS
Absence of peristalsis (involuntary muscular movement of the digestive tract).

APEX
The top of a body, organ or part.

APEXCARDIOGRAPHY
A procedure in which a transducer is applied to the apex of the heart, to

identify abnormal heart sounds in such conditions as heart valve disease or tumor of the heart muscle.

APGAR RATING
System of scoring a newborn infant's physical condition one and five minutes after birth.

APHAGIA
Inability to swallow.

APHAKIA
Absence of the clear lens of the eye.

APHALANGIA
Congenital absence of fingers or toes.

APHASIA
A defect or loss of language function, in which the comprehension or expression of words is impaired as a result of injury to the language centers in the cerebral cortex of the brain.

APHEMIA
Inability to utter words, due to emotion orpsychoneurosis.

APHONIA
Inability to utter sounds, owing to defect or disease of the larynx.

APHRODISIAC
Anything contributing to sexual excitement.Aphrodisiacs may be external (touch, sight, etc.) or internal (foods, drugs, etc.), the latter working usually by suggestion or, like alcohol and marijuana, by lowering inhibitions. Most foods traditionally regarded as aphrodisiac depend for their supposed efficacy merely on their chance genital shape.

APHTHA
A small ulcer occurring usually in the mouth.

APHTHONGIA
Inability to utter words, because of muscular spasm in the tongue.

APHTHOUS ULCER
White, often painful ulcer, usually appearing asclusters on the lower lip.

APICECTOMY
Excision of the apex of the petrous (hard) part of the temporal bone protecting the inner ear, or the apex of a tooth.

APIS MELLIFICA
Homeopathic drug prepared from live honey bees. The drug has been used successfully to treat hot, red swellings in any part of the body; the ill effects of swallowing hot things; sore throat; nettle rash; dropsy; white swelling of knee; and inflammation of the eyes, skin and kidneys.

APLASIA
Congenital absence or defective development of a tissue or organ.

APLASTIC ANEMIA
Anemia characterized by a drastic fall in theproduction of all blood cells in the bone marrow.

APNEA
Temporary cessation of breathing.

APOCRINE SWEAT GLAND
Gland exhibiting that type of secretion in which the free end of the secreting cell is cast off along with the secretory product.

APONEUROSIS
A white, very resistant membrane surrounding the voluntary muscles and large arteries, and covering the skull beneath the scalp.

APOPHYSIS
Bony outgrowth that has never been entirely separated from the bone of which it forms a part.

APOPLEXY
Another name for stroke: abolition or sudden diminution of sensation

and voluntary movement, resulting from clotting in or rupture of the blood vessels of the brain.

APOSTASY
An abandonment of what one has professed; a total desertion or departure from one's faith or principles.

APP
Brand name of a compound drug for certain disorders of the gastrointestinal tract, containing as active ingredients homatropine (an antispasmodic drug), bismuth (an antiulcer drug), and calcium carbonate, magnesium carbonate, magnesium trisilicate, and aluminum hydroxide.

APPENDECTOMY
Surgical excision of the vermiform appendix.

APPENDICITIS
Acute or chronic inflammatory process of the appendix.

APPENDICOLYSIS
Surgical cutting of adhesions about the appendix.

APPENDICULAR
Relating to an appendage or limb.

APPENDIX
Usually referring to the vermiform appendix, a small hollow blind organ located where the small and large intestines meet.

APPERCEPTION
In the original sense, clear perception, in particular where there is recognition or identification. Nowadays in the psychology of education, it is taken as the fundamental process in acquiring knowledge, and the part played by existing knowledge.

APPETITE
Immediate desire, commonly associated with food, sexual feelings, etc.; used also to describe an insistent impulse, inherited or acquired and, when congenital, frequently classed as an instinctive impulse.

APPETITE SUPPRESSANT
Medicine used in the short-term (a few weeks) treatment of obesity. For a few weeks (6 to 12), these medicines in combination with dieting, exercise, and changes in eating habits can help patients lose weight. However, since their appetite-reducing effect is only temporary, they are useful only for the first few weeks of dieting until new eating habits are established. They are not effective for continuous use in diet control.

APPLIED PSYCHOLOGY
The branch of psychology which seeks to apply to practical problems and practical life the methods and results of pure and (especially) experimental psychology. The term is somewhat broad, including industrial, clinical and educational psychology.

Sometimes the term psychotechniques is used, but in a narrower, and more technical sense, to describe the actual practice, particularly in the industrial field.

APPRECIATION
The quick grasp of a situation or set of actions; the first stage of comprehension.

APPREHENSION
Mental perception or understanding.

APPREHENSION SPAN
The largest numbers of objects that can be remembered after a limited period of seeing them.

APPROACH-APPROACH CONFLICT
A conflict existing within a person who, with two or more desirable but mutually exclusive goals, is temporarily torn between them.

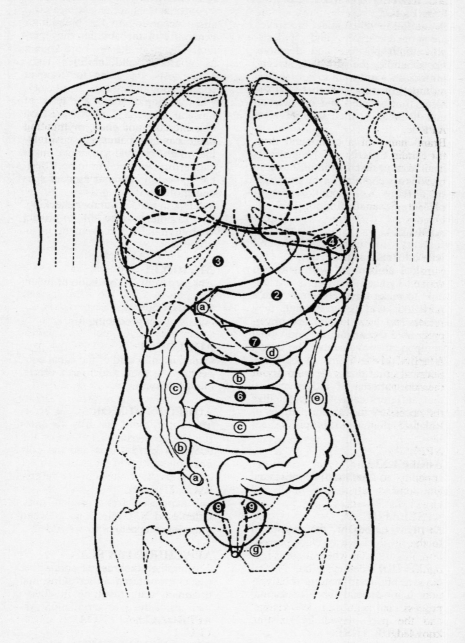

Localization of the appendix in the abdominal cavity.
1. heart and lungs; 2. stomach; 3. liver, 4. spleen; 6. small intestine (a. duodenum; b. jejunum; c. ileum); large intestine (a. appendix; b. cecum; c. ascending colon; d. transverse colon; e. descending colon; f. sigmoid; g. rectum); 9. urinary bladder.

APPROACH-AVOIDANCE CONFLICT

A conflict in which many incentives are at oncedesirable and undesirable, both positive and negative. For example, the girl likes sweets, but she does not want to get fat. The attitude toward a goal that is at the same time wanted and not wanted and disliked, is called an ambivalent attitude.

APPROBATION

That state or disposition of the mind in which we assent to the propriety of a thing with some degree of pleasure or satisfaction.

APRAXIA

Inability to execute purposeful learned movements despite the physical ability and willingness to do so. Typically, sufferers are unable to make themselves move in a particular way, even though they understand how to and are physically able to execute the individual component movements. The defect is apparently an injury in the nerve pathways that retain the memory of learned patterns of movement, so that sufferers cannot conceptualize the necessary movement patterns or translate them into purposive action.

APROSEXIA

Inability to maintain concentrated attention.

APSELAPHESIA

Disorganization of the sense of touch.

APTITUDE

Natural ability to acquire relatively general or special types of knowledge or skill.

APTITUDE TEST

A test that predicts performances not yet obtained. The items in the test consist of samples of achievements, that is, of what can be accomplished now.

Aptitude tests are sometimes classified according to the breadth or generality of the abilities they predict. Therefore the tests are known as aptitudes and abilities tests. Many tests are given to discover special aptitudes.

For example, there are tests of musical aptitude - tests based on discrimination of pitch, rhythm and other aspects of musical sensitivity that might be able to predict musical performance and training. Clerical aptitude is another kind of special aptitude.

A test in simple number checking, for example, may be able to predict an individual's achievement in an office job.

APYREXIA

Absence of or intermission of fever.

APYROGEN

An agent not producing fever.

AQUEDUCT

Canal, usually said of the canal connecting the third and fourth ventricles of the brain.

AQUEOUS HUMOR

The watery fluid that fills the anterior and posterior chambers of the eye between the lens and the cornea.

ARACHIS OIL

Oil expressed from ground nuts. Often used in injections, when drugs such as penicillin are added.

ARACHNODACTYLY

An inherited disorder of connective tissue transmitted as an autosomal dominant trait, resulting in abnormalities of the eyes, circulation system and skeleton.

ARACHNOID MEMBRANE

The semi-transparent, thin middle membrane that covers the brain and spinal cord.

ARBOVIRUSES
Viruses that are maintained in nature through transmission between vertebrates and hematophagous arthropods (bloodsucking insects); they multiply in both the vertebrates and the arthropods. Examples of arboviruses are yellow fever and dengue, which are transmitted by mosquitoes.

ARCHETYPE
Carl Jung's term for the content of the collective unconscious. It is used in the sense of the inherited unconscious patterns that Jung held to constitute the fundamental structure of the mind.

Archetypes can be observed only through their effects, e.g. images recurring in dreams, behavior patterns, etc.

ARCUS SENILIS
The opaque white ring that appears in old age around the cornea of the eye because of cholesterol deposits.

ARDS
Abbreviation for "acute respiratory distress syndrome," respiratory failure with life-threatening respiratory distress and hypoxemia (too little oxygen in the blood), associated with various acute injuries to the lungs.

ARENAVIRUSES
Lymphocytic choriomeningitis and structurally related viruses that are transmitted by rodents and can show man-to-man transmission.

AREOLA
A small area or space; the colored circle or halo surrounding the nipple.

ARGININE
An amino acid occurring in proteins.

ARGYLL ROBERTSON PUPIL
One which reacts to accommoda-tion - that is, it contracts when the eyes converge on a near object - but not to light. It is a diagnostic sign in syphilis.

ARM
The part of the upper limb between wrist and shoulder.

ARNICA
(Arnica montana) Plant, the flowers and rootstock of which are used for

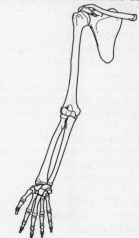

Skeleton of the right arm and shoulder girdle, anterior view. From top to bottom: shoulder blade and collar bone, upper arm (*humerus), fore arm (radius and ulna) and hand.

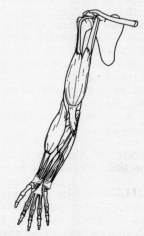

Major muscle of the right arm, anterior view.

medicinal purposes. The horizontal, dark brown, branched rootstock of the plant sends up a slightly hairy, simple or lightly branched stem that reaches a height of 0.30 to 0.60 m (1-2 ft). Arnica is primarily for external use. Used as a tincture in salve, it helps promote the healing of wounds, bruises and irritation. However, only very dilute solutions of tincture should be used, since it can cause blistering and inflammation when applied.

ARRECTOR PILLI

The minute muscles arising in the skin connected to the hair follicles, which contract when stimulated by cold or fright, causing the hair to stand on end and resulting in the condition called "goose-flesh."

ARRHENOBLASTOMA

A tumor of the ovaries that results in the development of masculine physical characteristics.

ARRHYTHMIA

Absence or disturbance of rhythm, as in the heartbeat.

ARSENIC POISONING

The acute condition - that is, when a large dose is taken at one time - may result in shock and death, with skin rashes, vomiting, diarrhea, abdominal pain, muscular cramps and swelling of the eyelids, feet and hands. The chronic form is due to ingestion of small amounts of arsenic over long periods, and is marked by skin pigmentation, peripheral neuropathy (inflammation of the nerves in the outer parts of the body) and confusion.

ARSENICUM ALBUM

Homeopathic drug derived from arsenic. Among the leading general indications for this drug are prostration, restlessness, sudden sinking, extreme weakness, burning, great thirst, physical condition that is worse at rest and when cold.

ARTERIAL HYPERTENSION

Elevation of systolic and/or diastolic blood pressure, either from unknown causes (primary or essential hypertension) or known causes (secondary hypertension). The condition needs specific treatment.

ARTERIALIZATION

To change venous blood to arterial blood by oxygenation.

ARTERIECTOMY

Removal of an artery or part of an artery by surgery.

ARTERIOGRAPHY

The visualization of an artery or arterial system by X-ray after the injection of a radio-opaque medium.

ARTERIOLE

A small muscle-walled artery.

ARTERIOPLASTY

An operation to repair or reconstruct an artery.

ARTERIOSCLEROSIS

Disease of the arteries in which their walls become thickened and rigid, and blood flow is hindered. Arteriosclerosis is a generic term for a number of blood vessel diseases, atherosclerosis being the mostimportant.

ARTERIOSCLEROTIC DEMENTIA

Dementia attributable, because of physical signs (on examination of the central nervous system) to degenerative disease of the arteries of the brain. Symptoms suggesting a particular lesion (e.g., tumor) in the brain are common.

There may be a fluctuating or patchy intellectual defect that the sufferer is aware of, and it is common for this to come and go. It is very difficult or impossible to differentiate between this and senile or presenile dementia, both of which may co-exist with it.

ARTERIOSTENOSIS
Temporary or permanent narrowing of the interior of an artery.

ARTERIOVENOUS
Relating to the arteries and veins.

ARTERIOVENOUS FISTULA
An abnormal connection between an artery and a vein, causing symptoms of a lack of oxygen in the blood, ulceration due to embolization and ischaemia, or symptoms related to the veins not working properly due to the high-pressure arterial flow within the involved veins.

ARTERIOVENOUS MALFORMATION
Abnormal, tangled collection of dilated blood vessels that are congenitally malformed, so that the blood from arteries flows directly into veins without the usual resistance of an intervening capillary bed.

ARTERITIS
Inflammation of an artery.

ARTERY
Blood vessel which carries blood from the heart to the tissues.

ARTHRALGIA
Pain, especially neuralgic pain, in a joint.

ARTHRECTOMY
Excision (cutting out) of a joint.

ARTHRITIS
Inflammation of one or more joints, causing pain, swelling, and restriction of movement.

ARTHRODESIS
Surgical fusion of a joint.

ARTHRODYNIA
Pain in a joint.

ARTHROGRAPHY
The inside of a joint shown by X-rays. It is usually necessary to inject

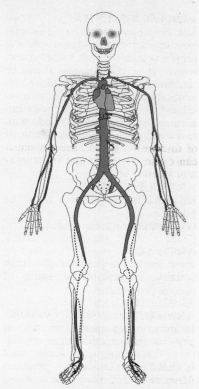

Distribution of the major arteries in the body.

the joint with a substance opaque to X-rays.

ARTHROPATHY
General term for any disease or disorder of a joint.

ARTHROPLASTY
(1) Surgical repair of a joint.
(2) The making of an artificial joint.

ARTHROSCOPY
Direct examination of the interior of a joint by means of an instrument called on arthroscope.

ARTHROSIS
Any disease causing degeneration of a joint.

ARTHROSYNOVITIS
Inflammation of the membrane lining of a joint.

ARTHUS REACTION
The development of an inflammatory lesion, which occurs when a person is injected with something to which he or she is overly sensitive (an antigen) that is then attacked by antibodies. The reaction is characterized by the area of the body becoming hard and fluid-filled, with hemorrhage and necrosis (death of tissue) within hours after the injection.

ARTICULATION
(1) A joining or juncture, as of the bones.
(2) Distinct and clear speech.

ARTIFACT
Term applied to products of human activity, as against the results of natural processes.

ARTIFICIAL INSEMINATION
Introduction of sperm into the vagina by means other than copulation. The technique is widely used forbreeding livestock as it produces many offspring from one selected male. It has a limited use in treating human impotence and sterility.

ARTIFICIAL RESPIRATION
A method by which air is rhythmically forced into and out of the lungs of a person whose breathing hasceased.

ARYTENOID
Ladle-shaped; usually referring to the two cartilages of the larynx to which the vocal cords are attached.

ASBESTOSIS
A diffuse fibrous pneumoconiosis resulting from the inhalation of asbestos dust. The risk of developing asbestosis is related to the dose of asbestos dust to which the worker has been exposed. The process is progressive and symptoms (cough, wheezing) become more severe in association with advancing physical abnormalities.

ASCARIASIS
Infection with the roundworm Ascaris lumbricoides. After being taken into the body, the larvae migrate first to the lungs, then to the intestines.

ASCARICIDE
An agent that destroys ascarids (roundworms).

ASCHOFF'S NODE
A white mass of Purkinje fibres (a specific impulse-conducting system) found in the heart at the base of the interatrial septum and forming the beginning of the atrioventricular "bundle of His."

ASCHOFF'S NODULE
Nodule in myocardium (heart muscle) and connective tissue in rheumatoid arthritis.

ASCITES
The presence of free fluid in the peritoneal cavity of the abdomen.

ASCORBIC ACID
Vitamin C.

ASEMASIA
Pathological inability to use or understand language.

ASENDIS
Brand name of a tricyclic antidepressant drug containing amoxapine as the active ingredient.

ASEPSIS
Absence of micro-organisms; prevention of sepsis.

ASEXUAL
Without sex, sexless. In biology it is used in the sense of reproduction by other than sexual action, without the union of male and female germ cells.

ASIAN INFLUENZA
An epidemic form of influenza, probably originating in China.

ASIATIC CHOLERA
A form of cholera.

ASPERGILLOMA
Fungus ball; a characteristic form of aspergillosis, which appears on chest X-rays as a dense round ball, capped by a curved sliver of air, in a cavity.

ASPERGILLOSIS
An infectious disease of the lung, with occasional spread through the blood, caused by certain fungi of the genus Aspergillus. The fungus appears after antibacterial or antifungal therapy in bronchi damaged by bronchitis, bronchiectasis or tuberculosis.

ASPERITY
Roughness or harshness to touch, taste, hearing or feelings.

ASPERMIA
Failure to produce or ejaculate sperm.

ASPHYXIA
The complex of symptoms due to inability to take oxygen into or excrete carbon dioxide from the lungs. The commonest causes are drowning, suffocation orstrangling; inhalation of poisonous gases, obstruction of larynx, trachea or bronchi of the lungs (which can occur in severe cases of croup and asthma). Early artificial respiration is essential.

ASPIRATE
Fluid drawn by suction from the body for laboratory examination, or to reduce excess fluid.

ASPIRATION
Ambition. The term aspiration is also used in the following two senses:
(1) the pronunciation of an aspirate (such as the letter H) or the sign that marks one;
(2) the action or use of an aspirator.

ASPIRATOR
A device that uses suction to remove air, liquids or granular substances from a cavity of the body.

ASPIRIN
Acetylsalicylic acid, an effective painkiller, which reduces fever and inflammation and also affects blood platelets so that blood does not clot as readily. It is useful in headache, minor feverish illness,menstruation pain, rheumatic fever, inflammatory arthritis, and may also be used to prevent thrombosis (blood clots). Aspirin may cause gastrointestinal irritation and hemorrhage, and should be avoided in cases of peptic ulcer.

ASSERTIVITY TRAINING
A behavior therapy technique by which the anxiety felt by many people in interpersonal situations is overcome by encouraging them to express other spontaneously felt emotions in the actual situation.

ASSIMILATION
In the general sense, becoming like, or being like. The term has various technical senses according to context:
(1) Sociologically, becoming in thought and behavior like the social milieu;
(2) Physically, using food material to build up organic substances such as cells, or merely the building up of complex molecular structures;
(3) Psychologically, interpreting a new fact or experience by bringing it into relation with already existing knowledge, or as the result of a process akin to complication, the combining into a whole of direct and reproduced items of immediate experience.

ASSOCIATION
Used generally to describe the way a person may find a connection between ideas, feelings or movements in such a way that this calls them

readily to mind. This principle and process has been recognized since the time of Aristotle. The laws, in accordance with which connections are established, are known as the laws of association.

The term association is also used as an adjective in the following senses:
(1) of areas of the cerebral cortex of the brain, whose functions have not been determined;
(2) of fibers connecting one area to another within the same hemisphere of the brain;
(3) of experiments, or tests, in the field of learning, thought, etc.
(4) of time, in reaction experiments, where the response involves the functioning of associative connections.

ASSOCIATION AREAS
Portions of the cerebral hemispheres of the brain other than the projection areas. Because their function is unknown, the assumption is made that these areas serve some sort of integrative or associative function.

ASSOCIATIONISM
The name given to a psychological theory, which takes association to be the fundamental principle of mental life, in terms of which even the higher thought processes are to be explained.

It is usually combined with sensationalism, and is opposed to theories emphasizing an independent activity of the mind.

ASSOCIATION PSYCHOLOGY
A pre-experimental branch of psychology, whose basic explanatory principle is the association of ideas.

ASSOCIATION TESTS
Tests, usually verbal, where the subject responds to a word with another word. Where the subject can respond with the first word that comes to mind regardless of whatever word it is, this is known as a "free" or "chance" test. Where the subject is instructed to respond by giving the antonym or synonym, etc. of the presented word, this test is known as a "controlled association" test.

ASSOCIATIVE THINKING
Relatively uncontrolled and undirected thinking as in free association, reverie and dreams.

ASTASIA
Unsteadiness or tremor, in the contraction of a muscle, or in maintaining a position.

ASTEATOSIS
Any disease in which there is a loss of activity of the sebaceous glands of the skin or scantiness of their secretions.

ASTEREOGNOSIS
Inability to recognize by touch the form of solid objects.

ASTHENIA
Lack or impairment of strength, as in neurasthenia or psychasthenia.

The word asthenic is used to describe depressive feelings or emotions, or of a type of physical build with a small trunk and long limbs.

ASTHENIC REACTION
A psychoneurotic reaction characterized by chronic aches, pains, physical and mental fatigue.It usually occurs in young adults and is believed to result from sustained emotional stress which the individual cannot cope with.

ASTHENOPIA
Weakness of the eye muscles or visual power because of fatigue.

ASTHMA
A reversible obstruction of the airways not due to any other disease. Asthma is a respiratory disorder characterized by unpredictable periods of breathlessness and wheezing; often an allergic disorder.

ASTIGMATISM

A malformation of the lens of the eye, such that rays of light are not brought to converge at the same point.

ASTRINGENT

An agent that contracts the organic tissues and canals of the body, thereby checking or diminishing bleeding or excessive discharges.

Astringents are used in a number of antiperspirants and skin tonics because they remove excessive moisture from the skin surface. They are also used in ear drops for outer-ear inflammation because they promote healing of the inflamed tissue.

ASTROCYTE

A star-shaped supporting cell in the central nervous system.

ASTROCYTOMA

A tumor formed by astrocytes, usually of a malignant nature.

ASYLUM

An institution for receiving and maintaining persons laboring under certain bodily defects or mental maladies.

ASYMBOLIA

Inability, owing to a brain disorder, to use or understand language.

ASYMMETRY

When the two sides of the body do not match, particularly with respect to paired members such as the hands, but also used of vision, where one eye operates more strongly than the other in convergence.

ASYMPTOMATIC

Showing or causing no symptoms.

ASYNERGIA

Inability, owing to a disorder of the cerebellum of the brain, to carry out complex actions depending on the coordination of different muscle groups.

ASYSTOLE

Faulty contraction of the ventricles of the heart, preventing it from performing a complete systole (contraction).

ATARAX

Brand name of hydroxyzine hydrochloride, an anti-anxiety drug.

ATAVISM

The inheritance by an individual of characteristics not shown by its parents. Once thought to be throwbacks to an ancestral form, atavisms are now known to be primarily the result of the random reappearance of recessive traits, though they may also result from aberrations in the development of the embryo or from disease.

ATAXIA

Impaired coordination of body movements resulting in unsteady gait, difficulty in fine movements and speech disorder. Caused by a disease of the cerebellum of the brain or the spinal cord, ataxia occurs with multiple sclerosis, certain hereditary conditions and in the late stage of syphilis.

Static ataxia is the form where an individual tries to maintain a fixed position or posture. Ataxic writing is writing showing a lack of coordination in the writing movements.

ATAXIA TELANGIECTASIA

A hereditary progressive disease characterized by ataxia from a disease of the cerebellum of the brain, telangiectasias (abnormally dilated small arteries and capillaries), recurrent infections andvariable defects of the immune system.

ATELECTASIS

A shrunken and airless part or all of the lung; the disorder may be acute or chronic, complete or incomplete.

Atelectasis is often accompanied by infection. The atelectatic lung or lobe is a complex mixture of airlessness, infection, bronchiectasis (dilation of the airways), destruction and fibrosis.

ATHEROEMBOLIC RENAL DISEASE

A clinical syndrome involving either rapid deterioration of renal (kidney) function or a more slowly progressive renal failure, depending on the amount of fibro-fatty atheromatous material that obstructs the blood vessels of the kidneys.

ATHEROSCLEROSIS

A common disorder of the arteries in which plaques of material (mostly cholesterol and lipids) form on the inner arterial walls, making them thick and inelastic, and narrowing the opening of the vessel, thus causing decreased flow of blood to those organs supplied by the artery.

ATHETOSIS

A condition in which the hands and feet continually perform involuntary, slow, irregular movements, due to brain damage.

ATHLETE'S FOOT

Ringworm of the feet, a contagious disease caused by a fungus that grows in wet or damp areas.

ATHROMBIA

Defective clotting of the blood.

ATLAS

The first vertebra of the neck.

ATONIC CONSTIPATION

Another name for colonic inertia.

ATONY

Defect of muscular power. The term is also used in the sense of weakness of every organ.

ATOPIC DERMATITIS

A chronic, itching, superficial inflammation of the skin, usually occurring in individuals with a personal or family history of allergic disorders.

ATOPY

An inherited tendency to develop asthma, hay fever and other allergies to things that usually provoke no immune reactions in most persons.

ATP

Acronym for adenosine triphosphate.

ATRACURIUM

Generic name of a drug used to relax the muscles in general anesthesia.

ATRESIA

Closure of a normal body opening, such as anus or vagina, caused by failure of development or disease.

ATRIAL FIBRILLATION

An abnormal heart rhythm which results from the continuous and chaotic re-entry of electrical impulses within the muscle of the atrium of the heart.

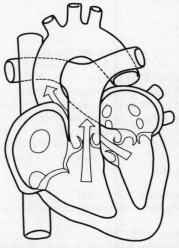

Illustration of the open heart. The left and right atrium are located above the large ventricles.

ATRIAL FLUTTER
An abnormal heart rhythm in which continuous electrical activity within the atrium of the heart comes in regular cyclic waves, producing an atrial rate of between 240 and 400 contractions per minute.

ATRIOVENTRICULAR BLOCK (A-V BLOCK)
A heart disorder characterized by the electrical impulse (which causes the heart to beat) being blocked between the muscle of the atrium and that of the ventricle, because of abnormal conduction across the atrioventricular node.

ATRIUM
Either of the two chambers of the heart that receive blood from outside the heart.

ATROPHY
Wasting or withering away or failure to develop normally, from lack of food or use.

ATROPINE
A poisonous crystalline alkaloid used in medicine. Atropine is an ingredient in many gastrointestinal and ophthalmic preparations as well as being contained in plants such as jimsonweed and deadly nightshade (belladonna). The fatal dose for adults is usually estimated to be 0.1 g, but adults have recovered from single doses of as much as 1.0 g; 0.01 g of atropine will usually produce severe distress in adults. The estimated lethal dose for children (extremely sensitive) is 0.01 g. Intoxication in young children has been reported from administration of eye drops containing it.

ATS
Anti-tetanus serum; serum to produce artificial passive immunity against tetanus.

ATTACHMENT
The act of attaching one thing to an other; a bond of affection or friendship.

ATTACHMENT BEHAVIOR
An outward expression of a young child's need to re-establish contact and reaffirm the bond with the primary caregiver. Attachment is most often displayed when the child is confronted with unfamiliar circumstances.

ATTACK
A sudden episode affecting a person in apparently good health, or a sudden worsening of a chronic condition.

ATTACK, CATAPLECTIC
A sudden and very brief slumping of the body affecting part or all of the body's muscles and occurring in certain narcoleptic subjects independently of any epileptic mechanism.

ATTACK, EPILEPTIC DROP
An atonic epileptic seizure in which the muscles holding the body upright lose their strength partially or completely for a very short time. Depending on whether the loss of tone involves all the postural muscles or only those of the head and neck, the subject either slumps to the ground or his head suddenly falls on to his chest. He gets up again immediately after the fall, which may be violent enough to cause injury, particularly when his head strikes an object in its path.

ATTENTION
The process of mental selection in which the individual concentrates on certain elements by considering them apart from their environment. Active attention is a voluntary reaction to outside stimuli.

ATTENTION DEFICIT HYPERACTIVITY DISORDER (ADHD)
Developmentally inappropriate degrees of inattention, impulsiveness,

and hyperactivity. People with the disorder generally display some disturbance in each of these areas, but to varying degrees.

Manifestations of the disorder usually appear in most situations, including at home, in school, at work, and in social situations, but to varying degrees. Some people, however, show signs of the disorder in only one setting, such as at home or at school.

Symptoms typically worsen in situations requiring sustained attention, such as listening to a teacher in a classroom, attending meetings, or doing class assignments or chores at home.

In pre-school children, the most prominent features are generally signs of gross motor overactivity, such as excessive running or climbing. The child is often described as being on the go and "always having his motor running." Inattention and impulsiveness are likely to be shown by frequent shifting from one activity to another.

In older children and adolescents, the most prominent features tend to be excessive fidgeting and restlessness rather than gross motor overactivity. Inattention and impulsiveness may contribute to failure to complete assigned tasks or instructions, or careless performance of assigned work.

In adolescents, impulsiveness is often displayed in social activities, such as initiating a diverting activity on the spur of the moment instead of attending to a previous commitment (e.g., joy riding in stead of doing homework). In approximately half of the cases, onset of the disorder is before age four. Frequently the disorder is not recognized until the child enters school.

Central nervous system abnormalities, such as the presence of neurotoxins, cerebral palsy, epilepsy, and other neurologic disorders, are thought to be predisposing factors. Disorganized or chaotic environments and child abuse or neglect may be predisposing factors in some cases.

ATTENUATED VIRUS VACCINES
Liquid products of killed germs used for injections to prevent certain diseases.

ATTIC
That portion of the ear lying above the tympanic cavity.

ATTRIBUTE
A fundamental aspect or characteristic of a sensation, with the vanishing of which the sensation vanishes; for example, all sensations must have quality, intensity and duration.

ATYPICAL SOMATIFORM DISORDER
Another name for hypochondriasis.

AUDICORT
Brand name of an anti-infective preparation used for ear inflammatory processes, and containing benzocaine, neomycin, and triamcinolone as active ingredients.

AUDIOGRAM
Graphic record of an individual's hearing ability through the range of audibility.

AUDITORY
Relating to hearing or to the sense or organs of hearing.

AUDITORY NERVE
The nerve of hearing (part of the eighth cranial nerve), going from the organs of hearing and the semicircular canals of the ears to the brain.

AUDITORY PROJECTION AREA
The area in the superior temporal

convolution of the cerebral cortex of the brain where the auditory nerve terminates and where hearing is perceived.

AURA

Subjective feelings preceding an attack of epilepsy or migraine. Historically, a term introduced by the 2nd-century Greek physician Galen to describe the sensation of a breath (from the Latin aura, a breath or puff of air) felt by some subjects prior to the start of an epileptic seizure.

In present usage, a muscular, sensory, autonomic or psychological symptom constituting the initial manifestation of
- a partial epileptic seizure that subsequently becomes generalized;
- a partial epileptic seizure of complex symptoms that does not go on to the second stage of convulsions;
- a feeling of unusual well-being or, more commonly, visual symptoms (blurriness, flickering lights) preceding an attack of classical migraine.

AURAL ECZEMATOID DERMATITIS

Eczema, characterized by itching, redness, discharge, descaling and even fissuring leading to secondary infection, frequently involving the pinna (outer ear) and ear canal.

AURICLE

Also called the pinna: the external ear, or that part which is prominent from the head.

AURISCOPE

An instrument for examining the eardrum.

AUROTHERAPY

The use of gold salts in the treatment of a disease, especially rheumatic diseases.

AUSCULTATION

A method of listening to body sounds for diagnostic purposes, particularly the heart, lungs and fetal circulation. A stethoscope is used for auscultation.

AUSTRALIAN ANTIGEN

An antigen often found in the serum of people who have hepatitis; the blood test for this antigen is used to detect serum hepatitis (Type B), and to differentiate it from Type A hepatitis.

AUTISM

Usually in the sense of infantile autism, a syndrome present from birth or beginning almost invariably in the first 30 months of life. Responses to auditory and visual stimuli are abnormal and there are usually severe difficulties in the understanding of spoken language.

Speech is delayed in developing; if it does develop, it is characterized by echolalia (meaningless, repetitive speech), the reversal of pronouns, immature grammatical structure and the inability to use abstract terms. There is generally an impairment in the social use of both verbal and body language. Problems in social relationships are most severe before the age of five years and include an impairment in the development of eye-to-eye contact, social attachments and cooperative play.

Ritualistic behavior is usual and may include abnormal routines, resistance to change, attachment to odd objects and stereotyped patterns of play. The capacity for abstract or symbolic thought and for imaginative play is diminished. Intelligence ranges from severely subnormal to above normal. Performance is usually better on tasks involving rote memory than on those requiring symbolic or linguistic skills.

AUTISTIC THINKING

Mental activity which is controlled by the wishes of the individual, as contrasted with reality thinking, controlled by the conditions imposed by the real nature of objects and events.

AUTO-ANTIBODY
An antibody that acts like a foreign substance (antigen) and may react against normal tissues to cause disease.

AUTO-ANTIGEN
Some substance within the body capable of imitating the production of auto-antibodies.

AUTOCHTHONOUS
Literally "belonging to the soil;" employed to describe ideas which rise in the mind, independently of the train of thought at the time, and foreign to the normal mode of thought - exemplified in schizophrenia.

AUTOCHTHONOUS TUMOR
Tumor arising in the same host.

AUTOCLAVE
A machine that sterilizes objects and equipment using pressurized steam.

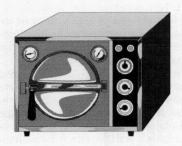

Modern autoclave for the sterilization of objects and instruments for surgery.

AUTO-DIGESTION
Digestion of tissues or destruction of cells by their own secretions.

AUTO-EROTISM
Refers either to a pleasurable activity in which the self is used as an object (e.g. masturbation) or to a li-bidinal attitude, orientation or stage of development. In the former case, the term is used objectively to describe observable behavior; in the latter it is used to describe a hypothesis about a person's or infant's disregard of external objects.

According to classical instinct theory, infants are auto-erotically oriented, i.e. their attitude towards their mother is based solely on self-love and their need for her is based on the capacity of the mother to provide them with gratification. When used in this sense, "auto-erotic" is synonymous with "narcissistic."

Object-theory is opposed to the idea of an auto-erotic phase in infancy and takes the view that the infant is mother-related from the very beginning, that the infant is "object-seeking, not pleasure-seeking." According to this view, auto-erotic behavior is substitutive, the subject using part of himself as a symbolic equivalent of someone else.

AUTOGENOUS VACCINE
A vaccine produced by culturing a person's own bacteria; the hepatitis vaccine is an example of this.

AUTOGRAFT
Transfer of tissue from one location to another in the same individual.

AUTO-HEMOTHERAPY
Injecting a person with his own blood.

AUTO-HYPNOSIS
Self-induced hypnosis.

AUTO-IMMUNE DISEASE
A disorder characterized by an abnormal immune reaction of unknown cause. In most cases it is directed against a constituent, often protein in nature, of the person's own body. this constituent is regarded as a foreign body by the person's own immune and defense system which forms antibodies (auto-

antibodies) against the constituent as it would against any foreign invader. Examples of auto-immune disease are:

(1) Systemic lupus erythematosus (rash, pains in joints, inflammation of lungs, damage to kidneys);

(2) Goodpasture's syndrome (severe kidney and lung disease);

(3) Hashimoto's thyroiditis (enlarged and inflamed thyroid);

(4) Myasthenia gravis (great muscular weakness);

(5) Rheumatoid arthritis (spreading inflammation and deformity of joints);

(6) Progressive systemic sclerosis (hardening of blood vessels and nerves).

Every person goes through life surrounded by potentially harmful microorganisms. Those that invade the body usually held at bay by the body's immune defenses, an elaborate system that stands guard to intercept and destroy foreign cells and substances. The system sometimes goes awry in such a way as to give rise to the diverse group of disorders known as auto-immune diseases.

Such disorders result when the immune system, which ordinarily distinguishes "self" from "non-self" with great precision, begins to attack certain of the body's own cells.

Auto-immunity is now accepted as being important in human disease. A survey of large university hospitals showed that some 20 percent of the patients suffered from a disease with significant immunological features. The understanding of some of these diseases has already been greatly strengthened by detailed experimental studies of auto-immunity. For example, the realization that auto-immunity plays a role in systemic lupus erythematosus has led to the use of immunosuppressive drugs (which damp down the immune system's responses) as an effective treatment of the disease, arresting what was once thought to be an inexorable and fatal process. In diagnostic laboratories tests for auto-antibodies are now a regular step in identifying many diseases, including systemic lupus erythematosus, thyroiditis, rheumatoid arthritis, some forms of progressive liver disease and even pemphigus, a severe and formerly fatal skin disorder.

AUTO-INFECTION
Infection transferred from one part of an infected body to one or more additional parts.

AUTO-INTOXICATION
Intoxication or poisoning by toxins developed by one's own body.

AUTOKINESIS
Significant shifts of judgment or subjective modifications or interpretations of objective data, through the operation of set, attitude or frame of reference.

AUTOLYSIN
Any agent or substance that produces autolysis.

AUTOLYSIS
Digestion or disintegration of tissue by enzymes generated in cells.

AUTOMATISM
Usually a complex act performed unconsciously, but in psychological research, sensory automatism is employed to describe the automatic functioning of the senses, which is seemingly of the nature of hallucination.

AUTOMATISM, EPILEPTIC
More or less coordinated and adapted involuntary motor activity occurring during a state of clouding of consciousness either in the course of or after an epileptic seizure, and usually followed by amnesia of the event.

The automatism may be simply a continuation of an activity that was going on when the seizure occurred or, conversely, a new activity that develops in association with the impairment of consciousness. Usually the activity is commonplace in nature, often provoked by the subject's environment or by his sensations during the seizure; exceptionally, fragmentary, primitive, infantile or antisocial behavior is seen.

From the point of view of symptoms, the following are distinguished:
- eating automatism, such as chewing, swallowing;
- automatisms of mimicry, expressing the subject's emotional state, usually of fear, during the seizure;
- gestural automatisms, simple or complex, directed towards either the subject or his environment;
- ambulatory automatisms, characterized by walking or running;
- verbal automatisms.

AUTONOMIC NERVOUS SYSTEM
That part of the nervous system that regulates involuntary vital functions, such as the activity of the heart and smooth muscle.

AUTOPHOBIA
Morbid fear of solitude.

AUTOPLASTY
The repairing of injured or diseased parts of the body with tissue from another part of the same body.

AUTOPROTHROMBIN
Any of several blood factors formed in the conversion of prothrombin to thrombin.

AUTOPSY
Dissection and inspection of a body after death to determine the cause of death.

AUTO-PSYCHOSIS
Mental disorder in which all ideas are centered round the self.

AUTOREGULATION
The maintenance of relative constancy of a physiological process by a bodily part or system under varying conditions; especially the maintenance of a constant supply of blood to an organ in spite of varying arterial pressure.

AUTOSCOPE
A device for recording or magnifying small involuntary movements of the body.

AUTOSCOPY
Visual hallucination of an image of one's body.

AUTOSERUM
A serum used to treat the same patient from which it was taken.

AUTOSITE
The larger part of a double fetal monster that is usually capable of independent existence and nourishes both itself and the parasite twin.

AUTOSOMES
Those chromosomes that are not sex chromosomes. Humans each have 22 pairs of autosomes.

AUTOSUGGESTIBILITY
The quality or state of being subject to autosuggestion.

AUTOSUGGESTION
Suggestion, arising from the individual himself. The process of influencing one's conduct, or state of mind or body, by an idea which one keeps constantly in mind, e.g. to help oneself to get to sleep by telling oneself that one is sleepy.

AUTOTELIC
A term employed to describe a type of character or character trait to indicate the predominance of aims towards self-defense, self-protection and self-development in an individual's system of purposes.

AUTOTHERAPY
The treatment of disease using the person's own body secretions.

AUTOTOMY
Reflex separation of a part from the body especially in an invertebrate.

AUTOTOPAGNOSIA
Loss of the power to recognize or orient a bodily part due to a brain lesion.

AUTOTOXEMIA
Self-poisoning by absorption of a poisonous substance produced in the body.

AUTOTOXIN
A poisonous substance formed within the body and acting against it.

AUTOTRANSFUSION
The replacement into a person of the actual blood lost by hemorrhage, especially when it occurs into the abdominal cavity.

AUTOTRANSPLANTATION
The action of autotransplanting; the condition of being autotransplanted.

AUTOTROPHY
The condition of being autotrophic; the process by which an autotrophic organism obtains energy from carbon dioxide or carbonates and inorganic substances.

AUTOVACCINATION
Vaccination of an individual by material from his own body or with a vaccine prepared from such material.

A-V BLOCK
Short name for atrioventricular block

AVERSION
A feeling of repugnance toward something with a desire to avoid or turn from it; The term is also used to describe a tendency to extinguish a behavior or to avoid a thing or situation.

AVERSION THERAPY
A method of treatment used in behavior therapy with the emphasis on deconditioning. Effective in some forms of addiction and abnormal behavior.

AVITAMINOSIS
A disease caused by vitamin deficiency.

A-V MALFORMATION
Short name for arteriovenous malformation.

AVOIDANCE-AVOIDANCE CONFLICT
A conflict based on two unattractive alternatives. There is a strong tendency to escape the dilemma by doing something else. Children who are told to eat their spinach or go right to bed may play with their fork or stare out the window. If their choice is forced, they take longer to decide and vacillate more than in the choice between two attractive alternatives.

AVOIDANT DISORDER
An excessive shrinking from contact with unfamiliar people that is of sufficient severity to interfere with social functioning in peer relationships. This is in children and adolescents coupled with a clear desire for social involvement with familiar people, such as peers the person knows well and family members.

Relationships with family members and other family figures are warm and satisfying.

A child with this disorder is likely to appear socially withdrawn, embarrassed, and timid when in the company of unfamiliar people and will become anxious when even a trivial demand is made to interact with strangers. When social anxiety is severe, the child may be inarticulate or mute, even if his or her communication skills are unimpaired.

AVOIDANT PERSONALITY DISORDER

A pervasive pattern of social discomfort, fear of negative evaluation, and timidity, beginning by early adulthood and present in a variety of contexts.

Most people are somewhat concerned about how others assess them, but those with this disorder are easily hurt by criticism and are devastated by the slightest hint of disapproval. They generally are unwilling to enter into relationships unless given an unusually strong guarantee of uncritical acceptance; consequently, they often have no close friends or confidants (or only one) other than first-degree relatives. Social or occupational activities that involve significant interpersonal contact tend to be avoided.

AVULSION

A pulling or tearing apart or off, as by surgery or injury.

AWARENESS

Mere experience of an object or idea, sometimes equivalent to consciousness.

AXILLA

The armpit, the cavity under the upper part of the arm or shoulder.

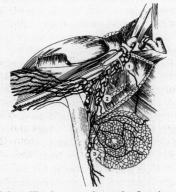

Right axilla. 1. pectoral muscle; 2. veins; 3. breast.

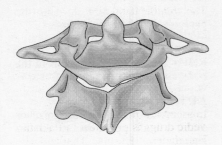

The upper two cervical; vertebrae: atlas and axis.

AXIS

The pivotal vertebra of the neck on which the head turns.

AXON

A long, single nerve fiber that carries transmitted nerve signals away from the body of the nerve cell.

AXONOTEMESIS

Nerve damage (as from compression or crushing) that affects axons but does not completely sever the surrounding endoneural sheath so that regeneration can take place.

AYURVEDA

Naturopathic system of medicine that originated in India and is still widely practiced in Asia. The word "Ayurveda" is composed of two terms, ayus meaning life and veda meaning knowledge or science. Medicine apart, various other aspects of life come within the purview of Ayurveda. In its broadest perspective, it deals with the health and treatment of diseases of man, animals and even plants.

Ayurveda provides rational means for the treatment of many internal diseases that are considered to be obstinate and incurable in other systems of medicine. Simultaneously it lays a great deal of emphasis upon the maintenance of the positive health of an individual. It thus aims at both the prevention and cure of diseases. Ayurveda also studies basic human nature and natural urges such as hunger, thirst, sleep, sex, etc., and provides measures for a disciplined, disease-free life.

Ayurveda is not only practiced in India, Sri Lanka and Nepal (in these countries more than 400,000 Ayurveda doctors practice), but in a modified form, the practice of ayurvedic drugs is prevalent in Pakistan, Bangladesh, Burma, Thailand, Indonesia, Malaysia, Tibet, China, Mongolia, Japan and some of the Arab countries.

AZATHIOPRINE
Generic name of an immuno-suppressive drug. It is prescribed as part of the treatment of any disease where it is desirable to suppress the normal immune response of the body. Without azathioprine the body would see a transplanted organ as a foreign object and soon destroy it. People taking this drug are unusually susceptible to infection and must be constantly alert to any changes. Normal responses (fever, etc.) may not be present or may be delayed by treatment with this drug. Possible side effects include:
- rapid heart rate;
- sudden fever;
- muscle or joint pain;
- cough;
- shortness of breath;
- infection or low blood count causing chills;
- back pain;
- painful urination;
- nausea and vomiting;
- appetite loss.

AZIDOTHYMIDINE (AZT)
Generic name of a drug used in the treatment of AIDS. The drug is prescribed for the treatment of selected adult patients infected with HIV (human immunodeficiency virus), AIDS (acquired immune deficiency syndrome) and advanced ARC (AIDS-related complex). The drug does not cure the infection.

Possible side effects include:
- lip or tongue swelling;
- pale skin;
- severe headache;
- nausea;
- strange taste;
- vomiting;
- insomnia;
- diarrhea;
- sweating, fever;
- appetite loss;
- abdominal pain;
- numbness in hands and feet;
- shortness of breath;
- nervousness;
- itching;
- mouth sores.

AZOOSPERMIA
Absence of spermatozoa in the semen.

AZOTEMIA
A large accumulation of urea and other nitrogenous waste in the blood resulting from a kidney malfunction.

AZOTURIA
An excess of urea and other nitrogenous substances in the urine.

AZT
Abbreviation of azidothymidine, drug used in the treatment of AIDS.

AZYGOGRAPHY
X-ray examination of the azygos vein (unpaired vein in the chest) after injection of contrast medium.

AZYGOS VEIN
Any of a system of three veins which drain the thoracic wall and much of the abdominal wall and which form a collateral circulation when either the inferior or superior vena cava is obstructed; especially a vein that receives blood from the right half of the thoracic and abdominal walls, ascends along the right side of the vertebral column, and empties into the superior vena cava.

B

BABCOCK TEST
Test for determining the fat content of milk and milk products.

BABESIOSIS
A cosmopolitan infection of animals by parasites of the genus Babesia. The disease is rare in humans.

The organisms are transmitted by hardbodied ticks and produce hemolytic anemia (in which the red blood cells break up) with fever. Treatment is usually not required for those with intact spleens.

BABINSKI REFLEX
Also called Babinski's sign: an abnormal reflex found in certain diseases of the nervous system in which the foot flexes upwards when the sole is stroked. It is also found quite normally in newborn babies.

BABKIN REFLEX
When pressure is applied to an infant's palms and its head turns to midline.

BABY
An extremely young child; especially an infant. Each newborn is classified as either premature, full-term or postmature, depending on when in the mother's pregnancy it was born (gestational age).

This permits anticipation of medical problems, since how mature the baby's organs are is primarily determined by how long it was in the womb. The neonate is also classified as either large, appropriate or small for gestational age.

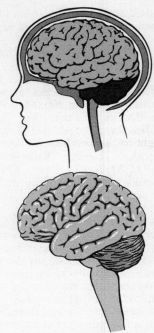

The brain of a baby or infant as compared to the brain of an adult.

BABY BOOM
Steep increase in the US birthrate following World War II. During 1946-64, 76 million people were born, accounting for nearly one-third of the US population in 1980. In the 1970s the birth rate dropped. The resulting uneven age distribution had has a multitude of social effects on educational systems and so on.

BABY TALK
(1) The syntactically imperfect speech or phonetically modified forms used by small children learning to talk.
(2) The consciously imperfect or mutilated speech or prattle often used by adults in speaking to small children.

BACCHANAL
From Bacchus, the god of wine; revelling in or characterized by intemperate drinking.

BACILLARY
Related to or caused by bacilli

BACILLEMIA
The presence of bacilli in the blood.

BACILLURIA
Presence of bacilli in the urine.

BACILLUS
Straight-rod-shaped bacteria.

BACK
The posterior part of the trunk; the hind part of the body in humans and the upper part in other mammals.

BACKACHE
Lower back pain; also called lumbago. What can go wrong in the back to produce backache? One or more of the bones in the spine may be injured or fractured. The site of the pain, its severity and how dangerous it is will depend on which bone is hurt. The back is vulnerable to most forms of arthritis, but the commonest is the kind caused over the years by wear-and-tear-osteo-arthritis. Where you feel the pain will depend on what part of the spine is involved.

BACKBONE
The vertebral column; the spine.

BACKING
The metal portion of a dental crown, bridge, or similar structure to which a porcelain or plastic tooth facing is attached.

BACK PRESSURE-ARM LIFT METHOD
Artificial respiration in which the operator kneels at the head of the prone victim, compresses the chest manually by pressure on the back, and then pulls up the elbows thereby expanding the lungs.

BACKWARDNESS
The quality or state of being dull, not quick of apprehension.

BACTEREMIA
Invasion of the circulatory system by bacteria.

BACTERIA
Any of numerous unicellular (one-celled) micro-organisms of the class Schizomycetes, occurring in a wide variety of forms, existing either as free-living organisms or as parasites, and having a wide range of biochemical, often pathological, properties.

Bacteria do not produce disease by their mere presence in the tissues; their effects in humans are due to reactions of the host (the body) to specific bacteria and their products.

Micro-organisms, like other living creatures, can be classified into orders, families, etc. However, there is at present no standard international classification of bacteria. The true bacteria are conveniently divided into a higher group, the members of which resemble the fungi in their morphology (form), and into a lower group of simpler organisms. The spirochetes and rickettsiae form other separate groups. The organisms belonging to the lower group are generally pathological to humans.

The simpler unicellular structures can be divided into four groups:
(1) cocci when the cells are spherical;
(2) bacilli when they are straight and cylindrical in shape;
(3) vibrios when they are curved and comma-shaped;
(4) spirilla when they are spiral rods.

Some 300 species of bacteria are pathogenic (disease-causing) to humans. There are many bacteria with which everyone comes into contact: saprophytes in the environment and relatively benign parasites living on the skin and in the gut and respiratory passages which are normally non-pathogenic. Of these, a few become pathogenic under certain circumstances. In addition, many bacteria are primarily pathogenic parasites of animals other than humans, and those of us who come into close contact with the susceptible animals may become infected.

Bacteria in body fluids can be detected with light and electron microscope. To determine the susceptibility for certain drugs, a definite diagnosis rests on how the bacteria react when introduced to the drug in a culture.

BACTERIAL
Pertaining to or caused by bacteria.

BACTERIAL ENDOCARDITIS
Bacterial infection of the inner lining of the heart, characterized by symptoms of infection throughout the body, the growth of warty nodules on the heart valves and the breaking off of parts of these nodules, the resulting fragments carried by the blood to different parts of the body where they can cause blockage.

BACTERIAL VACCINE
An emulsion of killed, living or attenuated (weakened) bacteria, used for raising the immunity of a person suffering from infection by the same germ.

BACTERICIDAL
Destructive to bacteria;term used to describe a drug that kills bacteria.

BACTERIOLOGIST
One who studies and is skilled in the science of bacteriology, using chemical and physical methods.

BACTERIOLOGY
Study of bacteria, viruses and fungi that cause disease.

BACTERIOLYSINS
Antibodies that dissolve bacteria when complement is present. Complement is a normal body protein needed for antigen-antibody reaction.

BACTERIOLYSIS
The process of dissolving or destruction of bacteria.

BACTERIOPHAGE
A submicroscopic, usually viral, organism that destroys bacteria.

BACTERIOPHOBIA
A morbid fear of bacteria and other microbes.

BACTERIOSTASIS
An arrest or retardation of growth of the bacteria.

BACTERIOSTATIC
A term used to describe a drug that stops the growth or multiplication of bacteria.

BACTERIOTHERAPY
Treatment of a disease or disorder by introduction of bacteria into the bloodstream.

BACTERIOTROPIC
Directed toward bacteria or affecting them in a specific way.

BACTERIURIA
The presence of bacteria in the urine.

BACTEROIDACEAE
A family of extremely varied gram-negative bacteria that usually live in the alimentary canal or on mucous surfaces and are sometimes associated with acute infective processes.

BAGASSE
Plant residue (as of sugercane or grapes) left after a product (as juice) has been extracted.

BAGASSE DISEASE
An industrial disease characterized by:
- cough;
- difficult breathing;
- chills;
- fever;
- prolonged weakness.

The disease is caused by the inhalation of the dust of bagasse.

BAGASSOSIS
A chronic inflammatory lung disorder induced by the dust of bagasse derived from sugar cane and used in board-making.

BAG OF WATERS
The double-walled fluid-filled sac that encloses and protects the fetus in the mother's womb and that breaks releasing its fluid during the birth process.

BAINBRIDGE REFLEX
A homeostatic reflex mechanism that causes acceleration of heartbeat following the stimulation of local muscle spindles when blood pressure in the venae cavae and right atrium is increased.

BAKER'S ITCH
Form of dermatitis caused by handling yeast and dough.

BAL
Abbreviation of British Anti-Lewisite. Brand name of dimercaprol.

BALANCE
In general sense, maintenance of equilibrium or posture; in the field of esthetics, used to describe the equivalence of value or weight, on the right and left sides of a picture.

BALANITIS
Inflammation of the glans penis.

BALANUS
Bulbous tip of the penis, the glans of the penis.

BALDNESS (Alopecia)
Loss of hair, usually from the scalp, due to disease of hair follicles. "Male-pattern baldness" is an inherited tendency, often starting when a man is in his 20s. Alopecia areata is a disease of unknown cause producing patchy baldness, though it may be total. Prolonged fever, lupus erythematosus and ringworm may lead to temporary baldness, as may certain drugs and poisons.

BALKAN BEAM
Wooden beam attached to a hospital bed whereby a Thomas's bed splint can be slung up, with pulleys and weights attached.

BALL-AND-FIELD TEST
One of the tests in the Binet-Simon series, in which subjects are asked to show the track they would pursue to find a ball lost in a circular field.

BALLISM
Violent, flinging limb movements caused by injury in the area of the subthalamic nucleus of the brain, usually a small stroke. The head is sometimes also affected. The repeated violent movements incapacitate and may exhaust the sufferer.

BALLOON CATHETER
A catheter that has two lumens and an inflatable tip which can be expanded by the passage of gas, water, or a radiopaque medium through one of the lumens and that is used to measure blood pressure in a blood vessel or to expand a partly closed or obstructed bodily passage or tube (as a coronary artery).

BALLOTTEMENT
Diagnostic sign of pregnancy elicited by the doctor placing a finger in the vagina just below the cervix and giving the presenting part of the fetus a slight push, so that it floats away and returns to touch the examining finger.

BALNEOTHERAPY
Treatment of disease by medicinal baths, the standard treatment offered at various spas.

BALSAM
Mixture of oils and resins derived from certain plants and trees.

BANDAGE
Piece of material used to bind up wounds, hold dressings in place or support injured limbs. Variously shaped pieces of sterilized crêpe, muslin, gauze, cotton, linen or elastic fabric are used.

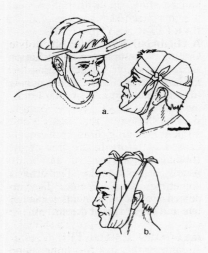

Methods (a and b) for bandaging a fracture of the jaw.

BAND KERATOPATHY
Calcium deposition in Bowman's membrane and the stroma of the cornea that appears as an opaque gray streak and occurs in hypercalcemia and various chronic inflammatory conditions of the eye.

BANKHART'S OPERATION
Operative procedure for recurrent dislocation of the shoulder joint, in which the defect of the glenoid cavity is repaired.

BANTING
A method of dieting for obesity by avoiding sweets and carbohydrates.

BANTI'S SYNDROME
Clinical syndrome characterized by gastrointestinal bleeding, anemia, leukopenia (a great increase of white cells in the blood) and thrombocytopenia (few or no platelets in the blood).

BAPTISIA TINCTORIA
Homeopathic medicine derived from wild indigo. It is prescribed for chills, with aching pains in head, back and limbs. Furthermore it is used for diarrhea with no pain, and for chronic slight fevers.

BARANY CHAIR
A chair for testing the effects of circular motion especially on airplane pilots.

BARBER'S ITCH
Another name for sycosis.

BARBITURATES
A class of drugs acting on the central nervous system which may be sedatives, anesthetics, or anticonvulsants. They act on the brain and central nervous system to produce effects which may be helpful or harmful. This depends on the individual patient's condition and response and the amount of medicine taken.

Barbiturates are taken by mouth, given by injection, or used rectally. They may be used to treat insomnia (sleeplessness) by helping patients fall asleep. Also, they may be used to relieve anxiety or tension. Some of the barbiturates are used as anticonvulsants to help control convulsions or seizures in certain disorders or diseases, such as epilepsy.

If barbiturates are used regularly (for example, every day) for insomnia, they usually are not effective for longer than 2 weeks. Also, if too much of a barbiturate is used, it may become habit-forming. These medicines are available only with your doctor's prescription.

BARBOTAGE
Method of spinal anesthesia; the production of spinal anesthesia by repeated injection and removal of fluid.

BARITOSIS
Pneumoconiosis caused by inhalation of dust composed of barium or its compounds.

BARIUM ENEMA
The use of barium sulphate and air as contrast media to help with visualization of the interior of the stomach and intestines in X-ray studies.

BARIUM MEAL
A solution of barium sulphate that is swallowed by a patient to facilitate fluoroscopic or roentgenographic diagnosis.

BARLOW'S DISEASE
Another name for infantile scurvy.

BAROTITIS MEDIA
Damage to the middle ear due to pressure changes in the environment. During a sudden increase in pressure, as in a descent of an aeroplane or in deep sea diving, air moves from the nasopharynx at the back of the throat into the middle ear to maintain equal pressure on both sides of the tympanic membrane (eardrum). Very severe pressure differences cause bleeding into the middle ear and rupture of the tympanic membrane.

BAROTRAUMA
Injury due to change in atmospheric or water pressure.

BARR BODY
The sex chromatin mass in sex cells of the female.

BARRIER NURSING
Isolation nursing technique; a method of preventing the spread of infection from an infectious patient to the others in an open ward.

BARTHOLINITIS
Inflammation of Bartholin's glands.

BARTHOLIN'S DUCT
Duct opening into the floor of the mouth from a gland lying beneath the tongue. It is one of the glands that produce saliva.

BARTHOLIN'S GLANDS
Glands situated in the walls of the vagina that produce and excrete the lubricating fluid that makes sexual intercourse possible.

BARTTER'S SYNDROME
A combination of fluid, electrolyte and hormonal abnormalities characterized by the kidney excreting too much potassium and salt, low levels of potassium in the blood, hyperreninemia (too much of the protein renin produced by the kidneys) and normal blood pressure.

BASAL
At the base of, or forming the basis on which something rests; used to describe mental age, for the level at which an individual passes all the tests; also describes metabolism, representing the energy requirements in the vital functions alone when the person is resting but not asleep.

Also to describe the masses of nerves or ganglia at the base of the cerebrum of the brain.

BASAL ANESTHESIA
Partial anesthesia produced by injecting a drug in order to reduce the amount of anesthetic that needs to be inhaled to produce complete anesthesia.

BASAL BODY TEMPERATURE
The temperature of the body under conditions of absolute rest.

BASAL MENTAL AGE
In individual tests of the Binet type, the highest age level at which, and below which, all tests are passed.

BASAL METABOLIC RATE
The minimum production of body heat after 12 hours of fasting and while lying completely at rest.

BASE EXCESS
A test of the body's acid-base balance, measured as bicarbonate.

BASEMENT MEMBRANE
A thin layer of connective tissue cells underlying the epithelium, the lining of the organs.

BASIC TRUST
The underlying effects of good experiences of mothering.

BASIPHOBIA
Pathological fear of walking.

BASOPHIL
Cells or tissues easily stained with basic dyes.

BASTARD
A child conceived and born out of wedlock; an illegitimate child.

BACHELOR PLASTER
A type of double plaster, with the legs encased from groin to ankles, in full abduction and medial rotation - that is, fixed so that both legs remain as far to either side as possible.

BATHOPHOBIA
Pathological fear of looking down from high places.

BATTERED CHILD SYNDROME
Child abuse: psychopathological disorder of one or both parents. The child is beaten and abused, and sometimes death is the result.

BATTERED PARENT SYNDROME
Abuse of one of the parents by an older child or adult. A survey by the National Institutes of Health has shown, in a nationwide random sample of 2134 families, that in any given year, 3 out of every 100 children aged 3 to 18 have committed severe acts of physical aggression against their parents. This syndrome is also known to occur among adults forced to care for aged parents.

BATTLE FATIGUE
State of physical and emotional exhaustion caused by stress during active combat or other hardships of war. It acts as a precipitating factor in causing a variety of behavior disorders.

B CELL
A lymphocyte, a type of white blood cell probably derived from bone marrow in humans, which is responsible for the production of antibodies in body fluids.

BCG
Abbreviation for Bacillus Calmette-Guérin, a vaccine used to immunize against tuberculosis.

BEARD
Growth of hair on a man's skin, cheeks and neck, regarded by many races as a symbol of strength and virility. Among the ancient Egyptians, Assyrians and Chinese, the beard had a ritual significance. The religious cult of the beard is still prevalent in Eastern cultures. Indian Sikhs are forbidden to remove a hair from their bodies; Hindus are usually clean-shaven. The Western habit of shaving became common with the Romans.

BEARING DOWN
A pseudonym for the expulsive pains in the second stage of labor.

BED-CRADLE
Apparatus to keep the weight of the bedclothes off the sick person's legs and feet.

BED-DISABILITY DAY
A day on which a person stays in bed for more than half of the daylight hours (or normal waking hours) because of a specific illness or injury.

BEDPAN
A utensil for urination or defecation by bedridden persons.

BEDREST
Therapeutic measure in a number of diseases to assist rapid recovery.

BEDSIDE MANNER
The solicitous or reassuring manner of a doctor; the attitude and approach of doctors towards patients.

BEDSIDE RADIOGRAPHY
X-ray studies performed at the bedside when the patient is too ill to be removed.

BED SORE
Ulceration of the skin on the back of a person who is allowed to remain for too long in one position. Pressure of the bed against the skin first squeezes out the blood supply and then, by friction, breaks down the tissues into an ulcer (sore) that causes no pain.

BED TRACTION
Any form in which the patient is, of necessity, confined to bed.

BEDWETTING
Another name for enuresis.

BEEF WORM INFECTION
An infection of the intestinal tract that usually produces no symptoms, which is caused by the cestode (ribbon-like intestinal worm) Taenia saginata. Sometimes pain in the abdomen just over the stomach, diarrhoea and weight loss may occur. Treatment consists of a single 2-g dose of niclosamide.

BEHAVIOR
Those activities of an organism that can be observed by someone or by an experimenter's instruments. A child eats breakfast, rides a bicycle, talks, blushes, laughs and cries - all these verbs describe forms of behavior. Observation of behavior may be made unaided, as in watching a child at play, or it may be aided by instruments.

A distinction is sometimes made between molecular and molar behavior. Molecular behavior refers to such things as isolated muscular movements or glandular secretions, such as might be studied when investigating problems of the physiology of a nerve or muscle. Such behavior is called 'molecular' because it is fragmentary and segmental.

Molar behavior, by contrast, refers to behavior organized into meaningful sequences or patterns into activities that satisfy the organism's needs, bring it closer to its goals or help it to avoid danger. A dog digging up a buried bone is exhibiting molar behavior; the movements of the dog's stomach as he digests the bone after gnawing it provide an example of molecular behavior.

Innate behavior in humans
A variety of inborn behavior seems to exist in humans. If a baby had to learn how to coordinate its breathing and swallowing while suckling at its mother's breast, it would choke repeatedly and probably starve.

Deaf-blind children grow up in eternal darkness and silence; yet later in life, they laugh and cry without ever being able to imitate such behavior. When angry, these same children crease their brows and stamp their feet. Such complicated movements develop, in other words, through maturation. While it is undeniably possible that mimicry can be the result of touching, say, the faces of others, this exposure cannot be of primary importance, since thalidomide children born deaf, blind and without arms also laugh and cry in the same way.

Children have an innate ability to integrate visual and tactile impressions. In recent experiments, images of objects were projected on a screen in front of a young subject. The subject grasped for the object and showed surprise at its failure, as registered by an increased pulse rate. In contrast, no change in pulse rate was measured when the infant was allowed to catch hold of the object reached for. We can only conclude that there is an inborn expectation of tactile consequences arising from certain optical impressions.

The sense of smell is also marked by evolutionary adaptation. Women react more sensitively than men, for example, to the odor of certain musk substances, perceiving these substances even when they are diluted to a point where men can no longer smell them. However, women do not acquire this ability until puberty, and they lose it at menopause. Furthermore, the perceptual threshold fluctuates cyclically: the capacity to smell the musk is greater at the time of ovulation. This leads us to conclude that hormonal factors play a primary role here. Indeed, men can be made to smell the very diluted musk by injecting them with the female hormone estrogen.

BEHAVIORAL SCIENCES
Those sciences dealing with human activity, individually or socially. The term, which is sometimes treated synonymously with social sciences, embraces such fields as physical and, in particular, cultural and social anthropology, psychology and sociology.

BEHAVIOR DETERMINANT
Any variable that may be considered a cause of a particular kind of behavior.

BEHAVIORISM
School of psychology based on the proposal that behavior should be studied empirically -by objective observations of reactions - rather than speculatively. It had its roots in animal behavior studies, defining behavior as the actions and reactions of a living organism (and, by extension, humans) in its environment, and, more specifically, in the work of Pavlov in such fields as conditioned reflexes.

BEHAVIOR SYSTEM
A set of habits or customs of a person motivated by a common inborn or acquired drive and leading to common satisfactions. The behavior system can be traced throughout the life history of the individual; it is thus much more comprehensive than a single motivated sequence of behavior.

BEHAVIOR THERAPY
The types of methods for changing habits that are based on experimentally established techniques.

BEHAVIOR, TYPE A AND TYPE B
Two kinds of behavior patterns, as recognized in medicine. Type A behavior is characterized by high degrees of competitiveness, aggressiveness and awareness of the pressure of time. This type of behavior is thought by some cardiologists (heart specialists) to be a risk factor in the development of coronary heart disease. Individuals with the converse type B behavior are more easy-going and contemplative and more easily satisfied.

BEHCET'S SYNDROME
An inflammatory disorder that may involve the genitals, eyes, joints, blood vessels, central nervous system and gastrointestinal system. The cause is unknown. The syndrome is generally mild, but there may be periods of remission and relapse extending over several decades.

BEJEL
Non-venereal syphilis.

BELCH
To involuntary expel wind from the

stomach in a noisy manner.

BELLADONNA
Deadly nightshade; poisonous bushy herb, native to Europe and parts of Asia. Its dried leaves and roots provide the belladonna drug from which medicinal alkaloids such as atropine are produced. Modern synthetic drugs are more reliable and are superseding belladonna alkaloids.

BELLADONNA ALKALOIDS
Medicines belonging to the group of drugs known as antimuscarinics. They are taken by mouth or given by injection. Scopolamine, one of the brand names, is used also by transdermal disk (a small patch that is applied to the skin).

Belladonna alkaloids are used to relieve cramps or spasms of the stomach, intestines, and bladder. Some are used in the treatment of peptic ulcer together with antacids or other medicine. Others are used to prevent nausea and vomiting and motion sickness. In Parkinson's disease, belladonna alkaloids may be used to decrease stiffness and tremors.

BELL'S PALSY
Disorder of the function of the seventh cranial nerve (facial nerve) resulting in weakness of the face muscles. The cause is unknown; the disorder is thought to be due to a virus infection of the facial nerve in the facial canal but no virus has ever been isolated from these patients. Bell's palsy occurs most often in young men.

It begins suddenly and is often associated with a dull ache in the parotid area behind the jaw. There is weakness of all muscles supplied by the facial nerve. The forehead is smooth on one side, the fold between the nose and mouth is less prominent and the mouth pulled over towards the non-paralysed side. Because of muscular weakness the eye cannot be tightly closed nor can the lips be pursed as for whistling.

In the majority of cases, power begins to return to the paralysed muscles within ten days or so and there is usually complete recovery. However, there are an unfortunate few in whom partial or complete paralysis exists.

The doctor will prescribe corticosteroids in high dosage as soon as possible after the onset of the disorder in order to reduce the incidence of persistent facial weakness.

BELL'S SPASM
A facial tic, a habit spasm.

BELLY
That part of the human body which extends from the breasts to the tops of the thighs; the abdomen.

BELONEPHOBIA
Pathological fear of sharp-pointed objects.

BENCE JONES PROTEIN
A protein excreted in urine in the presence of various conditions, such as multiple myeloma.

BENDS
Another name for decompression sickness.

BENEDICT'S TEST
Test for sugar in the urine. Benedict's solution and a sample of urine are boiled in separate test-tubes and then added together; if the urine contains sugar, the resulting solution turns a bright orange.

BENIGN
Harmless, not malign, not severe.

BENIGN TUMOR
A tumor that grows by expansion, does not exhibit the features of malignant tumors that invade other tissues, and is not likely to recur after removal.

BENNET
Also called wood avens: perennial plant of which the rootstock and herb is used for medicinal purposes. As an astringent, bennet is useful for diarrhea, and it also makes a good gargle for gum problems and halitosis (bad breath). It promotes appetite and acts as a tonic during convalescence. A wine extract of the root promotes digestion in older people and can also be used for chronic bronchial catarrh and for intermittent fever.

To make a decoction: add 1 teaspoon dried root or herb to 230 ml (8 fl. oz) of water. Take this amount each day.

BENZODIAZEPINES
Medicines belonging to the group of drugs called central nervous system depressants that slow down the nervous system. Brand names include: Librium, Rivotril, Rival, Valium, Paxipam, Centrax, Restoril, Halcion.

They are taken by mouth or given by injection. Some are used to relieve nervousness or tension. Others are used in the treatment of insomnia or sleeplessness. However, if used regularly (for example, every day) for insomnia or sleeplessness, they are usually not effective for more than a few weeks. Also, one of the diazepines, is used to relax muscles or relieve muscle spasms. Benzodiazepines should not be sued for nervousness or tension caused by the stress of everyday life. If too much is taken, it may become habit-forming (causing mental and physical dependence).
Side effects may include:
- clumsiness;
- unsteadiness;
- drowsiness;
- constipation;
- blurred vision;
- false sense of well-being;
- headache;
- nausea;
- vomiting;
- problems with urination;
- slurred speech;
- unusual tiredness.

BENZOIN TINCTURE
A resin used in inhalations for sinusitis and nasal congestion.

BENZTRONE
Brand name of a hormonal drug containing oestradiol as active ingredient. Possible side effects are:
- nausea;
- weight gain;
- headache;
- depression;
- breast enlargement;
- rashes;
- skin pigmentation;
- changes in sexual drive;
- abnormal blood clotting.

BENZTROPINE MESYLATE
Anti-cholinergic drug. It is prescribed for treatment of Parkinson's disease and for prevention or control of muscle spasm caused by other drugs. Benztropine mesylate has an action on the body similar to that of atropine sulphate, but side-effects are less frequent and less severe.

The drug should be used with caution if one has narrow-angle glaucoma, stomach ulcers, obstructions in the gastrointestinal tract, prostatitis or myasthenia gravis.
Possible side effects are:
- difficulty in urination;
- constipation;
- blurred vision;
- increased sensitivity to strong light.
The usual dose is 0.5 to 6.0 mg per day, depending upon the disease being treated and patient response.
Side-effects of dry mouth, constipation and increased sensitivity to strong light may be relieved by, respectively, chewing gum or sucking on hard sweets, taking a stool softener and wearing sunglasses. Such side effects are easily tolerated in the absence of undesirable drug in-

teraction.

BEREAVEMENT, UNCOMPLICATED

Normal reaction to the death of a loved one. A full depressive syndrome frequently is a normal reaction to such a loss, with feelings of depression and such associated symptoms as poor appetite, weight loss, and insomnia. However, morbid preoccupation with worthlessness, prolonged and marked functional impairment, and marked psychomotor retardation are uncommon and suggest that the bereavement is complicated by the development of a major depression.

In uncomplicated bereavement, guilt, if present, is chiefly about things done or not done by the survivor at the time of the death; thoughts of death are usually limited to the person's thinking that he or she would be better off dead or that he or she should have died with the deceased person.

The person with uncomplicated bereavement generally regards the feeling of depressed mood as "normal,"
although he or she may seek professional help for relief of such associated symptoms as insomnia or anorexia.

The reaction to the loss may not be immediate, but rarely occurs after the first two of three months. The duration of normal bereavement varies considerably among different cultural groups.

BERIBERI

Deficiency disease caused by lack of vitamin B_1 (thiamine); it may occur as a result of malnutrition or alcoholism or as an isolated deficiency. Neuritis (nerve inflammation) leading to sensory changes, and foot or wrist drop, palpitations, edema (excess fluid) and heart failure are features; there may be associated dementia. Onset may be gradual or acute. Treatment is thiamine replacement; thiamine enrichment of common foods prevents beriberi.

BERYLLIOSIS

A disease of the lungs, caused by inhalation of dust or fumes containing beryllium compounds and products. The acute condition is characterized by difficulty in breathing, cough, weight loss and a highly variable chest X-ray pattern, usually indicating the blocking of the alveoli (air sacs) of the lungs. Prognosis in the acute disease is good, but the chronic form often results in progressive loss of respiratory function.

BERYLLIUM DISEASE

Another name for berylliosis.

BETA-ADRENERGIC BLOCKING AGENT

Another name for a beta-blocker.

BETA-BLOCKER

Agent that influences the transmission of signals at beta receptors, which are part of the sympathic portion of the autonomic nervous system. At beta receptors, adrenaline provides the transmission of signals from the nerve fibers to the organs to which they are attached.

A beta-blocker or beta-adrenergic blocking agent prevents this stimulation and reduces the oxygen needs of the heart, and is therefore prescribed in conditions such as angina pectoris.

BETAHISTINE HYDROCHLORIDE

Generic name of a drug for treatment of dizziness, nausea and vomiting.

BETALOC

Brand name of a drug containing metoprolol tartrate as the active ingredient. The drug is a beta-blocking agent for reduction of oxygen needs of the heart by reducing the

rate of the heart activity. Mainly used in the treatment of angina pectoris.
Possible side effects are:
- nausea;
- insomnia;
- diarrhea;
- weariness.

BETA RHYTHM
A pattern of brain waves observed on an electroencephalograph (EEG) in which the waves are faster and of less amplitude than alpha rhythm. The prevailing frequency is 16-30 per second.

BETAXOLOL
Generic name of a drug used in the eye to treat certain types of glaucoma. It works by lowering the pressure in the eye.

BETEL NUT
The kernel of the betel palm. Enclosed in betel leaves and mixed with an aromatic paste, it is chewed extensively in Africa and the East.

BETHANECHOL CHLORIDE
Generic name of a drug with laxative properties.

BETHANIDINE SULPHATE
Generic name of a drug for the treatment of high blood pressure. Possible side effects are:
- low blood pressure;
- faintness;
- dizziness;
- diarrhea;
- sexual impotence.

BETHANECHOL
Generic name of a parasympathicomimetic drug for urinary retention and paralytic ileus.

BEZOAR
Certain concretion (hard mass) found in the intestines of some animals, formerly used as an antidote to poison.

BICARBONATE
A constituent of carbonic acid; blood levels of bicarbonate provide an index of the body's alkali reserve.

BICEPS
Having two heads. The term is applied to various muscles, notably the biceps muscles in the arm and thigh.

BI-CONCAVE
Concave or hollow on both surfaces.

BI-CONVEX
Having two convex (rounded, elevated) surfaces.

BICUSPID
Having two cusps (sharp, raised points); term used of heart valves.

BIDET
Low-set, trough-like basin in which the area between the legs can be immersed, while the legs are outside and the feet on the floor.

BI-DIRECTIONALITY
Occurring in two directions; refers to the notion that parents influence children as well as children influence parents in their relationships.

BIFOCAL
Having a double focus. Bifocal spectacles are those that have two lenses, one for distance vision and one for close vision.

BIFURCATION
Divided into two branches.

BILE
A yellow-brown fluid secreted by the liver and containing salts derived from cholesterol. Stored and concentrated in the gallbladder and released into the duodenum after a meal, the bile emulsifies fats and aids absorption of fat-soluble vitamins A, D, E and K.

Other constituents of bile are, in fact, waste products. Yellow bile and black bile were two of the humors of Hippocratic medicine.

BILE ACID
An acid found in bile that promotes the digestion of fats and acids in the absorption of many water-insoluble, organic substances.

BILE DUCT
The tube through which the liver secretion passes as it leaves the gallbladder.

BILHARZIA
Parasitic worm that enters the body and causes bilharziasis.

BILHARZIASIS
Disease caused by a parasitic worm that results in bloody urine and other symptoms, and is the 'Bill Harris' disease that was familiar to troops in the Middle East in World War II. Also called schistosomiasis.

BILIARY CIRRHOSIS
Cirrhotic condition of the liver that may be of unknown cause and characterized by chronic obstructive jaundice or may be the result of obstruction of the extrahepatic bile ducts by stones, tumors, scars or congenital atresia .

BILIOUS
Pertaining to the bile or to bilious attacks, so called because of the presence of bile in the vomit.

BILIRUBIN
One of the bile pigments, derived from hemoglobin, the red pigment of red blood cells.

BILIRUBINEMIA
Increased concentration of bilirubin in the blood.

BILIRUBINURIA
Presence of bilirubin in the urine.

BILIVERDIN
A greenish pigment found in bile chiefly in herbivores and birds, although a small amount is present in humans.

BILLROTH'S OPERATION
Partial removal of the stomach. Billroth I: excision of the lower part of the stomach, part of the remainder closed, with the duodenum attached to the part of the stomach that has been left open. Billroth II: excision of the lower part of the stomach, with the cut ends of the stomach attached directly to the jejunum.

BIMANUAL
Involving the use of both hands.

BINET'S TEST
Properly called the Binet-Simon scale. A series of graded intelligence tests in which an individual's intelligence level is compared with his chronological age.

BINOCULAR VISION
The use of two eyes, set a small distance apart in the head and aligned approximately parallel, to view a single object. Owing to the different angles, the images in the two eyes are slightly different, which enables what is seen to be perceived in three dimensions and so allows the person to judge distance, size and shape. Only humans and some higher animals possess binocular vision.

BIOASSAY
Quantitative determination or estimate of the biological activity or potency of a substance, such as a hormone, by observation of its action on a test organism.

BIO-ASTRONAUTICS
The study of the biological, behavioral and medical effects of flight and space travel.

BIOAVAILABILITY
The amount of a drug that enters the blood stream and so reaches the tissues throughout the body, usually expressed as a percentage of the dose given.

Injection of a drug directly into a vein produced 100 percent bioavailability.

BIOCATALYST
A substance, such as a hormone, that accelerates or modifies a physical process.

BIOCIDE
Destruction of living organisms by such effects of "civilization" as pollution, nuclear fallout and pesticides.

BIOCLIMATOLOGY
The science and study of effects of weather and climate on living organisms - plants, animals, humans.

BIOGENESIS
Origin and evolution of living forms. The law of biogenesis is the principle that all living organisms are derived from a parent or parents. The law of biogeny is the principle that the development of each individual repeats the evolution of the race.

BIOLOGICAL CLOCKS
The mechanisms that control the rhythm of various activities of plants and animals. Some activities, such as mating, migration and hibernation, have a yearly cycle; others, chiefly reproductive functions follow the lunar month. The majority, however, have a period of roughly 24 hours, called a circadian rhythm. As well as obvious rhythms such as the patterns of leaf movement in plants and the activity/sleep cycle in animals, many other features such as body temperature and cell growth oscillate daily. Although related to the day/night cycle, circadian rhythms are not directly controlled by it. Organisms in unvarying environments will continue to show 24-hour rhythms, but the pattern can be changed and the clock "reset."

BIOLOGISM
The type of theory that takes biological use as the universal and ultimate explanatory principle in dealing with life at all levels.

BIOMEDICINE
A field of medical science concerned with the ability of a human being to live and function in abnormal environments.

BIOMETRY
The branch of biological science concerned with the quantitative statistics of the properties and phenomena of living organisms.

BIONIC LIMB
Artificial arm or leg powered by an electric motor or other devices that are stimulated by nerve impulses from the user's limb.

BIONICS
The science of designing artificial systems which have the desirable characteristics of living organisms. These may be simple imitations of nature, or systems that embody a principle learned from nature. Examples of the latter include radar, inspired by the echo-location system of bats, or the development of associative memories in computers that resemble those in the human brain.

BIONOMICS
The branch of biology which studies the relations of organisms to their environment.

BIOPHYSICS
A branch of biology in which the methods and principles of physics are applied to the study of living things. It has grown up in the 20th

century alongside the development of electronics. Its tools include the electroencephalograph and the electron microscope, its techniques those of spectroscopy and X-ray diffraction, and its problems the study of nerve transmission, bioluminescence and materials transfer in respiration and secretion.

BIOPSY
Removal of a piece of living tissue from the body and its examination in various ways, such as under a microscope, to determine its structure and the presence or absence of disease.

BIOSOCIAL
Used to describe those social relationships that are determined mainly by social factors, or to describe organisms that have social significance for the human being, e.g. animals as pets.

BIOSPHERE
The region inhabited by living things. It forms a thin layer around the earth, including the surface of the lithosphere, the hydrosphere and the lower atmosphere. The importance of the concept was first pointed out in the early 19th century by the French biologist, Lamarck.

BIOSYNTHESIS
The biochemical reactions by which living cells build up simple molecules into complex ones.

These reactions require energy, which is obtained from light or from ATP, a nucleotide present in all cells that is produced in degradation reactions.

BIOTIC POTENTIAL
The highest possible rate of population increase, resulting from maximum birth rates and minimum death rates.

BIOTIN
A member of vitamin B complex; also known as vitamin H and as coenzyme R.

BIOTYPE
Applied to a group of organisms of common descent, with the same complex of hereditary factors.

BIPARA
Woman who has had two separate pregnancies and been delivered of one or more children from each pregnancy.

BIPAROUS
Giving birth to twins.

BIPLANE CEREBRAL ANGIOGRAPHY
X-ray studies of the blood vessels in the brain after injection of contrast medium, showing the structures from the side and front-to-back.

BIPOLAR DISORDER
Psychological disorder characterized by one or more manic episodes usually accompanied by one or more major depressive episodes.

In a bipolar disorder the initial episode that occasioned hospitalization is usually manic. Both the manic and major depressive episodes are more frequent than the depressive episodes in a major depression.

There is evidence that cases of a bipolar disorder with a mixed or rapid cycling episode have a much more chronic course than those without this type of episode.

It is estimated that from 0.4% to 1.2% of the adult population have had a bipolar disorder. Recent epidemiological studies in the US indicate that the disorder is equally common in males and in females, unlike a major depression, which is more common in females.

BIPOLAR VERSION
Turning a baby in the womb, performed by manipulating both the

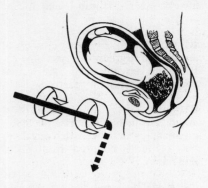

Primary phase in the birth of a child. Uterine contractions gradually open the cervix of the uterus.

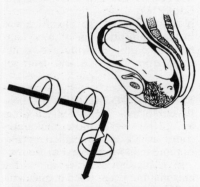

Next phase in the birth of a child. The cervix is fully dilated and the baby's head is showing. The second stage does not last very long - probably one to two hours. The baby's head moves down the vagina until it "crowns", that is, when about half of the head can be seen at the vaginal opening.

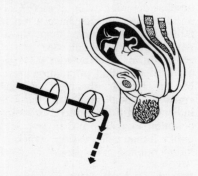

Once the head is born, most of the hard work for the mother is over. With one more gentle push, the rest of the body will be born.

head and pelvis of the baby.

BIRTH
The condition to which a person is born; delivery.

BIRTH CONTROL
Prevention of unwanted births, by means of contraception, abortion, sterilization and, in the past, infanticide.

It is medically advisable if the child is likely to be defective. At family level, birth control can help to prevent poverty, while globally it could help prevent mass starvation.

BIRTHMARKS
Skin blemishes, usually congenital. There are two main types: pigmented nevuses, or moles, which are usually brown or black and may be raised or flat; and vascular nevuses, local growths of small blood vessels, such as the "strawberry mark" and the "port-wine stain." Although harmless, they are sometimes removed for cosmetic reasons or if they show malignant tendencies.

BIRTH PALSY
Form of paralysis caused by damage to the baby during birth.

BIRTH RATE
The number of live births in a given period by the population resident in an area during that period. The rate may be restricted to births to women of specific age, race, marital status or geographical location, or may be related to the entire population.

BIRTHRIGHT
Any right or privilege to which a person is entitled by birth.

BIRTH SYMBOLISM
Employed in psychoanalytic literature for a symbolic representation, which stands for the first separation from the love object as experienced

in the separation of the newborn child from its mother.

BIRTH TRAUMA
Injury from a traumatic or difficult delivery.

BISEXUALITY
The term is only used occasionally to refer to persons who are bisexual in the sense of engaging in both heterosexual and homosexual relations, but usually to the presence of masculine and feminine psychological attributes in a single person. Psychoanalytical theory has always assumed that all human beings are constitutionally psychosexually bisexual. Contemporary theory, however, tends to explain psychosexual bisexuality by reference to the fact that children identify with both parents.

The theory of bisexuality assumes that it is possible to attach a sexual connotation to non-sexual functions and to designate passive, submissive, masochistic, intuitive and receptive behavior as feminine, and active, assertive, sadistic, intellectual and penetrative behavior as masculine, and that shifts in attitude imply changes in sexual orientation. The problem of bisexuality is bedeviled by social preconceptions about male and female roles.

BISHOP SCALE
Scoring method used to evaluate the readiness of a woman's body for labor or induction; includes states of cervical dilation, effacement, consistency and position, as well as the position of the baby.

BISMUTH
White crystalline metal with a reddish tint. The insoluble salts of bismuth are commonly used in stomach mixtures to act as an inert protective covering for an irritable or ulcerated lining of the stomach or duodenum. As an injection, bismuth salts were formerly used in the treatment of syphilis.

BISTOURY
A small, narrow surgical knife, used for minor incisions.

BITOT'S SPOTS
Collections of dried epithelium, flaky masses and micro-organisms at the sides of the cornea of the eye, caused by vitamin A deficiency.

BITTERNESS
The state or quality of being bitter in all its senses, whether to the taste, feelings or mind.

BLACK DEATH
Name for an epidemic of bubonic plague that swept through Asia and Europe in the mid-14th century, annihilating whole communities and perhaps halving the population of Europe. Originating in China, it was carried by flea-infected rats on vessels trading to the West. Its economic effects were far-reaching, and also fanned the flames of superstition and religious prejudice. European Jews, accused of poisoning wells, were massacred, and the idea that the plague was punishment for sin led to a wave of fanatical penance.

BLACK EYE
An eye with the surrounding flesh or skin discolored by a blow or bruise.

BLACKHEAD
Also called a comedo. Skin blemish consisting of a blackish fatty secretion in a follicle.

BLACK INDURATION
Fibrosis of the lung in miners suffering with anthracosis.

BLACK LUNG DISEASE
Another name for anthracosis.

BLACKOUT
Result of diminished blood circula-

tion to the brain and retina of the eye. The most common causes are epilepsy and syncope (fainting).

The very first symptoms are important and often have to be patiently extracted from patients who are often so overwhelmed by the embarrassment and surprise of 'fainting' that they may have forgotten the preceding chest pain and palpitations (an abnormal heart rhythm that they were aware of), the unreal fragment of memory, and nausea rising from the stomach during the dream-like aura and visual blurring before syncope, and the pins–and–needles and tightness around the throat during hysterical overbreathing.

Occasionally syncope or epilepsy occurs during a migraine and, very rarely, a blackout with a severe headache can be due to acute hydrocephalus (an abnormal accumulation of fluid within the skull).

BLACK VOMIT
Condition due to bleeding occurring in the stomach or intestines. Being partly digested, the blood changes from red to black and is then vomited.

BLACKWATER FEVER
Severe form of malaria associated with bloody urine.

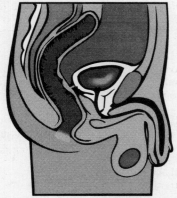

Side view of the male genital apparatus. The location of the urinary bladder is clearly seen between the symphysis and rectum.

BLADDER
A membranous sac, such as one serving as receptacle for a secretion, especially the urinary bladder.

BLADDER CANCER
Malignant tumor of the urinary bladder.

BLADDER STONE
Calculus (hard mass) in the cavity of the urinary bladder.

BLALOCK'S OPERATION
Anastomosis (joining together) of the pulmonary artery to a branch of the aorta. Most often performed for Fallot's tetralogy of the heart.

BLASTEMA
The mass of undifferentiated cells from which an organ or a body part is evolved during embryonic development.

BLASTOCYST
The blastula, having a knob of cells at one side that develops into the embryo, the remainder developing into the placenta.

BLASTODERM
Germinal membrane of an egg which forms the growing embryo.

BLASTOGENESIS
The theory of the transmission of hereditary characteristics by genes.

BLASTOMA
Tumor originating in immature or embryonic cells.

BLASTOMYCOSIS
An infectious disease caused by the fungus Blastomyces dermatitides, primarily involving the lungs and occasionally spreading hematogenously (via the blood), characteristically involving the skin.

BLASTULA
A hollow sphere composed of a single layer of cells, formed by the di-

viding of a fertilized ovum; the first stage in the development of the embryo. In mammals, a singular cluster, the blastocyst, is formed, which has an inner cell mass and a spherical envelope, the latter developing into the placenta.

BLEEDER
Person who suffers with hemophilia, a condition in which the blood lacks the ability to clot.

BLEEDING TIME
The time it takes for a needle prick, usually in the ear lobe, to stop bleeding. In normal persons, it is usually one to three minutes, but in those suffering from hemophilia, the time may be indefinite.

BLEMISH
A noticeable defect, flaw or imperfection, usually on the skin.

BLENNORRHAGIA
Any profuse mucous discharge from anywhere in the body, particularly the profuse gonorrheal discharge from the penis or the vagina.

BLENNURIA
An excess of mucus in the urine.

BLEPHARECTOMY
Excision of a portion of an eyelid.

BLEPHARISM
Spasmodic twitching of the eyelids.

BLEPHARITIS
Inflammation of the margins of the eyelids. In a run-down child it may be due to unhealthy and poor living conditions, and is sometimes associated with seborrhea of the scalp that produces dandruff, and this infects the eyelids.

BLEPHARON
The eyelid.

BLINDNESS
Severe loss or absence of vision, caused by injury to the eyes, congenital defects or diseases including cataract, diabetes, glaucoma, leprosy, trachoma and disease of the blood vessels. Malnutrition (especially vitamin A deficiency) may cause blindness in children. Infant blindness can result if the mother had rubella (German measles) early in pregnancy; it was also formerly caused by gonorrheal infection of a baby's eyes at birth, but routine use of silver nitrate reduced this risk. Transient blindness may occur if one is exposed to a vertical acceleration of more than five Gs (as in a spacecraft at blast-off).

Cortical blindness is a disease of the higher perceptive centers in the brain concerned with vision: the person may even deny blindness despite severe disability.

Blindness due to cataract may be relieved by removal of the eye lens and the use of glasses. Prevention or early recognition and treatment of predisposing conditions are essential to saving sight, as established blindness is rarely recoverable.

BLIND SPOT
The area of the retina of each eye where the optic nerve and blood vessels enter, about 2 mm (1/10 in) in diameter; it has no light-sensitive receptors. In binocular vision, the two spots do not receive corresponding images, and so are not noticeable.

BLISTER
Bleb, vesicle or fluid-filled swelling arising within and on the skin.

BLOCK DESIGN TEST
Intelligence test, where colored cubes have to be assembled to make a given design.

BLOCKING
Experience of being impeded, or brought to a standstill, in a train of association or thought. The major

feature of this phenomenon is the interruption of a train of speech before a thought or idea has been completed. After a period of silence, which may last from a few seconds to minutes, the person indicates that he or she cannot recall what he or she has been saying or meant to say. Blocking should be judged to be present only if the person spontaneously describes losing his or her train of thought or upon questioning by an interviewer, gives that as the reason for pausing.

BLOCKING ANTIBODY
An antibody that can block the combination of an antigen with another antibody.

BLOOD
A thick red fluid filling the heart and blood vessels. It consists of plasma, a transparent fluid, that contains minute solid particles or corpuscles (blood cells) in it.

BLOOD BANK
An institution for storing and processing blood or blood plasma received from donors.

BLOOD-BRAIN BARRIER
The membranes between the circulating blood and the brain. Some drugs can pass from the blood to the cerebrospinal fluid; others cannot.

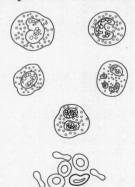

Drawings of various types of blood cells. Upper rows: leukocytes. Bottom row: erythrocytes and platelets.

BLOOD CELL
A basic structural unit of the blood, also called a blood corpuscle.

BLOOD CIRCULATION
The movement of blood from the heart through the arteries, capillaries and veins and back to the heart. The circulatory system has two distinct parts: the pulmonary circulation, in which blood is pumped from the right ventricle of the heart through blood vessels to the lungs (where the blood is oxygenated and carbon dioxide is eliminated) and then through blood vessels into the left atrium of the heart; and the systemic circulation, in which the oxygenated blood is pumped from the left ventricle through all the blood vessels of the body tissues (where - in the capillaries - the blood is deoxygenated and carbon dioxide is taken up) and then to the right atrium of the heart. As it leaves the heart, the blood is under considerable pressure - about 120 mm of mercury maximum (systolic pressure, when the heart contracts) and 80 mm of mercury minimum (diastolic pressure, when the heart relaxes). Sustained high blood pressure, or hypertension, occurs in kidney and hormone diseases and in old age, but generally its cause is unknown. It may lead to arteriosclerosis and heart, brain and kidney damage. Low blood pressure occurs in shock and trauma.

BLOOD CLOT
The jelly-like mass formed as liquid blood congeals when blood vessels are injured.

BLOOD CORPUSCLE
A red or white blood cell. Red blood corpuscles are called erythrocytes, white ones leukocytes.

BLOOD COUNT
Number of red and white blood cells found in a standard sample of blood.

BLOOD CULTURE
The incubation of a blood sample in nutrient material to determine the growth and type of infection-causing micro-organisms.

BLOOD DONOR CENTER
An establishment in which blood and/or blood components are obtained from donors.

BLOOD DYSCRASIA
General term for any blood disease.

BLOOD GASES
Gases dissolved in the blood that maintain its acid-alkali balance.

BLOOD GROUP
Typing of blood according to the specific antigen or antigens on each red blood cell surface.

BLOODLETTING
The act of letting blood or bleeding, as by opening a vein, as a remedial measure.

BLOOD PLASMA
Also called blood serum: the clear, almost colorless fluid of the blood that results when it is separated from blood cells by centrifuging.

BLOOD PLASMA, FRESH FROZEN
A plasma frozen within six hours of donation and stored below zero degree centigrade.

BLOOD PLASMA, FROZEN
A plasma obtained from whole blood within a specified time (but no longer than six hours) of collection and maintained in a frozen state below minus 20 degrees centigrade.

BLOOD PLASMA, SPECIFIC IMMUNE
A plasma that can be used either for passive immunization (making someone immune to a disease by injecting them with plasma from another who is already immune) or for

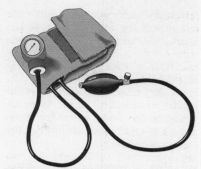

Transportable apparatus for measuring blood pressure.

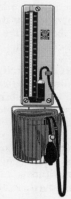

Fixed apparatus for measuring blood pressure, as used in a hospital.

the manufacture of specific immunoglobulins.

BLOOD PLASMAPHERESIS
Procedures by which whole blood is separated by
physical means into components and one or more of them returned to the donor.

BLOOD PLATELET
A minute, circular or oval body found in blood, necessary for blood clotting.

BLOOD POISONING
A disease condition of the blood caused by the presence of toxic matter or micro-organisms.

BLOOD PRESSURE
The pressure of blood within the ar-

teries, primarily maintained by contraction of the left ventricle of the heart.

BLOOD PRESSURE, DIASTOLIC

Pressure (usually recorded in millimeters of mercury) in the large arteries of the body when the heart muscle is relaxed and filling for the next contraction.

BLOOD PRESSURE, SYSTOLIC

Pressure (usually recorded in millimeters of mercury) in the large arteries of the body at the instant the heart muscle contracts.

BLOOD PROCESSING

Any procedure used after collection and before compatibility testing with a prospective recipient.

BLOOD SERUM

Also called blood plasma: the yellowish, clear liquid remaining after all solid constituents of the blood have been removed.

BLOODSHOT

Red and inflamed because of excessively dilated capillaries; said of the eye.

BLOODSTREAM

The blood flowing through the circulatory system.

BLOOD SUGAR

Sugar normally found in the blood and burned for energy.

BLOOD TRANSFUSION

The procedure of transferring blood or a component of blood from a donor to a recipient.

BLOOD TYPE

The type and subtype of an individual's blood; specified as A, B, AB or O; Rh-negative or Rh-positive, and including a number of subtypes. It is important to determine the blood type when a woman is pregnant, to make sure her blood is not incompatible with her unborn baby's, or when a patient needs a transfusion, to avoid a dangerous reaction with an incompatible type.

BLOOD UREA

The amount of urea (the end product of protein metabolism) in the blood; varies within the normal range of 20 to 40 mg per 100 ml of blood.

BLOTCH

An inflamed eruption or discolored patch on the skin.

BLUE BABIES

Babies having a blueness of skin (cyanosis) caused by insufficient oxygen in the arterial blood. This often indicates a heart defect, but may have other causes such as premature birth or impaired breathing.

BLUE DEVILS

A colloquial phrase for dejection, hypochondria or lowness of spirits.

BLUE SCLEROTICS

Intense blue coloration of the sclerotic membranes (the whites of the eyes) occurring in osteogenesis imperfecta, an hereditary disease characterized by extremely brittle bones.

BLUE-YELLOW BLINDNESS

Rare form of color-blindness in which the individual is unable to recognize the difference between blue and yellow.

BOBATH METHOD

System of physical exercises, developed by Bertha and Karl Bobath, used for the treatment of spastic conditions in children and adults. Inhibition of reflexes, rather than utilization, is the basic principle of the system.

The Bobaths feel that the abnormality of muscle tone and the display of primitive reflex patterns of movement are common to all those with cerebral palsy, even though masked by the involuntary movements found in these people. Lack of coordination in those who are brain-damaged is thought to be due to lack of muscle tone.

Treatment is based on the following principles:

- The inhibition of abnormal postural reflex activity to reduce muscle spasm in the spastic child.

- The facilitation of potential normal postural and movement patterns on the basis of a more normal muscle tone, in order to maintain and secure normal tone qualities obtained by inhibition.

- The increase of postural reflex tone and the regulation of reciprocal muscle inhibition.

The term facilitation of movement has been chosen to define techniques of obtaining inherent automatic movement patterns in response to handling, in contrast to movements performed at request.

BODY
The physical substance of a human being or animal.

BODY-BUILD INDEX
An index of constitutional types that groups individuals according to the value obtained from multiplying 100 times their height by six times their transverse chest diameter.

BODY-BUILDING
Development of the muscles to increase strength or improve the physique. Body-building is undertaken by sportsmen and women to strengthen particular parts of the body within the context of its overall development. The chief method uses training with weights, gradually increasing the heaviness of the weights and the number of times an exercise is done. This results in hypertrophy, or an increase in size of the muscles.

BODY DYSMORPHIC DISORDER
Preoccupation with some imagined defect in appearance in a normal-appearing person. The most common complaints involve facial flaws, such as wrinkles, spots on the skin, excessive facial hair, shape of nose, mouth, jaw, or eyebrows, and swelling of the face. More rarely the complaint involves the appearance of the feet. hands, breasts, back, or some other part of the body. In some cases a slight physical anomaly is present but the person's concern is grossly excessive. A history of repeated visits to plastic surgeons or dermatologists in an effort to correct the imagined defect is common. A depressive syndrome and obsessive compulsive personality traits are frequent. Often there is avoidance of social or occupational situations because of anxiety about the imagined defect.

The most common age at onset is from adolescence through the third decade. The disorder usually persists for several years.

BODY IMAGE
The image in an individual's mind of his or her own body. Distortions of this occur as a result of emotional disorders, parietal lobe tumors or injuries in the brain.

BODY LANGUAGE
The expression of thoughts, emotions, etc. through movements of the body.

BODY SALTS
Compounds of various minerals that are present in such body fluids as blood, urine, and sweat, and within cells. These salts play an important role in regulating water balance, acidity of the blood, conduction of nerve impulses, and muscle contraction.

BODY-SENSE AREA
A projection area of the cerebral

cortex of the brain lying behind the central groove. Electrical stimulation of the area commonly results in the report of sensory experiences.

BOILS
Another name for furuncles.

BOLUS
A soft, round mass of anything medicinal to be swallowed at once; larger and less solid than an ordinary pill.

BONDING
The development of a deep emotional attachment between parent and child.

BONE
The hard tissue that forms the skeleton. Bone supports the body, protects its organs, acts as anchors for muscles and as levers for the movement of limbs, and is the main reserve of calcium and phosphate in the body. Bone consists of living cells (osteocytes) embedded in a

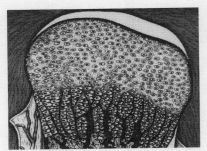
Development of bone. The microscopic preparation shows numerous osteoblasts and osteoclasts.

matrix of collagen fibers, with calcium salts similar in composition to hydroxyapatite deposited between them. Some carbonates are also present. All bones have a shell of compact bone in concentric layers (lamellae) around the blood vessels that run in small channels (Haversian canals). Within this shell is porous or spongy bone, and in the case of long bones, there is a hollow cavity containing marrow. The bone is enveloped by a fibrous membrane, the periosteum, that is sensitive to pain, unlike the bone itself, and which has a network of nerves and blood vessels that penetrate the bone surface.

BONE GRAFT
The transplantation of a piece of bone from one part of the body to another, or from one person to another.

BONE MARROW ASPIRATION
Removal of bone marrow from the breastbone or hip bone through a needle. The blood cells produced by the bone marrow are evaluated as to number, appearance, development and presence of infection. This procedure is performed when leukemia, severe anemia or other disease affecting the bone marrow is suspected.

BONE MARROW DEPRESSION
Disorder of the bone marrow char-

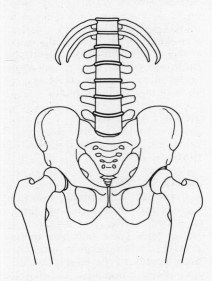
The skeleton is made of more than 200 bones. The bones of the pelvis, part of the vertebral column and the proximal parts of the femur are shown.

acterized by a decrease in blood cell development. Many drugs taken for long periods of time in high doses can cause toxicity to the blood-producing capacity of human bone marrow.

BONE SCAN
A scan of the bones after injection of radioactive material into a vein. An increased concentration of radioactive material in a given area may indicate cancer, arthritis, fracture or other disease conditions.

BONE X-RAY
X-ray studies of bone to determine if fracture or disease is present.

BONJELA GEL
Brand name for choline salicylate, a drug that works in a similar way as aspirin.

BORAX
Biborate of soda that acts in much the same way as boric acid, but does not have its acid reaction.

BORBORYGMUS
The rumbling sound caused by the movement of gas or fluid in the large intestine.

BORDERLINE
A patient who is on the border between neurosis and psychosis, i.e. either one whose psychopathology defies categorization or one whose behavior does not warrant his being treated as psychotic.

The usage arises from the fact that diagnostic systems assume that neurosis and psychosis are mutually exclusive while clinical observation shows they are not.

It is also used in the sense of individuals who are near the line division between two classes as, for example, sanity and insanity, but more specifically, in mental tests to describe cases near, but not below, the dividing line between dull, normal and subnormal, i.e. IQ 70 to 75.

BORDERLINE PERSONALITY DISORDER
A pervasive pattern of instability of self-image, interpersonal relationships, and mood, beginning by early adulthood and present in a variety of contexts.

A marked and persistent identity disturbance is almost invariably present. This is often pervasive, and is manifested by uncertainty about several life issues, such as self-image, sexual orientation, long-term goals or career choice, types of friends or lovers to have, or which values to adopt.

The person often experiences this instability of self-image as chronic feelings of emptiness or boredom.

Interpersonal relationships are usually unstable and intense, and may be characterized by alternation of the extremes of overidealization and devaluation. These people have difficulty tolerating being alone, and will make frantic efforts to avoid real or imagined abandonment.

Recurrent suicidal threats, gestures, or behavior and other self-mutilating behavior (e.g., wrist-scratching) are common in the more severe forms of the disorder. This behavior may serve to manipulate others, may be the result of intense anger, or may counteract feelings of "numbness" and depersonalization that arise during periods of extreme stress.

BORIC ACID
An acid derived from boron trioxide, a white crystalline acid occurring in nature, or prepared from borax and used as a weak antiseptic. It should never be used on infants and young children.

BORNHOLM DISEASE
Another name for epidemic pleurodynia.

BOTTLE FEEDING
Dried cows' milk given to babies

instead of breastfeeding. Prepackaged infant formulas are readily available, usually coming in powdered form to which boiled (and cooled) water is then added.

They are all fortified with vitamin D, and many contain other vitamins; they have all been modified to reduce the high levels of sodium and phosphate found in cows' milk. All equipment used in bottle feeding (bottle, teats, etc.) must be sterilized before a baby is fed, until the child is about one year old. The infant should be offered water between feedings, particularly in hot weather or in a hot, dry environment.

BOTULISM
Usually fatal type of food poisoning caused by a toxin produced by the anaerobic bacteria Clostridium botulinum and C. parabotulinum, which normally live in soil but may infect badly canned food. The toxin paralyses the nervous system. Thorough cooking destroys both bacteria and toxin.

BOUGIE
A slender, flexible instrument for dilating or opening passages of the body.

BOWEL OBSTRUCTION
A condition in which the passage of the contents of the intestines is arrested or seriously impaired. The small or large intestine may be obstructed by a physical blockage, or the movement of the bowel may have ceased for some reason.

BOWLEG
An outward curvature of the legs, causing a separation of the knees when the ankles are in contact.

BOXING INJURY
Injury acquired during fighting with fists. The commonest boxing injuries are cuts around the eyes from either a punch or an accidental clash of heads. The immediate effect is to create the impression of a gory mess; however, they are easily dealt with after the contest is over. Careful stitching by a competent doctor followed by six to eight weeks' rest from sparring or boxing allows even the deepest cuts to heal properly. The only danger from a cut around the eye is that the blood flowing profusely may impair the boxer's vision temporarily and therefore disturb his concentration and ability to avoid his opponent's punches. Other eye injuries are not common. The cauliflower ear is virtually unknown today, due to the extreme vigilance of referees in preventing injury and the immediate treatment of any swellings as they arise. Occasionally a boxer receives a direct blow to the ear and as a result sustains a traumatic perforation of the eardrum.

Lacerations of the lips and mouth are not common. So long as the boxer has adequate dental care and wears a well-fitting gum shield, he is unlikely to suffer injury to his mouth.

BOYLE'S ANESTHETIC MACHINE
An apparatus by which chloroform, ether, nitrous oxide gas and oxygen may be administered.

BRACE
A wire device for straightening the teeth.

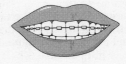

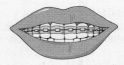

Two types of braces used to correct the position of the teeth in children.

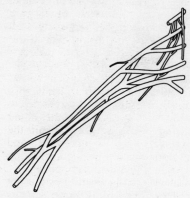
Schematic drawing of the brachial plexus.

BRACHIAL
Pertaining to the arm.

BRACHIALGIA
Pain arising in the arm.

BRACHIAL PLEXUS
Network of nerve fibers formed by the union of the ventral branches of the lower four cervical nerves in the neck and the greater part of the ventral branch of the first thoracic nerve leaving the spine at the top of the shoulders.

In the neck, the brachial plexus lies in the posterior triangle between the collarbone and the lower part of the posterior border of the sternocleidomastoid muscle, being covered by skin, platysma (plate-like muscle) and deep bands of fibrous tissue. When the arm is by the side, it can be felt as a bunch of tense cords. The brachial plexus gives rise to the nerves of the arm and part of the chest wall.

BRACHIOCEPHALIC
Pertaining to the arm and the head.

BRACHIUM
The arm, especially the arm above the elbow.

BRACHYCEPHALIC
Having a disproportionately short head, denoting a skull with a cephalic index over 80 - that is, its width is at least four-fifths its length.

BRACHYDACTYLY
Abnormal shortness of the fingers or toes.

BRADFORD FRAME
A stretcher-type of bed used for immobilizing the spine and preventing deformity.

BRADYCARDIA
Slowness of the heartbeat and pulse, usually defined as a rate under 60 beats per minute.

BRADYKINESIA
Exaggerated slowness of movement, usually caused by a disorder or disturbance of brain function.

BRADYKININ
A substance found in blood plasma that is important for many reactions in the body, particularly inflammation.

BRADYIGNORE
Abnormal slowness of articulation, due to brain lesion.

BRADYLOGIA
Slowness of speech, due to functional, and not organic, disorder or defect.

BRADYPNEA
Slow or labored breathing.

BRADYURIA
Extremely slow passing of urine.

BRAILLE
System of writing devised for the blind by Louis Braille. It employs patterns of raised dots that can be read by touch.

Braille typewriters and printing presses have been devised for the mass-production of books for the blind.

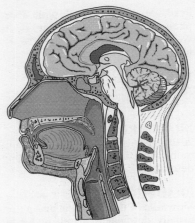

Medial view of the head and central nervous system. The brain is protected by the bony cranium of skull.

BRAIN
A complex organ that, together with the spinal cord, comprises the central nervous system and coordinates all nerve-cell activities.

BRAIN ABSCESS
An encapsulated collection of pus in the brain. It is usually due to an extension from a bacterial infection outside the brain.

BRAIN CASE
The cranium or skull that surrounds the brain.

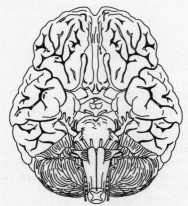

Side view of the brain to show the gyri and sulci of the hemispheres. The cerebellum is located below the hemispheres. Part of the brain stem is seen below.

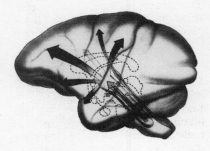

Brain stem with a schematic drawing of the ascending reticular formation.

BRAIN DEPRESSANTS
Any drug that depresses brain function, such as tranquilizers, narcotics, alcohol, barbiturates.

BRAIN FEVER
A disease in which the major symptoms are severe headache, high temperature and vomiting. An important feature of the disease is that it apparently only occurs during the winter and spring. Modern antibiotic treatment has cut short this disease process and largely abolished the serious complications that used to occur.

BRAIN SCAN
A scan of the brain after injection of radioactive material into a vein. An increased concentration of radioactive material in a given area indicates a possible disease.

BRAIN STEM
All of the brain except the cerebrum and cerebellum.

BRAINWASHING
The manipulation of an individual's will, generally without his or her knowledge and against his or her wishes. Most commonly, it consists of a combination of isolation, personal humiliation, disorientation, systematic indoctrination and alternating punishment and reward.

BRAIN WAVES
The spontaneous and rhythmic electrical discharges of the living brain, particularly of the cerebral cortex. These can be recorded on an electroencephalogram (EEG).

BRAXTON-HICKS CONTRACTIONS
Intermittent contractions of the uterus increasing in frequency as pregnancy nears completion. Unlike true labor contractions, Braxton-Hicks contractions do not progress in terms of length or strength.

BREAST
The front of the chest, especially the modified cutaneous, glandular structure it bears - the mamma or mammary gland.

BREASTBONE
Also called the sternum: a narrow, flat bone shaped like a dagger with a handle, blade and tip. The first seven costal cartilages of the ribs are attached to it on either side. It is attached by joints to the clavicles (collarbones) above.

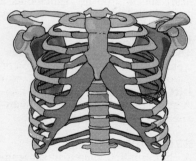

Skeleton of the thorax. The breastbone is located in the middle. The collar bones form joints with the breastbone; furthermore many ribs are attached to it.

BREATHING
The normal rate of breathing is 16 breaths per minute.

BREATH SOUND
The sound heard over the chest by the stethoscope during respiration.

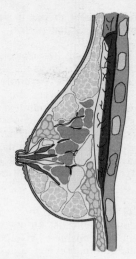

Side view of the female breast.

BREECH DELIVERY
The birth of a baby with the buttocks appearing first.

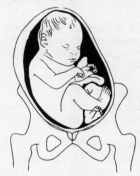

Position of the fetus in a case of breech delivery.

BREGMA
The point of junction of the sagittal and coronal sutures of the skull.

BRIEF REACTIVE PSYCHOSIS
Sudden onset of psychotic symptoms of at least a few hours', but no more than one month's, duration, with eventual full return to premorbid level of functioning. The psychotic symptoms appear shortly after one or more events that, singly or together, would be markedly

stressful to almost anyone in similar circumstances in that person's culture.

The precipitating event(s) may be any major stress, such as the loss of a loved one or the psychological trauma of combat. Invariably there is emotional turmoil, manifested by rapid shifts from one intense affect to another, or overwhelming perplexity or confusion, which the person may acknowledge or which can be judged from the way he or she responds to questions and requests.

BRIGHT'S DISEASE
Also called nephritis: kidney degeneration accompanied by imperfect uric acid elimination and high blood pressure.

BRILL'S DISEASE
An acute infectious disease milder than epidemic typhus but caused by the same rickettsia.

BRILL-ZINSSER DISEASE
Reappearance of epidemic typhus, occurring years after an initial attack.

BRIQUET'S SYNDROME
Another name for somatization disorder.

BRITTLE BONES
Also called osteogenesis imperfecta: a rare hereditary condition that can cause severe deformity. During childhood, trivial falls can result in serious fractures. The liability to fracture diminishes with age. If there have been repeated fractures, the lower limbs may not develop normally and the person affected may have to rely totally on a wheelchair.

BROADBENT'S SIGN
Visible movement of the left side and back, in the region of the lower ribs, that occurs with each heartbeat and is due to adhesions between the pericardium (membrane that surrounds the heart) and diaphragm.

BROAD BETA DISEASE
Another name for hyperlipoproteinemia type III.

BROAD LIGAMENTS
Double fold of parietal peritoneum (membrane that lines the abdominal cavity) that hangs over the womb and supports the outstretched Fallopian tubes.

BROCA'S SPEECH AREA
A portion of the left cerebral hemisphere of the brain said to control the muscles that produce speech. That the area has these precise functions is doubtful.

BROMIC ACID
An unstable, strongly oxidizing acid, occurring only in solution or in a salt: used as an oxidizing agent in the manufacture of medicines.

BROMIDE
A salt of hydrobromic acid, especially potassium bromide, that acts as a depressant of the brain and the heart and is used in medicine as a sedative and a hypnotic.

BROMIDROSIS
The secretion of foul-smelling perspiration.

BROMINISM
A group of symptoms caused by excessive use of bromides.

BROMODERMA
A skin eruption caused in susceptible persons by the use of bromides.

BRONCHADENITIS
Inflammation of the lymph glands in the chest.

BRONCHI
The main branches of the trachea (windpipe); the plural form of bronchus.

BRONCHIAL ARTERY
Any branch of the descending aorta or first intercostal artery that accompanies the bronchi.

BRONCHIAL ASTHMA
A respiratory disorder characterized by inflammation of the bronchi and causing difficulty in breathing.

BRONCHIAL CARCINOMA
Malignant tumor of the branches of the windpipe. Lung cancer is the more common name for this disease.

BRONCHIAL OBSTRUCTION
A condition most often caused by inhalation of vomit, by a foreign body or by a malignant tumor of the lung.

BRONCHIAL RESPIRATION
The sound of breathing as heard over the main air passages in health.

BRONCHIAL SOUND
The harsh sound produced by air passing through the bronchial tubes.

BRONCHIAL TUBE
A bronchus (one of the air passages within the lungs).

BRONCHIAL VEIN
Any vein accompanying the bronchi and their branches and emptying into the azygos and superior intercostal veins.

BRONCHIECTASIS
Condition that sometimes follows diseases such as whooping cough, in which there is dilation of the bronchi or bronchioles.

BRONCHIOLE
Minute endbranch of a bronchus; a minute thin-walled branch of a bronchus.

BRONCHIOLITIS
An acute viral infection of the lower respiratory tract, characterized by

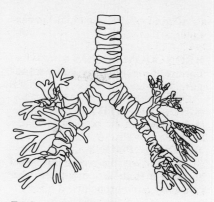
Trachea and main bronchi.

respiratory distress, difficulty in breathing out, and wheezing, and affecting infants and young children.

BRONCHITIS
Inflammation of one or more bronchi; may be acute or chronic.

BRONCHOCONSTRICTOR
A substance that causes the airways in the lungs to narrow. An attack of asthma may be caused by the release of bronchoconstrictor substances such as histamine or certain prostaglandins.

BRONCHODILATORS
A group of drugs used to dilate the bronchial tubes to treat such problems as asthma, emphysema, bronchitis, allergies and others.

BRONCHOGENIC
Relating to, or arising in or by way of the air passages of the lungs.

BRONCHOGRAPHY
Radiography of the lungs after injection of an opaque medium in the bronchi.

BRONCHOLITHIASIS
A condition in which concretions are present in a bronchus.

BRONCHOMOTOR
Relating to or affecting contraction

or dilation of the bronchial air passages.

BRONCHOMYCOSIS
Form of bronchitis caused by a fungus.

BRONCHOPATHY
Any disease of the bronchi.

BRONCHOPHONY
The sound of the voice as heard through a stethoscope applied over a healthy large bronchus.

BRONCHOPLASTY
Surgical repair of a bronchial defect.

BRONCHOPNEUMONIA
Inflammation of the lungs commencing in the bronchi, sometimes patchy and localized. In lobar pneumonia, a whole lobe of a lung is affected.

BRONCHOPULMONARY
Pertaining to or affecting both bronchi and lungs.

BRONCHORRHEA
Excessive discharge of mucus from the air passages of the lungs (bronchi).

BRONCHOSCOPE
Instrument that is passed down the main airway to examine the lungs and air passages.

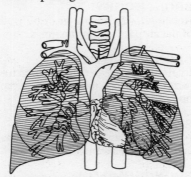

Distribution of the main bronchi in the various lobes of the lungs.

BRONCHOSCOPY
Inspection of the interior of the bronchus with a bronchoscope.

BRONCHOSPASM
Spasmodic contraction of the smooth muscles of the bronchi, as occurs in asthma.

BRONCHOSPIROMETRY
Determination of vital capacity, oxygen intake and carbon dioxide excretion of a single lung.

BRONCHOSTENOSIS
Narrowing of the inner diameter of a bronchus.

BRONCHOTRACHEAL
Relating to both bronchi and trachea.

BRONCHUS
One of the main branches of the trachea, the main airway of the chest.

BRONTOPHOBIA
Pathological fear of thunder.

BROW PRESENTATION
That position in which the brow of a baby shows first in childbirth.

BROWN FAT
A mammalian heat-producing tissue occurring especially in human embryos and newborn infants and in hibernating animals.

BROWN INDURATION
Chronic passive congestion and fibrosis of the lung due to pigmentation by an iron-containing blood pigment.

BRUCELLA AGGLUTININS
Antibodies elevated in blood of patients with brucellosis.

BRUCELLOSIS
Also called undulant fever: an infectious disease characterized by a first stage of high fever, sweats, joint pain and headaches, and a

chronic stage with relapses of fever, weakness, sweats and vague aches and pains. It is caused by the bacterium Brucella abortus, a parasite carried by cattle.

BRUDZINSKI'S REFLEX
In meningitis, when flexion of the patient's head also causes flexion of the ankle, knee and hip.

The test can also be performed by flexing one leg at the hip joint, which causes the other leg to flex automatically.

BRUISE
Also called a contusion: superficial injury to the skin or soft tissues in which the minute blood vessels are broken causing slight bleeding into the tissues, and producing the characteristic blue staining.
First aid: Rest injured part. Apply cold compresses for 30 minutes, making sure that no ice touches the skin. If bruising is extensive or complicated with abrasions and/or cuts, consult a doctor.

BRUIT
Any sound heard within the body, as by means of a stethoscope.

BRUNNER GLAND
Any of the compound racemose glands in the submucous layer of the duodenum that secrete alkaline mucus and a potent proteolytic enzyme; also called duodenal gland, gland of Brunner.

BSR
Blood sedimentation rate.

BUBO
An inflammatory swelling of the lymphatic gland, especially in the groin or armpit.

BUBONIC PLAGUE
One type of plague; a plague caused by a bacterium of the genus Yersinia and characterized especially by the formation of buboes.

BUCCA
Mouth or cheek.

BUCCAL
Pertaining to the mouth or cheek.

BUCCAL OCCLUSION
Position of a premolar or molar tooth that is outside the line of occlusion (in which both jaws meet).

BUCCAL GLAND
Any of the small racemose mucous glands in the mucous membrane lining the cheeks.

BUCCAL SMEAR
Cells scraped from the inside of the cheek to detect abnormalities of sexual development.

BUCCINATOR
A thin broad muscle forming the wall of the cheek and serving to compress the cheek against the teeth and to retract the angle of the mouth.

BUCCOLINGUAL
Relating to or affecting the cheek and the tongue.

BUCCOPHARYNGEAL MEMBRANE
A membrane in an early embryo composed of ectoderm and endoderm and separating the head end of the gut from the stomodeum..

BUD
An outgrowth from the body of an organism that differentiates into a new individual.

The term is also applied to a primordium having potentialities for growth and development into a definitive structure.

BUERGER'S DISEASE
Also called thromboangiitis obliterans: a disease of unknown cause, characterized by acute inflammation with thrombosis (blood clotting) affecting both arteries and veins prin-

cipally in the lower leg. Seen chiefly in young or middle-aged men, it affects almost exclusively heavy tobacco smokers.

BUFFER SOLUTION
A solution prepared from a weak acid, or a weak base (non-acid) and a salt of the weak base, which resists any appreciable change in the pH (acid-alkali balance) on the addition of small amounts of acid or alkali or by dilution with water.

BULBOCAVERNOSUS
A muscle that in the male surrounds and compresses the bulb of the penis and the bulbar portion of the urethra and in the female divides into lateral halves that extend from immediately behind the clitoris along either side of the vagina to the central tendon of the perineum and serve to compress the vagina.

BULIMIA
Insatiable hunger related to both increased appetite as well as increased intake of food, often observed in psychotics but now realized to be more common than was once thought. It is related to anorexia nervosa and primarily affects women.

BULLA
A large blister; a cutaneous vesicle filled with serous fluid.

BULLOUS PEMPHIGOID
A chronic, benign, blister-like eruption seen chiefly in the elderly. The eruption usually improves with treatment by prednisone.

BUNDLE OF HIS
A slender of modified cardiac muscle that passes from the atrioventricular node in the right atrium to the right and left ventricles by way of the septum.

It maintains the normal sequence of the heartbeat by conducting the wave of excitation from the right atrium to the ventricles.

BUNION
Swelling over the outer side of the big toe due to wearing, for many years, shoes that are too narrow and pointed.

BURKITT'S LYMPHOMA
A highly undifferentiated B-cell lymphoma (tumor of lymphoid tissue) that tends to involve sites other than the lymph nodes and reticuloendothelial system.

BURN
Bodily injury resulting from exposure to heat, caustics, electricity, or some radiations, marked by the varying degrees of skin destruction and hyperemia often with the formation of watery blisters and in severe cases by charring of the tissues, and classified according to the extent and degree of injury.

BURSA
Pocket of fibrous tissue containing fluid interposed between muscles or between muscle and bone, to reduce friction.

BURSECTOMY
Surgical removal of a bursa.

BURSITIS
Inflammation of a bursa.

BUTTONHOLE INCISION
Small straight cut made into an organ or cavity.

BYPASS
Installation of an alternate route for the blood to bypass an obstructed vital artery. The operation is frequently applied to the heart.

BYSSINOSIS
Lung disease caused by inhaling cotton dust over a long period. It is also called stripper's asthma, grinder's asthma and cotton card room asthma.

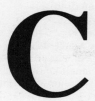

CACHET
Capsule in which disagreeable-tasting drugs are enclosed so that they can be swallowed without unpleasantness. The cachet is soluble and dissolves in the stomach.

CACHEXIA
A morbid condition of general feebleness.

CACHOU
A pill or pastille for sweetening the breath.

CACIDROSIS
Excessive, offensive sweating.

CADAVER
A dead body, especially of a human being used for dissection.

CADAVEROUS
Pertaining to a dead body; especially having the appearance or color of a dead body.

CADDY STOOLS
Those resembling fine, dark, sandy mud, as seen in yellow fever.

CAECAL
Also spelled cecal; relating to the caecum (cecum), the first part of the large intestine.

CAECORECTOSTOMY
Surgical operation to permit intercommunication between the caecum (cecum, the blind pouch-like commencement of the large intestine) and the rectum (the lower part of the large intestine).

CAECOSTOMY
Also spelled cecostomy, operation in which a part of the caecum (cecum) is brought to the surface of the abdomen, so that the intestinal contents will emerge through the abdominal outlet, not through the back passage.

CAECUM
Also spelled cecum; blind pouch that lies in the right lower region of the abdomen (the right inguinal area, or right iliac fossa). The ascending colon commences at the top of the caecum, and at its lower end is the insertion of the small intestine, the appendix being attached close to this.

CA.EDTA
An abbreviation for calcium disodium versenate, a substance used in the treatment of lead poisoning.

CAESAREAN (CESAREAN) SECTION
Surgical incision through the abdomen and uterus for removal of a fetus, performed when conditions (e.g., maternal hemorrhage, fetal distress, baby too large for passage through mother's pelvis) for normal vaginal delivery are deemed hazardous for mother or baby.

CAFERGOT
Brand name of a drug containing ergotamine tartrate and caffeine as active ingredients. The drug is prescribed for the treatment of migraine.
Possible side effects are:
- drowsiness;
- nausea;
- stomach ache.
It should not be used by pregnant or breastfeeding women.

CAFFEINE
A slightly bitter alkaloid used as a stimulant and diuretic and found in coffee, tea, etc.; poisonous when taken in large doses.

CAFFEINE INTOXICATION
Disorder characterized by symptoms causes by recent use of caffeine-containing substances, usually in excess of 250 mg. At least five of the following signs have to present in a case of real caffeine intoxication:
- restlessness;
- nervousness;
- excitement;
- insomnia;
- flushed face;
- diuresis;
- gastrointestinal disturbance;
- muscle twitching;
- rambling flow of thought and speech;
- tachycardia or cardiac arrhythmia;
- periods of inexhaustibility;
- psychomotor agitation.

Complications include developing or aggravating gastrointestinal and heart disease.

Caffeine can produce epigastric distress and, occasionally, peptic ulcer and hematemesis. In addition to arrhythmia with extremely high dose, the substance can cause marked hypotension and circulatory failure.

CAFFEINISM
Caffeine intoxication.

CAISSON DISEASE
A painful, sometimes fatal condition in which, because of a rapid drop in outside pressure, nitrogen bubbles form in the body and cause pain, disorientation, and faintness, as when a diver ascends too quickly. Treatment is by return to a higher pressure environment and gradual decompression in a special chamber.

CAJUPUT
A pungent, volatile oil, obtained from the cajuput tree of the Moluccas island group of Indonesia. It is used for rubbing over painful joints, and a spirit of cajuput may be given for severe colic.

CALABAR SWELLINGS
A symptom of loiasis.

CALAMINE
A pink, water-insoluble powder consisting of zinc oxide or carbonate and a small amount of ferric oxide, used in lotions and ointments to treat skin disorders.

CALCANEUS
The largest bone of the tarsus (foot); the bone that forms the heel.

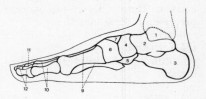

Side view of the skeleton of the foot.
1. tibia; 2. talus; 3. calcaneus; 4: navicular bone: 5: cuboid bone; 6, 7 and 8: cuneiform bones; 9: metatarsal bones; 10: proximal digits of the toes: 11: middle digits of the toes: 12: distal digits.

CALCAREA CARBONICA
Homeopathic medicine derived from carbonate of lime. The medicine is prescribed for scrofula, goiter, headache with cold feet, eczema, incipient consumption, dyspepsia, mental or physical overwork, interrupted convalescence.

CALCAREA PHOSPHORICA
Homeopathic medicine derived from phosphate of lime. It is especially useful in late development of teeth, bone disease, anemias, after acute diseases and chronic wasting illnesses.

CALCAREOUS
Having the nature or the qualities of or containing calcium carbonate.

CALCARIURIA
Presence of abnormal amounts of calcium salts in the urine.

CALCICOSIS
Pneumoconiosis (severe lung disease) from the inhalation of limestone dust.

CALCIFEROL
Vitamin D_2, created by the action of ultra-violet light on ergosterol. Occurs naturally in milk and fish-liver oils.

CALCIFICATION
A process in which tissue becomes hardened as the result of the depositing of calcium salts (lime), especially calcium carbonate and phosphate.

It is the most important process in the formation of bone, but can be harmful, as when it occurs in old scars.

CALCINOSIS
A condition characterized by abnormal deposition of calcium salts in the tissues.

CALCIPENIA
Absence or deficiency of calcium salts in body fluid.

CALCIUM
An element, the fifth most abundant in the human body, found primarily in bone but also present in body fluids and soft-tissue cells.

It is important for nerve impulse transmission, muscle function, blood coagulation, teeth and bone formation.

CALCIUM CARBONATE
A colorless crystal or gray powder (chalk) used as an antacid. Calcium carbonate is a medicine taken by mouth to relieve heartburn or acid stomach by neutralizing excess stomach acid.

When used for this purpose, it is said to belong to the group of medicines called antacids. It may be used to treat the symptoms of stomach or duodenal ulcers.

Calcium carbonate may also be used to prevent or treat hypocalcemia (not enough calcium in the blood). In addition, it may be used as a dietary supplement for patients who are unable to get enough calcium in their regular diet or have need for more calcium, when recommended by their doctor.

Calcium carbonate is available without a prescription; however, your doctor may have special instructions on the proper use and dose for your medical problem.

CALCIUM CHANNEL BLOCKING AGENTS
Agents like diltiazem, nedipine, and verapamil that are taken by mouth or given by injection to relieve and control angina (chest pain).

Calcium channel blocking agents affect the movement of calcium into the cells of the heart and blood vessels.

As a result, they relax blood vessels and increase the supply of blood and oxygen to the heart while reducing the work load.

Possible side effects are:
- breathing difficulty;
- coughing;
- wheezing;
- irregular heartbeat;
- skin rash;
- swelling of ankles, feet, or lower legs;
- fainting.

CALCIUM GLUCONATE
A well-tolerated calcium salt used for the treatment of disorders characterized by calcium deficiency. It is water-soluble and so can be injected.

CALCIUM HYDROGEN PHOSPHATE
Substance used as a source of calcium to treat and prevent the occurrence of disorders resulting in calcium deficiency.

CALCIUM LACTATE
Substance used as a source of cal-

cium to treat and prevent the occurrence of disorders resulting in calcium deficiency.

CALCIUM SUPPLEMENTS
Supplements used to increase calcium concentration in the blood in an attempt to make bones denser (as in osteoporosis). These supplements include calcium citrate, calcium gluconate, calcium glycerophosphate and calcium lactate, etc.

CALCULUS
A stone-like mass sometimes formed in the gallbladder, kidneys or other organs or ducts of the body.

CALDWELL-LUC OPERATION
Surgical procedure for drainage of the interior of the maxilla (upper jawbones) in cases of abscess formation.

CALENDULA
(Calendula officinalis) Also called pot marigold: annual plant of which the flowers and leaves are used for medicinal purposes. An infusion of the flowers (either the ray florets alone or the whole head) can be used for such gastrointestinal problems as ulcers, stomach cramps, colitis and diarrhea.

It is also useful taken internally for fever, boils, abscesses and to prevent recurrent vomiting. The fresh juice of the herb or flowers can be substituted for the infusion.

For external use, a very good salve for wounds can be made from the dried flowers or leaves, from the juice pressed out of the fresh flowers, or from a tincture.

CALF
Fleshy part of the leg at the back of the shin bone below the knee.

CALISTHENICS
The act or practice of taking exercise for health, strength, or grace of movement.

CALLIPER
Device for supporting any part of the body from the hips down; instrument inserted into the lower end of a fractured long bone for traction purposes.

CALLOSITY
Any thickened or hardened part on the surface of the human body (e.g. a corn) or a new growth of bony matter between the extremities of fractured bones.

CALLOSUM
Short name for corpus callosum, the bundle of nerve fibers connecting the hemispheres of the brain.

CALLOUS
Hardened, as portions of the skin exposed to friction.

CALLUS
Another name for callosity. Also, hard tissue that forms at the site of a broken bone, eventually becoming new bone.

CALOR
Heat, one of the classic signs of inflammation, the others being pain, swelling, redness, malfunction.

CALORIC TEST
A test of the inner ear in which hot water or ice water is placed in the ear and eye movement observed; performed on patients with ear disease or injury, or symptoms of dizziness or fainting.

CALORIE
The amount of heat needed to raise one gram of water one degree on the Celsius scale.

CALORIMETER
Any of several apparatuses for measuring quantities of heat absorbed or produced by the body.

CALVARIA
The cranium; skull.

CALYX
A cup-like part, such as one of the funnel-shaped structures that enclose the tips of the pyramids in the interior of the kidneys.

CAMPHOR
A white crystalline compound distilled from the wood and young shoots of a species of laurel tree (Cinnamonum camphora).

Camphor has a strong characteristic odor that repels insects.

It is also used medicinally - internally as a pain-killer and antispasmodic, and externally in liniments. In large doses it is a narcotic poison.

CAMPHOR ICE
An ointment composed chiefly of camphor, white wax, spermaceti and castor oil, used for chapped or blemished skin.

CANAL
Any cylindrical or tubular cavity in the body through which solids and/or liquids pass.

CANALICULOTOMY
Surgical term applied to the formation of a drainage canal in the lacrimal canaliculus (the canal through which the fluid washing the eye flows).

CANALICULUS
A small tubular or canal-like passage or channel, as in a bone.

CANALIZATION
Tendency of children to return to their growth curve trajectories after their growth rate has been deflected for a brief time by environmental factors.

CANCELLATION
A test, employed in the experimental study of perception, attention or work, in which the subject is required to discriminate and mark particular figures, letters or forms, irregularly distributed in a mass of similar figures, letters or forms.

CANCER
An abnormal, malignant growth of cells that invade nearby tissues and often spread to other sites in the body, interfering with the normal function of the affected sites.

CANCEROCIDAL
Agent, drug or method lethal to cancer.

CANCEROGENIC
Capable of causing cancer, such as certain chemical or physical agents.

CANCEROPHOBIA
Pathological fear of having cancer or getting cancer in the near future.

CANCROID
Term in cancerology with two different meanings:
(1) Resembling a cancer, as in certain tumors.
(2) A form of cancer of the skin and intestinal tract.

CANDIDIASIS
An infection caused by a Candida species of fungus, affecting most often the skin, mouth, and vagina, and causing itching, peeling, whitish exudate, and sometimes easy bleeding.

CANESTEN
Brand name of a drug containing clotrimazole as the active ingredient. The drug stops the growth of fungi in and on the body.

CANICOLA FEVER
Infection by Leptospira canicola, characterized by high fever, headache, conjunctivitis with swelling, jaundice, muscular pains and vomiting.

The symptoms slowly disappear in two weeks. The infection is common among rats, dogs, foxes and possibly cats.

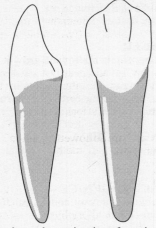

Side view and posterior view of a canine.

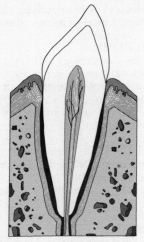

Canine in its bony socket in the lower jaw.

CANINE
Resembling a dog; term applied to four teeth, two in each jaw, situated between the incisors and the premolars.

CANKER SORE
An ulcerated sore of the lips or membranous lining of the mouth.

CANNABIS
Ancient and mildly hallucinogenic drug originally obtained from the flowering tops of the Indian hemp plant (Cannabis sativa), which grows in mild climates in many parts of the world. One of the least understood of all natural drugs, cannabis also is known by many other names.

The term marihuana (or marijuana) is often used to refer to any part of the hemp plant or to its extract.

Among other names for the crude drugs are:
- hashish;
- charas;
- dagga;
- bhang;
- ganja;
- kif.

CANNABIS ABUSE
Episodical use of Cannabis. The person shows evidence of maladaptive behavior, such as driving while impaired by Cannabis intoxication.

CANNABIS DEPENDENCE
Disorder characterized by daily, or almost daily, use of the substance. Cannabis is regarded by many people as a substance of low abuse potential that is extremely unlikely to cause any problems with continued use. For that reason, many people start using the substance without any appreciation of its capacity to induce dependence.

Since impairment in social and occupational functioning and the development of related physical disorders in Cannabis dependence are less than those typically seen with other psychoactive substances, such as alcohol, cocaine, and heroin, people with Cannabis dependence and abuse rarely seek treatment for these disorders Cannabis dependence usually develops with repeated use over a substantial period of time; rapid development following initial use is rare.

Tolerance may develop to some of the substance's psychoactive effects and thus promote increased levels of consumption.

Typically, it is the frequency

rather than the absolute amount of Cannabis used that increases over time. With chronic heavy use there is often a diminution or loss of the pleasurable effects of the substance. There may be a corresponding increase in dysphoric effects, but this is not seen as frequently as in chronic heavy use of amphetamine or cocaine.

CANNABIS DELUSIONAL DISORDER
Organic delusional syndrome usually with persecutory delusions, developing shortly after Cannabis use. Marked anxiety, emotional lability, depersonalization, and subsequent amnesia for the episode can occur. Associated physical symptoms are the same as those seen in Cannabis intoxication.

CANNIBALISM
(Anthropophagy) Consumption by humans of human flesh, common throughout the world at various times in the past and still occasionally practiced, though now generally taboo.

Among primitive man, the motive appears to have been the belief that eating an enemy or a respected elder transferred to the eater the strength, courage or wisdom of the dead.

CANNULA
A small tube of metal or the like that draws off fluid from or injects medicine into the body.

CANTHARIDIS
Also called Spanish fly: agent prepared from the dried Spanish beetle Cantharis vesicatoria, causing damage to the skin (blisters) and mucous membranes. In the past, it has been erroneously used as an aphrodisiac.

CANTHARIDISM
A morbid state caused by the use of cantharis.

CANTHARIS
Homeopathic medicine derived from the Spanish fly Cantharis vesicatoria.

The medicine is prescribed for inflammatory conditions of the urinary tract or genital organs.

Cantharis is useful for scalds and burns, with rawness and smarting, that are relieved by cold applications and are followed by undue inflammation.

CANTHUS
The angle or corner on each side of the eye formed by the junction of the upper and lower lids.

CAPIAT
An instrument for removing a foreign substance from the uterus or other body cavities.

CAPILLARY
A tiny bloodvessel connecting arterioles and venules. Through the one-cell-layer-thick walls (approximately 0.008 mm diameter) of capillaries oxygen and nutrients are passed from arterioles to body tissues and carbon dioxide and other wastes are passed from body tissues to venules.

CAPILLARY ACTION/ATTRACTION
Phenomenon that allows fluid to rise in a tube of very small diameter because of the adhesive force between the liquid and the side walls of the tube.

CAPILLARY FRAGILITY TEST
A test to measure the fragility of small blood vessels near the skin, done with the cuff of a blood pressure apparatus. Fragility of these vessels is indicative of various blood vessel diseases.

CAPILLARY PULSE
A pulsation that can be seen in the skin capillaries under the fingernails

or on the forehead. It is common in aortic regurgitation (backflow of blood into the heart).

CAPITALIUM
The rounded, raised area at the lower end of the upper arm bone or humerus.

CAPITATUM
One of the small bones, the capitate bone, in the hand.

CAPLAN'S SYNDROME
Combination of severe lung illness (pneumoconiosis) and rheumatoid arthritis. The disease occurs in workers exposed to coal.

CAPOTEN
Brand name of a drug containing captopril as the active ingredient.

CAPOZIDE
Brand name for a drug containing captopril (an ACE inhibitor) and hydrochlorothiazide (a thiazide diuretic) as active ingredients.

CAPSICUM
The pod of the cayenne pepper plant which, when dried and prepared, is used in medicine as an irritant and a stimulant.

CAPSULE
A membranous structure enveloping an organ or any other part, or a joint; also called a capsula. Also, a gelatinous case enclosing a dose of medicine.

CAPSULECTOMY
Surgical removal of the capsule of a joint or the lens of the eye.

CAPSULITIS
Inflammation of the capsule of a joint, generally not caused by microorganisms.

CAPTIVATION
The act of gaining or winning over one's affections.

CAPUT
(1) The head.
(2) Any head, or expanded or rounded extremity of an organ or other anatomical structure.

CAPUT SUCCEDANEUM
Swelling found on a baby's scalp after it is born, caused by pressure during childbirth. It quickly disappears and should cause no anxiety.

CARACE
Brand name for an ACE inhibitor containing lisinopril as an active ingredient.

CARAWAY
(Carum carvi) Biennial or perennial plant of which the seed is used for medicinal purposes. The hollow, furrowed, angular, branched stem grows in the second year from a white, carrot-shaped root. The leaves are bi- or tripennate and deeply incised, the upper ones on a sheath-like petiole. The small white or yellow flowers appear in May and June, forming a compound umbel with rays of unequal length. The fruit is dark brown, oblong, flattened and two-seeded. The seeds may be chewed, or the following preparations used:
Infusion: add 3 teaspoons crushed seeds to 115 ml (4 fl. oz) water.

CARBAMAZEPINE
Generic name of a drug with anticonvulsant properties. The drug is prescribed for certain types of epilepsy and the treatment of trigeminal (facial) neuralgia. It must not be used for other aches or pains.
This medicine may also be used for other conditions as determined by your doctor. Carbamazepine is available only with your doctor's prescription.
Possible side effects are:
- nausea;
- diarrhea;
- dizziness;
- skin rashes;

- jaundice or icterus

It should not be taken during the first three months of pregnancy.

CARBAMINOHEMOGLOBIN

A compound formed between carbon dioxide and hemoglobin. It is a physiological mechanism by which part of the carbon dioxide is carried in the blood.

CARBOHYDRATE

Any of a group of organic compounds (containing the elements carbon, hydrogen, and oxygen), including starches and sugars, that are the chief energy sources of the body.

CARBOHYDRATE INTOLERANCE

A disorder characterized by diarrhea and abdominal distention, and caused by inability to digest carbohydrates because of a lack of one or more intestinal enzymes.

The disorder is readily controlled by a lactose-free diet, or often simply by abstaining from milk drinks.

CARBOLURIA

The presence of carbolic acid in the urine, as in poisoning. The urine turns green or dark.

CARBON DIOXIDE

A colorless, odorless gas given off from the lungs as a waste product of respiration.

CARBONIC ANHYDRASE INHIBITORS

Drugs used to treat glaucoma and seizures and to prevent high altitude sickness.

CARBON MONOXIDE

A colorless, odorless, very poisonous gas, which burns with a pale blue flame and is a component of coal gas, exhaust fumes and most smoke (including cigarette smoke). It may cause severe brain damage.

CARBON MONOXIDE POISONING

Poisoning by inhalation of carbon monoxide, which attaches to the hemoglobin in the blood and thus deprives the body of oxygen.

Toxicity varies with length of exposure, concentration inhaled, respiratory and circulation rates.

The symptoms vary with the percentage of carboxyhemoglobin in the blood. They include:
- headache;
- vertigo;
- shortness of breath;
- confusion;
- bright pink complexion;
- dilated pupils;
- convulsions;
- coma.

CARBO VEGETABILIS

Homeopathic medicine derived from vegetable charcoal. The medicine is prescribed for stagnation of blood supply, slow digestion, flatulence and offensive discharges. It is also useful in old people with venous congestions and states of collapse in severe diarrhea.

CARBOXYHEMOGLOBIN

A compound of carbon monoxide and hemoglobin.

CARBOXY-HEMOGLOBINEMIA

The presence of carboxy-hemoglobin in the blood in an excessive amount, as seen in carbon monoxide poisoning.

CARBOXY-HEMOGLOBINURIA

The presence of carboxy-hemoglobin in the urine, usually due to severe kidney disease.

CARBUNCLE

Infection under the full thickness of the skin caused by the pus-forming germ Staphylococcus. It produces a large infected area from which the pus escapes by making numerous openings for itself through the skin, producing a sieve-like appearance.

CARCINECTOMY
The surgical removal of a cancerous growth, such as a malignant tumor.

CARCINOEMBRYONIC ANTIGEN
An antigen measured in blood serum and sometimes other body fluids, to detect the presence or recurrence of cancer in such sites as the colon, pancreas, lung, breast or prostate.

CARCINOGEN
Any substance or agent capable of producing a cancer.

CARCINOGENESIS
The development of a malignant (cancerous) tumor or growth.

CARCINOMA
A malignant tumor or new growth (neoplasm) derived from epithelial and glandular tissues; a form of cancer.

CARCINOMATOPHOBIA
Dread of cancer.

CARCINOMATOSIS
General spread of cancer throughout the body. A state in which numerous carcinomas, disseminated from a primary source, grow in the body at the same time.

CARCINOMATOUS
Cancer-like, pertaining to malignant growth.

CARCINOSARCOMA
A malignant tumor having the elements of both carcinoma and sarcoma.

CARDAMON
(Elettaria cardamomum) A perennial plant of which the seed is used for medicinal purposes. The simple erect stem of the plant grows to a height of 1.80 to 3.05 m (6-10 ft) from a thumb-thick, creeping rootstock.

The leaves are lanceolate, dark green. The small, yellowish flowers grow in loose racemes on prostrate flower stems. The fruit is a three-celled capsule holding up to 18 seeds. These are useful for flatulence, but they are usually used to increase the efficacy of other remedies.

CARDIA
The region of the stomach that opens into the esophagus, and lies immediately behind the heart.

CARDIAC
Relating to the heart.

CARDIAC ARRHYTHMIA
Irregular action of the heart. There are many types.

CARDIAC ASTHMA
Asthmatic attack that comes on suddenly, often in the middle of the night, due to spasm of the lungs from heart disease.

CARDIAC CATHETERIZATION
A primarily diagnostic technique in which a flexible catheter is passed along veins or arteries into the heart, in order to explore the heart structure, to measure pressures and bloodgas levels in the heart chambers and associated blood vessels, and to inject dyes for angiography.

CARDIAC CYCLE
Succession of beats of the chambers of the heart.

CARDIAC FAILURE
Inability of the heart to maintain the circulation; its inability to pump sufficient blood into the main vessels.

CARDIAC GLYCOSIDE
Type of drug that has the ability to

increase the strength and to help regulate the rate of the heartbeat.

CARDIAC INDEX
Volume of blood that flows per minute per square meter of the body surface.

CARDIAC MASSAGE
A manual technique for stimulating and reviving cardiac arrest (a stopped heart) by rhythmically pressing upon and releasing the lower part of the breast bone at the rate of 60 to 80 times a minute.

CARDIAC MURMUR
Abnormal sound heard over and produced within the heart. These murmurs, or added sounds, have been clearly classified as either innocent or a sign of a disorder. There are many types and each is diagnostic of the disorder present.

CARDIAC NEUROSIS
A psychological disorder characterized by complaints of pain near the heart, accompanied by severe palpitations, which are not due to heart disease. Sometimes called effort syndrome.

CARDIAC REHABILITATION
Rehabilitation of patients with heart diseases.

CARDIAC SPHINCTER
Ring of muscle between the esophagus and the stomach at the level of the diaphragm, which regulates the flow of food into the stomach, and prevents the contents of the stomach from returning to the esophagus.

CARDIAC TAMPONADE
Symptoms of pressure on the heart caused by a backflow of blood, and due to disease in the chest resulting in obstruction of the flow of blood.

CARDIALGIA
Heartburn, an uncomfortable burning sensation in the upper stomach.

CARDIASTHENIA
Neurasthenia with cardiac symptoms such as palpitations.

CARDIOGENIC
From the heart or caused by the heart. The term is also applied to shock brought on by lowered activity of the heart such as in myocardial infarction (heart attack).

CARDIOGRAM
Record of the heartbeat taken through the chest wall.

CARDIOGRAPH
Instrument for recording the heartbeat graphically.

CARDIOLOGIST
A medical specialist in the study of the heart and its structure and functions.

CARDIOLOGY
The science of the heart, including the study of its diseases and functions.

CARDIOMEGALY
Enlargement of the heart due to a congenital malformation or an acquired condition.

CARDIOMYOPATHY
Severe pathological condition of the muscle of the heart.

CARDIOMYOTOMY
Surgical procedure consisting of cutting off the muscle encircling the entrance to the stomach, performed when there is a stricture of the junction between the esophagus and the stomach.

CARDIONEUROSIS
Another term for cardiac neurosis.

CARDIOPATHY
Term for any diseased condition of the heart, regardless of cause.

CARDIOPERICARDITIS
Inflammation of the heart and the sac surrounding it.

CARDIOPHOBIA
Fear of heart disease.

CARDIOPLASTY
Surgical procedure consisting of correction of the cardiac sphincter of the stomach.

CARDIOPULMONARY
Pertaining to the heart and the lungs.

CARDIOPULMONARY RESUSCITATION
The restoration of heartbeat and breathing by external cardiac massage and mouth-to-mouth breathing.

CARDIOSCLEROSIS
Hardening of the heart muscle due to the depositing of fibrous tissue.

CARDIOSPASM
Spasm of the valve of the stomach (cardiac sphincter) preventing the proper passage of food from the gullet to the stomach.

CARDIOTHORACIC
Pertaining to the heart and the chest cavity.

CARDIOTOMY
Surgical incision into the heart or the cardia of the stomach.

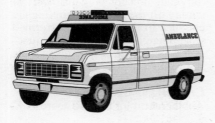

Cardulance equipped with special apparatus to regulate heart activity.

CARDIOVALVULITIS
Inflammation of the valves of the heart.

CARDIOVASCULAR SYSTEM
Body parts, including the heart and blood vessels, involved in the pumping of blood and transport of nutrients, oxygen and waste products throughout the body.

CARDIOVERSION
The application of very brief discharges of direct-current electricity across the chest and into the heart muscle in order to stop a cardiac arrhythmia and allow the normal heart rhythm to take over.

This technique is most often used as an emergency measure, but can also be used to correct chronic conditions.

CARDIOVERTER
An instrument capable of delivering a brief direct-current electric shock to the heart, and used to terminate certain cardiac arrhythmias.

CARDITIS
Inflammation of the inner lining of the heart (endocarditis), the muscle wall (myocarditis), or of the outer lining (pericarditis).

CARD SORTING
A type of experiment, used for various purposes - as a learning experiment, for the study of interference, as a test of efficiency of discrimination and motor response.

CARDULANCE
Special ambulance for the transport of patients with myocardial infarction. This type of ambulance is equipped with special apparatus to stimulate the heart activity in case of a severe disorder of the heart rhythm or complete stop of the heart function.

CARFECILLIN
Generic name of a penicillin prepa-

ration, which is prescribed for the treatment of infections of the urinary tract.

CARIES
The breakdown and death of tooth tissue, resulting in soft, discolored areas. Studies suggest that eating sugary foods tends to produce tooth decay as does failure to brush the teeth and remove food particles.

CARLINE THISTLE
(Carlina vulgaris) Perennial plant of which the rootstock is used for medicinal purposes. The finger-thick rootstock is brown on the outside, lighter and fissured on the inside and has an unpleasant, pungent odor when dried.

Carline thistle has been recommended in some herbals of the past for kidney and stomach problems, dropsy, impotence, and fever related to gastric problems. It is now mostly used externally. The rootstock applied in this way is said to remove scars, and a decoction of it, prepared with white wine or wine vinegar, is used for washing wounds and for skin problems.

CARMINATIVE
Term used to indicate the property of a drug or agent capable of relieving flatulence and associated colic.

CARMUSTINE
Generic name of an alkylating agent for the treatment of certain symptoms of Hodgkin's disease and solid tumors.

CARNOPHOBIA
Pathological fear of eating meat; in a number of cases an early sign of Hodgkin's disease.

CAROB
The seed pods of the Mediterranean tree, Ceratonia scilicet; also known as St John's bread and honey locust. Carob is rich in calcium, potassium and phosphorus.

It is used as a natural sweet to take the place of sugar, chocolate and cocoa. In addition to the pods themselves, carob is also available as tablets, powder, syrup and wafers, as well as in ready-made "natural" sweets.

CAROTENE
A precursor of vitamin A. Yellow pigment found in carrots, green vegetables, yellow and orange fruits, milk, animal fat, capable of being converted into vitamin A.

CAROTID
Principal artery, found on each side of the neck, that carries blood from the heart to the brain and the tissues of the head and neck.

CAROTID ARTERIOGRAPHY
X-ray studies of the neck arteries after injection of contrast medium into the carotid artery.

CAROTID SINUS
That area where the carotid artery divides into the internal and the external carotid arteries, and which is richly provided with nerves.

CAROTID SINUS SYNDROME
Attacks of giddiness, fainting and sometimes convulsions associated with a fall in blood pressure and slowing of the pulse, and caused by excessive irritability of the carotid sinus.

The attacks may occur without warning, follow an emotional upset or be caused by pressure over the carotid sinus.

CARPAL
Relating to the carpus, or wrist. Carpal is any bone of the carpus, or wrist.

CARPAL TUNNEL SYNDROME
A common disorder of the wrist and hand, caused by compression of the median nerve in the wrist area and

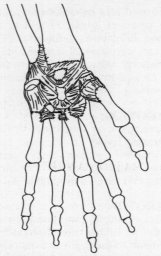

The carpus, located between the forearm and the metacarpal bones of the hand. The muscles of the carpus are shown.

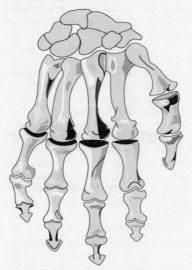

Dorsal view of the skeleton of the carpus, located between the forearm and the metacarpal bones of the hand.

manifested by pain, tingling, burning, and muscular weakness, sometimes spreading to arm and shoulders.

CARPOMETACARPAL
Pertaining to the carpal and metacarpal bones of the wrist and hand.

The term is also applied to the joints between them and the ligaments.

CARPOPEDAL SPASM
A spasm of the hands and feet associated with tetany, a condition of muscle spasm caused by too little calcium in the blood.

CARPUS
The part of the skeleton between forearm and hand; the wrist.

CARRIER
An individual who carries a recessive gene, either autosomal or sex-linked, together with its normal allele, but who does not show any significant clinically detectable effects of the gene.

CARRIER PROTEIN
Protein to which a hapten (a specific protein) can become attached, enabling the hapten to induce an immune response.

CAR SICKNESS
Nausea caused by motion, especially when riding in a car.

CARTILAGE
(1) An elastic tissue composing most of the skeleton in unborn babies, then largely being converted into bone.
(2) The gristle or specialized connective tissue between bones.

CARUNCLE
A small, fleshy nodule.

CARYLDERM
Brand name for an antiparasitic preparation used in the treatment of head lice. The drug contains carbaryl as active ingredient.

CASCARA
Laxative drug containing the dried bark of Rhamnus purshiana. The drug increases large bowel movements by irritating the lining and/or

stimulating the bowel muscles to contract.

The drug may color the urine red, cause excessive loss of fluids and, if taken for a long time, may cause patchy pigmentation of part of the bowel.

CASE
An individual occurrence or specific instance of a disease.

CASEATION
Deterioration of tissue, as in tuberculosis, into a soft, crumbly, cheese-like substance.

CASE HISTORY
A biography obtained for scientific purposes; the material is sometimes supplied at one interview, sometimes collected over the years.

CASEIN
The principle protein in milk.

CASEINOGEN
Substance in milk that, combining with lime salts, forms casein.

CASE RECORD
Information gathered about an individual or group of individuals to serve as a psychological biography in social work, psychiatry, medicine and sociology.

CASE WORK
A detailed study of persons in need of social assistance, which can be used for diagnosis and treatment.

CASSIA
A tropical plant, Cassia senna, that yields senna, used as a laxative.

CAST
(1) Fibrous matter that takes the shape of the organ in which it is formed and is ejected from the body.
(2) A mould made of plastic or plaster of Paris, usually applied for immobilization, as in fractures, dislocations and other injuries.

CASTOR OIL
A thick oil obtained from the castor bean, used as a purgative.

CASTRATION
Surgical removal of the gonads (sex organs): in the male, removal of the testes; in the female, removal of the ovaries.

CASTRATION ANXIETY
According to classical psychoanalytical theory, all men and male children are liable to castration anxiety, though what the precise nature of this dread is has been subject to both controversy and elaboration. The concept only rarely refers to castration in its anatomical sense, but more frequently to:
- a loss of the penis, as in castration threats used to deter little boys caught masturbating;
- loss of the capacity for erotic pleasure;
- demoralization in respect of the masculine role.

CASTRATION COMPLEX
The fear concerned with possible or threatened loss of the reproductive organs, especially the penis. The term is used analogously to describe fears of loss of sexuality or the capacity for erotic pleasure in either males or females.

CASTROPHRENIA
A delusion that occurs sometimes in schizophrenic persons, that their enemies are depriving them and/or controlling their thoughts.

CASUALTY
Accident, mishap, disaster, especially one resulting in death or bodily injury.

CATABOLISM
A breaking down of complex molecules into simpler ones, accompanied by a release of energy.

CATABOLITE
One of the breakdown products produced in the metabolism of the body.

CATALEPSY
Trance-like state associated with hysteria and schizophrenia, and a stage of self-hypnotic sleep. In localized catalepsy, a single muscle or group of muscles is affected and the subject will keep, say, an arm raised for an indefinite period without apparent fatigue.

CATALEPTIC STATE
The retention of limbs in positions into which they are placed, such as occurs in hypnosis or catatonia.

CATALYST
Agent or substance capable of speeding up a chemical reaction in the body.

CATAMNESIS
A person's medical history taken during or after recovery from an illness.

CATAPHASIA
A disorder in the ability to use language, caused by brain injury or disease and characterized by frequent and uncontrollable repetition of the same words or phrases without reference to their meaning.

CATAPHORA
State of coma punctuated by brief lucid intervals.

CATAPHORESIS
Diffusion of electrically charged drugs through a mucous membrane.

CATAPHORIA
Condition in which the visual axis of each eye tends to incline below the horizontal plane.

CATAPLASIA
A reversion of cells or tissues to an earlier or more primitive stage.

CATAPLEXY
Muscular weakness affecting the whole body, as a result of fear or shock, or as a defensive reaction.

CATARACT
An eye disorder in which the lens becomes less transparent (more opaque) so that light rays cannot reach the retina and there is progressive painless loss of vision. Most cataracts are caused by degenerative changes after age 50, but some may be caused by trauma to the eye or exposure to certain chemicals; some are hereditary and some congenital (due perhaps to viral infection during pregnancy).

Treatment is removal of the lens and use of special contact lenses or eyelenses or the implantation of an intraocular lens.

CATARRH
Mild inflammation of a mucous membrane, associated with a copious secretion of mucus. Medically speaking, this refers to any mucous membrane in the body, but popularly refers to nasal or bronchial catarrh.

CATARRHAL JAUNDICE
Also called infectious hepatitis: acute disease characterized by jaundice coming on a few days after what appears to be a gastrointestinal upset, and accompanied by loss of appetite, diarrhea and, sometimes, a raised temperature. The urine is colored orange-yellow by the presence of bile pigments, and the absence of bile pigments from feces leaves them a light yellow color. It sometimes occurs in epidemic form and is caused by a germ or a virus that produces inflammation and blockage of the bile ducts in the liver. It is the commonest type of jaundice.

CATATONIA
Symptom of mental illness, usually schizophrenia, in which limbs are retained in a posture for long peri-

ods. For instance, if the subject's arm is placed above his/her head, he/she will keep it there for a period which, in a normal person, would be impossible owing to fatigue and pain.

CATATONIC BEHAVIOR
Marked motor anomalies, generally limited to disturbances within the context of a diagnosis of a nonorganic psychotic disorder.

CATATONIC EXCITEMENT
Excited motor activity, apparently purposeless and not influenced by external stimuli.

CATATONIC NEGATIVISM
An apparently motiveless resistance to all instructions or attempts to be moved. When passive, the person may resist any effort to be moved; when active, he or she may do the opposite of what is asked - for example, firmly clench jaws when asked to open mouth.

CATATONIC POSTURING
Voluntary assumption of an inappropriate or bizarre posture, usually held for a long period of time.

CATATONIC RIGIDITY
Maintenance of a rigid posture against all efforts to be moved.

CATATONIC SCHIZOPHRE-NIA
A form of schizophrenia in which the victim retreats into a totally inattentive, completely preoccupied and virtually stuporous state, sitting or standing in a grotesquely contorted position for hour after hour, without moving a muscle, sometimes without even blinking an eye. Catatonic schizophrenics may remain in this weird, dream-like condition for days or even weeks, paying no attention to food, sometimes even retaining control over urine or feces to a point that is far beyond the normal. Then, suddenly, they erupt into a wildly "excited" phase, breaking out into a frenzy of purposeless motion until they drop from exhaustion. Appearances are deceptive here although this would seem the most alarming of all forms of schizophrenia, treatment quite often leads to long periods of remission during which the sufferer can live a normal life.

CATATONIC STUPOR
Marked decrease in reactivity to the environment and reduction in spontaneous movements and activity; sometimes to the point of appearing to be unaware of one's surroundings.

CATECHOLAMINES
Compounds, such as adrenaline and noradrenaline, produced by the medulla of the adrenal glands and at the endings of some peripheral and central nerves. The drugs are used to treat excess catecholamine production (often a cause of hypertension). These drugs include dopamine, norepinephrine and epinephrine.

CATECHU
A strong, astringent substance prepared from the wood of various tropical Asiatic plants and used in medicine with prepared chalk to treat diarrhea.

CATGUT
Thread made from the intestines of sheep and other animals. It is used for stitching up inside the body or as ligatures around blood vessels. In time, catgut is absorbed by the body.

CATHARSIS
In psychoanalysis (where it is also generally termed abreaction), the bringing into the open of a previously repressed memory or emotion, thus, hopefully, relieving unconscious emotional stress. Play, which can be viewed as working off

atavistic (primitive) impulses, is sometimes described as cathartic. In medicine, the term is used for the artificial induction of vomiting.

CATHARTIC
A drug that stimulates bowel action to produce a soft or liquid bowel movement.

CATHETER
Slender, flexible tube made of metal, rubber or plastic, passed into body organs for investigation or treatment.

Urinary catheters are used for relief of bladder outflow obstruction and sometimes for the loss of nervous control of the bladder; they also allow measurement of bladder function and special X-ray techniques. Cardiac catheters are passed through arteries or veins into the chambers of the heart to study its functioning and anatomy.

CATHEXIS
Accumulation of mental energy on some particular idea, memory or line of thought or action, much used in this sense by psycho-analysts.

CATMINT
(Nepeta cataria) Also called catnip: a perennial herb of the mint family, that is used for medicinal purposes. Catmint tea is taken for upset stomach, colic, spasms, flatulency and acid. It can also be used as an enema.

CAT SCAN
An abbreviation for computerized axial tomography scan, a painless diagnostic procedure in which hundreds of X-ray pictures are taken as a camera revolves around a body part - for instance, chest, head, pelvis. The pictures are fed into a computer, which integrates them to reveal structures within the body.

CAT-SCRATCH DISEASE
A fever characterized by enlarge-

ment of the glands. About half of the cases can be traced back to a scratch from a cat. A few days after a minor scratch (or a puncture wound from a thorn or splinter), a lump or blister develops at the site. Swelling of lymph glands near the wound develops within two weeks. Encephalitis is a rare but severe complication, usually occurring one or more weeks after onset. Treatment with tetracycline may shorten the course of the illness, and spontaneous node regression usually occurs within four weeks; prognosis is excellent.

CAUDA
Tail or tail-like termination.

CAUDAL ANESTHESIA
A type of anesthesia that blocks the transmission of pain and is produced by the injection of a local anesthetic into the peridural space (near but not in the spinal canal) through the sacral hiatus (tailbone of the spine).

This numbs the person from the waist down, and is sometimes used for pain relief in childbirth.

CAUL
A portion of the amniotic sac (the membrane enveloping the fetus), sometimes encompassing the head of a child at birth.

CAULIFLOWER GROWTH
Type of malignant growth, for instance, of a certain type of stomach cancer.

CAUSALGIA
Burning pain present in injuries of the sensory nerves, particularly those nerves supplying sensation to the skin of the palms and soles of the feet, and sometimes associated with changes in the tissues of the hands and feet.

CAUSTICUM
A homeopathic medicine, pre-

scribed for complaints in old, bro-ken-down constitutions suffering from chronic diseases; only occa-sionally is it used in acute diseases.

CAUTERIZATION
The application of a cautery agent or cautery knife to tissue to burn it away with a chemical or red-hot in-strument, or by means of diathermy (microwave electrical current). The method is often used for the re-moval of warts.

CAUTERY
A burning or searing, as of diseased tissue, by a hot iron or by caustic substances; the instrument or drug employed in cauterizing.

CAVA VEINS
Collecting veins of the systemic cir-culation, through which blood is re-turned to the heart.

All the veins of the systemic cir-culation flow into either the supe-rior vena cava or inferior vena cava. They in turn empty into the right atrium.

CAVERN
A cavity, especially an excavation caused by the loss of pulmonary tis-sue in tuberculosis.

CAVERNOMA
Tumor composed of large vessels, usually blood vessels.

CAVERNOUS
Containing hollow spaces.

CAVERNOUS RESPIRATION
A blowing breath sound of low pitch, alternating with gurgling and emerging from a cavity in the lung.

CAVERNOUS SINUS SYN-DROME
Paralysis of the muscles supplied by the third, fourth and sixth cranial nerves due to thrombosis of the cav-ernous sinus (a widened blood ves-sel at the base of the brain).

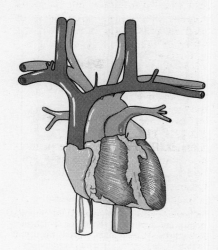

Heart with the superior cava vein in front of the aortic arc, emptying into the right atrium.

CAVITATION
The formation of a cavity as a hol-low abscess in the lung.

CAVITY
Defect or loss of tooth structures produced by tooth decay (caries).

CAYENNE
(Capsicum frutescens) Perennial plant of which the fruit is used for medicinal purposes. The ripe fruit, or pepper, is a many-seeded pod with a leathery exterior in various shades of red and yellow. In powder or tablet form, cayenne is used as a general stimulant and to build up re-sistance at the beginning of a cold.

CEPHALOSPORINS
Drugs belonging to the general fam-ily of medicines called antibiotics. Antibiotics are medicines used in the treatment of infections caused by bacteria. They work by killing bacteria or preventing their growth. Cephalosporins will not work for colds, flu, or other virus infections.

Cephalosporins are taken by mouth or given by injection to treat infections in many different parts of

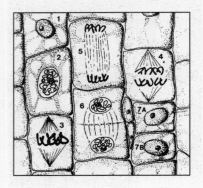

In normal cell division (mitosis) the chromosomes are duplicated so that each daughter cell retains the same number of as the parent cell. Mitosis proceeds in a number of phases.
1. Cell with nucleus and nucleolus.
2. The chromosomes become visible. At the beginning the chromosomes duplicate, shorten and thicken. The two centrioles separate drawing out a mass of fibers called the spindle.
3. The chromosomes migrate to the equator of the spindle.
4. The chromosomes divide.
5. The chromosomes move rapidly to the poles of the spindle.
6. The cell splits down the equator; the new nuclear membrane is formed.
7. The cell divides completely. Two separate cells exists (7A, 7B).

the body. They are sometimes given with other antibiotics. Some cephalosporins are also given by injection to prevent infections before, during, and after surgery.

CELANDINE
(Chelidonium majus) Biennial or perennial plant of which the rootstock and herb is used for medicinal purposes. Use with extreme caution, preferably with medical direction.

Taken internally, celandine has a special effect on the digestive system, and its anti-spasmodic properties make it useful for asthmatic symptoms; it is also used for water retention. Externally, made into an ointment or a poultice, celandine can be used for skin diseases such as herpes, eczema and ringworm.

The rootstock should be gathered in spring, before the plant flowers. The dried plant is less active than the fresh.

CELIBACY
Abstention from sexual relations.

CELL
An individual living unit, the basic structure for tissues and organs, made up of an outer membrane (cell membrane), the main mass (cytoplasm), and the nucleus, which controls the cell's metabolism and reproduction.

CELL-MEDIATED
Pertaining to those aspects of the immune response that are under the control of thymus-dependent cells.

CELL MEMBRANE
The thin, semi-permeable membrane enclosing the cytoplasm of a cell.

CELLOPHANE
Transparent, impermeable material derived from cellulose and used in surgical dressings.

CELLULAR
Pertaining to or characterized by having cells; composed of cells.

CELLULAR IMMUNE SYSTEM
That portion of the immune system, involving the T-cells (lymphoid cells arising in the thymus), that is responsible for delayed skin tests, delayed hypersensitivity and graft rejection, and acts as an important defense against malignant cells, viral infection and some bacteria. The specific type of immune response is mediated by small lymphocytes in humans, and in most animals is dependent upon the presence of the thymus gland at birth.

CELLULASE
An enzyme that breaks down cellu-

lose-like polysaccharides, including cellulose itself; obtained from a fungus and used in medicine.

CELLULITIS
Inflammation of tissue, especially that below the skin, characterized by redness, pain, and swelling. Treatment is by antibiotics.

CELLULOSE
Also called dietary fiber and roughage: the main constituent of the cell walls of higher plants, many algae and some fungi; for example, cotton is 90 percent cellulose. Cellulose is a carbohydrate with a similar structure to starch. In its pure form it is a white solid that absorbs water until completely saturated, but dissolves only in a few solvents.

It can be broken down by heat and by the digestive tracts of some animals, but it passes unchanged through the human digestive tract, where it is valuable in stimulating movement of the intestines.

CELOM
The general body cavity in the adult.

CEMENTUM
The layer of bony tissue forming the outer surface of the root of the tooth within the gum.

CENOGENESIS
The introduction of new features in the development of an individual, absent from the early evolution of the species.

CENSOR
The psychological influence that prevents unconscious thoughts and wishes coming into consciousness; term applied by Sigmund Freud to describe the resistance that prevents repressed material re-entering the conscious mind.

CENSORSHIP
Term employed by Sigmund Freud,

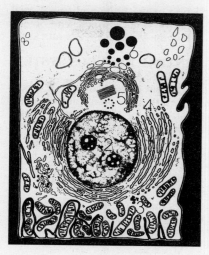

Schematic drawing of a cell (at the electron-microscopic level of magnification) with the main constituents:
1. cell membrane;
2. nucleus with nucleoli;
3. mitochondria;
4. endoplasmic reticulum;
5. Golgi-apparatus;
6. fat droplets.

to express figuratively the influence of a psychological selective agency that functions as a barrier to prevent repressed impulses, memories and ideas from coming into the consciousness.

CENTIGRADE
One hundred divisions or degrees of the Celsius scale, in which the freezing point of water is fixed at 0 degrees and the boiling point at 100 degrees.

CENTRALIS POSITION
A theoretical position held by certain psychologists who believe that thinking can best be explained as processes going on inside the brain or nervous system, with muscular movements as mere accompaniments or facilitators of the central processes.

CENTRAL NERVOUS SYSTEM
The part of the nervous system con-

sisting of the brain and spinal cord with their nerves and end-organs within the skull and vertebral canal.

CENTRAL NERVOUS SYSTEM DEPRESSANTS
Drugs that cause sedation or otherwise diminish brain activity and other parts of the nervous system; for example, anesthetics, anticonvulsants, antidepressants, benzodiazepines, etc.

CENTRAL NERVOUS SYSTEM STIMULANTS
Drugs that cause excitation, anxiety and nervousness or otherwise stimulate the brain and other parts of the central nervous system.

CENTRAL PHASE
The stage of the immune response concerned with the formation of antibody.

CENTRAL VISION
Vision with the macula of the retina.

CENTRIFUGAL
Moving away from a center, as when a nerve signal moves away from the center of a neuron to the periphery.

CENTRIFUGE
Machine in which centrifugation (the process of separating particles in a solution) takes place, for instance, in the analysis of body fluids.

CENTRIPETAL
Moving towards the center, as when a nerve signal moves towards the center of a neuron from the periphery.

CENTROMERE
The constricted portion of the chromosome, which is the point of attachment to the equatorial plane of the mitotic or meiotic spindle during cell division.

CENTROSOME
A specialized area of condensed cytoplasm in the cell believed to be concerned with the division of the nucleus.

CEPHALALGIA
Another name for headache.

CEPHALIC
(1) Of or pertaining to the head.
(2) Situated or directed towards the head.

CEPHALIC INDEX
In anthropometry, an index used originally in attempts to classify race, now used mainly to indicate possible relationships between small groups. The index is given by: maximum head breadth x 100/maximum head length

Peoples with broad heads (cephalic index over 80) are classed as brachycephalic; those with long heads (less than 76) as dolichocephalic; and those in between as mesocephalic (mesaticephalic).

CEPHALIC PRESENTATION
That in which any part of the head presents at the mouth of the womb during childbirth.

CEPHALIC VERSION
A procedure in which an unborn baby is gently moved manually to ensure that it will be born head first.

CEPHALIZATION
In the evolution of animals, the tendency for sense organs and associated nervous tissue to be concentrated at one end of the body - the end that "faces" the environment. Cephalization has led to the development of a distinct head in most animals.

CEPHALOCAUDAL PRINCIPLE
Principle of development stating that growth proceeds from the head to the lower part of the body.

CEPHALOCELE
Protrusion of a part of the contents of the cranial cavity through the skull.

CEPHALHYDROCELE
Collection of cerebrospinal fluid situated beneath the scalp, which can only arise in cases of skull fracture when a wound penetrates to the spaces of the brain occupied by cerebrospinal fluid.

CEPHALOMETRY
Measurement of the dimensions of the head in order to detect disorders of growth or hydrocephalus.

CEPHALOSPORINS
Group of broad-spectrum antibiotics, most of which are derived from the penicillin-like cephalosporin C that was discovered in sewage in Sardinia.

They act against the same bacteria as natural penicillin and some semisynthetic penicillins. They can produce allergic reactions, especially in those sensitive to penicillin.

CEREBELLAR FIT
Seizure associated with tumors of the cerebellum, and characterized by sudden loss of consciousness and falling, dilated and immobile pupils and rigid extension of the body.

CEREBELLAR GAIT
Unsteady gait in which there is dissociation of movement between the body and legs. The body either lags behind or is thrust forward, resulting in a "drunken" walk.

CEREBELLUM
A large section of the brain, also called the small brain, that is the coordinating center for voluntary movements, equilibrium and posture. The cerebellum is composed of a central lobe and two lateral lobes, and is located at the back of and underlying the cerebrum.

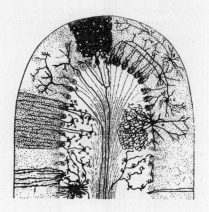

Various types of neurons in the cortex of the cerebellum.

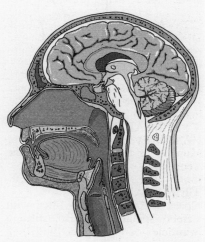

Location of the cerebellum below the hemispheres in the back of the head.

CEREBRAL
(1) Pertaining to the cerebrum or brain.
(2) Expressing an appeal to or use of the intellect.

CEREBRAL ACCIDENT
A sudden injury occurring inside the brain, such as a hemorrhage.

CEREBRAL ANGIOGRAPHY
X-ray studies of cerebral blood vessels after injection of contrast medium.

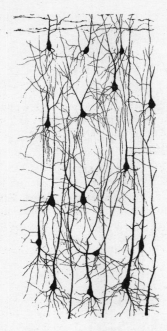

Nerve cells or neurons in the cerebral cortex of the human brain.

CEREBRAL BLINDNESS
An inability to see due to disease or damage in the visual area of the cerebrum.

CEREBRAL CAVITY
Space within the brain filled with cerebro-spinal fluid; also called a ventricle.

CEREBRAL CORTEX
The surface area of the cerebral hemispheres in higher animals, including humans. It is commonly called gray matter because its many cell bodies give it a grey appearance in cross-section, in contrast to the nerve fibers that make up the white matter.

CEREBRAL DIPLEGIA
Disease affecting persons who are popularly called "spastics." The child has a spastic paralysis of the limbs, usually the legs, often associated with convulsions and varying degrees of mental deficiency. The condition is also called spastic diplegia and Little's disease.

CEREBRAL DOMINANCE
The fact that one brain hemisphere is dominant over the other in the control of body movement, for example, resulting in a person being right- or left-handed.

CEREBRAL HEMISPHERES
Two large masses of nerve cells and fibers constituting the bulk of the brain in humans and other higher mammals. The hemispheres are separated by a deep fissure, but connected by a broad band of fibers.

CEREBRAL EDEMA
Edema (swelling) of the brain, due to toxic (poisonous) nutritional causes. It is usually associated with delirium, convulsions or coma.

CEREBRAL PALSY
A diverse group of conditions caused by brain damage around the time of birth and resulting in a variable degree of nonprogressive physical and mental handicap; sufferers are commonly called "spastics." While abnormalities of muscle control are the most obvious, loss of sensation and some degree of deafness are common accompaniments.

Speech and intellectual development can also be impaired but may be entirely normal. Spastic paralysis of both legs with mild arm weakness (diplegia), or of one half of the body (hemiplegia), are common forms. A number of cases have abnormal movements (athetosis) or loss of power in governing movements (ataxia).

Common causes include:
- birth trauma;
- anoxia (lack of oxygen);
- prematurity;
- Rhesus incompatibility;
- cerebral hemorrhage.

CEREBRAL THROMBOSIS
A clot forming in a blood vessel of the brain.

CEREBRAL VASCULAR ACCIDENT
Sometimes called cerebro-vascular accident, apoplectic stroke, or simply stroke.

An impeded blood supply to some part of the brain, generally caused by one of the following four conditions:
(1) A blood clot forming in the vessel (cerebral thrombosis).
(2) A rupture of the blood vessel wall (cerebral hemorrhage).
(3) A piece of clot or other material from another part of the vascular system which flows to the brain and obstructs a cerebral vessel (cerebral embolism).
(4) Pressure on a blood vessel, such as by a tumor.

CEREBRATION
Mental activities associated with the higher nervous centers.

CEREBROSPINAL
Of or pertaining to the brain and spinal cord, or to these coupled with the spinal and cranial nerves.

CEREBROSPINAL FLUID
Normally clear liquid, produced in ventricles of the brain, that fills and protects the cavities in the brain and spinal cord. In the adult there is normally about 140 milliliters of the fluid.

CEREBROSPINAL SYSTEM
All the nerves of the central nervous system of the body except those associated with the autonomic nervous system.

CEREBROVASCULAR
Pertaining to the blood vessels of the brain and cranial cavity.

CEREBRUM
The principal portion of the brain, including practically all parts within the skull except the brain stem and cerebellum.

CERTIFIED
Term used in relation to severe psychological disturbances (psychoses) of patients who cannot leave a mental hospital of their own accord. Generally the term "detained" is used.

CERULOPLASMIN
A protein with which most of the blood's copper is combined. Elevated levels may occur in liver disease and heart attack. Decreased levels occur in other forms of liver disease and in nutritional deficiencies.

CERUMEN
Wax secreted in the outer ear.

CERUMOL
Brand name of a drug containing turpentine oil, paradichlorobenzene and chlorbutol as active ingredients. It is mainly used to dissolve ear wax.

CERVICAL
Pertaining to the neck, to the neck of the womb, or to a neck-like structure.

CERVICAL RIB
Excessive enlargement of one side of the seventh cervical vertebra in the spine, which sticks out resembling a rib and causes pressure on nerves and blood vessels, producing attacks of pins–and–needles in the arms and hands.

CERVICAL RIB SYNDROME
One type of thoracic outlet obstruction syndrome.

CERVICAL SYNDROMES
A spectrum of acute and chronic neuromuscular disorders affecting the cervical region of the spinal cord (in the neck), the distribution

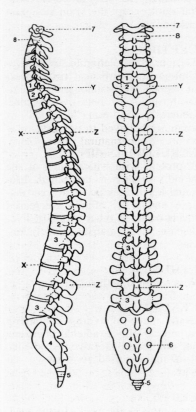

Side view (left) and posterior view (right) of the spine or vertebral column.
1. cervical vertebra; 2. dorsal vertebra; 3. lumbar vertebra; 4. sacral bone; 5. coccyx; 6. foramen; 7. atlas; 8. axis.
X. intervertebral disc; Y. vertebral joint; Z. spinous process.

of the cervical nerve roots, or both. Acute cervical syndromes are common and range in seriousness from non-specific painful muscle spasms in the back of the neck to acute painful attacks with defects of muscular and sensory activity.

CERVICAL VERTEBRA
Either of seven constituents of the cervical part of the spine or vertebral column. The bodies of cervical vertebrae are smaller than those of the thoracic vertebrae. The arches, however, are larger. The spinous processes of the second through sixth cervical vertebrae are often bifid, having a cleft. Each cervical vertebra contains an opening, the transverse foramen. The vertebral artery and its accompanying vein and nerve fibers pass through it.

CERVICECTOMY
Surgical removal of the cervix of the womb.

CERVICITIS
Inflammation of the neck of the womb.

CERVIX
The neck or necklike part of an organ, esp. the neck of the uterus, that part of the uterus that extends into the vagina.

CERVIX UTERI
Neck of the womb. It is frequently referred to as the cervix without qualification.

CHAIN REFLEX
A series of reflexes so related that the completion of the action of one initiates the next, and so on in a chain.

CHALAZION
Chronic swelling of the Meibomian gland on the eyelid, caused by the blockage of its duct, often following inflammation of the gland.

CHAMOMILE
(Anthemis nobilis) A perennial plant of which the flowers are used for medicinal purposes. The solitary, terminal flowerheads, rising 20 to 30 cm (8-12 in) above the ground, consist of prominent yellow discs and silver-white ray florets. The flowering time is June and July.

Chamomile tea is good for flatulent colic, dyspepsia, and for fever and restlessness in children. It also makes a good wash for open sores and wounds. Chamomile oil can be taken internally for colic, spasms and stomach cramps.

CHANCE
In a statistical sense, the theoretical probability of the occurrence of an event, calculated on the basis of the mathematical theory of probability; in a biological sense, a variation that appears random or unpredictable.

CHANCRE
The sore that is the first symptom of syphilis.

CHANCROID
Soft sore that appears on genitals in a similar situation to a syphilitic chancre but is not syphilitic in origin.

CHARACTER
Employed in a biological sense to describe any feature of an organism in respect of which it can be compared with other organisms. Psychologically, employed to describe that integration of habits, sentiments and ideals that renders an individual's actions relatively stable and predictable; special features in this integration, or revealing themselves in action, are designated "character traits," and tests devised to bring out such features are "character or personality tests."

CHARACTERIZATION
Description of the main features of an object or a personality; in a more special sense, used to describe the development of character through social interaction.

CHARACTER NEUROSIS
Neurotic symptoms that have become accepted by the ego and incorporated into the personality.

CHARCOAL
The residue after burning organic substances in an enclosed vessel. Activated charcoal is used as a general-purpose antidote to poisons, because of its adsorptive power.

CHARCOT'S JOINTS
Another name for neurogenic arthropathy.

CHARM
Anything believed to possess some occult or supernatural power, such as an amulet or spell or some mystic observance. The term is also used in the sense of attraction, fascination.

CHAUFFEUR'S FRACTURE
Fracture of the lower end of the radius (the bone on the thumb side of the forearm) and styloid process (a projection on the outer end of the radius), so called because it can be caused by the movement of a car as it backfires when started using the handle.

CHEDIAK-HIGASHI SYNDROME
A progressive genetic disorder characterized by partial albinism, severe recurrent bacterial infections leading to abscesses, and development of a lack of white blood cells.

CHEEK
Either side of the face below the eye and above the lower jawbone.

CHEEKBONE
Bone or bony prominence below the outer angle of the eye; the zygomatic bone.

CHEEK TOOTH
One of the molar teeth that act as grinders of the food.

CHEILITIS
Inflammation of the lips. The usual symptoms are dryness, cracking and tenseness of the lips, causing severe discomfort. Several factors are involved: infection with an accompa-

nying fever, dehydration and antibiotic therapy. Cheilitis may be
caused by sunlight or cold, but is
more commonly due to a combination of the two. Alcohol in combination with a particular foodstuff,
such as shellfish, is a common
cause. The treatment consists of a
soft lipstick, elimination of the
known cause and/or application of a
1 percent hydrocortisone ointment.

CHEILOSIS
A condition in which fissures and
ulcers appear at the angles of the
mouth, usually caused by vitamin B
deficiency.

CHELATING AGENT
Soluble organic compound capable
of combining with a metal in complexes. Such an agent is used to
treat metal poisoning. A chelating
agent acts by combining with the
metal to form a less poisonous substance and in some cases increases
excretion in the urine. Penicillamine
is a commonly-used chelating
agent.

CHELIDONIUM MAJUS
Homeopathic medicine derived
from celandine. It is a prominent
liver remedy, covering many of the
direct reflex symptoms of that organ. The jaundiced skin, and especially the constant pain under the
inferior angle of the right shoulder
blade are certain indications, as are
a yellow tongue, a bad taste in the
mouth, jaundice, constipation, hard
stools.

CHELOID
Unnatural amount of scar tissue, the
scar becoming heaped up, hard and
unsightly.

CHEMICAL INTEGRATION
The way in which the body is organized to deal efficiently with
chemical substances transmitted via
the bodily fluids, especially the hormones.

CHEMICAL SENSE
Generally a sense which is affected
by a chemical reaction produced in
the receptor by a stimulus substance.

CHEMOPROPHYLAXIS
The prevention of disease by
chemical drugs or agents.

CHEMORECEPTION
The physical response of a sense organ to the reception of chemical
stimuli.

CHEMORECEPTOR
A receptor organ or sensor sensitive
to stimulation by certain chemical
substances.

CHEMOSIS
Edema (swelling) of the conjunctiva
of the eye.

CHEMOTAXIS
Enhanced migration of cells in the
presence of chemical substances,
usually towards the substance. Leukocyte (white blood cell) chemo-
taxis, which occurs in response to
substances released during an immune reaction, is a part of the inflammatory response.

CHEMOTHERAPY
The use of chemical substances to
treat disease. More specifically, the
term refers to the use of non-antibi-
otic anti-microbials and agents for
treating cancer. The drug must interfere with the growth of bacterial,
parasitic or tumor cells, without significantly affecting normal cells in
the body.
    In anti-microbial chemotherapy,
the work of Paul Ehrlich on aniline
dyes and arsenicals (resulting in the
drug Salvarsan) and of Gerhardt
Domagk on Prontosil led to the development of the anti-bacterial sulphonamides. Many useful synthetic
compounds are now available for
bacterial and parasitic disease, although antibiotics are often pre-

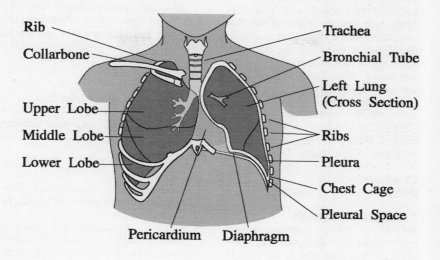

Rib

Collarbone

Upper Lobe

Middle Lobe

Lower Lobe

Trachea

Bronchial Tube

Left Lung
(Cross Section)

Ribs

Pleura

Chest Cage

Pleural Space

Pericardium   Diaphragm

Localization of the lungs in the chest.

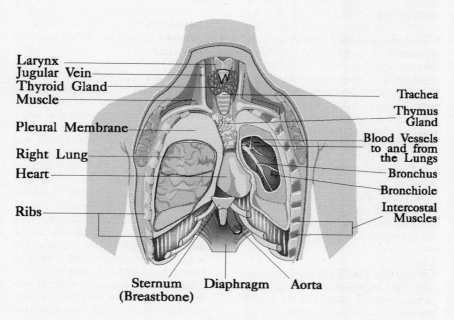

Larynx
Jugular Vein
Thyroid Gland
Muscle

Pleural Membrane

Right Lung

Heart

Ribs

Trachea

Thymus
Gland

Blood Vessels
to and from
the Lungs

Bronchus

Bronchiole

Intercostal
Muscles

Sternum   Diaphragm   Aorta
(Breastbone)

Cross section of the chest

ferred for bacteria. Cancer chemotherapy is especially successful in leukemia and lymphoma; in carcinoma, it is usually reserved for disseminated tumor. Nitrogen mustard, alkaloids derived from the periwinkle, certain antibiotics and agents interfering with DNA metabolism are used, often in combination and usually with steroids.

CHEROMANIA
Mental disorder characterized by excessive cheerfulness.

CHEROPHOBIA
Fear of rejoicing or pleasure.

CHERRY ANGIOMA
Bright red, raised tumors, a few millimeters in diameter, on the trunk; common in elderly persons.

CHERVIL
(Anthriscus cerefolium) Annual plant of which the flowering herb is used for medicinal purposes. The round, finely grooved, branched stem grows 0.30 to 0.60 m (1-2 ft) high from a thin, whitish root. The leaves are opposite, light green and bipennate, the upper sessile on stem sheaths.

The juice pressed out of the fresh flowering herb is popularly used for various purposes, including scrofula, eczema, gout stones (tophi), abscesses, water retention, and women's abdominal complaints.

CHESS-BOARD ILLUSION
A visual illusion of depth produced by a black-and-white check pattern in a circle, the checks becoming progressively larger towards the circumference.

CHEST
Upper part of the trunk, between the neck and abdomen. The chest wall consists of ribs jointed at the spinal column, the sternum (breastbone) and the related muscles. The diaphragm separates the chest from the abdomen. The lungs fill much of each side of the chest while the heart, the aorta and other large vessels lie centrally, the heart slightly to the left; the trachea (windpipe) and esophagus pass into the chest from the neck.

CHEST X-RAY
An X-ray to detect lung diseases, or determine the size and position of the heart, ribs or other internal structures of the chest.

CHEYNE-STOKES RESPIRATION
Rhythmical breathing that starts with small breaths, each breath becoming deeper up to a climax, after which the breaths become progressively shallower until breathing practically stops, this cycle being repeated again and again. It occurs in grave disorders of the nervous system, heart and lungs, and in uremia (the result of kidney failure), and is frequently a sign of impending death.

CHIASMA
A crossing, such as of two tendons or two nerves.

CHIASMA SYNDROME
Impaired vision, headache, giddiness and limitation of the visual fields due to a lesion in the optic chiasm (the point at which the two optic nerves cross just outside the brain).

CHICKEN POX
An acute viral disease of children, usually ushered in by mild symptoms that are followed shortly by a skin eruption appearing in crops and characterized by red pimples that become fluid-filled vesicles, which then burst and crust over.

Mild cases require only treatment of symptoms, e.g. calamine lotion to relieve the itching. Local or systemic antihistamines may be used in severe cases. Affected children should be kept at home until the vesicles have crusted over, as they are contagious until then. Chicken pox is usually a relatively mild disease in childhood.

CHICKWEED
(Stellaria media) Herb known for its high vitamin C content. It is used most often to treat scurvy. Also used in the treatment of constipation, hemorrhoids, rheumatism and some respiratory disorders.

CHICORY
(Cichorium intybus) Perennial plant of which the rootstock and flowering herb is used for medicinal purposes.

The rootstock is light yellow outside, white inside, and contains a bitter, milky juice. The stiff, angular, branching stem bears lanceolate leaves that are coarsely toothed near the bottom of the plant but appear entire higher up. The light-blue to violet-blue, axillary or terminal flowerheads feature rays that are toothed at the ends.

Chicory is often recommended for jaundice and for spleen problems. The juice of the leaves and a tea made from the flowering plant promotes the production of bile, the release of gallstones and the elimination of excessive internal mucus.

CHIGGER
Also called a chigoe or harvest mite: an insect closely resembling the common flea, but of more minute size, which burrows beneath the skin and, becoming distended with eggs, produces a troublesome ulcer.

CHILBLAINS
Reaction to cold with pain, itching and bluish-redness, that can lead to the formation of blisters and ulcers. The lesions are particularly common on fingers, toes, shins, nose and ears, but may occur on other sites. They are caused by poor cir-

culation and being exposed to the cold and damp. Chilblains are most common in children and young women. They tend to recur every winter, but usually disappear after a few years. They can be avoided by keeping the body (particularly the extremities) warm and dry, and by massaging the areas most likely to be affected by chilblains.

CHILD ABUSE
Physical, emotional or sexual maltreatment of a child, often resulting in serious and often permanent injury or impairment and sometimes in death.

CHILD ANALYSIS
The psychoanalysis of children. This differs technically from the analysis of adults in that play replaces free association. It differs theoretically in that parents and parent-substitutes are still actual, external figures in the person's life, and in that dependency on them is a social and biological fact, not a neurotic symptom. It differs morally in that the relationship between analyst and patient is not one between consenting adults; the decision to have treatment is not made by the patient but by his or her parents.

CHILDBEARING
Pregnancy and childbirth. Term often applied to the age at which women are capable of these, i.e. after puberty and before the menopause.

CHILDBED FEVER
An infection of the mother occurring at childbirth; puerperal fever.

CHILD GUIDANCE
A development of methods, carried out chiefly at state-run clinics, for dealing with behavior and educational problems in children.

CHILDHOOD
The total life period from birth up

to but not including adolescence.

CHILDHOOD AVOIDANT DISORDER

Excessive shrinking from contact with unfamiliar people that is of sufficient severity to interfere with social functioning in peer relationships and that is of a considerable duration. This is coupled with a clear desire for social involvement with familiar people, such as peers the person knows well and family members. Relationships with family members and other familiar figures are warm and satisfying.

A child with this disorder is likely to appear socially withdrawn, embarrassed, and timid when in the company of unfamiliar people and will become anxious when even a trivial demand is made to interact with strangers. When social anxiety is severe, the child may be inarticulate or mute, even if his or her communication skills are unimpaired.

CHILDHOOD DISEASES

Characteristic diseases that may occur during childhood: mumps, chicken pox, measles, diphtheria, rubella (German measles), pertussis (whooping cough), scarlet fever.

CHILDHOOD REACTIVE ATTACHMENT DISORDER

Markedly disturbed social relatedness in most contexts that begins before the age of five and is not due to mental retardation or a pervasive developmental disorder, such as autism. The disturbance is presumed to be due to grossly pathogenic care that preceded the onset of the disturbance.

The disturbance may take the form of either persistent failure to initiate or respond in an age-expected manner to most social interactions or - in an older child -indiscriminate sociability, e.g., excessive familiarity with relative strangers, as shown by making requests and displaying affection. Some severe forms of this disorder, in which there is lack of weight gain and motor development, have been called "failure to thrive" or "hospitalism.".

CHILDHOOD SCHIZOPHRENIA

Diagnostic category for those children exhibiting a schizophrenic state, including such symptoms as withdrawal from people and reality, escape into a fantasy world, disturbance in their ability to make contact with the world through the emotions, autistic thought processes, becoming mute. There exists also excessive impulsiveness or inhibition, identification with animals or objects, stereotyped gestures, impassivity or extreme outbursts of rage and anxiety, bizarre posturing, etc.

CHILD-PARENT FIXATION

A child's emotional attachment of love, hate or both towards one of his/her parents which is so firm as to interfere with his/her forming other relationships.

CHILD PSYCHOLOGY

A branch of psychology which studies the human being in development from birth to maturity.

CHIMERA

An individual who has received a transplant of genetically and immunologically different tissue, either of the same or of another species. From Greek mythology, the monster with a lion's head, goat's body and serpent's tail.

CHIMNEY SWEEP'S CANCER

Malignant growth of the tissues of the scrotum (scrotal epithelioma), occurring as an occupational hazard. This was the first occupational disease to be identified.

CHIROGNOMY

Attempt to read character from the lines on the hand.

CHIROGRAPHY
The study of handwriting.

CHIROPODIST
One who treats ailments and irregularities of the feet.

CHIROPODY
The science dealing with the treatment of foot ailments and irregularities.

CHIROPRACTIC
A health discipline based on the theory that disease results from misalignment of the vertebrae of the spine. Manipulation, massage, dietary and general advice are the principal methods used. It was founded by Daniel D. Palmer in Davenport, Iowa, in 1895 and has a particularly substantial following in the US.

CHIROSPASM
Writer's cramp.

CHIVE
(Allium schoenoprasum) A perennial plant of which the leaves are used for medicinal purposes. The leaves are hollow, cylindrical, closed at the top and dilated to surround the stem at the bottom. These should always be used fresh, and heating them should be avoided. The common method of chopping them fresh and sprinkling them over food just prior to serving is best.

Chive helps to stimulate appetite and to promote the digestive processes. The plant also contains iron (as well as arsenic in harmless amounts) and may therefore be helpful for anemia.

CHLOASMA
Condition in which pigment is deposited in the skin in patches of various shapes and sizes and of any color from yellow, brown to black. Often associated with some disorder of the endocrine glands, it can also be a side-effect of taking the combined contraceptive pill.

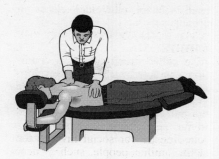

Application of chiropractic treatment for disorder of the spine.

CHLOASMA UTERINUM
Pigmented areas occurring on the forehead, temples, cheeks, nipples and abdomen that may become more marked during menstrual periods or during pregnancy (when it is called the "mask of pregnancy"). May also occur with tumors or disorders of the ovaries.

CHLORAL
Trichloroacetaldehyde, a colorless, oily liquid made by the reaction between chlorine and ethanol or acetaldehyde, used chiefly in the manufacture of DDT.

CHLORIDE
A compound of chlorine with an element or radical; a salt of hydrochloric acid.

CHLORINE
A greenish-yellow gaseous element, highly irritating to the organs of respiration, occurring naturally combined in table salt. As chlorinated lime, it is used as a disinfectant.

CHLOROFORM
Trichloromethane, dense, colorless, volatile liquid made by chlorination of ethanol or acetone. One of the first anesthetics in modern use (by Sir James Simpson in 1847), it is now seldom used except in tropical countries, despite its potency, since it has a narrow safety margin and is highly toxic in excess. It is also

used in cough medicines and as an organic solvent.

CHLOROMA
Also called green cancer: a condition characterized by the development of multiple, localized, pale green or green-yellow masses of abnormal cells, especially in relation to the periosteum (membrane surrounding bone) and ligaments of the skull.

CHLOROPHENOTHANE
An insecticide (DDT), known to cause severe side-effects and chronic poisoning.

CHLOROPHYLL
The green coloring matter of plants and leaves, used in the manufacture of carbohydrates.

CHLOROSIS
A form of irondeficient anemia, characterized by a great reduction in hemoglobin. The condition is observed chiefly in girls, from puberty until they reach their 30s.

CHOANA
The paired openings between the nasal cavity and the nasopharynx at the back of the throat; any funnel-shaped opening.

CHOCK
Uncoordinated response elicited by a sudden stimulus for which the individual has not been prepared by immediately preceding experience.

CHOICE REACTION
A form of reaction experiment, where the subject is instructed to react differently to two or more different stimuli; may also be made the basis of a learning experiment, either with animal or with human subjects.

CHOKE
To stop the breath, by stricture of or obstruction in the windpipe.

CHOKED DISC
Swelling of the cup or disc in the back of the eyeball. Fluid extension causes blurring and blindness.

CHOLEMIA
The presence of bile or bile pigments in blood, causing jaundice.

CHOLAGOGUE
Drug or substance causing an increase in the flow of bile into the intestine.

CHOLANGIOGRAPHY
X-ray examination of the gallbladder, done after the subject eats a prepared fatty meal, and swallows a contrast agent that outlines the gallbladder and nearby structures.

CHOLANGIOHEPATITIS
Inflammatory process affecting the liver and bile ducts.

CHOLANGIOMA
Tumor or malignant growth arising from the cells of the bile ducts.

CHOLANGITIS
Inflammation of the bile ducts, characterized among others by the occurrence of jaundice.

CHOLECYSTECTOMY
Surgical removal of the gallbladder.

CHOLECYSTITIS
Inflammation of the gallbladder, usually of the mucosal lining of the gallbladder.

CHOLE-CYSTO-DUODENOS-TOMY
Surgical operation in which the duodenum and gallbladder are joined together, usually in cases of obliteration or stricture of the main duct between the gallbladder and duodenum.

CHOLE-CYSTO-GASTROS-TOMY
Surgical joining together of the

gallbladder and the stomach to secure the flow of bile to the intestine in cases of obliteration or stricture of the duct between the gallbladder and the duodenum.

CHOLECYSTOGRAPHY
X-ray visualization of the gallbladder by administering drugs that, when stored in the gallbladder, are opaque to X-rays.

CHOLECYSTOLITHIASIS
The presence or formation of gallstones.

CHOLECYSTOSTOMY
Surgical operation that brings the gallbladder to the surface of the abdomen so that bile is discharged through the abdominal opening. Performed to permit drainage of the gallbladder.

CHOLELITHIASIS
Gallstones, concretions in the gallbladder.

CHOLELITHOTOMY
Removal of gallstones via a surgical incision into the gallbladder.

CHOLERA
Acute infection with the bacteria Vibrio cholerae, characterized by severe diarrhea and vomiting, often leading to dehydration, electrolyte imbalances and, if untreated, death.

Spread by water and food contaminated with the feces of infested persons, it is endemic in some parts of the world and frequently occurs at times of natural disasters.

CHOLERIC
Particular type of temperament, the possessor being subject to wild attacks of rage and irritability. In ancient times it was thought such people possessed or made too much bile. Hence the term choleric comes from the Greek khole, meaning "bile".

CHOLESTASIS
Stagnation of bile in the liver that results when bile flow is impaired.

CHOLESTEATOMA
Tumor occurring in the ear as a result of chronic middle ear disease and constant discharges of pus. Also a rare form of brain tumor, sometimes called a "pearl tumor," arising from remnants of embryonic cells.

CHOLESTEROL
A complex chemical present in all animal fats and widespread in the body, especially in bile, the brain, blood, adrenal glands and nerve-fiber sheaths. In the body cholesterol is involved in the synthesis of certain hormones and vitamin D. Many studies indicate that excessive cholesterol levels in the blood can clog arteries and predispose to heart attacks and strokes.

CHOLESTEROLOSIS
A condition resulting from a disturbance in the metabolism of lipids, characterized by deposits of cholesterol in tissues, especially in the inner lining of the gallbladder.

CHOLINE ESTERASE
A catalytic enzyme that hydrolyses acetylcholine into choline and acetic acid.

CHOLINE MAGNESIUM TRISALICYLATE
Generic name of a drug with properties similar to those of aspirin, used in the treatment of arthritic conditions.

CHOLINE SALICYLATE
Generic name of a drug with properties similar to those of aspirin used in the relieving of pain of mouth disorders.

CHOLINERGIC
Relating to nerve fibers or medicines that cause effects similar to

those induced by acetylcholine.

CHOLINERGICS
Chemicals or drugs that facilitate passage of nerve impulses through the parasympathetic nervous system.

CHOLINESTERASE INHIBITORS
Drugs that prevent the action of cholinesterase (an enzyme that breaks down acethylcholine in the body).

CHOLURIA
The presence of abnormal amounts of bile in the urine.

CHONDRALGIA
General term for pain in or around a cartilage.

CHONDRITIS
Inflammation of a cartilage, especially the cartilage of a joint.

CHONDROCALCINOSIS
A specific joint disease with intermittent attacks of acute arthritis and X-ray evidence of calcinosis of the articular cartilage. Calcinosis is a condition characterized by abnormal depositing of calcium salts in the tissues, here in the cartilage of joints.

CHONDROMA
A tumor, either malignant or benign, in a cartilage.

CHONDROMALACIA
Softening of any cartilage, as sometimes occurs in certain rheumatic diseases.

CHONDROMATOSIS
The presence of multiple tumor-like foci in cartilage.

CHONDRO-OSTEODYSTROPHY
Childhood condition characterized by interference with the growing ends of bone, resulting in disturbances of height and growth.

CHONDROSARCOMA
A malignant growth or neoplasm derived from cartilage cells.

CHORDA
Any cord, tendon or nerve filament; the notochord, that part of the embryo which gives rise to the spinal column.

CHORDAE TENDINAE
Fibrous bands attached to the atrioventricular valves (the valves between the upper and lower chambers of the heart).

CHORDITIS
Inflammation of the vocal chords.

CHORDOTOMY
Surgical cutting of the anterolateral tracts of the spinal cord to give relief from severe and intractable pain. The anterolateral tracts convey pain impulses from the peripheral nerves to the brain.

CHOREA
Abnormal, non-repetitive involuntary movements of the limbs, body and face. It may start with clumsiness, but later uncontrollable and bizarre movements occur. It is a disease of the central nervous system.

Sydenham's chorea or chorea minor (formerly called St Vitus's dance) is a childhood illness associated with streptococcus infection and rheumatic fever; recovery is usually full.

Huntington's chorea is a rare hereditary disease, usually coming on in middle age and associated with progressive dementia.

CHOREA GRAVIDARUM
Chorea-like movements developing during pregnancy. It is quite rare, usually occurring in the first pregnancy and during the first trimester.

Treatment is tempered by concern for the developing fetus. Sedation with barbiturates is safest.

CHOREA MINOR
Another name for Sydenham's chorea.

CHOREIFORM
Movement, situation etc. resembling chorea.

CHORIOCARCINOMA
Another name for trophoblastic disease.

CHORION
Outermost layer of the membrane within which the unborn baby lives.

CHORIONEPITHELIOMA
Extremely rare malignant tumor arising from the cells of the thread-like projection from the chorion, left in the womb after childbirth or abortion.

CHORIONIC VILLI
Projections from the outermost of the foetal membranes through which diffusion of gases, nutrients and waste products occurs.

CHORION SOMATOMAMMOTROPIN
A hormone, produced by the placenta, that is essential for the production of breastmilk.

CHORIORETINITIS
Inflammation of the choroid and the retina of the eye.

CHORIORITIS
Inflammation of the iris membrane of the eye.

CHOROIDITIS
Inflammation of the middle coat of the eye, between the sclera and the retina, containing blood vessels.

CHOROID PLEXUS
Fringelike growth of blood vessels that projects into the cavities of the brain and creates the cerebrospinal fluid.

CHOROMANIA
Frenzied dancing, appearing as a social epidemic, belonging with a number of other social phenomena that can be regarded as a phenomenon of mass suggestion and imitation.

CHRISTIAN SCIENCE
A religious movement, the major tenet of which is the belief in the power of Christian faith to heal sickness. It was founded by Mary Baker Eddy, who organized the first "Church of Christ, Scientist" at Boston, Mass., in 1879. There are now many affiliated churches throughout the world.

CHRISTMAS DISEASE
Blood clotting disturbance caused by a hereditary deficiency of clotting factor IX (Christmas factor).

CHROMAFFIN
Giving a brownish-yellow reaction with chrome salts, denoting certain cells in the medulla of the adrenal glands.

CHROMAFFIN TUMOR
A tumor of the sympathetic nervous system, most often discovered in the adrenal glands, but occasionally in other sites. It is made up of chromaffin cells that have a strong affinity for taking up chrome salts. May be accompanied by high blood pressure.

CHROMATID
One of a pair of chromosomal strands formed when a chromosome duplicates during cell reproduction.

CHROMATIN
The substance in cell nuclei and chromosomes that stains intensely with basic dyes, composed of DNA combined with protein.

CHROMATIN-NEGATIVE
Refers to nuclei that lack the sex chromatin mass, or Barr body. Characteristic of the normal human male.

CHROMATIN-POSITIVE
Refers to nuclei containing the distinctive sex chromatin mass. Characteristic of the normal human female.

CHROMATOPSIA
Seeing colorless objects as a result of an abnormal condition of vision, as in snow-blindness.

CHROMATOSIS
Abnormal pigmentation of the skin.

CHROMESTHESIA
Association of particular colors with sounds or, less frequently, with sensations from other senses.

CHROMIC ACID
Acid derived from chromium used as a astringent in a 5 percent solution. The agent is also used in the treatment of warts.

CHROMOBLASTOMYCOSIS
Another name for chromomycosis.

CHROMOMYCOSIS
Also called chromoblastomycosis: an infectious disease caused by Hormodendrum pedrosoi and characterized by warty skin nodules that slowly develop into large wart-like vegetations that tend to ulcerate. Incidence is worldwide, but highest in the tropics. The disease is prevalent from the ages of 30 to 50, primarily in men.

CHROMOPROTEIN
A protein compound, such as hemoglobin, made up of a protein usually combined with a pigment.

CHROMOSCOPY
The procedure for testing color vision.

CHROMOSOME
Threadlike structure in every cell nucleus that carries the inheritance factors (genes). They are composed of DNA, the gene material and a protein. A human cell normally contains 46 chromosomes or 22 homologous pairs and 1 pair of sex chromosomes; one member of each pair of chromosomes is derived from each parent.

CHROMOSOME NUMBER
The number of chromosomes found in the somatic cells of an individual or of a species; normally 46 in humans.

CHROMOSOME TESTS
Those performed to determine the true sex should this be in doubt or, more commonly, to discover whether certain congenital defects are liable to be passed on to future offspring. It is a painless procedure in which a few cells are scraped from the inside of the cheek for microscopic examination. The test is also required for women athletes in international sports events.

CHRONAXY
The shortest duration of an effective electric stimulus having a strength equal to twice the minimum strength required for excitation.

CHRONIC
Applied to disorders that persist over a long period.

CHRONIC CHOLECYSTITIS
Chronic inflammation of the gallbladder; the commonest type of gallbladder disease.

CHRONIC DISCOID LUPUS ERYTHEMATOSUS
A form of discoid lupus erythematosus.

CHRONIC FICTITIOUS ILLNESS
A form of Munchausen's syndrome.

CHRONIC GLOMERULONEPHRITIS
Another name for slowly progressive glomerular disease.

CHRONIC GRANULOCYTIC LEUKEMIA
Also called chronic myeloid leukemia: abnormal accumulation of the granulocytic elements of the blood, usually progressing slowly, and responsive to treatment during the major period of the disease. The disease, slightly more prevalent in males, occurs at any age but chiefly in the 30s and 40s.

CHRONIC GRANULOMATOUS DISEASE
A disorder characterized by repeated infections with granuloma (tumors made up of formative cells) and abscess formation, resulting from the inability of phagocytes (white blood cells) to destroy certain microorganisms after they have attacked them. The disease occurs primarily in boys as an X-linked trait.

CHRONIC HEPATITIS
A spectrum of liver disorders that merge, on the one hand, into acute hepatitis and, on the other, cirrhosis. Hepatitis lasting more than six months is generally defined as chronic, though this is arbitrary.

CHRONIC LYMPHOCYTIC LEUKEMIA
Abnormal accumulation of immature lymphocytes (a type of white cell formed in lymphoid tissues) in the blood when normally these are present only in small numbers.

The disease, almost three times more common in males, occurs chiefly from age 50 to 70, but may appear at any age.

CHRONIC MUCOCUTANEOUS CANDIDIASIS
An uncommon form of candidiasis (commonly called thrush), characterized by chronic infection of the skin, nails, scalp and mucous membranes, usually developing in infancy, and often but not invariably caused by the inability of T-lymphocytes (a type of white blood cell) to react to certain antigens.

CHRONIC MYELOID LEUKEMIA
Another name for chronic granulocytic leukemia.

CHRONIC OBSTRUCTIVE PULMONARY DISEASE
Clinically significant, irreversible, generalized obstruction of the airways associated with varying degrees of chronic bronchitis, abnormalities in small airways and emphysema.

CHRONIC OPEN-ANGLE GLAUCOMA
A disorder characterized by a gradual rise in the pressure inside the eyeball, causing slowly progressive loss of vision, and when uncontrolled, late loss of central vision and ultimate blindness.

CHRONOLOGICAL AGE
Age from birth; calendar age.

CHVOSTEK'S SIGN
Neurological reaction elicited by tapping the facial nerve and resulting in excessive twitching of the face.

CHYLE
A white milky fluid in the intestines, made up of fats broken down into a fine emulsion. It is taken up by the lacteal vessels, joins the lymph system and finally enters the blood via the thoracic duct.

CHYLOCELE
Presence of fatty lymph under the membrane covering the testicle, seen as a result of rupture of lymphatics in elephantiasis.

CHYLOTHORAX
Accumulation of chyle in the pleural cavities of the chest.

CHYLURIA
The presence of digested fats in the urine due to the obstruction anywhere between the intestinal lymphatics and the thoracic duct.

CHYME
The pulpy mass of partially digested food as it enters the intestines from the stomach and before the chyle is extracted from it.

CHYMOTRYPSIN
Enzyme found in the intestines with action similar to that of trypsin, acting on certain peptide linkages.

CICATRICIAL STENOSIS
Contracture or narrowing produced by a scar.

CICATRIN
Trade name of a skin preparation containing antibiotics (neomycin and bacitracin), amino-acetic acid and some amino acids. The medicine is prescribed for the treatment of skin infections.

CICATRIX
A scar, formed from connective tissue; the fibrous tissue left after the healing of a wound.

CICLACILLIN
Generic name of a semi-synthetic penicillin preparation.

CILIA
Eyelashes; also the hair-like projections protruding from the cells of the lining of the upper respiratory tract, which move in a rhythmical pattern to pass on, in a sweeping action, dust, germs and mucus.

CILIARY MUSCLE
Muscle that adjusts the shape of the eye lens enabling the eye to focus between near and far objects.

CILIOSIS
Twitching of the eyelid.

CINCHONA
Any of the trees or shrubs constituting the genus Cinchona and cultivated for the bark, which yields quinine and other alkaloids.

As a homeopathic medicine, it is prescribed for weakness and debility resulting from any drain on the system, loss of blood or vital fluids, diarrhea, etc., as well as for pale face, sunken eyes with dark rings about them, sweats and headache, chronic liver and spleen diseases, dyspepsia with cold stomach.

CINCHONINE
An alkaloid obtained from the bark of several species of Cinchona, along with quinine, and used to reduce fever.

CINCHONISM
A disturbed condition of the body characterized by dizziness, ringing of the ears, temporary deafness and headache, the result of overdoses of quinine.

CINE-ANGIOGRAPHY
The photographic recording of X-ray images of the blood vessels by motion picture techniques.

CINERADIOGRAPHY
The photographic recording of X-ray images of internal organs (for instance, the heart) by motion picture techniques.

CINERADIOLOGY
Discipline of the radiological sciences with the emphasis on the interpretation of pictures obtained by cineradiography.

CINNAMON
The inner bark of a tree of the laurel family, used as a spice or in medicine as a digestion stimulant and for dyspepsia.

CIRCADIAN RHYTHM
Rhythmic physical changes that occur during a period of 24 hours. Also called the "biological clock."

CIRCLE OF WILLIS
A circle of arteries at the base of the brain, formed by the union of the branches of the internal carotids (anterior and medial cerebral arteries) with the branches of the basilar artery (posterior cerebral artery) and three communicating arteries.

CIRCULATION
The continuous movement of blood through the vessels of the body maintained by the pumping action of the heart.

CIRCUMCISION
Generally refers to the removal of the foreskin of the penis, either as a religious requirement (notably among Jews and Muslims) or as a surgical measure for sanitary or other reasons (for example, to relieve tightness of the foreskin). In ancient Egypt, circumcision was regarded as a initiation into puberty. For the Jews it symbolizes an infant's induction into the covenant between God and Abraham. In some cultures, notably in Africa, young girls are circumcised by having their clitorises removed. This practice is now considered barbaric.

CIRCUMDUCTION
Circular movement of a limb or the eye.

CIRCUMSTANTIALITY
A term used to describe speech that is indirect and delayed in reaching the point because of unnecessary, tedious details and parenthical remarks. Circumstantial replies or statements may be prolonged for many minutes if the speaker is not interrupted and urged to get to the point. Circumstantiality is common in an obsessive compulsive personality disorder and in many people without a mental disorder.

CIRCUS MOVEMENTS
Movements in which the organism tends to move in a circle, owing either to a one-sided brain injury or to continuous one-sided stimulation.

CIRRHOSIS
A chronic deseased condition of the liver in which fibrous tissue and nodules replace normal tissue, interfering with blood flow and normal functions of the organ, including gastrointestinal functions, hormone metabolism, and alcohol and drug detoxification. A chief cause of cirrhosis if chronic alcoholism, and hepatitis.

CIRRHOTIC
Affected with or having the character of cirrhosis.

CIRSOTOME
Instrument for cutting varicose veins.

CIRSOTOMY
Multiple surgical incisions of veins as treatment for varicose veins.

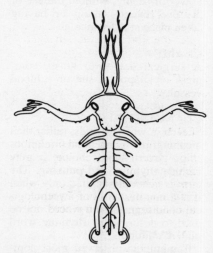

Circle of Willis; circular group of brain arteries located between brain and base of the skull.

STERNA
A closed space between the brain membranes, serving as a reservoir for cerebrospinal fluid.

CITRAMAG
Brand name for an osmotic laxative drug containing magnesium citrate as active ingredient.

CITRATES
Medicines taken orally to make urine more acid. Citrates include potassium citrate, potassium citrate and citric acid, potassium citrate and sodium citrate, sodium citrate and acid, tricitrates.

CITRIC ACID
The acid derived from lemons and similar fruits or obtained by fermentation of carbohydrates, used to flavor foods, beverages and drugs and to condition water.

CLAIRAUDIENCE
Power of hearing sounds and words, conveying information of events at a distance, without the use of the ear.

CLAIRVOYANCE
Power of seeing, without the use of the eye, events taking or having taken place at a distance.

CLAMP
A surgical device to grasp, compress or support tissue or a blood vessel.

CLANGING
Speech in which sounds, rather than meaningful, conceptual relationships govern word choice; it may include rhyming and punning. The term is generally applied only when it is a manifestation of a pathological condition; thus, it would not be used to describe the rhyming word play of children.

Clanging is observed most commonly in schizophrenia and manic episodes.

CLAP
A slang term for the sexually transmitted disease, gonorrhea.

CLASS
A level of social stratification, e.g. upper, middle and lower class, but without the rigid boundaries characterizing caste, so that mobility between classes is possible.

CLASSICAL ANALYTICAL TECHNIQUE
Analysts are said to practice classical technique if they:
- see their patients on a daily basis;
- have them lie on a couch;
- eschew all giving of advice, prescribing of drugs, management of their lives;
- confine their own utterances to interpretations;
- instruct their patients to obey the fundamental or basic rule of free association.

It is possible to practice classical technique without subscribing to classical theory, since theory determines what is said by analysts and not the setting in which they say it.

Classical technique was designed for the treatment of adult psychoneurotics. Controversy exists as to whether, and if so how, classical technique should be modified when analyzing children, adolescents and psychotics.

CLASSICAL ANALYTICAL THEORY
Concept that implies that there exists a norm against which other theoretical positions can be placed, either as deviations from it or as advances on it.

As a result, the concept tends to be used in different ways, meaning either theory that is in line with Freud's basic insights or theory as understood by other, possibly old-fashioned analysts.

CLASSICAL CONDITIONING
Conditioned-response experiments

conforming to the pattern of Pavlov's experiment. The main feature is that one type of stimulus, through repeated pairing with another one, acquires the response originally given to the first stimulus.

CLASSIC TYPHUS
Another name for epidemic typhus.

CLASSIFICATION
The act of forming into a class or classes, so as to bring together those beings or things that most resemble each other, and to separate those that differ.

CLASSIFICATION TEST
A type of mental test, where the subject is required to classify words, designating objects belonging together, either by crossing out ones that do not belong, or by underlining those that do.

CLAUDICATION
Limping, used in the sense of intermittent claudication: pain, tension and weakness in the legs on walking, due to a degeneration of the arterial wall and thus an inadequate supply of blood to the muscles, as a result of atherosclerosis.

CLAUSTROPHOBIA
Fear of closed places, one of the major phobias.

CLAVICLE
Another name for collarbone: either of two slender bones each jointed to the sternum (breast bone) and a scapula (shoulderblade) and forming the front part of the shoulder.

CLAVICULAR
Pertaining to the clavicle.

CLAVULANIC ACID
A substance given with the antibiotic amoxylline to make it more effective.

CLAW-FOOT
A deformity of the foot where the arch of the foot is increased in height, with the toes becoming claw-like, and the foot turning inwards.

CLAW-HAND
Deformity resulting from paralysis and wasting of some of the small muscles of the hand.

CLEFT PALATE
A congenital malformation in which more or less of the palate is lacking, so as to leave a longitudinal gap in the upper jaw; often an accompaniment of hare lip.

If the defects are severe, they may prevent proper feeding, with the food entering the nose instead of being swallowed. The deformity needs surgical repair.

CLEIDOTOMY
Surgical operation in which both collarbones are cut in the unborn baby in order to narrow the shoulders and permit it to be born, in cases where the width of the baby is causing an obstructed labor.

CLEMASTINE
Generic name of an antihistamine drug. The drug is used in treatment of allergic rhinitis and allergic skin disorders.

CLEXANE
Brand name for enoxaparin, a drug used for the prevention of blood clotting.

CLIENT-CENTERED COUNSELLING
A method of psychological counselling designed to let clients learn to take responsibility for their own actions and to use their own resourcefulness in solving their problems.

CLIMACTERIC
The period of time during which the ovaries begin to fail, usually start-

ing some time before the menopause.

CLIMACTERIC PSYCHOSIS
A mental disorder formerly associated with the menopause. It is now
held in disrepute.

CLINDAMYCIN
Generic name of an antibiotic prescribed for serious infections caused
by bacteria that are generally found
to be susceptible to this drug. This
is one of the few drugs, given by
mouth, that is effective against anaerobic organisms (bacteria that
grow only in the absence of oxygen).
  Possible side effects are:
- stomach pain;
- vomiting;
- diarrhea;
- pain on swallowing.
Safety in pregnant women has not
been established. Since this drug is
transferred to the breastmilk of
nursing mothers, its use by them
should be carefully considered.The
usual dose for adults is 150 to 450
mg every six hours.

CLINIC
A medical institution in which a
group of doctors jointly examine
and treat patients.

CLINICAL
Relating to a clinic, or relating to
the signs of disease as observed by
a doctor. Also used when dealing
with the study of patients as opposed to laboratory experiments.

CLINICAL DIAGNOSIS
That made from recognition of
symptoms and signs alone.

CLINICAL STATUS
Representation of the contemporary
status of a disease, injury or other
condition.

CLINICIAN
A doctor who examines and treats

patients at the bedside.

CLITORIDECTOMY
Surgical removal of the clitoris.

CLITORIDITIS
Inflammation of the clitoris.

CLITORIS
A small cylindrical, erectile body,
situated at the front of the vulva
(the area between a woman's legs)
and projecting between the labia
majora. Like the male penis, it becomes erect on sexual stimulation.

CLOACA
The passage in animals through
which the discharge of feces takes
place. The theory frequently held by
children that birth takes place
through this appears in the writings
of psychoanalysts as the "cloaca
theory."

CLONAL PROLIFERATION
Asexual division of a single cell, resulting in a large number of prog-
eny cells (the clone) that are genetically identical to the original cell.

CLONE
The reproduction of a cell in its exact image.

CLONIC SPASM
A spasm in which the muscles or
muscle fibres rapidly contract and
relax alternatively, as in epilepsy.
The term is usually applied to a
condition that is the opposite of
tonic spasm.

CLONORCHIASIS
An inflammation of the liver resulting from ingesting cysts of the fluke
Clonorchis sinensis, an important
liver fluke in humans.
  It can live for 20 to 50 years in the
liver and passes eggs into the feces.
Light infections usually do not produce symptoms.
  Apparent cases occur mainly in
adults, when the worm load in-

creases to more than 500. Complications include cholangiocarcinoma (a type of cancer), liver disorders and chronic pancreatitis.

Thorough cooking of freshwater fish prevents infection. No treatment is advised for those showing no symptoms. No consistently effective treatment is known, although chloroquine shows results in some persons.

CLONUS
Rhythmic clonic (spasmodic) movements that occur in persons with a pyramidal syndrome on whom certain maneuvers are performed during neurological examination, e.g., ankle clonus, patellar clonus.

CLONUS, EPILEPTIC
A term used to describe the clonic phase of a convulsive seizure.

CLOSTRIDIUM
A genus of spore-bearing bacteria, some of which produce gas gangrene in wounds and tetanus.

CLOSURE
One of the principles emphasized by gestalt psychologists, describing the process by which percepts, memories, actions, etc. attain stability - namely, the subjective closing of gaps, or completion of incomplete forms, so as to constitute wholes.

CLOT
A coagulated mass of soft or fluid matter, as of blood or lymph.

CLOT REACTION TIME
The time it takes for a sample of blood to form a contracted clot, usually about one hour.

CLOTTING TIME
The time it takes a blood specimen to form a normal clot, usually five to eight minutes.

CLOUDING
Used to describe consciousness in states of psychosis, when there is some lack of orientation to a present situation.

CLOUDY SWELLING
Degeneration and swelling of the tissues arising during the course of inflammation.

CLOVE
(Eugenia caryophyllata) Evergreen tree of which the flowerbuds are used for medicinal purposes. Oil of cloves will stop the pain of a toothache when dropped into a cavity. A few drops of the oil in water will stop vomiting, and clove tea will relieve nausea. Eating cloves is said to be aphrodisiac.

CLOVER'S CRUTCH
Apparatus to maintain the position of certain organs (for instance vagina and rectum) after an operation.

CLUBBING
A pathological condition resulting from a disease of the heart or lungs, characterized by thickening of the fingertips and occasionally the tips of the toes.

The nails become unnaturally curved. Clubbing itself is harmless and needs no treatment, but the underlying ailment of the heart or lungs should be treated.

CLUB FOOT
Also called talipes: misshapen foot that is permanently bent at the ankle, the result of a congenital defect.

CLUB HAND
A misshapen hand of congenital origin.

CLYSIS
The administration of a solution to replace lost body fluid, for instance, by injection, and generally not by mouth.

COAGULANT
Agent that promotes clotting of the blood.

COAGULASE
An enzyme that speeds the clotting process in blood.

COAGULATION TIME
The time it takes for the many different coagulation factors in the blood to interact, ultimately resulting in the formation of an insoluble clot.

COAGULUM
A clot; any coagulated mass.

COAL TAR
The black substance obtained by the distillation of coal. The substance is used in the treatment of various skin diseases.

COAL TAR PREPARATIONS
Creams, ointments and lotions used on the skin for various skin ailments.

COARCTATION
Narrowing of the diameter of a vessel or canal.

COARCTATION OF THE AORTA
Congenital narrowing of the aorta (the main artery from the heart) so that blood pressure is raised on the side nearest the heart. The obstruction may occur between the points where the two arteries to the arms arise, causing blood pressure in the right arm to be higher than that in the left.

COARCTOTOMY
Surgical incision to cut a coarctation.

COBALT
Chemical element (atomic number 27) used as a source for radiation therapy. It is also a component of vitamin B_{12}.

COCA
A shrub, Erythroxylon coca, whose leaves contain various alkaloids, especially cocaine. Native to the Andes, it is widely cultivated elsewhere. The leaves have been chewed by South American Indians for centuries to quell hunger and to refresh. Cocaine-free coca extracts are used in making cola drinks.

COCAINE
A white, crystalline powder, derived from the leaves of the coca plant (Erythroxylon coca) or prepared synthetically, once used as a topical anesthetic, especially for eye, ear, nose and throat examination, but now a drug of abuse, used for its stimulating and anesthetic properties. Adverse effects include:
- restlessness;
- euphoria;
- tremors.

COCAINE INTOXICATION
Maladaptive behavioral changes and other specific signs due to the recent use of cocaine. The maladaptive behavioral changes may include:
- euphoria;
- fighting;
- grandiosity;
- hypervigilance;
- psychomotor agitation;
- impaired judgment;
- impaired social functioning;
- impaired occupational functioning.
The other specific signs may include:
- tachycardia;
- pupillary dilation;
- elevated blood pressure;
- perspiration or chills;
- nausea;
- vomiting;
- visual hallucinations;
- tactile hallucinations.
The maladaptive behavioral changes and other specific signs begin no later than one hour after administration, and may occur within

a few seconds. When the immediate psychoactive effects of high doses of cocaine have subsided, they are replaced by unpleasant rebound effects (the "crash"), including a dysphoric mood and a craving for cocaine.

The course of cocaine intoxication is usually self-limited, with full recovery within 48 hours.

COCAINE DELIRIUM
A state of high excitement with mental confusion that is the result of taking cocaine. Tactile and olfactory hallucinations may be present. Affect is often labile. Violent or aggressive behavior is common, and restraint may be required.

The delirium usually occurs within one hour of substance use and is over in about six hours. When the substance is taken intravenously, the onset is almost immediate. More rarely, the delirium follows a period of intoxication. When the other pharmacologic effects of the substance have worn off, the delirium disappears completely.

COCAINE DELUSIONAL DISORDER
An organic delusional syndrome with rapidly developing persecutory delusions as the predominant clinical feature, appearing shortly after use of cocaine.

COCAINE DEPENDENCE
Disorder associated with two different patterns of use: episodic, and chronic daily, or almost daily, use. In episodic use, the cocaine use tends to be separated by two or more days of nonuse, e.g., it may be used on weekends and once or twice during the week. "Bingeing" is a common form of episodic use consisting of compressed time periods of continuous high-dose use; e.g., consumption of several grams or more of cocaine during a single 48-hour period.

Chronic daily, or almost daily, use may be at high or low doses. Use may be throughout the course of a day or be restricted to certain hours, e.g., only during working hours or only during the evening. In this pattern there are usually no wide fluctuations in the amount of cocaine used on successive days, but there is often a general increase in doses used over time.

Cocaine smoking and intravenous administration of cocaine tend to engender rapid progression from infrequent use to cocaine abuse or dependence, often within only a few weeks or months.

Cocaine abuse and dependence are usually associated with a progressive tolerance of the desirable effects of the substance, which leads to use of increasing doses. With continuing use there is a progressive diminution in pleasurable effects and a corresponding increase in dysphoric effects.

Eventually, a point is reached at which the person still craves the cocaine despite the absence of substance-induced euphoria because of tolerance, and an accumulation of unpleasant adverse effects caused by the craving and urges for the substance rather than attempts to avoid or alleviate withdrawal symptoms.

COCAINISM
Mental and physical symptoms of a degenerative nature, caused by a morbid graving for cocaine.

COCAINE WITHDRAWAL
Dysphoric mood (e.g., depression, irritability, anxiety) and fatigue, insomnia or hypersomnia, or psychomotor agitation due to abrupt cessation of prolonged (several days or longer) heavy use of cocaine or reduction in the amount of cocaine used.

The symptoms persist more than 24 hours after cessation of the substance use.

COCCIDIOIDOMYCOSIS
An infectious disease, caused by the fungus Coccidioides immitis, occurring in a primary form as an acute, benign, self-limiting respiratory disease, or in a progressive form as a chronic, often fatal, infection of the skin, lymph glands, spleen, liver, bones, kidneys, meninges (membranes surrounding brain and spinal cord) and brain.

COCCULUS
Homeopathic medicine derived from the Indian ockle. The medicine is prescribed for motion sickness, headache, low back pain, vertigo, nausea, trembling of the hands.

COCCUS
(plural cocci) A globular or spherical bacterium, as in Staphylococcus, Streptococcus, Micrococcus.

COCCYGEAL
Relating to the coccyx (tail bone).

COCCYGECTOMY
Surgical cutting out of the coccyx (tail bone).

COCCYGODYNIA
Neuralgic or rheumatic pain in the region of the coccyx.

COCCYX
Also called the tail bone: bone situated at the end of the spine and between the buttocks. It is the remnant of the tail bone found in most other animals.

COCHLEA
Small structure, shaped like a snail shell, in the inner ear that is the fundamental organ of hearing.

COCOA
Seeds of Theobroma cacao, used as a beverage. The seeds contain theobromine and caffeine.

CO-CONSCIOUSNESS
Term used to designate dissociated

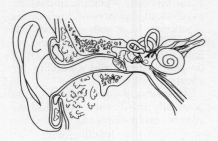

The cochlea is a winding cone-shaped tube forming a portion of the inner ear and containing the organ of hearing. The cochlea is situated in the right part of the illustration.

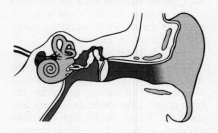

The cochlea is a winding cone-shaped tube forming a portion of the inner ear and containing the organ of hearing. The cochlea is situated in the left part of the illustration.

mental phenomena of the same order as conscious phenomena, but outside the individual's personal awareness. It is usually designated the subconscious and sometimes exhibits a high degree of organization, as in multiple personality.

CODE TEST
A type of mental test in which the subject is required either to translate, by the help of given clues, a secret code, or to write something in a code, the principles of its construction being given.

COELIAC (CELIAC) DISEASE
A chronic intestinal malabsorption disorder caused by intolerance to gluten, a protein in oats, wheat, rye and barley. This damages the mucous membrane of part of the small intestine, which in turn leads to an inability to absorb fats, calcium and

other nutrients. Symptoms usually start within a few weeks of the introduction of cereals into a baby's diet (at about four or five months). The baby starts to put on less weight (or even loses weight) and may have a poor appetite, which slows down progress even more. Several times each day he/she passes loose, pale, bulky, offensive-smelling feces, together with a lot of wind. The wind may make the baby's stomach swell, and this will contrast with his/her undernourished appearance. In some cases, ulcers develop in the mouth.

The diagnosis is confirmed on the basis of a biopsy of the lining of the small intestine. The principle treatment is to exclude wheat, rye and other grain gluten from the baby's diet.

If coeliac disease appears for the first time in an adult, the symptoms are abdominal pain and swelling, diarrhea, weight loss and a general lack of energy. Diagnosis and treatment of the disease is basically the same for adults as for children.

COELOSCOPY

Diagnostic investigation of the abdominal cavity, using a tube-like instrument called an endoscope.

COENESTHESIA

The general awareness of the body, as distinguished from the special sensations such as sight, smell, hearing, etc.

COENOTROPES

Types of acquired responses that may be regarded as the product of original nature and an environment shared in common with other organisms; alternatively, common behavior that results from common social motives.

CO-ENZYME

A compound produced by living cells that enhances or is necessary for the action of enzymes.

COERCIVE POWER

Ability to manipulate benefits and use rewards.

CO-FACTOR

A substance that is essential to the function of an enzyme.

COGENTIN

Brand name of benztropine mesylate, an anticholinergic drug used in the treatment of symptoms of Parkinson's disease.

COGNITION

A general term covering all the various modes of acquiring knowledge - perceiving, remembering, imagining, conceiving, judging, reasoning.

The cognitive function, as an ultimate mode or aspect of the conscious life, is contrasted with the affective and conative - feeling and willing.

COGNITIVE CONCEIT

Descriptive term of the child who believes that an adult who is wrong in one thing must be wrong in almost everything; but if the child is right in one thing, he/she must be correct in everything.

COGNITIVE STRUCTURE

The individual's organization of the world into a unified system of beliefs, concepts, attitudes and expectations.

COGWHEEL BREATHING

Form of jerky respiration usually seen in a neurotic person.

CO-HABITATION

Literally the living together of a man and a woman, but in legal circles, the term is used to indicate that a man and woman, living together outside marriage, have had sexual intercourse.

COITION

Copulation, sexual intercourse.

COITUS
The sexual union of a man and a woman in which the penis is inserted into the vagina, usually accompanied by excitement and often orgasm and ejaculation.

COLD, COMMON
Infection involving the nasal passages and upper part of the breathing system (not including the lungs) and including such symptoms as runny nose, watery eyes, and a sore throat. Caused by one of the many different viruses, a common cold may be treated with rest, decongestants, and increased fluids, but usually not with antibiotics, which do not affect viruses.

COLD INJURY
Injury of the extremities by cold, with secondary structural and functional disturbances of the smaller surface blood vessels, the nerves and the skin; or generalized lowering of body temperature. The old methods of slow rewarming or rubbing with or without snow should not be used.

The best treatment is by rapid local rewarming with unaffected hands or with a warm object.

COLD SORE
The common name for herpes simplex.

COLD SWEAT
A chill characterized by perspiration, often induced by a state of nervousness.

COLD URTICARIA
Hives that appear in areas of the body exposed to the cold.

COLECTOMY
Complete or partial removal of the large intestine (colon).

COLIC
Intermittent pain in the internal organs; generally experienced as bouts of severe pain with pain-free intervals. It is due to irritation or obstruction of certain organs - in particular, the gastrointestinal tract, ureter and gallbladder or bile ducts. In infants colic is often characterized by inconsolable crying, possibly due to abdominal discomfort.

Treatment of the cause is supplemented by painkillers and drugs that reduce smooth muscle spasm.

COLITIS
Inflammation of the colon.

COLITIS, ULCERATIVE
Chronic, recurring ulcers of the colon for unknown reasons.

COLLAGEN
Major component of connective tissue, constituting 70 percent of its dry weight. The fibrils making up the collagen fiber show characteristic transverse stripes under an electron microscope. These stripes are due to the arrangement of polypeptide chains like three-strand ropes. These contain a commonly occurring amino acid, glycine (each third amino acid is glycine), as well as two otherwise uncommon amino acids, hydroxyproline and hydroxylysine. The former is often used as a measure of collagen. Cross-links (consisting of an aldehyde formed from lysine) between collagen molecules further strengthen the fibrils. Collagen fibers of varying thickness are arranged in a loose mesh, which gives a low elasticity to the skin, i.e., skin can easily be dented or moulded, and these fibers are responsible for the high tensile strength of the skin. In tendons, the collagen fibers are parallel, and the elasticity of a tendon is high.

COLLAGEN DISEASE
Group of diseases whereby the collagen component of tissues is affected.
These include:

- discoid lupus erythematosus;
- vasculitis;
- systemic lupus erythematosus;
- polymyositis;
- dermatomyositis;
- some rheumatic diseases.

COLLAPSE
A more or less sudden failure of the body's vital functions; a sudden and complete failure of any kind.

COLLARBONE
Clavicle, part of the shoulder girdle.

COLLATERAL
Accessory, a small side branch, as of a blood vessel or nerve.

COLLECTING INSTINCT
Congenital impulse to obtain and hoard certain kinds of objects independently of their usefulness, the actual objects collected being, however, frequently determined by social imitation.

COLLECTIVE IMAGINATION
Imagination as represented by products such as myths that are definitely the result of cooperative or collective activity.

COLLECTIVE UNCONSCIOUSNESS
Term used, especially by Carl Jung, for those parts of the unconscious derived from racial, rather than individual, experience.

COLLES' FRACTURE
Fracture of the lower end of the radius (the forearm bone on the thumb side) giving the characteristic upward deformity said to resemble the back of a dinner fork.

COLLODION
A solution that dries to a flexible adhesive film, often used to seal slight wounds.

COLOBOMA
A congenital defect of the eye or any portion of it, usually a cleft or fissure of the iris.

COLOCYSTOPLASTY
Surgical formation of an enlargement of the urinary bladder by using part of the colon (large intestine).

COLOFAC
Trade name of a drug containing mebeverine as the active substance. The drug has atropine-like effects and is used to treat colic of the intestines.

COLON
The large intestine, from the cecum to (but not including) the rectum.

COLONIC INERTIA
Condition of the colon characterized by constipation, occurring in aged or invalid patients, especially the bedridden. Feces accumulate because the colon does not respond to the usual stimuli promoting evacuation, or because accessory stimuli provided by normal eating and physical activity are lacking. The use of drugs for associated medical conditions frequently compounds the problem. It sometimes occurs in patients whose rectal sensitivity to the presence of faecal masses is dulled by habitual disregard of the urge to defecate, or by prolonged dependence on laxatives or enemas, often initiated in childhood.

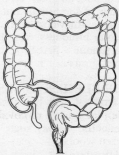

General schema of the colon with the ascending part (left), transverse part, descending part (right) and sigmoid (below).

COLONOSCOPY
Examination of the colon by inserting a flexible instrument called a fiber-optic endoscope.

COLON STASIS
Another name for colonic inertia.

COLONY
In bacteriology, a discrete group of microorganisms, such as a collection of bacteria in a culture.

COLOSTOMY
An artificial opening in the abdomen to enable the large intestine (colon) to empty into a plastic bag that is held in place by adhesive and a belt worn across the abdomen. The operation is often performed when there is cancer of the rectum, and sometimes when there is bowel incontinence, as in spina bifida, for example, or spinal injuries.

COLOSTRUM
The first thin watery fluid secreted by the breast after the birth of a child.

Although low in fat, it is rich in protein, including antibodies that are important in giving temporary passive immunity.

COLOTOMY
Incision into the large intestine.

COLOR BLINDNESS
Inability to discriminate between certain colors, an inherited trait. It is a disorder of the retina cones in the eye. The commonest form is red-green color blindness, usually found in men (about 8 percent), the other types being rare.

COLOR BLINDNESS TESTS
Three types of tests have been used for a rapid diagnosis of color defect:
(1) matching tests, such as the Holmgren wools.
(2) confusion tests in which the subject is required to recognize letters, numbers or forms, printed in confusion against a particular background.
(3) colored lights, presented under different conditions with respect to size and luminosity.

COLOR INDEX
The relative amount of hemoglobin, the red iron-containing pigment in red blood cells, expressed as the ratio of the percentage of hemoglobin to the percentage of red blood cells. The color index is a major indication for the detection of a particular type of anemia.

COLPITIS
Inflammation of the inner lining (mucous membrane) of the vagina.

COLPOCELE
Hernia protruding into the vagina.

COLPOCENTESIS
Withdrawal of blood through a small incision in the vagina.

COLPOCYSTOCELE
Protrusion of the urinary bladder into the vagina.

COLPOHYSTERECTOMY
Surgical removal of the womb via the vagina, occasionally used in cases of cancer of the uterus.

COLPORRHAGY
Hemorrhage from the vagina.

COLPORRHAPHY
Surgical procedure for repair of the wall of the vagina.

COLPOSCOPE
A special instrument with a lens (a type of endoscope) that can be inserted into the vagina to examine the interior. The method is useful for detection of disease-causing conditions of the cervix of the womb.

COLPOTOMY
Incision into the wall of the vagina.

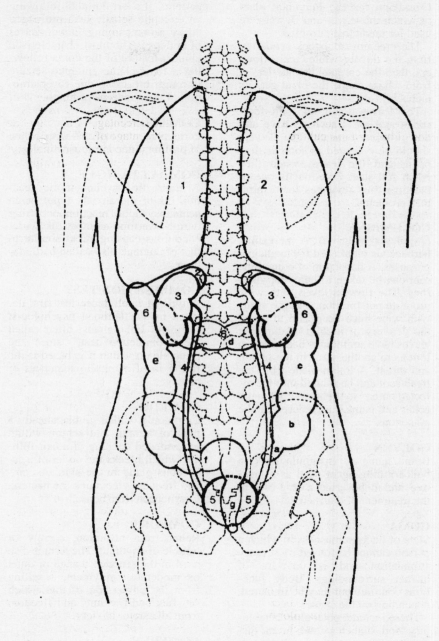

Back view of the trunk to show the location of the major abdominal and thoracic organs. 1. and 2. lungs; 3. kidneys; 4. ureters; 5. urinary bladder; 6. colon or large intestine (a. appendix; b. cecum; c. ascending colon; d. transverse colon; e. descending colon; f. sigmoid; g. rectum).

COLTSFOOT
(Tussilago farfara) Perennial plant of which the leaves and flowers are used for medicinal purposes.

The creeping rootstock sends up, first, the downy white, scaly flowers, then the cordate, dentate leaves from whose shape the plant gets its name.

The leaves stand on long footstalks and are glabrous above and downy white beneath. The flowers should be collected as soon as they open, and the leaves when they reach full size. Coltsfoot is one of the time-tried remedies for respiratory problems.

COLUMBINE
(Aquilegia vulgaris) A perennial, herbaceous plant used for medicinal purposes. A decoction of columbine root can be taken to help stop diarrhea. The flowers taken with wine promote perspiration, and the seeds with wine have been said to speed the delivery of a child. Columbine leaves have sometimes been used in lotions to soothe sores in the mouth and throat. A lotion made from the fresh root can be rubbed into the affected area to relieve rheumatic aches and pains. Large doses can be poisonous.

COLVEN
Brand name of ispaghula husk, a bulk-forming agent used as a laxative, and mebeverine, a drug used in the treatment of diarrhea.

COMA
State of unconsciousness in which a person cannot be roused by sensory stimulation and is unaware of his/her surroundings. Body functions continue but may be impaired, depending on the cause.

These include: poisoning, head injury and diabetes, and brain diseases, such as strokes and convulsions. Severe malfunction of the lungs, liver or kidneys may lead to coma.

COMA, EPILEPTIC
A coma of short duration following an epileptic seizure or a prolonged coma accompanying certain cases of epilepsy. The most characteristic clinical feature of the coma following a tonic-clonic epileptic seizure is rough breathing due to obstruction of the windpipe or lungs.

COMATOSE
Pertaining to or affected with a state of profound unconsciousness.

COMBAT FATIGUE
A traumatic psychoneurotic reaction (as of the anxiety type) or an acute psychotic reaction occurring during wartime combat or under conditions causing stress similar to that of combat; also called battle fatigue.

COMBINATION TEST
A type of intelligence test first devised by the German psychologist Hermann Ebbinghaus; often called the "completion test," since the principle on which it is based is the filling in of blanks in sentences or passages.

COMEDO
Commonly called a blackhead: a plug of keratin and sebum within the widened opening of a hair follicle, which blocks the outlet of a sebaceous gland in the skin. A comedo frequently contains the bacteria Corynebacterium acnes.

COMFORT
Relief from affliction, sorrow or trouble of any kind. The term is also used in the sense of a state of quiet or moderate enjoyment, resulting from the possession of that which satisfies bodily wants and freedom from all care or anxiety.

COMFREY
(Symphytum officinale) Perennial plant, common in moist meadows and other watery places, of which

the rootstock and the leaves are used for medicinal purposes. The rootstock is black outside, fleshy and whitish inside, and contains a glutinous juice.

A decoction of the rootstock makes a good gargle and mouthwash for throat inflammations, hoarseness and bleeding gums. It can be drunk to give relief to digestive and stomach problems, for intestinal difficulties, for excessive menstrual flow and to stop spitting blood.

COMMA BACILLUS
A bacterium of the genus Vibrio that causes Asiatic cholera.

COMMA TRACT
A small tract to the lateral cervical upper thoracic tract of the posterior white column of the spinal cord.

COMMENSAL
Living on or within another organism, and deriving benefit without harming or benefiting the host individual. Many such micro-organisms are adapted to grow on body surfaces and are potentially disease-causing.

COMMISSURE
(1) A tract of nerve fibers connecting, in the brain and nerve centers, two regions on opposite sides - the fibers are known as commisural fibers.
(2) A point or line of union or junction between two anatomical parts (as the lips at their angles or adjacent heart valves).

COMMISSUROTOMY
Surgical incision or disruption of the components of a commissure.

COMMON CAROTID ARTERY
The part of either carotic artery between its point of origin and its division into the internal and external carotid arteries.

COMMON COLD
An acute contagious disease of the upper respiratory tract caused by a virus and characterized by inflammation of the mucous membranes of the nose, throat, eyes, and eustachian tubes with a watery then purulent discharge.

COMMON-LEVEL TRAITS
Cluster of traits that are positively correlated with each other, giving rise to the interpretation that a superior individual tends to be generally superior, and an inferior individual generally inferior.

COMMON PERONEAL NERVE
The smaller of the branches into which the sciatic nerve divides passing obliquely outward and downward from the popliteal space and to the neck of the fibula where it divides into the deep peroneal nerve and the superficial peroneal nerve that supply certain muscles and skin areas of the leg and foot.

COMMON PURPURA
The most common bleeding disorder of the blood vessels, manifested by increased bruising, and representing increased fragility of the blood vessels.

COMMON SENSE
Apart from the popular use of this expression as meaning practical intelligence based on experience, it is also used to cover the ability to apprehend qualities common to various senses - the common senses - such as time, space, number.

COMMON TRAITS
Traits that are possessed to some degree by all individuals.

COMMUNICABLE DISEASE
A disease that can be transmitted from one person to another through direct contact, air vectors, food, body fluids or excreta.

COMMUNICATING ARTERY
Any of three arteries in the brain that complete the circle of Willis.

COMMUNICATION
Information or intelligence imparted by word or writing or any other means of transmitting information.

COMPARATIVE PSYCHOLOGY
The study of the relationship between species differences and behavior especially in reference to genetics and evolution.

COMPARTMENTALIZATION
Isolation or splitting off of part of the personality or mind with lack of communication and consistency between the parts.

COMPATIBLE
Medically, refers to two drugs that can be mixed together safely without one canceling out or enhancing the effect of the other.

COMPENSATION
A form of defense mechanism by which one attempts to cover up or balance failure in, or lack of talent for, one activity by a strenuous effort to excel in either a different or an allied activity.

COMPENSATORY TRAITS
The theory of trait organization, common in folklore, that good or desirable qualities balance poor undesirable ones, e.g., that beauty goes with stupidity, homeliness with intelligence.

COMPLEMENT
A complex series of 18 distinct enzymatic proteins, acting as nine functioning components, which are activated sequentially in a manner similar to the coagulation factors.

COMPLEMENT-DEPENDENT
Requiring the participation of activated complement components in blood.

COMPLEMENT FIXATION
The process of binding serum complement to the product formed by the union of an antibody and the antigen for which it is specific that occurs when complement is added to a mixture (in proper proportion) of such antibody and antigen.

COMPLEMENT-FIXATION TEST
A diagnostic test for the presence of a particular antibody in the serum of a patient that involves inactivation of the complement in the serum, addition of measured amounts of the antigen for which the antibody is specific and of foreign complement, and detection of the presence or absence of complement fixation by the addition of a suitable indicator system.

COMPLETED STROKE
The clinical condition manifested by brain damage of varying severity, usually abrupt in onset and either fatal or showing variable improvement, resulting from the interruption of blood flow to and death of brain tissue due to arteriosclerosis or high blood pressure.

COMPLETE LEARNING METHOD
Experimental method in the study of learning, where repetitions are carried out until complete reproduction is secured, an attempt to reproduce being made after each repetition.

COMPLEX
In psychological terms, an attitude accompanied by excessive emotion, often leading to neurotic types of response.

COMPLEXION
The temperament, habits, or natural disposition of the body or mind.

The term is also used in the sense of the color of the skin, particularly of the face.

COMPLICATION
In psychological terms, a mental process involving the combination of the sensations derived from the same object through different senses, in such a way that the experience of one of these sensations later tends to be accompanied by the partial revival of the others, as when the visual impression of an orange drags with it a partial revival of taste and smell sensations formerly experienced from an orange.

COMPLICATION EXPERIMENT
An experiment devised to illustrate the priority in time given to one of two simultaneous impressions to which attention is directed.

COMPOUND
Something formed by a union of elements or parts; a distinct substance formed by chemical union of two or more ingredients in definite proportion by weight.

COMPOUND FRACTURE
A bone fracture produced in such a way as to form an open wound through which bone fragments usually protrude.

COMPOUND NEVUS
A type of nevus (birthmark) that is a combination of a junctional nevus in which the pigmented cells lie in groups at the junction between the dermal and epidermal layers of the skin, and a dermal nevus, where the pigmented cells are situated entirely in the dermis.

COMPOUND REACTION
A type of reaction studied in reaction experiments, where the response is not the simple reaction to a stimulus, but a response depending on the performance of definite mental processes, such as discrimination, choice, etc. before the reaction takes place.

COMPREHENSION
Intelligent grasp of the meaning of a situation or an action. A test of comprehension is employed in the Binet scale, where the tested is asked what he/she would do in a given situation.

COMPRESS
A pad or bolster of folded linen or other material, applied with pressure, usually in the form of a wet dressing.

COMPRESSION
Act of pressing upon or together; the state of being pressed together. The act, process, or result of compressing especially when involving a compressing force on a bodily part.

COMPRESSION SYNDROME
The liberation into the bloodstream, because of severe crush injuries, of chemicals that affect the kidneys and produce profound symptoms of surgical shock.

COMPROMISE FORMATION
Any mental phenomenon that is the product of conflict and which partially expresses both parts of the conflict.

Typically, a symptom that refers to a compromise between the repressed impulse and the repressing agency.

COMPULSION
An irresistible unconscious force that makes an individual perform conscious thoughts or actions that he/she would not normally perform, perhaps even against his/her will. The force may also come from outside, i.e., from someone whose character dominates the individual.

COMPULSIVE PERSONALITY
A personality syndrome characterized by cleanliness, orderliness and obstinacy. In the extreme, behavior becomes repetitive and ritualistic.

COMPUNCTION
An uneasiness of mind or conscience.

COMPUTERIZED TOMOGRAPHY
Also called a CT or CAT (computerized axial tomography) scan: a new diagnostic method combining the technologies of radiology, computer processing and cathode ray tube display. The result is an image of the transverse of the body part studied that looks like an anatomical cross-section.

CONATION
Literally, "striving," used either as a general term inclusive of all experienced mental activity, or as the act of "striving" or "willing" being itself an ultimate type of experience, and not infrequently with confusion of these two senses.

CONCENTRATION
(1) The fixing of attention, or a high degree of intensity of attention.
(2) A crude active principle of a vegetable especially for pharmaceutical use in the form of a powder or resin.
(3) The relative content of a component (as dissolved of dispersed material) of a solution, mixture, or dispersion that may be expressed in percentage by weight or by volume, in parts per million, or in grams per liter.

CONCENTRATION CAMP SYNDROME
Post-traumatic stress syndrome; development of characteristic symptoms following a psychologically distressing event that is outside the range of usual human experience (i.e., outside the range of such common experiences as simple bereavement, chronic illness, business losses, and marital conflict). The stressor producing this syndrome would be markedly distressing to almost anyone, and is usually experienced with intense fear, terror, and helplessness.

The characteristic symptoms involve re-experiencing the traumatic event, avoidance of stimuli associated with the event or numbing of general responsiveness, and increased arousal.

CONCEPT
The properties or relationships common to a class of objects or ideas. Concepts may be of concrete things, e.g., the concept poodle referring to a given variety of dog, or of abstract ideas such as equality, justice, number, implying relationships common to many different kinds of objects or ideas.

CONCEPTION
Fertilization of the female egg cell by a male sperm; the beginning of pregnancy. The term is also used in the sense of the originating of a new idea.

CONCEPTUS
The products of conception, i.e., embryo/fetus, amniotic sac, umbilical cord, placenta.

CONCHA
The largest and deepest concavity of the external ear.

CONCRESCENCE
A growing together, especially convergence and fusion of the lateral lips of the blastopore to form the primordium of an embryo.

CONCRETE OPERATIONS
State of cognition, according to the Swiss psychologist Jean Piaget, that lasts from the age of seven to the age of ten or eleven.

CONCRETIO CORDIS
Adhesive pericarditis with the space between the layers of the pericardium mostly or completely obliterated by dense scar tissue.

CONCRETION
A tophus or other hard inorganic mass found in the body; a calculus.

CONCUBINE
An outdated term meaning a woman who cohabits with a man without being married to him.

CONCUSSION
Physical shock affecting head or spine, and usually producing brief unconsciousness with curious amnesic phenomena.

CONDENSATION
In psychology, the process by which two or more images combine or can be combined to form a composite image that is invested with meaning and energy derived from both. It is one of the primary processes characteristic of unconscious thinking, and is exemplified in dreams and symptom-formation.

CONDENSING OSTEITIS
Disorder of bone tissue usually involving the whole of a long bone and resulting in the marrow cavity filling with a dense bony mass, so that the bone becomes heavier and dense.

CONDITION
Something essential to the appearance or occurrence of something else; especially an environmental requirement for animal life.

CONDITIONED EMOTION
An emotional response acquired by conditioning, i.e. an emotion aroused by a stimulus that did not originally evoke it.

CONDITIONED REFLEX
One acquired as a result of repeated training. A famous example is the dogs trained by the Russian neurophysiologist Ivan Pavlov, which salivated when offered food at the simultaneous ringing of a bell. Eventually the mere sound of the bell was sufficient to cause the dogs to salivate.

CONDITIONED RESPONSE
The learned or acquired response to a conditioned stimulus, i.e., to a stimulus that did not evoke the response originally.

CONDITIONING
Term used to describe two quite different learning processes. In the first, a human or animal response is generated by a stimulus that does not normally generate such a response. In the second, animals (and, by extension, humans) are trained to perform certain actions to gain rewards or escape punishment.

CONDOM
A thin rubber sheath worn on a man's penis during sexual intercourse.

CONDUCT
Term used for that level of behavior that is presumably determined by foresight and volition.

CONDUCT DISORDER
Persistent pattern of conduct in which the basic rights of others and major age-appropriate societal norms or rules are violated. The behavior pattern typically is present in the home, at school, with peers, and in the community.

Physical aggression is common. Children or adolescents with this disorder usually initiate aggression, may be physically cruel to other people or to animals, and frequently deliberately destroy other people's property (this may include fire-setting). They may engage in stealing with confrontation of the victim, as in mugging, purse-snatching, extor-

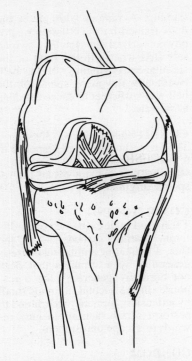

Frontal view of the knee joint; the large condyles of the femur are shown in the upper part of the illustration.

tion, or armed robbery. At later ages, the physical violence may take the form of rape, assault, or, in rare cases, homicide. Covert stealing is common.

This may range from "borrowing" others' possessions to shoplifting, forgery, and breaking into someone else's house, building, or car.

Lying and cheating in games or in schoolwork are common. The course is variable, mild forms frequently showing improvement over time and severe forms tending to be chronic.

Early onset is associated with greater risk of continuation into adult life as an antisocial personality disorder.

CONDUCTION
Used generally for the transmission of energy change along or through a body, and more particularly to de-

scribe the transmission of a nervous impulse along a nerve fiber. When a nerve impulse traverses a fiber in a direction opposite to the normal, this is spoken of as antidromic conduction. The passage of an impulse from one neuron to another is called synaptic conduction.

CONDUCTION DEAFNESS
Hearing loss or impairment resulting from interference with the transmission of sound waves to the organ of Corti.

CONDUCTIVITY
The quality or power of conducting or transmitting. The term is also used to describe the quality of living matter responsible for the transmission of and progressive reaction to stimuli.

CONDUCTOR
A substance or body capable of transmitting electricity.

CONDYLARTHROSIS
Articulation by means of a condyle (as that between the head and vertebral column involving the occipital condyles and the atlas.

CONDYLE
A protuberance on the end of a bone serving to form part of a joint with another bone. Examples are the projecting parts of bones at knees and elbows.

CONDYLECTOMY
Surgical removal of a condyle.

CONDYLOID FORAMEN
Foramen in front of each condyle of the occipital bone.

CONDYLOID JOINT
An articulation (as between the metacarpals of the hand and the first phalanx of the fingers) in which an ovoid head is received into an elliptical cavity permitting all movements except axial rotation.

CONDYLOID PROCESS
The rounded process by which the ramus of the mandible articulates with the temporal bone.

CONDYLOMA
Wart-like growth or tumor that usually arises near the anus or around the genital organs.

CONDYLOMATA ACUMINATA
Another name for genital warts.

CONE
(1) A solid having a circular base and sides that slope evenly to a point.
(2) One of the short sensory end organs of the vertebrate retina that function in color vision.
(3) Any of the numerous somewhat conical gastropod mollusks that include a few highly poisonous forms.

CONE BIOPSY
A surgical procedure in which a cone-shaped portion of the cervix is removed for examination under a microscope to determine whether or not there is disease.

CONENOSE
Any of various large bloodsucking reduvid bugs.

CONFABULATION
Unrestrained conversation; often shortened to 'confab'. The term is generally used for a pathological type of conversation in certain mental conditions.

CONFECTION
A preparation in which drugs are mixed with sugar or other substances.

CONFLICT
A painful state of consciousness due to clash between opposing emotional forces. In psychological medicine, the presence in the unconscious of two incompatible and contrasting wishes or emotions.

CONFRONTATION
Term occasionally used to describe analysts' communication in which they draw their patients' attention to some aspect of the latter's behavior without offering an explanation or interpretation of it.

CONFUSION
Disturbance of the mind in which the subject is unable to think clearly and is disorientated.

CONFUSION, EPILEPTIC
A term used to describe a confusional state, with or without agitation or delirium, likely to occur in epileptics either:
(1) during an epileptic seizure, of which it may be the only or main symptom;
(2) during generalized or partial non-convulsive status epilepticus;
(3) directly after a seizure;
(4) independently of any seizure, constituting thereby a psychiatric event apparently unrelated to true epilepsy.

CONGENITAL
Present at birth; not necessarily genetic or inherited.

CONGENITAL DEFECT
An abnormality, especially a structural one, present at birth; also called birth defect.

CONGENITAL DISABILITY
A disability, not necessarily hereditary, that is present at birth or shows itself soon after. A child may, for example, suffer an injury before birth and this is congenital although not hereditary.

CONGENITAL HEART DISEASE
Structural abnormalities of the heart, aorta and pulmonary artery present from birth.

CONGENITAL SCOLIOSIS
Sideways curvature of the spine due to a congenital defect of the development of the spine.

CONGENITAL SYPHILIS
Syphilis transmitted from the mother to the fetus via the placenta. The risk of this disease to the fetus is related to the stage of the mother's infection - i.e. untreated early syphilis is almost invariably transmitted, while the frequency is much less with the latent and tertiary stages. Congenital syphilis is preventable and occurs only in untreated pregnant women.

CONGESTION
Presence of abnormal amounts of fluids due to increased flow into the area, or decreased drainage.

CONGESTIVE
Characterized by excess accumulation of blood. In congestive heart failure, congestion occurs in the lungs, liver, kidney and other parts of the body to cause shortness of breath, swelling of the ankles and feet, rapid heartbeat and other symptoms.

CONGESTIVE HEART FAILURE
A clinical syndrome in which the heart fails to propel blood forward normally, resulting in congestion in the pulmonary artery and lungs and/or in the body's blood circulation and diminished blood flow to the tissues because of reduced cardiac output.

CONIZATION
Cutting out of a cone of tissue, as of the mucous membrane of the cervix.

CONJUGATED ESTROGENS
Generic name of female sex hormones prescribed for moderate to severe physical symptoms associated with menopause. There is no evidence that this drug is effective in relieving nervous symptoms or depression occurring during menopause.

Possible side effects are:
- breakthrough bleeding;
- changes in menstrual flow;
- candidiasis (thrush);
- cystitis-like symptoms;
- enlargement or tenderness of the breasts;
- nausea;
- vomiting;
- abdominal cramps;
- feeling of bloatedness;
- jaundice;
- skin rash;
- loss of scalp hair;
- development of new hairy areas.

The usual dose is 0.625 to 2.5 mg per day, depending on the symptoms and the woman's response.

Estrogens have been reported to increase the risk of developing certain types of pre-cancerous tissues in post-menopausal women taking such hormones for prolonged periods of time; this risk tends to depend upon the duration of treatment and on the dose of the estrogen being taken.

CONJUNCTIVA
Mucous membrane covering the inside of the eyelids and the front of the eyeball.

CONJUNCTIVAL REACTION
Result of placing a suspected substance into the eye to test whether the person is allergic to it. If positive, the white of the eye becomes pink and engorged.

CONJUNCTIVAL REFLEX
Automatic blinking of the eye when the white of it is touched.

CONJUNCTIVITIS
Inflammation of the mucous membrane lining of the eyelids and the front of the eye, caused by bacterial or viral infection, allergy, or irrita-

tion. The eyes look pink; the eyelids are stuck together in the morning, and there is discomfort, but usually not pain. Treatment depends on the cause; also called pinkeye.

CONNECTION
A wide general term, covering all kinds of relations between mental phenomena.

CONNECTIONISM
The theory that all mental processes may be regarded as involving the functioning of inherited or acquired connections between situation and response.

CONNECTIVE TISSUE
Material that supports and binds other tissues and parts of the body; it includes skin, bone, tendons, ligaments, and interlacing fibrils. Many diseases of connective tissue are difficult to cure, e.g., lupus erythematosus, rheumatoid arthritis, and sarcoidosis.

CONNECTORS
That part of the psycho-organic system whose function is to connect receptors and effectors.

CONNOTATION
A term in logic referring to the qualities, attributes and characteristics of an object designated by a word.

CONNOTATIVE MEANING
The suggestions and emotional meanings of a word or symbol, beyond its obvious meaning. Thus "naked" and "nude" refer both to an unclothed body (denotative meaning), but they have somewhat different connotations.

CONN'S SYNDROME
Primary aldosteronism; oversecretion of the hormone aldosterone by an adrenal adenoma (tumor), typically characterized by hypocalcemia (too little calcium in the blood), al-

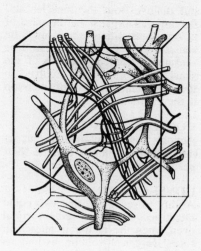

Schematic drawing of loose connective tissue showing the various types of fibers.

kalosis (increase in alkalinity of the blood) and high blood pressure.

CONSANGUINITY
The relation of persons by blood, the relation or connection of persons descended from the same stock or common ancestor.

CONSCIOUS
In psychoanalysis, the structure of the mind in which logical, conscious thought takes place. Because of confusion over the roles of conscious, consciousness, unconscious and unconsciousness (e.g., in dreams), the conscious is now often referred to as the ego.

CONSCIOUSNESS
Alertness, awareness; ability to perceive and respond.

CONSCIOUSNESS OF ACTIVITY
An unanalysable experience, such as in a psychotic disorder.

CONSCIOUSNESS OF EFFORT
An experience made up of sensations derived from various sources,

but mainly from the muscles and the internal organs. In the case of effort of attention, there may be sensations in the head, as well as sensations from adjustment of the sense organ or organs involved in the particular direction of attention at the moment.

CONSENSUAL ACTIONS
Actions that are involuntary, but accompanied by awareness of their performance.

CONSERVATION
Ability to recognize that two equal quantities of matter remain equal even when the matter is altered in form, weight or volume, as long as nothing is added or subtracted.

CONSOLIDATION
State of becoming solid. In lobar pneumonia the lobe of the lung that has become inflamed and collapsed is referred to as being consolidated.

CONSTANCY PHENOMENA
Phenomena of perception, where psychological laws seem to cut across physical laws, so that perceived objects retain to some extent certain characteristics in relative independence of change in the stimuli affecting the sense organ.

CONSTANT ERROR
A type of error occurring in psychological experiments, due to some factor that exercises a constant influence in a definite direction, and that, owing to the conditions under which the experiment must take place, cannot be eliminated.

CONSTANT REGION
The part of the polypeptide chain of a light or heavy chain of an immunoglobulin that ends in a free carboxyl group -COOH and that is relatively constant in its sequence of amino-acid residues from one immunoglobulin to another.

CONSTELLATION
Originally a grouping of ideas, determined by the operating of association, and usually round a main theme; the general usage in psychoanalysis now describes a group of emotionally colored and partially or wholly repressed ideas.

CONSTIPATION
Difficulty in having bowel movements because of loss of muscle tone in the intestine, very hard stools, or other causes.

CONSTITUTION
Total make-up of a person's character and personality. It also means an individual's ability to resist disease.

CONSTITUTIONAL REACTION
Generalized reaction of the body to an allergen other than the symptoms evoked at the site of injection.

CONSTITUTIVE
(1) Relating to, or being an enzyme or protein produced in relatively constant amounts of an organism without regard to cell environmental conditions (as the concentration of a substrate).
(2) Being chromatin of a chromosomal region that is condensed into heterochromatin in all cells of an organism rather that just some.

CONSTRAINED ASSOCIATION
A type of association experiment, where the subject's response must bear a certain defined relationship to the stimulus word.

CONSTRICTION
(1) An act or product of constricting.
(2) The quality or state of being constricted.

CONSTRICTOR
A muscle that contracts a cavity or orifice or compresses an organ.

CONSTRUCT

A term that some investigators have suggested as a substitute for "concept."

CONSTRUCTIVENESS

Behavior, sometimes instinctive behavior, that involves the utilizing of materials to build up objects relevant to the needs of the individual.

CONSULTANT

One who gives professional advice or services in the field of his special knowledge or training.

CONSUMPTION

A progressive wasting away of the body especially from pulmonary tuberculosis.

CONTAC-400

Brand name of an over-the-counter drug containing phenylpropanolamine and belladonna alkaloids as active substances. The drug is used in the treatment of the common cold.

CONTACT DERMATITIS

An acute or chronic inflammation, often sharply demarcated, produced by substances in contact with the skin.

CONTACT INFECTION

Infection or inflammation transmitted by direct contact with another person.

CONTACT INHIBITION

Cessation of cellular undulating movements upon contact with other cells with accompanying cessation of cell growth and division.

CONTACT LENS

A small lens worn directly on the cornea of the eye under the eyelid to correct defects of vision. Generally made of transparent plastic, they sometimes give better results than glasses and are certainly less noticeable.

CONTACT SENSATIONS

Light touch sensations, without the skin surface being dented due to pressure.

CONTAGION

The spreading of feelings or forms of behavior to other individuals through sympathy, imitation or suggestion.

CONTAGIOUS

A term applied to the spread of micro-organisms by personal contact and so causing disease or infection, in contrast to an indirect spread as in air or water.

CONTAGIOUS DISEASE

An infectious disease communicable by contact with one suffering from it, with a bodily discharge of such a patient, or with an object touched by such a patient or his bodily discharges. Micro-organisms are sources of contagious diseases.

CONTAGIUM

The medium by which a contagious disease is communicated, for example, a virus.

CONTAMINATION

A process of contaminating (infecting, soiling) or something that contaminates.

CONTEMPLATION

Term used specially of a phase of an experience that results from the very fact of having the experience, and involving a reaction of the individual in the form of attentive awareness of an object.

CONTIGUITY

The designation given to one of the primary laws of association, according to which, when two types of experiences have occurred together in time or place, the subsequent occurrence of one of them tends to bring the other to mind.

CONTINENCY
The restraint that a person imposes upon his desire and passions. The term is also used in the sense of the restraint of the passion for sexual enjoyment, and the ability of a person to control the action of the bladder and bowel.

CONTINGENCY
Probability of an association between two facts, qualities, occurrences or sets of data.

CONTINUITY
When the same laws regulate behavioral development within a particular age span or across the life span.

CONTRACEPTION
A process or technique for the prevention of pregnancy.

CONTRACEPTIVE
Agent that prevents conception/pregnancy.

CONTRACEPTIVES, ORAL
A group of hormonal preparations used to prevent ovulation, therefore preventing pregnancy. These hormonal preparations include both estrogens and/or progestagens.

CONTRACEPTIVES, VAGINAL
Topical medications or devices applied inside the vagina to prevent pregnancy.

CONTRACTED KIDNEY
Final stage of glomerulonephritis or chronic pyelonephritis.

CONTRACTED PELVIS
A pelvis that is abnormally small in one or more principal diameters and that consequently interferes with normal parturition.

CONTRACTILE
Having the property of being able to contract.

CONTRACTILE VACUOLE
A vacuole in a unicellular organism that contracts regularly to discharge fluid from the body.

CONTRACTILITY
A basic property of living tissue by which it contracts on stimulation.

CONTRACTION
The act of shortening, narrowing or lessening dimensions by causing the parts to approach nearer to each other.

CONTRACTURE
Abnormal condition of a muscle when it fails to return to its uncontracted condition, remaining contracted and, in certain cases, producing an anatomical deformity.

CONTRAINDICATION
Any special symptom or circumstance that renders the use of a remedy or the carrying out of a surgical procedure inadvisable. The term is also used to designate a factor in a person's current condition, medical history, or genetic make-up that may increase the risks of an adverse effect from a drug, to the extent that the drug should not be prescribed.

CONTRAST
An effect of intensifying the difference between two stimuli or sensations that are of the same type but differ markedly in quality and intensity.

CONTRAST MEDIUM
A liquid or semi-solid substance that is radio-opaque (i.e., will not allow the passage of X-rays through it); used to make internal structures visible during examinations using radiation and on X-ray film.

CONTRASUGGESTIBILITY
The tendency, characteristic of some individuals, to respond to attempts at suggestion by another person by taking exactly the opposite

view or course of action to that suggested.

CONTRE-COUP
Injury occurring on one side of an organ (as the brain) when it recoils against a hard surface (as of the skull) following a blow on the opposite side.

CONTROL
Generally the means taken to validate experimental results; employed to describe an experiment in which every condition is the same, except that which is under investigation.

For example, in drug trials, one set of people will be given the drug and another set (the control) will not, but both groups will be treated in exactly the same way.

CONTROLLED ASSOCIATION
The process in word-association experiments in which the subject is instructed to give a specific kind of associated word, e.g., a word meaning the opposite of the stimulus word.

CONTROLLED HYPOTENSION
Low blood pressure induced and maintained to reduce blood loss or to provide a bloodless field during surgery.

CONTUSION
A superficial, nonlacerating injury from a blow.

CONUS MEDULLARIS
A tapering lower part of the spinal cord at the level of the first lumbar segment.

CONVALESCENCE
Period of recovery after an illness. It is a gradual recovery of health and strength after disease.

The term is also used to designate the time between the subsidence of a disease and complete restoration to health.

CONVALESCENT CARRIER
A person or animal recovering from an infection but still harboring the disease-causing micro-organisms, and capable of transmitting them to others.

CONVALESCENT SERUM
The serum of a person who has recovered from an infection. It may be given to another person as a preventive measure as it may contain antibodies against the original infection.

CONVECTION
Transmission of heat from the hotter to the colder part; one of the systems of heat transfer in the body.

CONVERGENCE
Meeting or bringing to a central point, as in the coordinated movement of both eyes when fixing on a near object.

CONVERGENCE THEORY
The view that seeks to explain psychological phenomena in terms of convergence of specific congenital qualities with specific external situations, as against one-sided nativistic or empirical views.

CONVERSION
(1) In obstetrics: alteration of the position of the unborn baby in order to make it easier to deliver.
(2) In psychology: the process by which a complex of ideas, wishes, feelings, etc. is replaced by a physical symptom. According to Sigmund Freud, it is the emotion attaching to the complex that is converted into a physical phenomenon, not the complex itself.

CONVERSION DISORDER
An alteration or loss of physical functioning that suggests physical disorder, but that instead is apparently an expression of a psychological conflict or need. The symptoms of the disturbance are not intention-

ally produced and, after appropriate investigation, cannot be explained by any physical disorder or known pathophysiologic mechanism.

The most obvious and "classic" conversion symptoms are those that suggest neurologic disease such as:
- paralysis;
- aphonia;
- seizures;
- coordination disturbance;
- akinesia;
- dyskinesia;
- blindness;
- tunnel vision;
- anosmia;
- anesthesia;
- paresthesia.

Usually the symptom develops in a setting of extreme psychological stress and appears suddenly.

The usual age of onset is in adolescence or early adulthood, but the symptom may appear for the first time during middle age, or even in the later decades of life.

The course of this disorder is unknown, but probably is usually of short duration, with abrupt onset and resolution.

CONVERSION HYSTERIA
Form of psychoneurosis in which the symptoms are physical complaints.

Conversion symptoms differ from physical symptoms in that
(1) the loss of function corresponds to the subject's idea of how his body works and not to the facts of anatomy and physiology;
(2) the symptom can be demonstrated to fulfil a function in the subject's life;
(3) the subject adopts a curious attitude towards the symptom, typically either a histrionic one or one of indifference.

CONVERSION NEUROSIS
Neurosis in which a person converts his or her anxiety into a positive physical symptom unconnected with the real cause of anxiety.

CONVERSION REACTION
Another name for hysterical neurosis.

CONVERSION SYMPTOM
A loss or alteration of physical functioning that suggests a physical disorder, but that is actually a direct expression of a psychological conflict or need. The disturbance is not under voluntary control, and is not explained by any physical disorder.

Conversion symptoms are observed in conversion disorders, and may occur in schizophrenia.

CONVOLUTION
Folding of an organ upon itself; usually refers to the appearance of the surfaces of the brain.

CONVULSANT
A chemical substance, e.g. pentretrazol, bemegride or strychnine, the administration of which produces convulsions, especially epileptic convulsions.

CONVULSION
Classically, any involuntary contraction of the muscles of the body. Such contractions may be "tonic" or "clonic," according to whether they are continuous or spasmodic, and of either cerebral or spinal origin. Convulsions may be caused by lack of oxygen (e.g., convulsions during some bouts of fainting), toxic conditions (e.g., convulsions due to the poison strychnine), psychological factors (e.g., hysterical convulsions), or epilepsy. Nowadays, the term "convulsion" usually refers to discontinuous muscular contractions, either brief contractions repeated at short intervals or longer ones interrupted by intervals of muscular relaxation.

CONVULSIONS, FEBRILE
Convulsions during episodes of high fever. They are seen most frequently in young children (particularly up to about three years of age)

but may occur at any age.

Most febrile convulsions are epileptic in nature and are due to a sudden reinforcement of the body's predisposition towards them, which is most marked in childhood and can be reinforced by such factors as fever.

This explains why febrile convulsions frequently run in families and why they carry a good prognosis, the convulsions generally disappearing as the subject grows older and his or her convulsive predisposition diminishes.

Febrile epileptic convulsions must be distinguished from the epileptic seizures that coexist with certain brain lesions in persons with infectious diseases causing fever, and from epileptic seizures that develop into status epilepticus and cause a secondary rise in body temperature.

COOLEY'S ANEMIA
Also called thalassemia: hereditary hemolytic anemia marked by a defect in the production of normal hemoglobin.

COOMBS TEST
An agglutination test used to detect proteins and especially antibodies on the surface of red blood cells.

COOPER'S LIGAMENT
A strong ligamentous band extending upward and backward from the base of Gimbernat's ligament along the iliopectineal line to which it is attached.

COORDINATION
This term is used in two distinct senses:
(1) to describe two objects of the same class in the sense of having the same relation to a higher or including class;
(2) of muscular or motor regulation or the harmonious cooperation of muscles or groups of muscles, in a complex action or series of actions.

COPROLALIA
Uncontrolled or obsessive obscene speech. The use of obscene (as scatological) language as sexual gratification.

COPROPHAGIA
Eating of feces; the eating of excrement that is normal behavior among many animals but in man is a symptom of some forms of insanity.

COPROPHILIA
Tendency to be interested in feces.

COPROPHOBIA
Irrational dread amounting to phobia for feces.

COPULATION
Sexual intercourse or coitus.

CORIUM
Also called the dermis: the layer of the skin lying immediately beneath the epidermis. It consists of a dense bed of connective tissue and blood vessels and contains the nerves and terminal organs of sensation, the hair roots and sebaceous and sweat glands.

CORN
A painful cone of horny dead tissue found principally over toe joints and between the toes. It is the result of pressure from a badly fitting shoe.

CORNEA
The outer, transparent portion of the eye, consisting of five layers through which light passes to the retina.

CORNEAL GRAFT
Surgery of the cornea during which a diseased or damaged one is replaced by healthy, transparent human cornea from a donor.

CORNEOPLASTY
Another name for corneal graft.

CORNIFICATION
Conversion of the outer layer of skin, the epithelium, into horn or a horny substance or tissue.

CORNU
A hornlike excrescense or projection, such as cornu cutaneum, a horny excrescence on human skin.

CORONAL SUTURE
The crownlike transverse join between the parietal and frontal bones of the skull.

CORONARY ANGIOGRAPHY
X-ray studies of the coronary arteries of the heart after injection of contrast medium through a catheter.

CORONARY ARTERIES
The branches of the aorta that encircle the heart and supply its muscle with oxygenated blood.

CORONARY ATHERO-SCLEROSIS
Commonly called coronary heart disease. An irregular thickening of the inner layer of the walls of the arteries that conduct blood to the heart muscle. The internal channels of these coronary arteries become narrowed and the blood supply to the heart muscle is reduced.

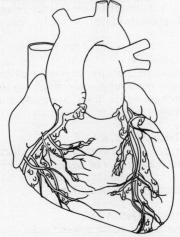

Location of the coronary arteries of the heart.

CORONARY BYPASS SURGERY
Surgery to improve the blood supply to the heart muscle when narrowed coronary arteries reduce flow of the oxygen-containing blood that is vital to the pumping heart. This reduction in blood flow causes chest pain (angina pectoris) and leads to increased risk of heart attack. Thus coronary bypass surgery involves constructing detours through which blood can bypass narrowed portions of coronary arteries to keep the heart muscle supplied.

Veins or arteries taken from other parts of the body where they are not essential are grafted on to the heart to construct these detours.

CORONARY CUSHION
A thickened band of extremely vascular tissue that lies at the upper border of the wall of the hoof of a horse.

CORONARY FAILURE
Heart failure in which the heart muscle is deprived of the blood necessary to meet the functional needs as a result of narrowing or blocking of one or more of the coronary arteries.

CORONARY HEART DISEASE
Also called coronary atherosclerosis, coronary artery disease and ischemic heart disease. Heart ailments caused by narrowing of the coronary arteries and therefore a decreased blood supply to the heart (ischemia).

CORONARY INSUFFICIENCY
A condition that occurs whenever the coronary arteries (which supply the heart muscle with blood) do not provide oxygen adequate to the needs of the pumping heart. This may produce chest pain (angina pectoris) or a heart attack, or no pain may occur at all. Acute coronary insufficiency is a term used to describe chest pain that is more se-

vere than that of angina pectoris, but in which no heart muscle damage is done (as there would be in a heart attack).

CORONARY LIGAMENT
(1) The folds of peritoneum connecting the posterior surface of the liver and the diaphragm.
(2) A part of the articular capsule of the knee connecting each semilunar fibrocartilage with the margin of the head of the fibula.

CORONARY OCCLUSION
An obstruction in a branch of one of the coronary arteries that hinders the flow of blood to some part of the heart muscle. This part of the heart muscle then dies because of lack of oxygen supply. Sometimes called a coronary heart attack or simply a heart attack.

CORONARY SCLEROSIS
Sclerosis of the coronary arteries of the heart.

CORONARY SINUS
A venous channel that is derived from the sinus venosus, is continuous with the largest of the cardiac veins, receives most of the blood from the walls of the heart, and empties into the right atrium.

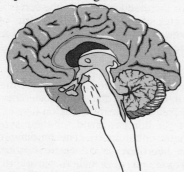

The corpus callosum consists of millions of gibers connecting the left and right hemispheres of the brain. The corpus callosum is located just below the hemispheres (just above the ventricle - shown in black).

CORONARY THROMBOSIS
Also called myocardial infarction, or heart attack, this is one of the commonest causes of serious illness and death in Western countries. The coronary arteries, which supply the heart with oxygen and nutrients, may become diseased with atherosclerosis that reduces blood flow. Significant narrowing may lead to the clotting of blood (thrombosis) in the artery, and this can cause sudden, complete obstruction and result in damage to a substantial area of heart tissue. This may end in sudden death, usually due to abnormal heart rhythm that prevents effective pumping.
Severe persistent pain in the center of the chest is common, and it may lead to shock or lung congestion. Characteristic changes may be seen in the electrocardiograph following myocardial damage, and enzymes appear in blood from the damaged heart muscle. Treatment consists of rest, painkillers and drugs to correct disordered rhythm or inadequate pumping, and some people must be carefully observed for development of rhythm disturbance. Recovery may be complete and normal activities resumed, but predisposing factors, including obesity, smoking, high blood pressure, excess blood fats and diabetes must be recognized and treated.

COR PULMONALE
Enlargement of the right ventricle of the heart that is secondary to malfunction of the lungs. This may be due to intrinsic pulmonary (lung) disease, abnormal chest bellows or a depressed ventilatory drive.

CORPUS
Body, main part of any organ.

CORPUS CALLOSUM
A mass or band of white matter joining the two halves of the brain. The corpus callosum is large, containing nearly two million fibers.

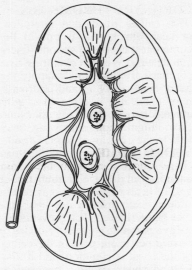

The cortex is the outer part of an organ such as that of the kidney (as shown here).

Despite its size, its functions are not clearly known, but it probably serves to allow both halves of the brain to share the experience of the other.

CORPUSCLE
Any small round body; minute end-organ of a sensory nerve; blood cell.

CORPUS LUTEUM
The yellowish endocrine tissue found in the ruptured Graafian follicle in the ovary after ovulation. It secretes the hormone progesterone for about ten days if the woman does not become pregnant; if she does, it persists for some time, being vital for readying the lining of the uterus to receive the fertilized egg.

CORRELATION
Relation between organs, structures, measurements, etc. that vary together. The most important technical use of the word in the psychological field is the statistical one, where it is applied to the tendency of two series of measurements to vary in the same way, in consequence of which knowledge of the one gives us the basis for drawing conclusions regarding the other.

CORROSIVE GASTRITIS
Degeneration of the inner mucous lining of the stomach caused by swallowing strong acids or alkalis, iodine, potassium permanganate or heavy metals. The degree of injury and the symptoms depend upon the nature and amount of the ingested substance. Gastric damage may range from only a mild blood congestion and edema (swelling) to severe necrosis (tissue death) of the mucosa.

CORSODYL
Brand name of a drug containing chlorhexidine as active compound. The drug has antiseptic and disinfectant properties and is used as gel and mouthwash.

CORTEX
The outer layer of an organ, used specially of the cerebrum and cerebellum of the brain and the adrenal glands. When the word is used alone, it always refers to the cerebral cortex.

CORTICALIZATION
An increased control by the cerebral cortex of processes of the brains of organisms that are highly placed in the phylogenetic scale.

CORTICOID
Any of the three hormones - cortisol, corticosterone and aldosterone - secreted by the outer region (cortex) of the adrenal gland, or their synthetic counterparts. The production of cortisol and corticosterone, which are also called glucocorticoids, is regulated by adrenocorticotropic hormone (ACTH) secreted by the pituitary gland.

Glucocorticoids promote the formation of glucose in the liver and are important in maintaining normal blood-sugar levels. Although the glucocorticoids also play a minor part in mineral regulation, it is the so-called mineralocorticoid action of aldosterone that primarily regulates sodium metabolism and promotes the excretion of magnesium in urine.

CORTICOSTEROID
Another name for corticoid.

CORTICOTROPHIN
Also called adrenocorticotrop(h)ic hormone (ACTH): the hormone of the anterior pituitary gland that especially stimulates the adrenal cortex to produce corticosteroids. Preparations from the anterior pituitary of mammals and synthetic varieties are available commercially for diagnostic testing of adrenocortical function and to stimulate hormone release in the treatment of certain diseases.

CORTICOTROPIN
Alternate spelling of corticotrophin.

CORTISOL
The major natural glucocorticoid hormone from the cortex of the adrenal gland.

CORTISONE
A steroid hormone of the adrenal cortex, now synthetically produced. It can be administered by mouth or by injection to cause remission, but not cure, of various inflammatory, allergic and rheumatic disorders. It must be used with caution, as long-term use can damage the adrenal glands, lead to changes in the metabolism of sugar, salt and protein, and reduce resistance to infection.

CORYZA
Acute inflammation of the mucous membrane of the nasal cavities; head cold.

COSMETIC
Any preparation or procedure that beautifies the skin or helps to improve appearance.

COSTA
A rib; *costal*: relating to the ribs.

COSTAL RESPIRATION
Breathing in which the chest movements predominate; the opposite of abdominal respiration.

COSTOTOME
A surgical instrument, such as a knife or shears, for cutting through a rib or cartilage.

COT DEATH
The common name for sudden infant death syndrome (SIDS).

CO-TENIDONE
Name of a generic drug containing atenolol (a beta-blocker) and chlorthiazide (a thiazide diuretic drug) as active ingredients.

CO-TWIN CONTROL
An experimental method employed in the study of maturation and learning in twins, the one twin being the subject and the other the control.

COTYLEDON
Any subdivision of the uterine surface of the placenta.

COUGH
A sudden, forceful and audible expulsion of air from the lungs that clears the air passages of irritants and helps to prevent aspiration of foreign particles into the lungs.

COUGH REFLEX
A cough caused by irritation of the lining of the larynx; also produced by syringing the ear.

COUNTEREXTENSION
Traction towards the body coincident with traction in the opposite direction, as with the pull of a fractured limb in opposition to the

pull of the extension apparatus.

COUNTERFEIT DRUG
A drug, or the container or labelling of which, that without authorization bears the trademark, trade name or other identifying mark, imprint or device, or any likeness thereof, of a drug manufacturer, processor, packer or distributor other than the person or persons who in fact manufactured, processed, packed or distributed such drug and which thereby falsely purports or is represented to be the product of, or to have been packed or distributed by such other drug manufacturer, processor, packer or distributor.

COURTESY
Polite manners, combined with kindness. The term is also used in the sense of polished manners or urbanity shown in behavior towards others.

COUVADE
A custom among some primitive peoples in which the father of a child being born is involved in acting out a labor. He usually remains in bed until the mother has recovered.

COWPER'S GLANDS
Bulbo-urethral glands; two small glands lying on either side of the urethra in males, below the prostate gland, and deep in the perineal membrane. They secrete lubricating fluid.

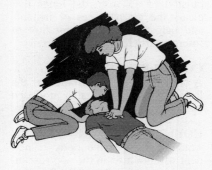

Application of cardiopulmonary resuscitation in case of choking.

COWPOX
A mild eruptive disease of milk cows caused by a virus. The disease is transmissable to humans. The lymph of those who have had cowpox is used in vaccination against smallpox.

COX or COXA
The joint of the hip.

COXALGIA
Pain in the hip or hip joint.

COXA VALGA
Deformity of the hip joint with increase in the normal angle between neck and shaft of the femur.

COXA VARA
Deformity of the hip joint with decrease in the angle between neck and shaft of the femur.

COXITIS
Inflammation of the hip joint.

COXSACKIE VIRUSES
Viruses named after the New York State village in which they were first identified. There are more than 30 of them, responsible for, among other things, herpangina, Bornholm disease and forms of meningitis.

CPR
Abbreviation for cardiopulmonary resuscitation; a procedure designed to restore normal breathing after cardiac arrest that includes the clearance of air passages to the lungs, heart massage by the exertion of pressure to the chest, and the use of certain drugs.

CRADLE CAP
A common form of seborrheic dermatitis in infants that causes the scalp to appear yellowish, scaly, and crusted.

CRAM
A method of preparing for an examination by memorizing the material immediately before the examination, mainly by repetitive methods.

CRAMP
Violent and painful contraction of a muscle or muscle group maintained for some time.

CRANIAL ARTERITIS
Another name for temporal arteritis.

CRANIAL CAVITY
Total space within the skull holding the brain and its membranes.

CRANIAL INDEX
The ratio of the full breadth of the skull to its length, multiplied by 100.

CRANIAL NERVES
The 12 pairs of nerves, each pair having sensory or motor functions, or both, that extend from the brain without passing through the spinal cord.

CRANIECTOMY
Surgical removal of a segment of the skull.

CRANIOLOGY
The science that deals with the size,

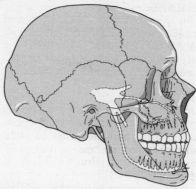

Location of the ganglion of the trigeminal nerve, one of the most important cranial nerves.

shape and other characteristics of skulls.

CRANIOMETRY
Measurement of the dimensions of the skull.

CRANIOPLASTY
Operative repair of a skull defect; any plastic operation of the skull.

CRANIOTOMY
Operation on the skull to remove a tumor, relieve pressure, evacuate blood or arrest hemorrhage.

CRANIUM
The skull or the part of the skull that encloses the brain.

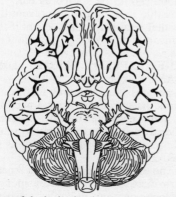

Base of the brain showing numerous cranial nerves emerging.

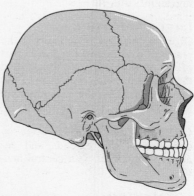

Side view of the cranium, the skull protecting the brain.

CRAZE
An effect of mass suggestion and imitation involving the uncritical, and often irrational, adoption of a style of dress, form of behavior etc., amounting sometimes to a mania.

CREATINE
Nitrogenous compound synthesized in the body; phosphorylated creatine is an important storage of high-energy phosphate.

CREATININE
The end product of creatine metabolism, found in muscle and blood and secreted in urine.

CREATINURIA
Increased concentration of creatinine in the blood; occurs in conditions in which muscle tissue is rapidly broken down.

CREATIVE THINKING
A form of directed thinking in which the subject seeks to discover new relationships, to achieve new solutions to problems, to invent methods or devices, or to produce new artistic objects or forms.

CREATIVITY
The capacity to arrive at novel but valid solutions to problems. The capacity to create imaginative products that are compelling, convincing, significant, etc.

CREDE'S METHOD
Obstetric method of delivering the placenta by rubbing the lower part of the uterus until it contracts, and then, by squeezing this part of the uterus, expelling the placenta into the vagina.

CREEPING ULCER
One that slowly extends and enlarges, sometimes with central healing.

CREMASTER
One of the fascia-like muscles in the scrotum, enveloping the testicles.

CREOSOTE
An antiseptic distilled from pine or beech.

CREPITATION
The sensation felt on placing the hand over the site of a fracture when the broken ends are moved. Also, the sound produced by broken ends of a bone, and the crackle produced by inflamed lungs.

CRESOL
Any one of three colorless, poisonous isomeric phenols, occurring in coal tar and wood tar, and mainly used as a disinfectant.

CRETINISM
Congenital disease caused by lack of thyroid hormone in late foetal life and early infancy, which interferes with normal development, including that of the brain. It may be due to congenital inability to secrete the hormone or, in certain areas of the world, to lack of dietary iodine (which is needed for thyroid hormone formation). The typical appearance, with coarse skin, puffy face, large tongue and slow responses, usually makes early diagnosis possible. It is crucial that replacement therapy with thyroid hormone should be started as early as possible to minimize or prevent the mental retardation that occurs if diagnosis is delayed.

CREUTZFELDT-JAKOB DISEASE
A progressive, inevitably fatal, slow virus disease of the central nervous system, characterized by progressive dementia and spasmodic muscle seizures, and affecting adults in mid-life.
    The disease is related to the "mad-cow-disease" (bovine spongy encephalopathy), in so far that both are caused by a small protein, called

prion. Treatment of the disease amounts to the relief of symptoms.

CRIBRIFORM PLATE
Bone in the skull perforated with numerous holes through which nerve filaments pass.

CRICOID CARTILAGE
The lowermost ring-shaped cartilage of the larynx.

CRI-DU-CHAT SYNDROME
A hereditary congenital syndrome characterized by microcephaly (abnormally small head), severe mental deficiency and a plaintive cat-like cry. One of the number 5 chromosomes is partly lost.

CRIMINAL PSYCHOLOGY
The branch of psychology which investigates the psychology of crime and of the criminal.

CRIPPLE
One who halts or limps, one who has lost or never enjoyed the use of his/her limbs.

CRISIS
The change of a disease or discomfort or disorder that indicates recovery or death. The term is also used in the sense of the decisive state of things, or the point of time when an affair has reached its height, and must soon terminate or suffer a material change.

CRISIS INTERVENTION
Intervention procedures designed to occur during any state or condition of an individual that is judged to be time-critical to avoid a consequent condition considered extremely undesirable.

CRISTA GALLI
Uppermost triangular portion of the thymoid bone.

CRITICAL PERIOD
Time when behaviors or the environment have a pronounced positive or negative effect more than at any other time.

CRITICAL SCORES
Scores based on experience with tests used for a given purpose, so that the persons scoring below the critical level are rejected as unlikely to succeed; e.g. a critical score on an examination is one below which no candidate is accepted for admission to a place of higher education.

CROHN'S DISEASE
Another name for regional enteritis.

CRO-MAGNON MAN
A race of primitive humans named for Cro-Magnon in France, dating from the Upper Paleolithic era and usually regarded as Aurignacian, although possibly more recent. Coming later than Neanderthal man, the Cro-Magnon people were dolichocephalic with high foreheads and large brain capacities, their faces rather short and wide. Males were probably around 1.70 m (5 ft 7 in) tall, powerfully muscled and robust.

CROSS ALLERGY
Sensitization to a particular substance that results in allergy to one or more chemically similar substances or to substances forming similar metabolites.

CROSS BIRTH
Birth in which the baby lies transversely across the womb with no part descending into the birth canal.

CROSS-CONDITIONING
A type of conditioning arising as a secondary result from entirely irrelevant stimuli received in the course of a response to primary conditioning.

CROSSED REFLEX
A reflex response on one side of the body, elicited by a stimulus on the other side.

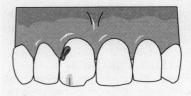

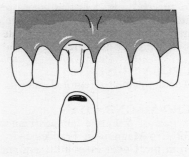

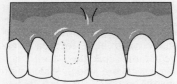

Artificial crown replacing the original crown in case of caries.

CROSS EDUCATION
Improvement in motor performances as a result of practice in that or a similar performance by one side or part of the body, produced in another side or part, itself unpracticed.

CROSS-EYES
Common name for strabismus.

CROSS INFECTION
Infection transmitted between persons with different types of germs.

CROSSING-OVER
The exchange of corresponding segments between maternal and paternal homologous chromosomes, occurring after fertilization, when maternal and paternal chromosomes are paired during prophase of the first meiotic division.

CROSSMATCHING
Determining the suitability of donor's blood with a recipient's blood prior to blood transfusion.

CROSS-OUT TEST
Test in which the tested is asked to cross out items, according to definite instructions or principles.

CROSS REACTION
The reaction between an antibody and an antigen with a non-homologous but very similar combining site.

CROTAMITON
A drug used against scabies. The solution should not be used on large skin areas in babies or near the eye. If dermatitis is also present, a specialist should be consulted.

CROTCH
The part of the human body where the legs meet.

CROUP
An acute viral inflammation of the upper and lower respiratory tracts, characterized by harsh breathing, swelling of the entrance to the larynx and respiratory distress that is most pronounced on breathing in.

CROWN
Portion of a tooth above the level of the gums. In cases of caries or tooth decay, the original, pathological crown is often replaced by an artificial crown of gold or porcelain.

CROWNING
Time during the second stage of labor when the fetal head (or crown) appears at the exit of the birth canal.

CRUDE DEATH RATE
The ratio of total deaths to total population during a given period of time, such as a year. It is calculated by dividing the total number of deaths during the year by the mid-

year population (estimated population on 1 July) of the same year.

CRUELTY
Disposition to take pleasure, or find satisfaction, in causing suffering to animals or to other human beings.

CRUISING
The act of taking steps while holding onto supports, such as furniture.

CRUSH SYNDROME
A condition resulting from damage to the renal tubules in kidneys following severe injury to muscle tissue in crushing accidents. The condition is characterized by: edema (excess fluid), oliguria (abnormally low excretion of urine) and other symptoms of renal failure.

CRUST
Dried serum, blood or pus. Crusting is encountered in a wide variety of inflammatory and infectious diseases.

CRUTCH
Staff with a cross-piece at the top, usually used in pairs by those with injured or disabled lower limbs; also, the part of the human body where the legs meet.

CRUTCH PALSY
Also called drop wrist: paralysis of the extensor muscles of wrist, fingers and thumb from repeated pressure of a crutch upon the radial nerve in the armpit.

CRYANESTHESIA
The inability to sense cold.

CRY, EPILEPTIC
A harsh cry lasting several seconds and caused by the passage of air through the upper respiratory tract at the beginning of the tonic phase (continuous muscle spasm) of most tonic - clonic epileptic seizures. This cry may be preceded by a hiccuping cry accompanying the mus-

cle spasm that sometimes occurs before such a seizure. It is always followed by sounds that are synchronous with each jerk in the clonic phase (interrupted muscle spasm), and by stertorous breathing noises after the seizure. More rarely, an epileptic cry may be uttered during tonic epileptic seizures.

CRYOGLOBULINS
Immunoglobulins that precipitate only in cold temperature; found mainly in the presence of blood vessel illness.

CRYOPEXY
Surgical fixation with freezing.

CRYOPROBE
Freezing probe; a flexible metal tube containing liquid nitrogen.

CRYOSURGERY
Surgery with special instruments using extreme cold to destroy or remove diseased tissue.

CRYOTHERAPY
Treatment of disease by means of cold.

CRYSTAPEN
Brand name for a penicillin drug containing the antibiotic penicillin G as active ingredient.

CRYPTESTHESIA
A general term covering the varieties of alleged supernatural modes of insensibility, such as telepathy, clairvoyance, clairaudience and the like.

CRYPTOMENORRHEA
The occurrence of menstrual symptoms without external bleeding, as in imperforate hymen.

CRYPTOMNESIA
Memory without identification or recognition of something as a previous experience, original experiences being forgotten or repressed,

and their reinstatement appearing as a new experience.

CRYPTORCHIDISM
Failure of the testicles to descend in the scrotum.

CRYSTALLINE LENS
Lens of the eye, situated behind the pupil. When this becomes opaque and milky in appearance, it is called a cataract.

CRYSTALLIZED INTELLIGENCE
Component of the intelligence that is developed through experience and is dependent upon a person's cultural and educational background.

CRYSTALLURIA
The appearance of crystals in the urine.

CT SCAN
Common name for computerized tomography.

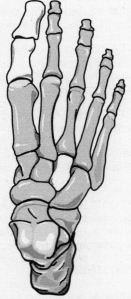

The cuneiform bones are part of the skeleton of the foot; they are located just in front of the calcaneus and talus.

CUBEB
(Piper cubeba) Perennial vine or shrub of which the unripe fruit is used for medicinal purposes. To make an infusion: steep 1 teaspoon cubeb berries in 230 ml (8 fl. oz) water. Take hot or cold, a mouthful three times a day or 115 ml (4 fl. oz) before bed. Cubeb is helpful for digestion, catarrh, bronchitis, coughs and lung problems. Cubeb oil is useful for urinary ailments and acts as an antiseptic against gonorrhea.

CUBITUS
The forearm or elbow.

CUBITUS VALGUS
Deformity of the elbow in which the forearm, when extended, deviates outwards in relation to the upper arm.

CUBITUS VARUS
The same as cubitus valgus but with the forearm deviating inwards.

CULDOCENTESIS
Aspiration of the pouch of Douglas (behind the rectum) for collection of fluid.

CULDOSCOPY
Visual examination of the female internal sexual organs through an endoscope introduced into the pelvic cavity through the posterior part of the vagina.

CULTURE
The propagation of microorganisms of living tissue cells in media conducive to their growth; the development of microorganisms on artificial media.

CULTURE-FAIR TESTS
Intelligence tests constructed to present situations and concepts common to various cultures.

CUNEIFORM BONE
Any of three wedge-shaped bones

of the foot that articulate with the navicular bone proximally and the bases of the first, second and third metatarsal bones distally.

CUNNILINGUS
A form of sexual behavior consisting of oral stimulation of the female genitalia.

CUPLEX
Brand name of a wart preparation containing copper acetate, lactic acid, and salicylic acid as active ingredients.

CUPPING
The application of a cupping glass - a small, bell-shaped glass in which the air is expanded by heating - on to skin to draw blood to the surface.

CUPRUM METALLICUM
Homeopathic drug derived from copper. It is prescribed for spasmodic conditions, cramps, convulsions, violent intermittent pain.

CURARE
A blackish, resin-like substance extracted from various tropical plants. Taken by mouth, it is practically inert. Used intravenously or intramuscularly, it produces muscular relaxation induced by the blocking of nerve impulses at the nerve endings in muscle.

A pure alkaloid derived from it is used as a relaxant before the giving of an anesthetic, enabling the dose of the latter to be as low as possible.

CURE
Most successful result of medical treatment.

CURETTAGE
Scraping with a curette.

CURETTE
A scoop-shaped surgical instrument for removing or scraping away foreign matter and granulations from the walls of a body cavity, such as the uterus.

CURRENT STATUS
Representation of the functional/dysfunctional processes and states that are operative at a given time.

CUSHING'S DISEASE
Excessive hormone stimulation of the cortex of the adrenal gland by a tumor of the pituitary gland, resulting in obesity, virilism (in females), high blood sugar and sugar in the urine, and high blood pressure.

CUSHING'S SYNDROME
A constellation of physical abnormalities due to chronic exposure to excess amounts of cortisol or related corticosteroids from the adrenal glands.

CUSP
A pointed or rounded projection, such as the crown of a tooth or the segment of a heart valve.

CUSTODIAL CASE
An individual requiring supervision and a measure of segregation, because of handicap, defect, mental disorder or criminality.

CUTANEOUS ABSCESS
Collection of pus on the skin causing fluctuating soft-tissue swelling that is congested with blood.

CUTANEOUS LUPUS ERYTHEMATOSUS
Another name for discoid lupus erythematosus.

CUTICLE
A layer of more or less solid substance covering the free surface of an epithelial cell in the outer layer of the skin.

CUTIS LAXA
A rare disorder characterized by lax skin hanging in loose folds. There is

no specific treatment, but plastic surgery considerably improves appearance.

CVA
The abbreviated term for cerebral vascular accident (commonly called 'stroke'), caused by cerebral hemorrhage, thrombosis or embolism, the consequence of which may be paralysis of one side of the body and/or speech disorders.

CYANOPIA
Vision in which all objects appear to be blue in color.

CYANOSIS
Bluish discoloration of the skin and mucous membranes, occurring when the oxygen in the blood is sharply diminished, as in carbon monoxide poisoning.

CYBERNETICS
The science of communication, information and feedback and control mechanisms in animals and machines.

CYCLICAL SYNDROME
Another name for pre-menstrual syndrome.

CYCLIMORPH 10
Brand name of a drug containing morphine as the active compound. It is used - under strict medical supervision - to treat severe pain syndromes.

CYCLITIS
Inflammation of the ciliary body of the eye.

CYCLOID
A personality type, characterized by oscillation between excitement and depression.

CYCLOPENTAMINE
Ephedrine-like drug used for the treatment of nasal congestion accompanying the common cold.

CYCLOPHORIA
Variety of muscular imbalance of the eyes, in which one eye tends to move slightly out of position round the horizontal axis. The eye is usually under control when it is fixed on one object, but the condition shows itself when the stimulus to focus is withdrawn.

CYCLOPLEGIA
Paralysis of the ciliary muscles of the eye, resulting in loss of the ability to change focus.

CYCLOTHYMIA
A chronic mood disturbance, of at least two years' duration, involving numerous hypomanic episodes and numerous periods of depressed mood or loss of interest or pleasure of insufficient severity or duration. The disorder usually begins in adolescence or early adult life.

CYLINDROMA
A tumor containing elongated twisted cords of hyaline material, found in malignant salivary gland and skin tumors.

CYMALON
Brand name of a drug containing sodium bicarbonate, citric acid, sodium citrate, and sodium carbonate as active ingredients. The drug is used in the treatment of inflammation of the urinary bladder.

CYST
A closed, fluid-filled sac embedded in tissue (as in the breast) that is abnormal or results from disease.

CYSTADENOMA
Growth containing an adenoma (tumor of a gland) and cysts.

CYSTATHIONINURIA
A hereditary disorder of cystathionine metabolism marked by increased concentration of cystathionine in the urine.

The disorder is characterized by

severe mental deficiency.

CYSTECTOMY
Surgical removal of a cyst, the cystic duct, part of the gallbladder or part of the urinary bladder.

CYSTICERCOSIS
Tropical disease caused by infection with cysticerci, a type of tapeworm. The illness is characterized by muscular pain, general muscular weakness, fatigue, loss of weight and nervous excitability.

CYSTIC FIBROSIS
An inherited disease, usually recognized in infancy or early childhood, in which the glands, esp. those of the pancreas, lungs, and intestines, become clogged with thick mucus.

CYSTINE
An amino acid, occurring among the hydrolytic products of protein, notably keratin and insulin.

CYSTINOSIS
Metabolic disorder in which cystine is deposited in the body. In childhood, osteomalacia (softening of the bones) may be the result.

CYSTINURIA
An inherited defect in the renal tubules in which resorption of the amino acid cystine is impaired, urinary excretion is increased and cystine calculi (stones) often form in the urinary tract.

CYSTITIS
Inflammation of the urinary bladder.

CYSTOCELE
Protrusion of the urinary bladder into the vagina. One of the forms of prolapse seen in some women following a series of pregnancies and deliveries.

CYSTOCOLOSTOMY
Operation in which the gallbladder is joined to the large intestine and a permanent communication is made between them.

CYSTODIATHERMY
The application of a cauterizing electrical current to the walls of the urinary bladder.

CYSTOGRAPHY
A diagnostic radiological method (using X-rays) of the urinary bladder achieved by passing a specific solution into the bladder. In this way, it is possible to make visible the interior of the urinary bladder.

CYSTOLITHIASIS
Formation of small stones in the urinary bladder.

CYSTOMETRY
The measurement of pressure in the urinary bladder.

CYSTOPEXIA
Surgical operation that fixes the urinary bladder to the abdominal wall.

CYSTOPLASTY
Surgical repair of the urinary bladder.

CYSTOSCOPY
Endoscopic method of examining the urinary bladder by passing a lighted tube through the urethra.

CYSTOSTOMY
Formation of an opening into the bladder by making a hole in the skin so that the urine passes through this aperture and not through the normal channel.

CYSTOTOMY
Incision into the urinary bladder.

CYSTO-URETHROGRAPHY
X-ray examination of the urinary bladder and the urethra.

CYSTO-URETHROPEXY
Forward fixation of the urinary

bladder and urethra to treat urine incontinence.

CYTODIAGNOSIS
Diagnosis based on the examination of cells.

CYTOGENETICS
A branch of genetics dealing with the cytologic basis of heredity; i.e., with the study of chromosomes.

CYTOLOGY
The study of cells, their origin, structure, function and pathology.

CYTOMEGALOVIRUS INFECTION
A virus infection occurring before or just after birth or at any age, and ranging in severity from a silent infection without consequences, through disease manifested by fever, hepatitis and severe brain damage in newborns, to stillbirth or perinatal death. There is no specific treatment.

CYTOPLASM
The living material of the cell outside to the nucleus.

CYTOPLEGIC
The action of paralysing the ciliary muscle in the eye. This muscle alters the shape of the lens when it contracts, enabling the eye to focus on objects. A cytoplegic drug prevents this action, and by doing so makes both examination of, and surgery on, the eye easier.

CYTOSTASIS
Arrest or hindrance of cell development.

CYTOTOXIC
A drug that kills or damages cells, most commonly used in the treatment of cancer. Although they primarily affect abnormal cells, they may also kill or damage healthy cells.

CYTOTOXIC ANTIBODIES
Antibodies that cause damage to antigenbearing cells, especially in the presence of complement.

CYTOTOXIC REACTION
Another name for type II hypersensitivity reaction.

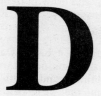

D

DA COSTA'S SYNDROME
Anxiety state in which palpitations are the most prominent symptom.

DACRYOADENITIS
Inflammation of a tear gland.

DACRYOCELE
Protrusion of a tear sac next to the eye.

DACRYOCYST
Lacrimal or tear sac.

DACRYOCYSTITIS
Inflammation in a lacrimal or tear sac, usually the result of abscess formation and obliteration of the tear duct.

DACRYOCYSTOTOMY
Surgical removal of a tear sac.

DACRYOLITH
Stony hardening of a tear sac.

DACRYORRHEA
Excessive flow of tears.

DACRYOSTENOSIS
Narrowing of a naso-lacrimal (tear) duct, often resulting from a congenital abnormality or an infection.

DACTYL
A finger or toe; *dactylate*: resembling a finger or toe.

DACTYLITIS
Inflammation of a finger or toe.

DACTYLOLOGY
Art of communication by means of signs with hands and fingers.

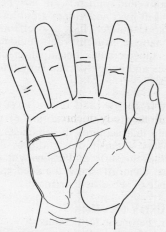

Dactylus is the professional medical term for finger or toe.

DACTYLOMEGALY
Abnormally large fingers or toes.

DACTYLOSCOPY
An examination of fingerprints, employed as a method of personal identification.

DACTYLOSPASM
Cramp in a finger or toe, usually due to decrease in blood flow to the end of the extremity.

DALTONISM
Color blindness, especially the inability to distinguish between red and green.

DANCING MANIA
An uncontrollable impulse, which has sometimes appeared in epidemic form, as a result of mass suggestion.

D&C
Abbreviation of dilatation and curettage.

DANDELION
(Taraxacum officinale) The leaves and root of this herb are useful as a

blood purifier. High in essential vitamins and minerals, it has been used in liver and kidney troubles as a blood builder. It is also effective for fatigue, skin disorders including age spots, cramps, constipation, diabetes and hypoglycemia (low blood sugar).

DANDRUFF
A harmless scaly condition of the scalp that acquires the character of disease when its unsightliness distresses the sufferer. Persons with severe dandruff show a raised incidence of seborrheic dermatitis.

DANDY FEVER
Another name for dengue.

DANERAL-SA
Trade name of an antihistamine drug containing pheniramine as the active ingredient.

DANGEROUS DRUGS ACT
Act designed to control the manufacture, sale, prescribing and dispensing of certain habit-forming drugs, to which an addiction may arise. The principal drugs concerned are: opium, cocaine, morphine, heroin, marijuana, cannabis.

DARIER'S DISEASE
Skin disease caused by an autosomal dominant gene. The findings are follicular papules ("gooseflesh") or brownish, greasy, odorous patches of overgrown horny skin, largely on the seborrhoea areas (where the skin is greasiest). Changes in and pitting of the fingernails may be present.

DARROW'S SOLUTION
Mixture of potassium chloride, sodium chloride and sodium lactate, used in gastroenteritis and other conditions in which a significant loss of salt occurs.

DARTOS
The muscular tissue beneath the skin of the scrotum, which is able to tighten up and draw in the organ, as in cold weather.

DARWINISM
The doctrine of Charles Darwin describing the origin and modifications of animals and plants. Its principle points are: there is a tendency towards variation in organic beings, so that descendants may differ very widely from progenitors; humans, animals and plants tend naturally to multiply rapidly; there is continuous struggle for existence among all organized beings; the strongest and best fitted for particular surroundings naturally survive.

DAYDREAMING
Type of fantasy, in which the individual allows his or her mind to wander aimlessly among pleasant imagery, gratifying wishes that are ungratified in real life.

DAYMARE
Acute anxiety seizure in the waking state.

DAY NURSE CAPSULES
Brand name of a drug containing dextramethorphan (a cough depressant) and paracetamol (a non-narcotic pain reliever) and phenylpropanolamine (a decongestant) as active compounds used for the relief of symptoms of severe congestion of mucous membranes.

DAY RESIDUES
Term used by Sigmund Freud and other psychoanalysts to describe emotional or worrying experiences of the preceding day that play a part in forming the contents of dreams.

DAY TREATMENT
The provision of a planned therapeutic program during most or all of the day for people needing broader programs than are possible through out-patient visits, but who do not require full-time hospitalization.

Physiotherapy, occupational therapy, medicines and other treatment methods are provided.

DDT
(dichloro-diphenyl-trichloroethane)
Also called dicophane: a chlorinated hydrocarbon insecticide. DDT is available as wettable powders of 25 percent to 75 percent concentrations; emulsified concentrated liquids of up to 50 percent; dusts of usually 10 percent. Most household sprays contained 5 percent solutions in liquid paraffin. DDT is no longer on the market for commercial use.

A single ingestion of 10 mg per kilogram of body weight will produce symptoms in some subjects.

Convulsions in humans are frequent with doses greater than 16 mg/kg taken by mouth, and a dose of 20 g in an adult produces severe symptoms lasting several weeks. Almost all fatalities have occurred from ingesting DDT in various solvents.

With many household sprays of low DDT concentration, the liquid paraffin solvent is responsible for most of the toxicity, i.e., hydrocarbon pneumonia.

Major symptoms are:
- nausea;
- vomiting;
- perspiration;
- tingling;
- pins–and–needles;
- central nervous system stimulation;
- tremor;
- seizures;
- confusion;
- apprehension;
- irregular pulse.
Death results from respiratory failure and/or abnormal heart rhythms.

DEAD HAND
Also called dead fingers: condition marked by disturbances of the circulation in the fingers in various diseases, but found especially in workers handling such vibrating tools as rotary cutters and pneumatic drills.

DEAF
Lacking the sense of hearing, either wholly or in part.

DEAF-AND-DUMB ALPHABET
A system of signs made with the hands for letters and some words.

DEAF-MUTE
A person who is both deaf and dumb, especially one whose dumbness dates from birth or early life.

DEAFNESS
Partial or complete loss of hearing in one or both ears, caused by the absence or incomplete development of the ear, the auditory nerve, or parts of the brain; by damage to the hearing apparatus; or by degeneration of the hearing apparatus.

DEAGGRESSIFICATION
The process by which the aggressive energy of infants loses its primitive, aggressive quality when the impulses to which it is attached are sublimated.

DEAMINATION
Removal of the amino group of a compound; this metabolic process occurs in the liver whereby amino acids are broken down.

DEATH
The state of the body in which brain function ceases and heart function can be maintained only artificially; the state at which loss of brain and heart function is not reversible.

DEATHBLOW
A blow causing death; anything that extinguishes hope or blights one's prospects.

DEATH FANTASY
Imagining oneself as being dead, and at the same time being aware of what is going on. Typical for

manic-depressives who often imagine themselves lying in a coffin while watching the reactions of their families and friends.

DEATH INSTINCT
According to Freud's theory, the impulses aiming at destruction, death or escape from stimulation on the part of the individual, as contrasted with the life instincts, and primarily appearing as the repetition compulsion, in consequence of which the individual must seek death only by repeating the normal life cycle.

DEATH MANIA
A form of psychomotor overactivity that may take place in conjunction with religious experience.

DEATH RATTLE
A rattling sound made by a person immediately before dying, caused by air passing through mucus in the throat.

DEBAUCHERY
Excessive indulgence in sensual pleasures of any kind, such as gluttony, intemperance, indulgence of lust.

DEBILITY
A state of general bodily weakness; feebleness.

DEBRIDEMENT
Surgical cleaning of a wound in which all damaged, infected and dead tissue is cut away.

DECALCIFICATION
The loss or removal of lime (calcium salts) from bones.

DECAPSULATION
Surgical stripping of the capsule (outer covering) of an organ, especially the capsule of a kidney that has stopped functioning, in an attempt to get it to secrete urine.

DECAY
The gradual process of losing original form, quality or value or falling into disrepair or great shabbiness.

DECEREBRATION
Elimination of cerebral function by cutting across the brain stem or by tying off the common carotid arteries and basilar artery at the center of the pons. The result is a state of deep unconsciousness.

DECHLORIDATION
Removal of sodium chloride from the body by restricting the dietary intake of salt.

DECIBEL
Tenth of a bell: the unit for measuring the volume of sound. A decibel is the lowest intensity of sound at which any given note can be heard.

DECIDUA
A membrane that develops in the upper layer of the mucous membrane lining the uterus, which is shed during each menstrual period or after childbirth.

DECIDUOMA
A uterine tumor.

DECIDUOUS TEETH
The first set of twenty teeth, which usually begin to erupt at about six months of age. Also called baby teeth or primary teeth.

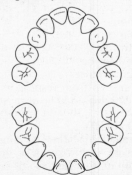

Deciduous teeth in the upper and lower jaw.

DECIDUOUS TOOTH
One of the 20 temporary milk teeth that are replaced by the permanent teeth between the ages of about seven and twelve.

DECLINE
A gradual decrease of physical power: wasting away of the body or the period of abatement in a disease.

DECOCTION
An extract obtained by boiling a medicinal plant.

DECOMPENSATION
Failure of compensation, usually refers to the heart and circulation failing, when the heart is unable to compensate for its deficiency.

DECOMPRESSION
Removal of pressure. Usually refers to a surgical operation performed to relieve pressure on the brain either by making burr holes in the skull or by raising a depressed fracture of the skull. It also refers to the slow process of bringing back to ordinary atmospheric pressure divers and caisson workers who have been operating under highly pressurized conditions.

DECOMPRESSION SICKNESS
Another name for caisson disease.

DECONGESTANT
An agent or drug that relieves congestion, especially in the mucous membrane of the nose. Decongestants are generally medicines that open nasal passages by shrinking swollen membranes lining the nose.

DECONGESTION
Relief of congestion or swelling.

DECONTAMINATION
Removing the clothes and cleaning the skin of individuals who have been exposed to toxic agents such as mustard gas, radiation, etc.

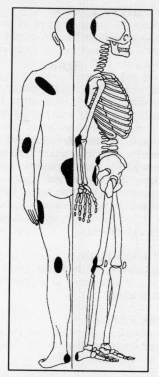

Occurrence of decubitus in preferred places of the body, where the bony structure of the skeleton is close to the surface.

DECORTICATION
Removal or stripping off the surface of an organ, as the removal of the capsule of the kidney.

DECORUM
Conformity to social standards of behavior and conduct, more particularly as regards the maintaining of one's personal dignity and self-respect in public.

DECREMENT
The period in the course of a muscle contraction when the force is subsiding.

DECRUDESCENCE
Decline in the severity of a disease.

DECUBITUS
Position when lying in bed.

DECUBITUS ULCER
Another name for bedsore or pressure sore: ischemic necrosis and ulceration of tissues overlying a bony prominence that has been subjected to prolonged pressure against an external object (e.g., bed, wheelchair, cast, splint). It is seen most frequently in patients who have diminished or absent sensations or are debilitated, emaciated, paralysed or otherwise long bedridden. The best treatment for pressure sores is prevention. A well-balanced diet, high in protein, is important. Blood transfusions may be needed for anemia. Most advanced ulcers require surgical treatment.

DECUSSATION
The crossing of two lines, rays or nerves, which meet in a point and then diverge.

DEEP REFLEX
A muscular reflex elicited by tapping the tendon of a muscle close to the attachment at the bone.

DEEP SENSIBILITY
Ability to feel sensations that depends on receptors lying deep in the skin.

DEER-FLY FEVER
Common name for tularemia.

DEFECATION
Act of opening the bowels; to void excrement from the bowels.

DEFEATISM
Mental acceptance of defeat before the real test takes place, thus making real defeat more likely.

DEFECTIVE DELINQUENT
A young delinquent, who is also mentally defective, and in whom the mental defect is a contributory factor in the delinquency.

DEFEMINATION
Loss of secondary female sexual characteristics, usually as a result of hormonal defects.

DEFENSE
A general designation for all the techniques that the ego makes use of in conflicts that may lead to neurosis. The function of defence is to protect the ego, and defences may be instigated by:
(1) anxiety due to bad instinctional tension.
(2) anxiety due to a bad conscience.
(3) realistic dangers.
The concept of defense is usually stated in terms that imply that the human ego is beset by threats to its survival emanating from the id, the super ego and the outside world, and that it is, therefore, perpetually on the defensive.

However, the concept should be regarded less negatively and taken to include all techniques used by the ego to master, control, channel and use forces that may lead to a neurosis. The concept also implies that neurosis is due to a failure of defense; according to this view, the inhibitions resulting from successful repression are not neurotic symptoms.

DEFENSE MECHANISM
Involuntary or unconscious measures adopted by an individual to protect him/herself against a painful emotion associated with some highly disagreeable physical or mental situation of frequent occurrence; may be employed to cover a wide range of the phenomena emphasized by analysts, from repressions and forgettings to mannerisms and the like, unconsciously assumed to cover a defect.

Defense mechanisms are patterns of feelings, thoughts, or behaviors that are relatively involuntary and arise in response to perceptions of psychic danger.

They are designed to hide or to alleviate the conflicts or stressors that give rise to anxiety. Some defense mechanisms, such as projection, splitting, and acting-out, are almost invariably mal-adaptive. Others, such as suppression and denial, may be either maladaptive or adaptive, depending on their severity, their inflexibility, and the context in which they occur.

DEFENSIVE REACTION
The resulting behavior of defense mechanisms. The term also includes defensive measures adopted more or less consciously to avoid exposing something that there is a strong desire to conceal.

DEFERENTITIS
Inflammation of the vas deferens of the male genital organs.

DEFERRED SURGICAL SHOCK
Shock that comes on only after an interval following an operation or accident.

DEFERVESCENCE
Cooling down of a feverish body to a more normal temperature.

DEFIBRILLATION
Stopping of the normal rhythm of the heart.

DEFIBRILLATOR
Agent or apparatus that arrests ventricular fibrillation (irregular heartbeat) and restores normal rhythm of the heart muscle.

DEFICIENCY DISEASE
An illness caused by the absence of certain necessary food elements in the diet, such as vitamins, minerals or some other normal constituent.

DEFICIENCY MOTIVATION
Needs for food, oxygen and water that motivate behavior. These needs must be satisfied before other needs, higher in the hierarchy, are considered.

DEFLECTION
Psychoanalytic term for the process of unconsciously evading attention to certain ideas or aspects of ideas.

DEFORMITY
A marked deviation from the normal due to development, accident or disease. Also applied figuratively to the mind or the personality.

DEGENERACY
Marked lowering of the level of social behavior or conduct of mental functions, either congenital or acquired.

DEGENERATION
Intellectual or moral deterioration. Also used in the sense of disintegration or structural change of a tissue or organ, or change of a tissue to a less specialized or functionally less active form.

DEGENERATIVE JOINT DISEASE
Another name for osteoarthritis.

DEGENERATIVE PSYCHOSIS
A psychosis in which the person becomes infantile in behavior.

DEGLUTITION
The act of swallowing, partly voluntary, partly involuntary.

DEHISCENCE
Bursting open, especially of a wound.

DEHLI SORE
Another name for Oriental sore.

DEHUMANIZE
The process by which someone is deprived of human characteristics.

DEHYDRATION
The loss or removal of water. Dehydration can become a serious problem in infants or adults with severe diarrhea.

DEHYDRO– EPIANDROSTERONE
A sex hormone secreted by the testes and adrenal glands that stimulates development of secondary sex characteristics.

DEJA VU
An illusion of recognition or type of paramnesia, when one experiences a new experience as if it all has happened before.

DELAYED
Used to describe an instinctive response or form of behaviour that appears only some considerable time after birth, or of a reaction, or reflex, that does not occur immediately on the stimulus, but only after a period of time (this is unusual for a reflex); sometimes also used to describe particular experiments.

DELAYED REACTION
An allergic reaction occurring hours or days after contact with an allergen. The reaction may be localized at the site of contact or generalized throughout the body.

DELICACY
In medicine, susceptibility to disease; constitutional weakness.

DELIRIUM
A usually brief state of incoherent excitement, confused speech, restlessness, and hallucinations.

DELIRIUM, COCAINE
Delirium developing within 24 hours of intake of cocaine. Tactile and olfactory hallucinations may be present. Affect is often labile. Violent or aggressive behavior is common, and restraint may be required.

The delirium usually occurs within one hour of substance use and is over in about six hours. When the substance is taken intravenously, the onset is almost immediate. More rarely, the delirium follows a period of intoxication. When the other pharmacologic effects of the substance have worn off, the delirium disappears completely.

DELIRIUM ABSTINENCE
A delirious state caused by the discontinuation of the habitual use of one or several drugs or alcohol.

DELIRIUM TREMENS
Specific delirium due to acute alcohol withdrawal in alcoholism. It occurs within days of drinking being stopped, and is often precipitated by injury, surgery or imprisonment, when drink is unavailable. The sufferer becomes restless, disorientated, extremely anxious and tremulous; fever and profuse sweating are usual. Characteristically, hallucinations of insects or animals cause abject terror. Constant reassurance, sedatives, well-lit and quiet surroundings are appropriate measures until the episode is over, and treatment of dehydration and reduction of high fever may be necessary. Deaths do occur from this.

DELIVERY
The state of being delivered of, or giving birth to, a child.

DELTOID
A large triangular muscle covering the joint of the shoulder, and serving to raise the arm at the side and to rotate the upper arm.

DELUSION
False opinion or belief that cannot be shaken by reason; if persistent, it is regarded as an insane delusion.

Delusion is a common sense, clinical concept that turns out to be unexpectedly difficult the moment psychiatrists ask two questions:
- How do the psychiatrists know their corresponding beliefs are true?
- In what sense do subjects believe their delusions?
The first question can be answered only if it is possible to discover the function of the beliefs in the minds

of the patient and the psychiatrist. The second question leads to the conclusion that the delusion is a manifestation of a thought disturbance - namely, loss of the capacity to distinguish between metaphorical and factual statements. If the correct mode can be discovered, delusional ideas can often be seen to show sense.

A delusion should be distinguished from a hallucination, which is a false sensory perception (although a hallucination may give rise to the delusion that the perception is true).

A delusion is also to be distinguished from an overvalued idea, in which an unreasonable belief or idea is not as firmly held as in the case with a delusion.

DELUSION, BIZARRE
A false belief that involves a phenomenon that the person's culture would regard as totally implausible. A man believed that when his adenoids had been removed in childhood, a box had been inserted into his head, and that wires had been placed in his head so that the voice he heard was that of the governor.

DELUSION, GRANDIOSE
A delusion whose content involves an exaggerated sense of one's importance, power, knowledge, or identity. It may have a religious, somatic, or other theme.

DELUSION, NIHILISTIC
A delusion involving the theme of nonexistence of the self or part of the self, others, or the world. A somatic delusion may also be a nihilistic delusion if the emphasis is on the body or part of the body.

DELUSION, SOMATIC
A delusion whose main content pertains to the functioning of one's body. Extreme valued judgments about the body may, under certain circumstances, also be considered somatic delusions. Hypochondriacal delusions are also somatic delusions when they involve specific changes in the functioning or structure of the body rather than merely an insistent belief that one has a disease.

DELUSION, SYSTEMATIZED
A single delusion with multiple elaborations or a group of delusions that are all related by the person to a single event or theme.

DELUSION OF BEING CONTROLLED
A delusion in which feelings, impulses, thoughts, or actions are experienced as being not one's own, as being imposed by some external force. This does not include the mere conviction that one is acting as an agent of God, has had a curse placed on him or her, is the victim of fate, or is not sufficiently assertive.

DELUSION OF PERSECUTION
An irrational belief held by certain individuals that they are victims of a conspiracy to kill them or to injure them or cause them to fail. It is most common in paranoid individuals where even seemingly innocuous events are taken as proof of the conspiracy.

DELUSION OF POVERTY
A delusion that the person is, or will be, bereft of all, or virtually all, material possessions.

DELUSION OF REFERENCE
The false belief of individuals that the behavior of others has malign and derogatory reference to the individuals when in fact they have no reference to them at all.

DEMARCATION
An outlining of the junction of, in medicine, diseases and healthy tissue. This process may occur in diseases of the blood vessels when gangrene exists.

DEMECLOCYCLINE
Generic name of a long-acting antibiotic drug.
Side effects may include:
- nausea;
- vomiting;
- diarrhea.

DEMENTIA
A progressive state of mental decline, especially of memory function and judgment, often accompanied by disorientation, stupor, and disintegration of the personality.

DEMENTIA APOPLECTICA
The dementia due to cerebral hemorrhage or softening of the brain tissue possibly due to cerebral arteriosclerosis.

DEMENTIA ARTERIOSCLEROTICA
Dementia due to cerebral arteriosclerosis or atherosclerosis.

DEMENTIA INFANTILIS
A degenerative disease of the nerve cells in the cerebral lobes occurring at about three years of age, which leads to a rapid loss of speech and some impairment of movement.

DEMENTIA, MULTI-INFARCT
A dementia due to significant cerebrovascular disease. There is a stepwise deterioration in intellectual functioning that, early in the course, leaves some intellectual functions relatively intact ("patchy" deterioration). Focal neurologic signs and symptoms are also present.
The onset is typically abrupt. The course is stepwise and fluctuating, with rapid changes, rather than uniformly progressive. The pattern of deficits is "patchy," depending on which regions of the brain have been destroyed. Certain cognitive functions may be affected early, whereas others remain relatively unimpaired.
The dementia typically involves disturbances of memory, abstract thinking, judgment, impulse control, and personality.
The focal neurologic signs seen include:
- weaknesses in the limbs;
- reflex asymmetries;
- extensor plantar responses;
- dysarthria;
- small-stepped gait.
Vascular disease is always presumed to be present and responsible for both the disease and the focal neurologic signs.
Evidence of cerebral and systemic vascular disease may be apparent on physical examination. Hypertension, fundoscopic abnormalities, or an enlarged heart may be present.

DEMENTIA PRAECOX
Another name for schizophrenia.

DEMENTIA SCHIZOPHRENIA
The final stage of deterioration in schizophrenia. The ego and superego no longer interfere with the action of the id, and personality structure breaks down.

DEMINERALIZATION
Abnormal loss of mineral salts from the body.

DEMON
A supernatural being or force not specifically evil.

DEMONISM
The belief in the existence and power of demons.

DEMONOMANIA
Popularly "demonic possession;" delusional disorder manifesting itself in the delusion on the part of an individual that he or she is under the influence of an evil spirit.

DEMONOPHOBIA
Irrational fear of demons.

DEMOPHOBIA
Morbid dread of crowds.

DEMORPHINIZATION
Treatment of addiction to morphine by a gradual diminution of the dose.

DEMULCENT
An oily medicine or application. The term is also used for a muci-laginous (thick) fluid that allays ir-ritation and soothes inflammation.

DEMYELINIZATION
The process by which certain nerve fibers lose their protective myelin sheaths, a condition found in such diseases as multiple sclerosis.

DENDRITE
One of the thread-like extensions of the cytoplasm of a nerve cell. It is the part of a nerve cell that trans-mits signals or impulses to the body of the nerve cell.

DENERVATION
Interruption of the nerve connection to an organ or part. The term usu-ally refers to the cutting into or out or blocking of a nerve.

DENGUE
Also called breakbone fever, three-day fever and dandy fever: an acute disease characterized by:
- sudden onset with headache;
- fever;
- prostration;
- severe joint pain;
- muscle pain;
- swollen glands.

A rash appears simultaneously with a second temperature rise following a period without fever. The virus is transmitted by the mosquito Aedes aegypti, and to prevent transmission to mosquitoes (thus perpetuating the cycle), sufferers in endemic ar-eas should be kept under mosquito netting until the second fever has abated. Treatment involves the re-lief of symptoms.

DENGUE HEMORRHAGIC FE-VER SYNDROME
An acute disease occurring in chil-

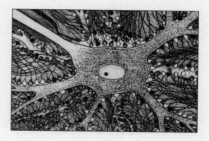

Large neuron of the spinal cord. The small branches of a nerve cell or neuron are called dendrites. The center of a nerve cell is the perikaryon, containing the nucleus and nu-cleic acids.

dren living where dengue is en-demic, and characterized by an abrupt onset of fever followed by internal hemorrhages and circula-tory collapse.

DENIAL
Defense mechanism by which either some painful experience is denied, or some impulse or aspect of the self is denied.

These two mechanisms are cer-tainly not the same process. Ac-cording to Freud, denial of the feel-ings produced by painful experi-ences is a general manifestation of a pleasure principle, the denial being part of hallucinatory wish-fulfill-ment. As a result, all painful per-ceptions have to overcome the re-sistance of the pleasure principle.

Denial of aspects of the self is something more complicated, since it is followed by splitting and pro-jection as a result of which the sub-ject denies that he or she has such feelings but goes on to assert that someone else does.

DENIS BROWN SPLINT
Splint used to correct certain foot deformities such as talipes equino-varus (club foot).

DENTAL
Of or pertaining to the teeth or to dentistry.

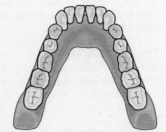

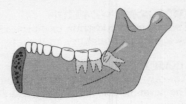

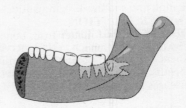

Method of flossing the teeth.

Presence of wisdom teeth in the upper jaw.

DENTAL FLOSS
A soft thread, sometimes coated with wax, used to clean between the teeth.

DENTAL HYGIENIST
One who assists a dentist in the minor functions of dentistry, such as cleaning teeth and taking X-rays.

DENTAL IMPACTION
Condition in which an unerupted tooth becomes wedged against the

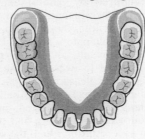

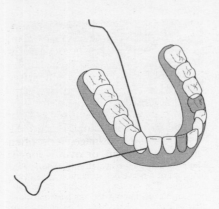

Dentition; permanent teeth in the upper and lower jaw.

tooth in front and is unable to grow out of the gum.

DENTAL PULP
The soft tissue filling the pulp chamber of a tooth and responsible for its vitality. It consists of connective tissue, blood vessels and nerves.

DENTAL TECHNICIAN
A specialist who makes dental appliances.

DENTIFRICE
A powder, paste or liquid used in cleaning teeth.

DENTINE
The hard calcareous tissue beneath the enamel and the cementum of a tooth, enclosing the pulp, and composing the greater part of the tooth.

DENTISTRY
The profession that deals with the diagnosis, prevention and treatment of malformations and diseases affecting the teeth and their related structures.

DENTITION
(1) The development and eruption of teeth;
(2) the number, type, and arrangement of teeth in the mouth.

DENTURE
Set of artificial teeth or the entire set of natural teeth.

DEODORANT
An agent for destroying odors; a preparation for checking or masking body odors.

DEOSSIFICATION
Loss of mineral matter from bones; absorption of bone.

DEOXYCORTICOSTERONE
One of the hormones excreted by the adrenal glands, which is concerned with electrolytes and water metabolism.

DEOXYGENATION
The act of depriving of oxygen; the removal of oxygen.

DEOXYRIBONUCLEIC ACID
Full name of DNA.

DEPENDENCE
Trust, reliance, depending on another for material or emotional support. Infantile dependence refers either to the fact that children are helpless and dependent on their parents, or to the fact that neurotics are fixated on their parents and imagine themselves to be dependent on them.

The term is also used to designate the physical or psychological dependence on a substance, or both. Psychological dependence produces physical withdrawal symptoms (sweating, shaking, abdominal pain, convulsions) if the substance is not taken. Dependence also implies loss of control over intake.

DEPENDENCE, PSYCHOACTIVE SUBSTANCE
A cluster of cognitive, behavioral, and physiologic symptoms that indicate that the person has impaired control of psychoactive substance use and continuous use of the substance despite adverse consequences. The following are the characteristic symptoms of dependence. It should be noted that not all nine symptoms must be present for the diagnosis of dependence, and for some classes of psychoactive substances, certain of these symptoms do not apply.

(1) The person often finds that when he or she actually takes the psychoactive substance, it is often in larger amounts or over a longer period that originally intended. For example, the person may decide to take only one drink of alcohol, but after taking this first drink, continues to drink until severely intoxicated.

(2) The person recognizes that the substance use is excessive, and has attempted to reduce or control it, but has been unable to do so (as long as the substance is available). In other instances the person may want to reduce or control his or her substance use, but has never actually made an effort to do so.

(3) A great deal of time is spent in activities necessary to procure the substance (including theft), taking it, or recovering from its effects. In mild cases the person may spend several hours a day taking the substance, but continue to be involved in other activities. In severe cases, virtually all the user's daily activities revolve around obtaining, using, and recuperating from the effects of the substance.

(4) The person may suffer intoxication or withdrawal symptoms when he or she is expected to fulfill major role obligations (work, school, homemaking). For example, the person may be intoxicated when working outside the home or when expected to take care of his or her children. In addition, the person may be intoxicated or have withdrawal symptoms in situations in which substance use is physically hazardous, such as driving a car or operating machinery.

(5) Important social, occupational,

or recreational activities are given up or reduced because of substance use. The person may withdraw from family activities and hobbies in order to spend more time with substance-using friends, or to use the substance in private.

(6) With heavy and prolonged substance use, a variety of social, psychological, and physical problems occur, and are exacerbated by continued use of the substance. Despite having one or more of these problems (and recognizing that use of the substance causes or exacerbates them), the person continues to use the substance.

(7) Significant tolerance, a markedly diminished effect with continued use of the same amount of the substance, occurs.

The person will then take greatly increased amounts of the substance in order to achieve
intoxication or the desired effect. This is distinguished from the marked personal differences in initial sensitivity to the effects of a particular substance.

(8) With continued use, characteristic withdrawal symptoms develop when the person stops or reduces intake of the substance. The withdrawal symptoms vary greatly across classes of substances. Marked and generally easily measured physiologic signs of withdrawal are common with the following substances:
- alcohol;
- opioids;
- sedatives;
- hypnotics;
- anxiolytics.

Such signs are less obvious with the following substances:
- amphetamines;
- cocaine;
- nicotine;
- cannabis.

No significant withdrawal is seen even after repeated use of hallucinogens; withdrawal from PCP and related substances has not yet been described in humans; although it has been demonstrated in animals.

(9) After developing unpleasant withdrawal symptoms, the person begins taking the substance in order to relieve or avoid those symptoms. This typically involves using the substance throughout the day, beginning soon after awakening. This symptoms is generally not present with cannabis, hallucinogens, and PCP.

DEPENDENT PERSONALITY DISORDER

A pervasive pattern of dependent and submissive behavior beginning by early adulthood and present in a variety of contexts. People with this disorder are unable to make everyday decisions without an excessive amount of advice and reassurance from others, and will even allow others to make most of their important decisions. A child or adolescent with this disorder may allow his or her parent(s) to decide what he or she should wear, with whom to associate, how to spend free time, and what school or college to attend.

This excessive dependence on others leads to difficulty in initiating projects or doing things on one's own. People with this disorder tend to feel uncomfortable or helpless when alone, and will go to great lengths to avoid being alone. They are devastated when close relationships end, and tend to be preoccupied with fears of being abandoned.

These people are easily hurt by criticism and disapproval, and tend to subordinate themselves to others, agreeing with people even when they believe them to be wrong, for fear of being rejected. They will volunteer to do things that are unpleasant or demeaning in order to get others to like them.

Frequently another personality disorder is present, such as schizotypal, narcissistic, or avoidant personality disorder. Anxiety and depression are common. People with this disorder invariably lack self-confidence.

They tend to belittle their abilities and assets. For example, a person with this disorder may constantly refer to himself or herself as "stupid." They may at times seek, or stimulate, overprotection and dominance in others.

DEPERSONALIZATION
In individuals, a more or less pathological state in which they lose their feeling of the reality of themselves, or of their bodies, or may feel that they are dead.

Also used of a philosophy of the universe, which no longer regards natural forces as manifestations of supernatural agents or gods.

DEPERSONALIZATION DISORDER
The occurrence of persistent or recurrent episodes of depersonalization sufficiently severe to cause marked distress.

The symptom of depersonalization involves an alteration in the perception or experience of the self in which the usual sense of one's own reality is temporarily lost or changed.

This is manifested by a feeling of detachment from and being an outside observer of one's mental processes or body, or of feeling like an automaton or as if in a dream. Various types of sensory anesthesia and a sensation of not being in complete control of one's actions, including speech, are often present. All of these feelings are ego dystonic, and the person maintains intact reality testing.

DEPERSONALIZATION SYNDROME
A neurosis characterized by an unpleasant state of disturbed perception in which external objects or parts of the person's own body are experienced as changed in their quality, unreal, estranged and devoid of their normal immediacy, and in which the individual may feel that his or her personality has changed or is unreal, remote or automatized.

The person is aware of the subjective nature of the change of experiences. Depersonalization may also occur as a feature of several mental disorders, including depression, obsessional neurosis, anxiety neurosis and schizophrenia.

DEPIGMENTATION
Loss of color or pigment.

DEPILATION
The removal of hair.

DEPILATORY
A substance employed to remove superfluous hair from the human skin.

DEPIXOL
Brand name of a tranquillizing drug containing flupenthixol as the active compound. The drug has antipsychotic and antidepressant properties.

DEPLETION
To empty the body of something, blood, for instance.

DEPLUMATION
Loss or falling out of eyelashes because of disease.

DEPOT INJECTION
Injection into a muscle of a drug that has been specifically formulated to provide a slow, steady absorption of its active ingredients by the surrounding blood vessels. The drug may be mixed with oil.

DEPRESSANT
Having the quality of depressing or lowering activity, physical, mental or emotional. Also a psychoactive drug belonging to the class of sedatives.

DEPRESSED FRACTURE
Fracture of a flat bone like that of the skull, in which a fragment is depressed below the surface and may touch the brain.

DEPRESSION
A dejected state of mind with feelings of sadness, discouragement and hopelessness, often accompanied by reduced activity and ability to function, unresponsiveness, apathy, and sleep disturbances.

DEPRESSION, ADOLESCENT
Mild depression often accompanied by hypochondria and anxiety, usually seen in young men and women.

DEPRESSION, AGITATED
A syndrome of abnormal behavior characterized by overactivity, restlessness and tension so that the person can remain still for only short periods of time.

DEPRESSION, ANACLITIC
Syndrome observed in infants who have lost their parents or guardians in which, due to the absence of the preferred objects, aggressive and sexual drives are turned inwards.

DEPRESSION, CYCLIC
A recurring mood disorder characterized by a severely depressed state and by a slowing down of mind and body; uneasiness, apprehension, perplexity and agitation may also be present.

DEPRESSION, MAJOR
Mental disorder characterized by at least five of the following symptoms that have been present during the same two-week period and represent a change from previous functioning. At least one of the symptoms is either depressed mood, or loss of interest or pleasure.
(1) Depressed mood (or can be irritable mood in children and adolescents) most of the day, nearly every day, as indicated either by subjective account or observations by others.
(2) Markedly diminished interest or pleasure in all, or almost all, activities most of the day, nearly every day (as indicated either by subjective account or observation by others of apathy most of the time).
(3) Significant weight loss of weight gain when not dieting (e.g., more than 5 percent of body weight in a month), or decrease or increase in appetite nearly every day (in children, consider failure to make expected weight gain).
(4) Insomnia or hypersomnia nearly every day.
(5) Psychomotor agitation or retardation nearly every day (observable by others, not merely subjective feelings of restlessness or being slowed down).
(6) Fatigue or loss of energy nearly every day.
(7) Feelings of worthlessness or excessive or inappropriate guilt (which may be delusional) nearly every day (not merely self-reproach or guilt about being sick).
(8) Diminished ability to think or concentrate, or indecisiveness, nearly every day (either by subjective account or as observed by others).
(9) Recurrent thoughts of death (not just fear of dying), recurrent suicidal ideation without a specific plan, or a suicide attempt or a specific plan for committing suicide.

DEPRESSION, REACTIVE
Also called psychogenic depression: a transient depression that is the result of some upsetting or saddening experience; individuals usually have no history of repeated depressions.

DEPRESSIVE EPISODE
Either depressed mood (or possibly, in children or adolescents, an irritable mood) or loss of interest or pleasure in all, or almost all, activities, and associated symptoms, for a

period of at least two weeks. The symptoms represent a change from previous functioning and are relatively persistent, that is, they occur for most of the day, during at least a two-week period.

The associate symptoms include:
- appetite disturbance;
- change in weight;
- sleep disturbance;
- psychomotor agitation;
- psychomotor retardation;
- decreased energy;
- feelings of worthlessness;
- inappropriate guilt;
- difficulty thinking;
- difficulty concentrating;
- recurrent thoughts of death;
- suicidal ideation or attempts.

DEPRESSOR
Any muscle that lowers or depresses a structure. Depressor is also the term used for the nerves that restrain or prevent certain functions such as hormone secretion, heart rate and blood pressure.

DEPRIVATION
The experience of receiving an inadequate amount of a necessary commodity. The verb to deprive means, in general, to withhold or take away something desirable or necessary from someone.

Psychoanalysis has concerned itself with two forms of deprivation: maternal and sexual. Both, but especially in recent years the former, have been suggested as causes of neurosis.

The maternal deprivation theory of neurosis exists in various degrees of sophistication, according to how the insufficient commodity is defined. For example, statistical theories of maternal deprivation have defined the deprivation in terms of how long the mother is physically absent.

Deprivation theories of neurosis imply that deprivation beyond a certain threshold produces relatively irreversible effects either by

retarding development or by initiating defenses.

DEPRIVATION DWARFISM
Condition whereby a child fails to grow in height because psychological stress creates a switching-off of growth hormones.

DEPTH PSYCHOLOGY
Term frequently applied to the explanation of experience and behavior in terms of phenomena of the unconscious.

DERADENITIS
Inflammation of a lymph gland in the neck.

DEREALIZATION
Psychiatric term for the symptom that leads to the person complaining that the world seems unreal.

DERIVED EMOTION
Such emotions as hope, disappointment, despair, etc.

DERMA
The corium, or true skin, beneath the epidermis.

DERMABRASION
Removal of extensive scars or marks on the skin by means of high-speed abrasive drills.

DERMAL NEVUS
Birthmark in which the pigmented cells are situated entirely in the dermis.

DERMANOPLASTY
Skin grafting.

DERMATITIS
Inflammation of the skin, accompanied by moderate to severe itching. In common usage, the term eczema has become somewhat imprecise in meaning, generally tending to refer to any chronic, non-specific form of skin inflammation, but when the term dermatitis is qualified by an

adjective, it denotes a particular form of skin inflammation.

DERMATITIS, ATOPIC

Refers to an allergic disorder of infants, children and young adults, characterized by a redness, thickening and scaling of the skin in patches, typically on the face, neck, hands and feet, in the crook of the elbow or behind the knee. The cause of atopic dermatitis is not known, but it tends to run in families and is more common in persons with other allergic manifestations. It often appears a few weeks after birth, lasting until about age two, when it disappears until puberty; thereafter most cases run a fluctuating course until the mid-20s, when inflammation tends to disappear permanently.

DERMATITIS, CONTACT

The most common form of dermatitis; the result of the skin being in contact with a substance to which it is hypersensitive.

These substances can be almost anything, but the most frequently troublesome are detergents, rubber (as found in the elastic of underwear), nickel (found in much "gold" jewellery, coins, zips, etc.), hair dyes, epoxy-resin adhesives, and cosmetics.

On contact with these, the skin may become reddened and itchy and develop small blisters and moist patches. The culprit substance has to be identified (it may be obvious or expert patch testing may be needed) and eliminated from the immediate environment.

DERMATITIS, EXFOLIATIVE

Also called erythroderma; a generalized redness and scaling of the skin that usually arises as a complication of a pre-existing skin disease or an allergy. More rarely, it may be indicative of a systemic disease, such as cancer of the lymphoid tissue. The onset of exfoliative dermatitis is gradual; initial single lesions coalesce into large patches of scaly, red skin that may extend over any part of the body until no healthy skin is left. Hair and nails may lose their luster and become brittle and fall.

Occasionally, a yellow secretion may ooze out of the skin, and itching is variable and may be intense. The continuous shedding of the scales results in a significant loss of body protein. The maintenance of body temperature is also affected, because of the plugging of a majority of sweat ducts; the person feels cold and feverish.

Treatment focuses on the underlying primary disease. Rest and a high protein diet are beneficial, and large doses of corticosteroids are often given. Exfoliative dermatitis is most common in middle life, affecting more men than women by a ratio of about three to one.

DERMATITIS HERPETIFORMIS

Chronic skin condition that can take the form of vesicles (areas of fluid under the top layer of skin), blisters, pimples and/or urticaria (nettle rash). There is severe itching, and the erupted skin is often torn by scratching. The changes are found on both sides of the body and are commoner on outer surfaces and the back than on inner surfaces; they are frequently found on elbows, knees, the lower back, the cleft between the buttocks, and the tops of the thighs. Bromides, iodides, saltwater fish and shellfish sometimes cause exacerbation, but it is the gluten found in various cereals (e.g., wheat, rye, oats) that seems to be the primary culprit; this is why the condition is often found in those suffering from celiac disease. The general condition of a person suffering just from this skin disorder is usually little affected, but the itching, frequently smarting or burning in character, may be incapacitating.

DERMATOFIBROMA
Also called fibrous histiocytoma: a firm, round, skin-colored or dark tumor about 1 cm (2/5 in) in diameter, level with the skin surface or slightly raised. It is most commonly found on the legs.

DERMATOGLYPHICS
The study of the patterns of ridges of the skin of the fingers, palms, toes and soles as a means of diagnosis of such congenital conditions as Down's syndrome and congenital heart disease.

DERMATOLOGIST
Specialist in the skin and its diseases.

DERMATOLOGY
Study and treatment of the skin and its diseases.

DERMATOLYSIS
Congenital laxity of the skin producing folds; small growth of the skin accompanied by lax, sagging skin.

DERMATOME
Instrument for cutting skin to produce a skin graft. Also the site of an embryonic somite, an area of skin supplied by a single spinal nerve.

DERMATOMYCOSIS
Any skin disease caused by a fungus, such as athlete's foot.

DERMATOMYOSITIS
A disease of collagen tissue affecting skin and muscles. The dermatitis component takes varying forms: characteristically, the skin on the face, especially round the eyes, is red and swollen, and red scaling is found on both sides of the body on the elbows and the backs of the fingers, particularly over the knuckles. The dermatitis heals with atrophy (wasting), giving an appearance of radiation damage. The myositis chiefly affects the muscles of the

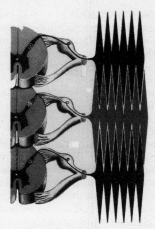

Three overlapping dermatome areas supplied by three spinal segments.

shoulder and pelvis, giving weakness and often atrophy. The intercostal (rib) muscles and diaphragm are also involved.

Treatment consists of the prescribing of prednisolone, 40-100 mg daily. The outlook varies greatly, with 20 percent of the sufferers dying within one year, but most children survive for long periods. Remission may occur after cancer treatment.

DERMATONEUROSIS
Skin disease secondary to anxiety and nervous irritability.

DERMATOPHOBIA
Pathologic fear of having or contracting a skin disease.

DERMATOPHYTE
A parasitic fungus infecting the skin, hair and nails of humans and animals, giving rise to various forms of skin disease, such as ringworm.

DERMATOPLASTY
The replacement of skin by skin grafting.

DERMATOSIS
General term covering any disease of the skin.

DERMIDEX CREAM
Brand name of a topical preparation containing chlorbutol, lignocaine, cetrimide, and aluminum chlorhydroxyallantoinate as active compounds used for the treatment of various skin disorders characterized by irritation.

DERMIS
Also called the corium: the inner layer of skin beneath the epidermis. It comprises a layer of connective tissue, one to four millimeters thick, that is thicker on the back than on the front of the body. The cells are most numerous just beneath the epidermis, the tissue being more fibrous in its deeper part. The boundary between dermis and epidermis is undulating, the waves being most pronounced where the skin is thick. The dermis contains many nerves, blood vessels and sweat glands. The raised parts of the dermis are called papillae, and at some sites, such as the finger tips, these are arranged linearly and produce characteristic patterns responsible for individual fingerprints.

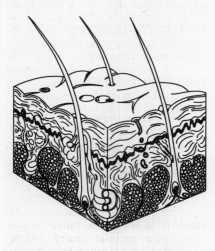

Cross section of the skin; the upper layer is called dermis. In the subcutaneous layer (below the dermis) the roots of hairs are implanted.

DERMOGRAPHIA
A condition in which weals occur on the skin after stroking or scratching of the skin with a dull instrument. The condition is seen in urticaria (nettle rash) and when the capillaries are highly unstable.

DERMOGRAPHISM
Harmless congenital phenomenon in which the slightest touch on the skin by a firm object leaves a red weal lasting for a few minutes.

DERMOID
Pertaining to or resembling skin; skinlike.

DES
Abbreviation of diethylstilbestrol.

DESENSITIZATION
Reduction of the abnormal sensitivity of the body to a substance.

DESERT SORE
Ulcer that appears on the face, hands and lower extremities in tropical climates.

DESEXUALIZATION
The process by which the sex drive in infants loses its primitive, erotic quality when the impulses to which it is attached are sublimated and the ego develops.

DESIGNER DRUG
A group of unlicensed substances whose only purpose is to duplicate the effects of certain illegal drugs of abuse or to provide even stronger ones.

Designer drugs differ chemically in some minor degree from the original drug, enabling the user and supplier to evade prosecution for dealing in, or possessing of, an illegal drug.

DESIRE
General term for appetite with clear consciousness of its object.

DESMOLOGY
The science of tendons and ligaments.

DESPAIR
An intensely unpleasant emotional state, associated with the abandoning of hope of success in one's efforts to attain an end or satisfy a desire. In mental illness, it occurs in schizoid and schizophrenic disorders, in which it appears to be the result of feelings of insurmountable alienation and ambivalence, and in the neuroses, in which it is a defensive attitude designed to reduce anxiety.

DESPONDENCY
An emotional attitude arising from failure, but not yet becoming despair.

DESQUAMATION
Shedding or peeling of the skin.

DETERGENT
An agent that purifies or cleanses. Such a substance is useful for removing greasy ointments from the skin.

DETERIORATION
Progressive impairment of function.

DETERMINATION
Decision in the mind; the mental habit of settling upon some line of action with a fixed purpose to adhere to it.

DETOXIFICATION
(1) Reduction of the toxic properties of a substance, e.g., vaccines.
(2) Treatment designed to assist in recovery from the toxic effects of a drug, e.g.,heroin and alcohol.

DETRITUS
Any disintegrated material, waste product or substance.

DETRUSOR
Muscle serving to expel something, such as the muscle attached to the pubis which, when it contracts, exerts pressure on the bladder and forces urine out.

DEUTERANOPE
A person who has a type of color blindness in which he or she cannot distinguish between green and red.

DEVELOPMENTAL ARITHMIC DISORDER
Marked impairment in the development of arithmic skills that is not explainable by mental retardation, inadequate schooling, or hearing or visual defects.

There are a number of different types of skills that may be impaired in this disorder. These include:
(1) linguistic skills, such as understanding or naming mathematical terms, understanding or naming mathematical operations or concepts, and coding written problems into mathematical symbols;
(2) perceptual skills, such as recognizing or reading numerical symbols or arithmetic signs, and clustering objects into groups;
(3) attention skills, such as copying figures correctly, remembering to add in "carried" numbers, and observing operational signs;
(4) mathematical skills, such as following sequences of mathematical steps, counting objects, and learning multiplication tables.

DEVELOPMENTAL DISORDER
Disorder characterized by a predominant disturbance in the acquisition of cognitive, language, motor, or social skills.

The disturbance may involve a general delay, as in mental retardation, or a delay as in failure to progress in a specific area of skill acquisition, or multiple areas in which there are qualitative distortions of normal development, as in the pervasive developmental disorders.

DEVELOPMENTAL EXPRESSIVE WRITING DISORDER

Marked impairment in the development of expressive writing skills that is not explainable by mental retardation or inadequate schooling and that is not due to a visual or hearing defect or a neurologic disorder. The impairment in the ability to compose written texts may be marked by spelling errors, grammatical or punctuation errors within sentences, or poor paragraph organization.

DEVELOPMENTAL INSANITY

Type of mental disorder related to definite periods of development such as is found in certain types of schizophrenia.

DEVELOPMENTAL PATHWAY

Representation of development as a succession of processes and states in relation to a time line.

DEVELOPMENTAL READING DISORDER

Marked impairment in the development of word recognition skills and reading comprehension that is not explainable by mental retardation or inadequate schooling and that is not due to a visual or hearing defect or a neurologic disorder.

Oral reading is characterized by omissions, distortions, and substitutions of words and by slow, halting reading.

DEVELOPMENTAL SEQUENCE

In the course of the development of an organism, there is a sequence of the appearance and development of structures in the organism. This sequence is, within limits, constant for all organisms of the same, or related, species.

DEVELOPMENTAL STAGE

A period in the life of an individual during which specific traits or behaviors become characteristic.

DEVELOPMENTAL TASKS

Achievements and skills obtained by the developing individual and regarded by a society or culture as appropriate and necessary to his or her level of development.

DEVIATED SEPTUM

The deflection, congenital or acquired by injury, of the cartilage partition between the nostrils.

DEVIATION

Variation, norm or standard of reference, used in two senses:
(1) visually, to describe one eye failing to assume its position in coordination with the other when staring at an object;
(2) statistically, to describe variation from the mean in a series, as mean or average deviation.

DEXTERITY

Smooth and rapid, or skilful, movement, usually of arm, hand or fingers.

DEXTRAD

Towards the right, usually of writing from left to right.

DEXTRAL

On, or belonging to, the right side of the body.

DEXTRALITY

Right-hand preference, right-handedness; sometimes used more generally for sidedness, and even inclusive of left-handedness.

DEXTROCARDIA

Congenital condition in which the heart is displaced to the right side of the chest as opposed to its normal position somewhat to the left side of the chest.

DEXTROSE

A form of glucose, the sugar found in blood and in many plants.

DEXTROSURIA
Presence of dextrose in the urine, caused by a metabolic disorder.

DIABETES
A complex and chronic disorder of metabolism due to total or partial lack of insulin secretion by the pancreas or to the inability of insulin to function normally in the body.

DIABETES INSIPIDUS
A rare disease, characterized by the passage of large amounts of urine, that is caused by a disorder of the pituitary gland.

DIABETES MELLITUS
Formal name of what is usually called simply diabetes.

DIABETIC GANGRENE
Gangrene due to the furring-up of the blood vessels, thus cutting off the blood supply, and usually affecting the extremities. It can be a complication of diabetes.

DIABETOGENIC
Producing diabetes.

DIABETOPHOBIA
Fear of diabetes.

DIABINESE
Brand name of chlorpropamide; an oral drug prescribed for the treatment of diabetes mellitus (sugar diabetes).

DIACETIC ACID
A ketone body (intermediate product of the breakdown of fat) produced in certain metabolic diseases such as uncontrolled diabetes; also known as acetonic acid.

DIAGNOSIS
The discrimination of diseases by their distinctive signs or symptoms.

DIAGNOSTIC DRUG
Agent used by a doctor to assist in the diagnosis of a disease.

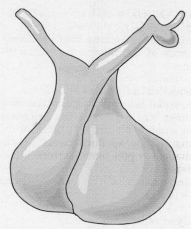

Diabetes insipidus: the origin of this disease may be located in a disorder of the posterior lobe (to the right) of the pituitary gland or hypophysis.

DIAGNOSTIC ULTRASONOGRAPHY
Commonly called ultrasound: the use of very high frequency pulse-echo imaging techniques to detect differences in tissue density within the body and thus display disease processes that are not adequately seen by other diagnostic procedures. It is also used to examine the fetus during pregnancy.

DIALYSIS
The process of separating elements in a solution by diffusion across a semipermeable membrane; a term usually used in respect of artificial kidneys.

DIAPEDESIS
The process by which the blood passes through the capillary walls into the tissues, one of the major signs of inflammation.

DIAPHORESIS
Profuse sweating.

DIAPHRAGM
Medical term used in three different meanings.
(1) A partition or septum.
(2) The muscular partition separat-

ing the chest cavity from the abdominal cavity.
(3) A device placed over the cervix (neck of the womb) for contraception.

DIAPHRAGMA SELLAE
A small horizontal fold of the dura mater that roofs over the sella turcica and is pierced by a small opening for the infundibulum.

DIAPHYSIS
The shaft of a long bone, between the epiphyses at either end.

DIAPOPHYSIS
A transverse process of a vertebra that is an outgrowth of the neural arch on the dorsal side; especially one of the dorsal pair of such processes when two or more pair are present.

DIARRHOEA
See Diarrhea.

DIARRHEA
Abnormally frequent excavation of watery stools.

DIARTHROSIS
A joint in which the bones move freely in every direction, as in the shoulder joint.

DIASCHISIS
The breaking up of a pattern of brain activity by a localized injury that temporarily throws the whole activity out of function through destroying only part of the structure.

DIASTASIS
Dislocation or separation of the end of a growing bone from the shaft without fracture.

DIASTOLE
The period between two contractions of the heart, when the chambers widen en fill with blood.

DIASTOLIC PRESSURE
The lowest arterial blood pressure of a cardiac cycle occurring during diastole of the heart.

DIASTROPHIC DWARFISM
An inherited dysplasia affecting bones and joints and characterized especially by club foot, deformities of the digits of the hand, malformed pinnae, and cleft palate.

DIATHERMY
The use of high-frequency, ultrasound or microwaves to raise the temperature of a part of the body; sometimes used to treat deep-seated pain.

DIATHESIS
Predisposition in a certain direction, as an inherited tendency towards a specific disease under certain environmental conditions.

DICHOTOMOUS KEY
A key for the identification of organisms based on a series of choices between alternative characters.

DICHROISM
The property of some crystals and solutions of absorbing one of two plane-polarized components of transmitted light more strongly than the other.

DICK TEST
A test to determine susceptibility or immunity to scarlet fever by an injection of scarlet fever toxin.

DICROTIC NOTCH
A secondary upstroke in the descending part of a pulse tracing corresponding to the transient increase in aortic pressure upon closure of the aortic valve.

DIENTAMOEBA
A genus of commensal amebas of the human intestine characterized by the presence of two nuclei in the trophozoite.

DIET

The customary amount and kind of food and drink taken by a person from day to day. More narrowly, a diet is defined as that which meets specific requirements of the individual, including or excluding certain foods.

DIETARY

The kinds and amounts of food available to or eaten by an individual group, or population.

DIETHYLSTILBESTROL (DES)

A nonsteroid manufactured chemical that has the properties of estrogen, a female sex hormone. It is used to treat problems of menopause and menstruation. It has been found to be associated with a higher-than-normal incidence of vaginal cancer in the daughters of women treated during pregnancy for threatened abortion.

DIETL'S CRISIS

An attack of violent pain in the kidney region accompanied by chills, nausea, vomiting, and collapse that is caused by kinking of the ureter and is usually associated with a floating kidney.

DIETOTHERAPY

A branch of dietetics concerned with therapeutic uses of food and diet.

DIFFERENTIAL BLOOD COUNT

Enumeration of the specific types of white blood cells found in a given volume of blood; used as an aid to diagnosis

DIFFERENTIAL DIAGNOSIS

A systematic method for diagnosing a disorder that lacks unique signs or symptoms.

DIFFERENTIATION

The process of changing from an original unspecialized form to a different, more specialized, form.

DIFFUSION

The movement of particles from an area of high concentration to an area of low concentration to produce an even distribution in the available space.

DIGASTRIC MUSCLE

Either a pair of muscles having two bellies separated by a median tendon that extend from the anterior inferior margin of the mandible to the temporal bone and serve to open the jaw.

DIGESTION

The conversion of food into chyme in the stomach and the separation from it of chyle that is then absorbed into the bloodstream.

DIGESTANT

A substance that digests or aids in digestion (as of a specific food substance).

DIGESTER

A medicine or an article of food that aids digestion.

DIGESTIBILITY

The fitness of something for digestion. The term is also used to describe the percentage of a foodstuff taken into the digestive tract that is absorbed into the body.

DIGESTIVE GLAND

Gland secreting digestive enzymes.

DIGESTIVE SYSTEM

Organs in the body that play a major role in the digestion of food, including the mouth, esophagus, stomach and bowls.

DIGIT

Any of the divisions in which the limbs of amphibians and all higher vertebrates including man terminate, which are typically five in number but may be reduced, and which typically have a series of phalanges bearing a nail.

DIGITAL
Pertaining to the fingers or toes.

DIGITALIS
Any of several drugs derived from foxglove plants, used to strengthen heart muscle contraction and regulate the beat of poorly functioning hearts.

DIGITALIZATION
The administration of digitalis (as in heart disease) until the desired physiological adjustment is attained.

DIGITATE
Having fingers or fingerlike projections.

DIGITAL NERVE
(1) Any of several branches of the median nerve and the ulnar nerve supplying the fingers and thumb.
(2) Any of the several branches of the medial plantar nerve supplying the toes.

DIGLYCERIDE
An ester of glycerol that contains two ester groups and involves one or two acids.

DILATATION
Expansion of an organ or vessel, or expansion of an orifice (opening), as in cervical dilatation.

DILATATION & CURETTAGE
Dilatation of the cervix of the uterus and scraping of the endometrium (lining) of the uterus.

DILUTION
Decrease in the amount of a substance in a solution for each unit of volume, usually the result of adding water to increase the volume.

DIMPLE
A slight natural indentation or hol-

low in the surface of some part of the human body.

DIOPTRICS
A branch of optics dealing with the refraction of light especially by lenses.

DIOXIDE
An oxide containing two atoms of oxygen in a molecule.

DIPEPTIDE
A peptide yielding two molecules of amino acid on hydrolysis.

DIPHASIC
Having two phases; as exhibiting a stage of stimulation followed by a stage of depression or vice versa.

DIPHTHERIA
An acute, contagious infection caused by the bacterium Corynebacterium diphtheriae, which produces a toxin affecting the whole body and characterized by severe inflammation of the throat and larynx with production of a membrane lining the throat, along with fever, chills, malaise, brassy cough, and, in some cases by impaired function of the heart muscle and peripheral nerves.

DIPLOE
Layer of bone of sponge-like appearance between the inner and outer walls of the bones of the skull.

DIPLOID
The normal complement of chromosomes; in humans, there are 22 pairs of homologous chromosomes and the sex chromosomes.

DIPLOPIA
Double vision; disorder of vision in which two images of a single object are seen because of unequal action of the eye muscles.

DIPROSALIC
Brand name of a skin preparation

containing as active compounds be-
tamethasone (a corticosteroid) and
salicylic acid (a karyolytic preparation that promotes peeling of the
skin).

DIPSOMANIA
An intense, persistent desire to
drink alcoholic beverages to excess;
alcoholism.

DIPSTICK
A chemically sensitive strip of cellulose used to identify the constituents (as glucose) of urine by immer-
sion.

DIRECTIVE
Of or relating to psychotherapy or
counseling in which the counselor
introduces information, content, or
attitudes not previously expressed
by the client.

DIRECTOR
An instrument grooved to guide and
limit the motion of a surgical knife.

DISABILITY
A weakness, defect, disorder, or
other impairment that results in reduction or loss of mental or physical function; an incapacity.

DISACCHARIDE
Any of a class of sugars yielding
two monosaccharide molecules after hydrolysis; sucrose is an example.

DISARTICULATION
Separation or amputation of a body
part at a joint.

DISC
Also called intervertebral disc: one
of the tough fibrous pads between
the vertebrae of the spine, which
cushion jolts and are flexible yet
strong.

DISCHARGE
A substance that is excreted from an
organ or part. The term is also used

in the sense of an electrical action
of a nerve cell.

DISCRIMINATION
The process by which two stimuli
differing in some aspect are re-
sponded to differently.

DISEASE
A disturbance of normal body function in the organism. The term is
used to designate an impairment of
the normal state of the organism or
of any of its components and is a response to environmental factors (as
malnutrition, industrial hazards, or
climate), to specific infective
agents, to inherent defects of the organism, or to combination of these
factors.

DISEQUILIBRIUM
Loss or weakness of balance.

DISHABITUATION
Restoration to full strength of a response that has become weakened
by habituation.

DISINFECTION
The destruction of all microorganisms by chemical or physical
means.

DISLOCATION
Displacement of an organ or joint.
In general, the term is used to indicate displacement of one or more
bones at a joint.

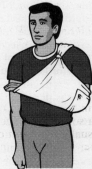

Dislocation. Armsling applied in dislocation
of the shoulder joint.

DISORDER
Disturbance or interruption of the functions of the body or the mind. The term is also used in the sense of "sickness."

DISORGANIZED TYPE SCHIZOPHRENIA
Mental disorder characterized by incoherence, marked loosening of associations, or grossly disorganized behavior, and, in addition, flat or grossly inappropriate affect. There are no systematized delusions, although fragmentary delusions or hallucinations, in which the content is not organized into a coherent theme, are common.
   Associated features include:
- grimaces;
- mannerisms;
- hypochondriacal complaints;
- extreme social withdrawal;
- other oddities of behavior.
The clinical picture is usually associated with extreme social impairment, poor premorbid personality, an early and insidious onset, and a chronic course without significant remissions.

DISORIENTATION
Mental confusion, characterized by a loss of awareness of space, time or personal identity; it may be caused by drugs, severe stress, or organic disease.

DISPLACEMENT
Unconscious transfer of feeling from an originally experienced object to another, more acceptable one. The term is also used to designate the substitution of another form of behavior for what is usual or expected especially when the usual response is nonadaptive.

DISPROPORTION
Absence of symmetry or the proper dimensional relationship, as between a large head and the average-size body.

DISRUPTIVE
Characterized by psychologically disorganized behavior

DISRUPTIVE BEHAVIOR DISORDER
Disorder characterized by behavior that is socially disruptive and is often more distressing to others than to the people with the disorders. Examples are:
- attention-deficit disorder;
- oppositional defiant disorder;
- conduct disorder.

DISSECT
To cut so as to separate into pieces or to expose the several parts for scientific examination.

DISSECTION
Separation of body tissues, usually along natural divisions, by cutting or probing, for visual or microscopic examination.

DISSOCIATION
In psychiatry, separation of certain ideas, thoughts or emotions from the consciousness, often as a defense mechanism.

DISSOCIATIVE DISORDER
Neurosis in which repressed emotional conflict causes a separation in the personality with confusion in identity. Marked by symptoms of amnesia, dream state, or multiple personality, it is treated with psychotherapy, hypnosis, and antianxiety drugs.

DISTAL
Away from the center; toward the far end of something.

DISTAL CONVOLUTED TUBULE
The convoluted portion of the nephron lying between the loop of Henle and the nonsecretory part of the nephron and concerned especially with the concentration of urine.

DISTEMPER
Disordered or abnormal bodily state.

DISTRACTIBILITY
Attention drawn too frequently to unimportant or irrelevant external stimuli.

DISTURBANCE
Agitation, disorder of thought. The term is also used in the sense of an interruption of a settled state of things.

DISULFIRAM
Generic name of a drug used in the treatment of alcoholism.

DISULFIRAM REACTION
When alcohol in the bloodstream interacts with disulfiram, it causes a flushed face, severe headache, chest pains, shortness of breath, nausea, vomiting, sweating and weakness. Severe reactions may cause death. A disulfiram reaction is the interaction of any drug with alcohol or another drug to produce these symptoms.

DIURESIS
An excessive flow of urine.

DIURETIC
A drug that promotes the production and excretion of urine. Diuretics are drugs that act on the kidneys to prevent reabsorption of electrolytes, especially chlorides.

They are used to treat edema, high blood pressure, congestive heart failure, kidney and liver failure and others.

DIURETIC, LOOP
Drug that acts on the kidneys to prevent reabsorption of electrolytes, especially chlorides.

The are used to treat edema, high blood pressure, congestive heart failure, kidney and liver damage and others.

These drugs include bumetanide, ethacrynic acid, furosemide.

DIURETIC, POTASSIUM SPARING
Drug that acts on the kidneys to prevent reabsorption of electrolytes, especially chlorides.

The are used to treat edema, high blood pressure, congestive heart failure, kidney and liver damage and others.

These drugs include amiloride, spironolactone, triamterene. This particular group of diuretics does not allow the unwanted side effect of low potassium in the blood to occur.

Since vital potassium may be lost, the potassium,-sparing diuretics increase the flow of urine but keep the potassium in the body tissues and cells.

DIURETIC, THIAZIDE
Drug used to treat high blood pressure. High blood pressure adds to the workload of the heart and arteries.

If it continues for a long time, they may not function properly. This can damage the blood vessels of the brain, heart, and kidneys, resulting in a stroke, heart attack, or kidney failure.

These problems may be avoided if blood pressure is controlled. Thiazide diuretics are also used to help reduce the amount of water in the body by increasing the flow of urine.

Possible side effects are:
- joint pain;
- flank pain;
- stomach pain;
- skin rash;
- sore throat;
- fever;
- stomach pain;
- diarrhea;
- dizziness;
- vomiting;
- loss of appetite;
- upset stomach;
- increased thirst;

- irregular heartbeats;
- mood or mental changes;
- muscle cramps or pain.

DIURNAL
Belonging to the period of daylight, as distinguished from night.

DIVERTICULITIS
Inflammation of an abnormal sac (diverticulum) at a weakened point in the digestive tract, especially the colon.

DIVERTICULOSIS
The presence of abnormal pouch-like sacs through the muscular layer of the colon.

DIVERTICULUM
A pouchlike herniation through the muscular wall of a tubular organ, especially the colon.

DIZZINESS
A sensation of unsteadiness, faintness or whirling in space, often with inability to maintain balance.

DNA
Widely used abbreviation for de-

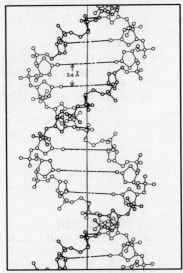

Basic spirally structure of DNA.

oxyribonucleic acid; one of two kinds of nucleic acids.

DOANS BACKACHE PILLS
Brand name of a drug containing the non-narcotic analgesics paracetamol and sodium salicylate as active pain-relieving compounds.

DO-DO-TABLETS
Brand name of a drug containing ephedrine, theophylline and caffeine as active compounds prescribed for severe cough and some nasal conditions.

DOMINANCE
(1) The ability of a specific genetic characteristic to appear at the expense of another.
(2) The fact or state of being dominant (exerting forcefulness or having dominance in a social hierarchy).
(3) Functional asymmetry between a pair of bodily structures (as the right and left hands).

DOMINATOR
A brightness receptor in the retina of the eye that is supposedly a group of cones linked to the terminals of a single nerve fiber.

DONNATAL
A fixed-combination drug, containing a sedative and several other agents, used to decrease gastrointestinal spasm.

DONOR
A person who gives living tissue (e.g., eye, blood, kidney) to be used in another person.

DOPAMINE
A chemical found in the brain and elsewhere in the body that functions as a neurotransmitter.

DORSAL
Pertaining to the posterior, or back, of an organ or the body.

DORSAL VERTEBRA
Thoracic vertebra; any of the 12 vertebrae dorsal to the thoracic region and characterized by articulation with the ribs.

DORSIFLEXION
The bending of a part backward.

DORSUM
The back part of any organ or the back itself.

DOSAGE
The amount and frequency by which a medicine is administered; the administration of medicine in doses.

DOSAGE COMPENSATION
The genetic mechanism by which the same effect on the phenotype is produced by a pair of identical sex-linked genes in the sex (as the human female) having the two sex chromosomes of different types or having only one sex chromosome.

DOSE
The amount of a medication or other substance, or of radiation, to be given at one time.

DOUBLE BIND
A psychological dilemma in which a usually dependent person (as a child) receives conflicting interpersonal communications from a single source or faces disparagement no matter what his or her response to a situation.

DOUBLE-BLIND STUDY
An experiment in which neither the investigator nor the subject knows whether the subject received the experimental variable (e.g., a drug) or a placebo, thus reducing any influence such knowledge might have on the reaction of the subject and the expectations or interpretations of the investigator. Only after the test is completed and the patients' responses are recorded is the identity

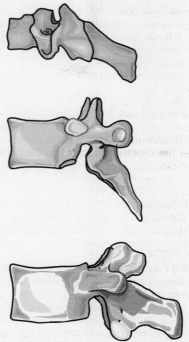

The twelve dorsal vertebrae make up the middle part of the spine or vertebral column. From top to bottom: cervical, dorsal and lumbar vertebra.

of those who received the new drug revealed. Double-blind trials are carried out for almost all new drugs.

DOUBLE HELIX
A helix or spiral consisting of two strands in the surface of a cylinder that coil around its axis; especially the structural arrangement of DNA in space that consists of paired polynucleotide strands stabilized by cross-links between purine and pyrimidine bases.

DOUBLE PNEUMONIA
Pneumonia of both lungs at the same time.

DOWN'S SYNDROME
A congenital defect, usually caused by the presence of an extra #21 chromosome (trisomy) and characterized by:
- mental retardation;

- oblique placement of the eyes;
- a small head flattened at the back;
- a large, furrowed tongue;
- short stature;
- bowel defects;
- heart abnormalities.

DRAGEE
A sugar-coated medicine.

DRAIN
A tube inserted into a body cavity, sometimes during surgery, to remove unwanted material.

DRAINAGE
The drawing off of fluid from a body cavity, usually fluid that has accumulated abnormally.

DREAM ANXIETY DISORDER
Repeated awakenings from sleep with detailed recall of frightening dreams. These dreams are typically vivid and quite extended and usually include threats to survival, security, or self-esteem. Often there is recurrence of the same or similar themes. The dream experience or the sleep disturbance resulting from the awakenings causes significant stress.

Dream anxiety episodes often increase with mental stress, less often with physical fatigue, and, in a few cases, with changes in the sleep environment.

Dream anxiety episodes occur during periods of REM sleep. Thus, although they may occur at almost any time during the night, they become more frequent toward the end of the night, when REM sleep is more abundant. During a typical dream anxiety episode, there is remarkably little autonomic agitation. Large body movements are rarely observed during the episode because the REM-related loss of muscle tone inhibits body movement, but they are often present during the awakening.

Upon awakening from the frightening dream, the person rapidly becomes oriented and alert. Usually, a detailed account of the dream experience can be given, both immediately upon awakening and in the morning. Many people who suffer nightmares have difficulty returning to sleep after awakening from a nightmare.

Over half the cases start before the age of 10, and in about two-thirds of cases, onset is before age 20. A major stressful event seems to precede the onset of the disorder in about 60% of cases.

The frequency of episodes is variable both within and among individuals. In many cases three or more nightmares per week are reported. Children frequently outgrow the disorder. If it begins in adulthood, the disorder often persists for decades.

DRIP
A non-medical term for an intravenous infusion.

DROMOMANIA
An exaggerated desire to wander.

DROP FOOT
A condition in which the foot is flexed toward the sole (plantar surface) or droops and cannot be voluntarily flexed toward a normal position.

DROOL
(1) To secrete saliva in anticipation of food.
(2) To let saliva or some other substance flow from the mouth. Most babies begin to drool at about four months.

DRUG
A substance used as medicine in treatment of disease, or a mood-altering substance, especially one that is addictive.

DRUG ABUSE
Use of a drug for nontherapeutic purposes (e.g., to alter one's sense

of awareness, as with LSD). Commonly abused substances include barbiturates, alcohol, sedatives, and amphetamines.

DRUG ADDICTION
A condition marked by an overwhelming desire to ingest or otherwise take a drug to which one has become habituated because of long-term use and by the development of withdrawal symptoms (mental and/or physical) if the drug is not taken. Heroin, cocaine and barbiturates are common addictive drugs.

DRUG DEPENDENCE
A condition in which one craves or depends on a particular drug that one is accustomed to taking.

DRY SOCKET
Inflammation at the site of an extracted tooth, characterized by pain, pus and frequently infection.

DUALISM
A theory that considers reality to consist of two irreducible elements or modes (as mind and matter).

DUCT
Tube or channel, particularly one carrying excretions or secretions.

DUCTLESS GLAND
Endocrine gland.

DUCTULE
A small duct, e.g., one of the small tubes found in the tear glands.

DUCTUS ARTERIOSUS
A blood vessel in the fetus connecting the pulmonary artery directly to the ascending aorta, thus bypassing the pulmonary circulation. It normally closes at birth.

DUCTUS ARTERIOSUS, PATENT
Failure of the ductus arteriosus to close at birth. This condition often requires surgical correction.

DUCTUS DEFERENS
Duct, about 18 inches (45 centimeters) long, leading from the testis, looping around the urinary bladder, and ending in the ejaculatory duct.

DUMPING SYNDROME
A group of symptoms, including nausea, dizziness, sweating, and faintness, occurring after a meal, particularly a meal rich in carbohydrates, in patients who have had stomach surgery; it is due to a too-rapid emptying of the stomach contents and the development of low sugar levels in the blood.

DUODENAL
Pertaining to the duodenum.

DUODENAL ULCER
An ulcer in the duodenum; it is the most common type of peptic ulcer.

DUODENUM
First part of the small intestine extending from the valve of the stomach to the jejunum.

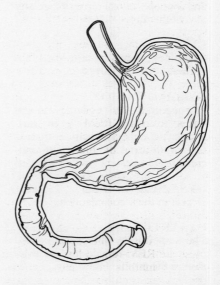

The first part of the intestinal tract is the duodenum. From the stomach the food is transported into the duodenum.

DUPUYTREN'S CONTRAC-TURE
A painless condition in which the fourth and fifth fingers bend into the palm of the hand and resist extension due to a progressive thickening of tissue beneath the skin in the palm. Of unknown cause, it primarily affects middle-aged men. Treatment involves surgical excision of the excess tissue.

DURA MATER
Outermost of the three membranes covering the brain and spinal cord.

DWARFISM
Underdevelopment of the body, characterized primarily by abnormally short stature, often with underdeveloped limbs and with other defects. Causes include genetic defects, pituitary or thyroid malfunctioning, kidney disease, and certain other disorders.

DYADIC
Pertaining to a relationship involving two persons, e.g., that of doctor and patient in therapy, especially psychotherapy.

DYS–
Combining form meaning bad, abnormal, difficult, adverse.

DYSADAPTATION
An impaired ability of the iris and retina to adapt properly to variations in light intensities that is often indicative of vitamin-A deficiency.

DYSAPHIA
Defect in the sense of touch.

DYSARTHRIA
The impairment of speech caused by central nervous disease or a lesion in the brain.

DYSCHEZIA
Difficulty in passing stools, usually from long-continued, voluntary suppression of the urge to defecate.

DYSCRASIA
Any diseased or imbalanced state of the body or its systems.

DYSCRASIA, BLOOD
Any abnormal condition of the blood.

DYSENTERY
Group of diseases characterized by inflammation of the colon resulting in pain, spasm of the rectum, intense diarrhea and the frequent passage of small amounts of mucus and blood.

DYSEQUILIBRIUM
Any abnormality in the sense of balance.

DYSFUNCTION
Bad performance or impaired function of some part of the body, such as the heart or nervous sytem.

DYSGENESIS
Defective development; malformation during embryonic development.

DYSGRAPHIA
An impairment of the ability to write correctly, due to a brain or motor disorder.

DYSKINESIA
Difficulty in carrying out voluntary movements.

DYSLEXIA
A condition in which an individual with normal vision has extreme difficulty in interpreting written language and therefore is, to a greater or lesser degree, unable to read.

DYSLOGIA
Impairment of the power to think logically and rationally.

DYSMENORRHEA
Painful menstruation.

DYSMENORRHEA, PRIMARY
Painful menstruation intrinsic to the process of menstruation and not the result of any other disease or condition.

DYSMENORRHEA, SECONDARY
Painful menstruation caused by a specific disorder (e.g., uterine tumor, pelvic inflammation, endometriosis).

DYSMETRIA
Impaired ability to estimate distance in muscular action.

DYSMORPHOPHOBIA
Preoccupation with some imagined defect in appearance in a normal-appearing person. The most common complaints involve facial flaws, such as wrinkles, spots on the skin, excessive facial hair, shape of nose, mouth, jaw, or eyebrows, and swelling of the face. More rarely the complaint involves the appearance of the feet, hands, breasts, back, or some other part of the body.

A history of repeated visits to plastic surgeons or dermatologists in an effort to correct the imagined defect is common. A depressive syndrome and obsessive compulsive personality traits are frequent. Often there is avoidance of social or occupational situations because of anxiety about the imagined defect.

The most common age of onset is from adolescence through the third decade.

DYSOSMIA
A condition in which the sense of smell is impaired.

DYSPAREUNIA
An abnormal condition in which sexual intercourse is painful; it may be caused by abnormality of the genital organs, psychophysiological reactions, inadequate sexual arousal, or other factors.

The disturbance is not caused by lack of lubrication or by vaginismus.

DYSPEPSIA
Indigestion, a disorder of the digestive function, marked by vague discomfort, heartburn, or nausea.

DYSPHAGIA
A condition in which swallowing is difficult or painful, due to obstruction of the esophagus or muscular abnormalities of the esophagus or pharynx.

DYSPHASIA
Loss of or deficiency in the power to use or understand language as a result of injury to or disease of the brain.

DYSPHONIA
Difficulty in speaking due to impairment of the voice.

DYSPLASIA
Formation of abnormal tissue; alteration in size, shape and organization of adult cells.

DYSPNEA
Breathlessness; shortness of breath.

DYSPRAXIA
A decrease in proper function (as of an organ) or of ability to coordinate muscular actions.

DYSREGULATION
Impairment of regulatory mechanisms (as those governing concentration of a substance in the blood or the function of an organ).

DYSRHYTHMIA
A disorder of the rhythm exhibited in a record of electrical activity of the brain or heart.

DYSSOMNIA
Sleep disorder characterized by a disturbance in the amount, quality, or timing of sleep. The dyssomnias

include three groups of disorders:
- insomnia disorders;
- hypersomnia disorders;
- sleep-wake schedule disorder.

In the insomnia disorders, sleep is deficient in the quantity or quality necessary for normal daytime functioning. In the hypersomnia disorders, the person feels excessively sleepy when awake, despite sleep of normal length. In sleep-wake schedule disorders, there is a mismatch between the person's sleep-wake pattern and the pattern that is normal for his or her environment.

DYSTHYMIA

A chronic disturbance of mood involving depressed mood (or possibly an irritable mood in children or adolescents), for most of the day, more days than not, for at least two years (one year for children and adolescents). In addition, during these periods of depressed mood there are some of the following associated symptoms:
– poor appetite or overeating;
– insomnia or hypersomnia;
– low energy or fatigue;
– low self-esteem;
– poor concentration;
– difficulty making decisions;
– feelings of hopelessness.

Dysthymia frequently seems to be a consequence of a preexisting, chronic, nonmood disorder, such as:
– anorexia nervosa;
– somatization disorder;
– psychoactive substance dependence;
– anxiety disorder;
– rheumatoid arthritis.

The disorder usually begins in childhood, adolescence, or early adult life, and for this reason has often been referred to as depressive personality.

The disorder usually begins without clear onset and has a chronic course. The impairment in social and occupational functioning is usually mild or moderate because of the chronicity rather than the severity of the depressive syndrome. Therefore, hospitalization is rarely required unless there is a suicide attempt or a superimposed major depression. In children and adolescents, social interaction with peers and adults is frequently affected.

DYSTOCIA

Abnormal labor, due to abnormal position of the fetus, contracted or obstructed birth canal, or other factor.

DYSTONIA

Abnormal muscle tone, especially sudden muscle spasms due to a rare inherited disease (dystonia musculorum deformans) or sometimes to drug reaction.

DYSTROPHIA

Defective or faulty nutrition. Usually applied to several neuromuscular disorders, e.g., muscular dystrophy.

DYSURIA

Painful or difficult urination; it may be caused by inflammation of the bladder or urethra.

E

EAR
The hearing organ, including three general structures: the outer (external ear); the middle ear, including the eardrum cavity and the three tiny bones that transmit the hearing vibrations; and the inner (internal) ear.

EARACHE
Pain in the ear; it may be caused by ear disease or by infection or disease of the nose, mouth region, throat, and other nearby areas.

EARDRUM
The tympanic membrane that separates the middle ear from the external ear.

EAR, SWIMMER'S
Ear infection caused by water remaining in the ear canal, containing microorganisms able to set up infection, with itching and pain. Once the infection develops, antibiotics are needed to eradicate it so one should see a doctor.

EAR WAX
Also called cerumen: a yellowish wax-like secretion from certain glands in the external acoustic meatus (auditory canal), which acts as a lubricant and stops dust from entering the ear.

EBURNATION
Polishing of the ends of bone due to the degeneration of cartilage, caused by osteoarthritis, which makes the bone become harder and denser.

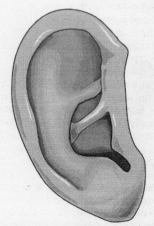

External ear with the entrance of the external meatus leading to the ear-drum.

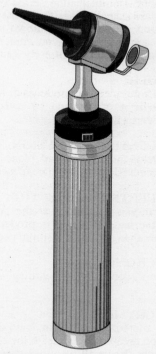

Otoscope for investigation of the external acoustic meatus and the ear-drum.

EBOLA VIRUS DISEASE
Viral disease with the following symptoms:
- sudden onset;
- general pains;
- fever;
- vomiting;
- watery diarrhea;
- rapid dehydration;
- prostration.

On the 5th-7th day the following additional symptoms may occur:
- maculopapular rash (may look like measles with conjunctivitis);
- pharyngitis;
- ecchymoses;
- petechiae;
- bleeding from the nose and gums;
- hematemesis;
- melena;
- metrorrhagia;
- circulatory failure;
- shock.

Death may occur between days 7 and 16. The fatality rate is about 50 percent. The incubation period is 2-21 days, usually 3-7. Transmission is probably from an unknown animal source. In 1995, an epidemic occurred in Congo (formerly Zaire).

EBOLIC
Any substance that produces or hastens labor or abortion by causing the uterus to contract.

ECCENTRIC OCCLUSION
Relation of the inclined planes of the teeth when the jaws are closed.

ECCENTRIC PROJECTION
Location of sensation at the point on the body where it is produced, rather than at the point stimulated.

ECCHONDROMA
Tumor consisting of cartilage tissue.

ECCHYMOSIS
Discolored patch of skin, caused by blood escaping underneath the skin. It later shows all the color changes seen in bruising.

ECCRINE
Any gland that delivers its secretion to the surface in the body, such as the sweat glands in the skin.

ECCRINE SWEAT GLANDS
Gland with the function to eliminate water, the evaporation of which regulates the body temperature.

Eccrine glands are simple, tubular glands distributed over the whole body (100-600 glands per square centimeter), with more in some areas and less in others.

The secretory part consists of a tangled knot of epidermal cells in the deep part of the dermis or in the upper part of the layer of subcutaneous fat.

The gland opens into a duct that first winds within this knot and then passes straight through the dermis and, in close spirals, through the epidermis.

ECCYESIS
Development of an embryo outside the uterus.

ECG
Abbreviation for electrocardiogram.

ECHINACEA
(Echinacea angustifolia) Plant of which the rootstocks are used for medicinal purposes. The stout, bristly stem bears hairy leaves that taper at both ends. The distinctive flower features 12 to 20 large, spreading dull-purple rays and a conical disc made up of numerous tubular purple florets. Echinacea is one of the blood-purifying plants used for conditions such as eczema, acne and boils, and it is thought to neutralize contaminants in the blood. It also promotes proper digestion and can be tried for fever. The rootstock may also help to dispel flatulence ("wind").

ECHINOCOCCIASIS
A tissue infection of humans caused by the larval stage of the tapeworm

Taenia echinococcus. It reaches humans primarily via dogs, but sheep are also common hosts.

The worms form hydatid cysts, the majority of which are found in the liver (although they can be situated in the brain, lungs and kidneys), where, after producing no symptoms for decades, they finally produce abdominal pain or a palpable mass.

Treatment involves the removal of the cysts by surgery.

ECHINOCOCCOSIS
An infection with a larval tapeworm (Echinococcus), usually transmitted through contact with infested dogs. It is characterized by cyst formation in tissue, especially the liver; symptoms depend on the tissue affected. Treatment involves surgical excision of the cysts.

ECHINOCOCCUS
Tapeworm that forms cysts in the brain, liver, kidney and lungs.

ECHINOSIS
A state in which the red blood cells have an irregular appearance.

ECHOCARDIOGRAM
Recording or a scan of the heart using ultrasound (very high frequency sound waves) to discover the structure, position and motion of the heart.

ECHOCARDIOGRAPHY
A diagnostic method by which pulses of ultrasound are transmitted into the body and the echoes returning from the surfaces of the heart and other structures are electronically plotted and recorded.

Stop-action or "real-time" images of the heart can be made into a record of the heart's movements.

ECHOENCEPHALOGRAPHY
A diagnostic procedure using ultrasound waves to study the brain; it may reveal expanding lesions or expansion of brain ventricles.

ECHOLALIA
In psychiatry, automatic and meaningless repetition of another's words, sometimes occurring in schizophrenia and other neurological and mental disorders.

ECHONDROMA
Growth composed of cartilage growing in tissue where cartilage is not ordinarily found, such as the interior of a bone.

ECHOPATHY
A general term, applied to a nervous disorder, characterized by senseless repetition of words and phrases.

ECHOPRAXIA
Automatic imitation of movements made by other people.

ECHOSCOPY
The use of ultrasound as a diagnostic method. Ultrasound waves are directed at the tissues and a record is made, as on an oscilloscope, of the waves reflected back through the tissues, which indicate interfaces of different acoustic densities and thus differentiate between solid and cystic structures.

ECHOVIRUS
Any of a group of small viruses, some of which are responsible for human illnesses.

ECLAMPSIA
A rare and serious pregnancy disorder. Eclampsia is characterized by:
- convulsions:
- coma:
- high blood pressure;
- protein in the urine;
- edema.

Once the convulsions are controlled and emergency treatment of the pregnant woman completed, delivery of the infant is usually necessary.

ECLECTICISM
A type of theory characterized by the attempts to reconcile inconsistent views, or improve on them, by the selective adoption of elements from each, and making of these a more or less self-consistent system.

ECOLOGY
The study of plants and animals in relation to their environment. The whole earth can be considered as a large ecological unit; the term biosphere is used to describe the atmosphere, each surface, oceans and ocean floors within which living organisms exist. However, it is usual to divide the biosphere into a large number of ecological sub-units, or ecosystems, within each of which the organisms making up the living community are in balance with the environment.

ECOMANIA
Pathological attitude and behavior towards members of one's family.

ECONOMIC
Used generally to describe motives involving earning a livelihood, the accumulation of wealth and the like. It is employed by psychoanalysts to describe the production, distribution and consumption of human energy in accordance with the principle of greatest utility for least expenditure or effort.

ECPHORIA
The revival of a memory trace or engram.

ECPHYMA
An excrescence, such as a wart.

ECSTASY
Rapture; in a special sense, extreme concentration of attention amounting to semi-trance, as a phenomenon or phase of prolonged contemplation of a limited field, in the case particularly of religious mysticism.

ECTASIA
Dilatation or distension of a part or organ, for instance, alveolar ectasia, abnormal expansion of the air sacs in the lungs.

ECTHYMA
A streptococcal or staphylococcal skin infection penetrating more deeply than impetigo, which it resembles, but shows little surface spread.

ECTODERM
Outer of the three primary germ layers of the embryo from which develops, among other tissues, the skin.

ECTOGENOUS
Capable of growth outside the body; usually refers to parasites or microorganisms.

ECTOMORPH
A person whose physique is thin, fragile, and generally nonmuscular.

ECTOMORPHY
The third of the three types of physique (the others being endomorphy and mesomorphy) in the theory of the psychologist Prof. W.H. Sheldon. In comprises delicacy of skin, fine hair, fragile frame and ultrasensitive nervous system.

ECTOPARASITE
A parasite living on the outside of the body on its host.

ECTOPIA
An abnormal positioning of a part or organ, especially at the time of birth.

ECTOPIC PREGNANCY
An abnormal pregnancy, occurring in about 2 percent of all pregnancies, in which the fertilized egg (conceptus, embryo) implants outside of the uterus, most often (90 percent) in the Fallopian tube, but occasionally in the ovary or ab-

dominal cavity. It is extremely rare for such a pregnancy to progress beyond the first two months of pregnancy. Because of the possibility of rupture and hemorrhage, when an ectopic pregnancy is suspected medical attention is required immediately. The embryo will be removed surgically, which usually results in one Fallopian tube being incapable of transporting further eggs.

ECTOPOTOMY
Surgical removal of an embryo that has been developing outside the uterus in an ectopic pregnancy.

ECTOTOXEMIA
Blood poisoning caused by introduction of a poison in the blood.

ECTRODACTYLY
Congenital absence of some fingers or toes.

ECTROGENY
Congenital absence of any body part or organ.

ECTROMELIA
Congenital absence of the whole or part of a limb or limbs.

ECTROPION
Turning of the inside of an edge or part outwards, especially of an eyelid.

ECZEMA
A collective term for many inflammatory conditions of the skin. An eczema causes one or more of the following physical changes to the skin:
- erythema (blood congestion);
- infiltration of plasma into the tissues;
- vesicles (blisters);
- papules.
  Secondary changes include:
- erosion of tissue;
- exudation of fluid onto the skin;
- crusts;
- lichenification (thickened areas of itchy skin);
- scaling.
The eczemas commonly show rapid changes in the clinical features and striking differences between different sites.

EDEMA
The abnormal collection of fluid in spaces between cells, especially just under the skin or in a given cavity or organ.
Causes include:
- injury;
- heart disease;
- kidney failure;
- cirrhosis;
- allergy.
Treatment depends on the cause.

EDENTULOUS
Without teeth, as when all the natural teeth have been removed.

EDIFICATION
Improvement and progress of the mind in knowledge, in morals or in faith and holiness.

EDUCATION
The act or art of developing and cultivating the various physical, intellectual, esthetic and moral faculties.

EDUCATIONAL AGE
Corresponding to the educational level of an average school child of any given chronological age, as determined by standardized educational tests.

EDUCATIONAL PSYCHOLOGY
Branch of applied psychology that is concerned with the application of psychological principles and findings, together with the psychological study of problems of education.

EDUCATIONAL QUOTIENT
The ratio of educational age to chronological age, expressed as a percentage.

EEG
Abbreviation for electroencephalogram.

EFFACEMENT
Shortening of the vagina and thinning of its walls as it is stretched and dilated during labor.

EFFECTOR
A motor nerve that transforms nerve impulses into physical action, such as the contraction of a muscle. The term is also used to describe muscles that contract or glands that secrete a particular substance upon stimulation by a motor nerve.

EFFEMINACY
Presence of feminine characteristics of physical structure, or the manifestation of feminine behavior characteristics in a man.

EFFERENT
Carrying away or going away from, such as a nerve carrying impulses away from the central nervous system or blood vessels carrying blood away from, say, an organ.

EFFLEURAGE
Rhythmic, firm or gentle, stroking, as in massage. Effleurage of the abdomen is commonly used in the Lamaze method of natural childbirth.

EFFLORESCENCE
A redness, rash or eruption of the skin.

EFFLUVIUM
Something flowing out in a subtle or invisible form, especially a noxious disagreeable exhalation.

EFFORT
An exertion of strength or power, whether physical or mental.

EFFORT EXPERIENCE
Sense of muscular effort in voluntary movement (kinesthesia) arising from the muscles involved in the effort, together with (according to some psychologists) direct experience or conation (the desire to perform an action).

EFFORT SYNDROME
Also called functional heart disease, da Costa syndrome and "disordered action of the heart": a group of symptoms (quick fatigue, rapid heartbeat, sighing breaths, dizziness) that do result from disease of organs or tissues and that are out of proportion to the amount of exertion required.

EFFUSION
The escape of any fluid out of the vessel containing it into another part. The term is also used in the sense of overflowing or demonstrative kindness.

EGERIS
Extreme alertness; abdominal wakefulness.

EGESTION
The voiding of the waste products of digestion.

EGG
Ovum; the sex cell (gamete) of the female, which, when fertilized by the male sperm, becomes a zygote.

EGO
A term used by Sigmund Freud and now generally accepted to mean the self, especially the conscious self. The ego represents what may be called reason and common sense.

"Ego" and "self" are often confused; they probably belong to different frames of reference, the ego belonging to an objective frame of reference that views personality as a structure, and the self belonging to a phenomenological frame of reference that views personality as experience.

EGO-ALTER THEORY
A theory seeking to account for the

growth of social consciousness and the development of social organization from the interaction between the self and the other.

EGO ANALYSIS
The intensive therapeutic study and analysis of the ways in which the ego resolved or attempts to deal with intrapsychic conflicts. Deals especially with the evolvement and employment of mental dynamics or mechanisms which the person unconsciously employs, and with the maturation of capacity for rational thought and action.

EGO ANXIETY
Anxiety arising from a threat to the ego, caused by the conflicting demands of the id, the ego and the superego.

EGO BOUNDARY
Psychological concept by which the distinction between self and not-self is imagined to be delineated. people are said to lack ego boundaries if they identify readily with others and so at the expense of their own sense of identity.

Analysts who hold that infants live in a state of primary identification with their mothers, postulate the gradual development of an ego boundary, i.e., the discovery that objects are not parts of oneself.

EGOCENTRIC
Selfish, focusing especially or exclusively on oneself. In association tests responses that are clearly personal are classified as egocentric responses. The fact that individuals can interpret the thoughts and acts of others only through their own experiences has been called the egocentric predicament.

EGO DEFENSE
Protection of the ego from unacceptable impulses of the id through the use of conscious defense mechanisms.

EGO DEVELOPMENT
The fact that psychoanalysis assumes that the psyche is divisible into an id and ego compels it to make a distinction between libidinal and ego development.

The former is the progress through various libidinal stages in which the sources and forms of sexual pleasure change, and the latter is the growth and acquisition of functions that enable individuals increasingly to master their impulses, to operate independently of parental figures, and to control their environment.

Attempts have been made to correlate phases of libidinal and ego development and to describe an oral ego, which is entirely pleasure-seeking and dependent on the mother, and an anal ego, which is concerned with control and mastery of impulses, etc.

Ego development may also refer to the process by which the ego differentiates out of the id.

EGO-DYSTONIC
Opposite of ego-syntonic: behavior and wishes are said to be ego-dystonic if they are incompatible with the subject's ideals or conception of himself; i.e., they refer to a value judgment by the subject himself.

EGO FAILURE
Failure of the ego to keep balance amid impulses coming from the id, demands of the superego, and external reality.

EGO FUNCTION
Anything that the subject can do. Since psychoanalysis ascribed all functions to the ego, anything that the subject can do is an ego function.

EGO IDEAL
A psychoanalytical concept, more or less a substitute for conscience, involving a standard of perfection

set up in the early life of the child, through identification with some admired person, e.g., the father.

EGO IDENTITY
A person's experience of himself as persisting essentially unchanged or as a continuous entity through time as a result of the function of the ego that synthesizes one's ideals, behavior and social role.

EGO INSTINCT
Term employed by psychoanalysts, meaning a type of instinct other than to a sex instinct.

EGO INTEGRITY
The last of the German-American psychoanalyst Eric Erickson's eight stages of man. The term is generally used in the sense of the serenity of old age and the acceptance of one's own death as natural as part of the order of things.

EGO INVOLVEMENT
Commitment to and absorption in a task so that success in it becomes important to self-esteem and failure leads to chagrin.

EGOISM
A system of ethical and social philosophy based on the view that the fundamental motive underlying all morality and all conduct is in the last resort self-interest; a characteristic of an individual exhibiting and illustrating this view in practice.

EGO LIBIDO
Libido that is invested in the ego.

EGOMANIA
Abnormally excessive self-regard.

EJACULATE
Sperm-containing fluid (semen) emitted during ejaculation. The fluid volume of each ejaculate is usually between 2 and 5 milliliters and it contains 50,000,000 to 150,000,000 spermatozoa.

EJACULATION
The prostate's pumping action and muscular contractions that send semen spurting through the urethra and from the penis. Most semen is ejaculated by the first five or six contractions.

EJACULATION, PREMATURE
Persistent or recurrent ejaculation with minimal sexual stimulation or before, upon, or shortly after penetration and before the person wishes it. The clinician will take into account factors that affect duration of the excitement phase, such as age, novelty of the sexual partner or situation, and frequency of sexual activity.

EJACULATORY DUCT
Duct, about 1 inch long, behind the bladder that transports sperm from the ductus deferens to the urethra.

ELASTOSIS
A condition in which elastic tissue breaks down.

ELBOW
The joint in the arm formed by the humerus above and the radius and ulna below. It is a common site of inflammation and injury (for instance, tennis elbow).

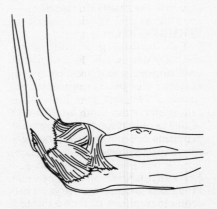

Anterior view of the elbow joint. Above: humerus; below: radius and ulna.

ELECTIVE

Decided on by the person and/or the physician, especially with relation to procedures (e.g., surgery) that are not essential.

ELECTIVE MUTISM

Persistent refusal to talk in one or more major social situations, including school, despite ability to comprehend spoken language and to speak.

The child with elective mutism may communicate via gestures, by nodding or shaking the head, or, in some cases, by monosyllabic or short, monotone utterances. Most commonly the child will not speak at school, but will talk normally within the home. Less commonly the child refuses to speak in nearly all social situations. Children with this disorder generally have normal language skills, though some have delayed language development and abnormalities in articulation.

Although onset is usually before age five, the disturbance may come to clinical attention only with entry into school.

ELECTRIC BURN

A burn caused by heat generated by an electric current.

ELECTRICAL HEALING

Use of electricity to increase the rate of natural repair of damaged tissue (e.g., fractures).

ELECTRIC SHOCK

A traumatic state caused by the passage of an electric current through the body. It usually results from accidental contact with exposed circuits in household appliances but may also result from contact with high-voltage wires or from being struck by lightening. The damage to the body depends on the type, intensity, and duration of the current; it commonly includes burns, heart rhythm abnormalities, and unconsciousness.

ELECTROANESTHESIA

Loss of sensation resulting from application of an electric current to the body or to a part.

ELECTROCARDIOGRAM (ECG)

A graphic recording, produced by an electrocardiograph, of the electri-

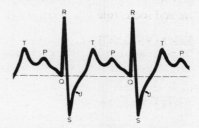

Normal electrocardiogram (ECG) characteristic PQRST-complex. J indicates a small, non-pathological deviation of the normal ECG.

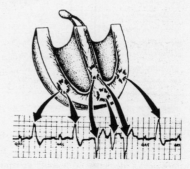

Abnormal electrocardiogram due to ectopic foci in the ventricle of the heart.

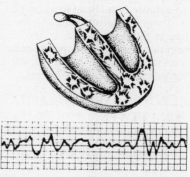

Abnormal electrocardiogram (ECG) due to fibrillation of the ventricle of the heart.

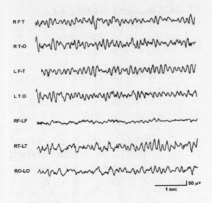

Normal electroencephalogram of a child of 12-years old.

Abnormal electroencephalogram of a person with a severe dementia with some epileptic activity.

cal activity of the heart.

Commonly referred to as an ECG, it allows the detection of abnormalities in the transmission of the heart impulse through the heart muscle and serves as an important aid in the diagnosis of heart ailments.

ELECTROCARDIOGRAPH
A device used to record the electrical activity of the heart.

ELECTROCAUTERY
The application of a needle or snare heated by an electric current to destroy tissue (e.g., to remove warts).

ELECTROCOAGULATION
Coagulation of tissues by an electrical current.

ELECTROCONVULSIVE THERAPY
Treatment of certain mental disorders, esp. severe depression, in which a brief convulsion is induced by passing an electric current through the brain.

ELECTROENCEPHALOGRAM (EEG)
A graphic recording, produced by an electoencephalograph, of the electrical activity of the brain. EEGs are helpful in detecting and locating brain tumors, circulatory disturbances, and in diagnosing epilepsy.

ELECTROENCEPHALO-GRAPH
A device for receiving and recording the electrical activity of the brain. In most cases electrodes are attached to various areas of the head and the patient is asked to remain quiet while the brain-wave activity is recorded.

ELECTROLYSIS
An electrical action that causes a chemical to break down into simpler forms. The term is also used for the passing of an electric current into a hair root to remove superfluous or unwanted hair.

ELECTROLYTE
Chemicals such as sodium, potassium, calcium and bicarbonate found in body tissues and fluids, which are vital for the maintenance of the correct balance of fluids in the cells.

ELECTROLYTE BALANCE
Equilibrium between electrolytes in the body that is essential for normal functioning, with a deficiency or excess of a particular electrolyte producing characteristic symptoms.

ELECTROMYOGRAM
A recording of the electrical activity occurring when voluntary (skeletal) muscles work; it is helpful in diagnosing muscle and nerve abnormalities.

ELECTRON MICROSCOPE
An instrument similar to a light microscope but which uses a beam of electrons, not light, to scan surfaces and create an image; magnification 2,000 times that of an optical microscope is possible.

ELECTROPHORESIS
The movement of charged particles in a liquid medium in response to changes in an electric field.

ELECTRORETINOGRAM
A graphic recording of the electrical activity of the retina; it is made by flashing a light into the eye and recording the effects on the retina with special devices attached to the eye and the back of the head.

ELECTROSLEEP
Sleep that is brought about by applying a controlled electric current to the head. The procedure has been used in treating mental and emotional disorders, e.g., anxiety, depression, and insomnia.

ELECTROSURGERY
Surgery performed using electrical devices (e.g., electrically wired needles).

ELEMENT
The simplest chemical form, in which only one kind of atom is contained.

ELEPHANTIASIS
A condition characterized by enormous enlargement of certain body parts, esp. the legs and scrotum, often with a thickening and coarsening of the skin.

It is the end stage of the disease filariasis and is due to the blockage of the lymphatic vessels by infiltration of filarial worms.

ELIMINATION
The process getting rid of a material, as of waste products through the urine.

ELIXIR
A sweetened, flavored liquid, usually containing a small amount of alcohol, used in compounding medicines to be taken by mouth.

An elixir often contains alcohol that forms the base for many liquid medicines such as those used to treat cough.

EMACIATION
Excessive thinness, due to disease or poor nutrition.

EMASCULATION
Surgical removal of the penis and/or testes. The term is also used in the sense of loss of a feeling of masculinity or of male characteristics.

EMBOLECTOMY
Surgical removal of an embolus.

EMBOLISM
The presence of substances other than liquid blood in the blood circulation, causing obstruction in arteries or interfering with the pumping of the heart.

EMBOLUS
Piece of foreign matter circulating in the bloodstream. It may be a blood clot, an air bubble, cancer cells, fat vegetation from a heart valve, clumps of bacteria or a foreign body.

EMBROCATION
An ointment rubbed on to the skin to relieve joint pain, muscle cramp or muscle injury. An embrocation usually contains a rubefacient, a preparation also known as counterirritant.

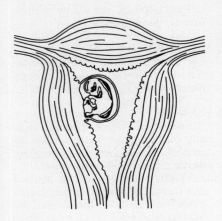

A two-month embryo in the uterus.

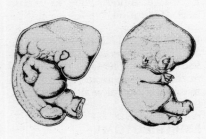

Left: embryo of about 6 weeks (ca. 5 mm).
Right: embryo of about 8 weeks (ca. 25 mm).

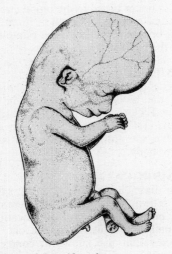

Embryo of about 12 weeks.

EMBRYO
The early developing organism, from the zygote to the fetal stage; in humans, from about week 3 to week 8 after conception, at which time the main organ systems have formed, at least in their early stages.

EMBRYOLOGY
The science of the development process of embryos.

EMESIS
Vomiting.

EMETIC
Any agent that causes vomiting. An emetic may work by irritating the lining of the stomach and/or by stimulating the part of the brain that controls vomiting.

EMETINE
An alkaloid with emetic and other medicinal properties.

EMISSION
Release of something, especially the uncontrolled discharge of semen during sleep (nocturnal emission).

EMMENAGOGUE
A medicine taken to promote the flow of menstrual blood.

EMMETROPIA
The normal refractive condition of the eye, in which rays of light are accurately focused on the retina and there is perfect vision.

EMOLLIENT
A substance that softens and soothes tissues that are inflamed. An emollient also has a moisturizing effect, preventing loss of water from the skin surface, by forming an oily film.

EMOTION
A state of the body and mind consisting of a subjective feeling that is either pleasurable or unpleasant but never neutral, that is accompanied

by expressive behavior or posture and by physical changes.

EMOTIONAL BLOCKAGE
Inability to remember or to think coherently due to strong emotions usually associated with fear.

EMOTIONAL CONFLICT
The clash which takes place between one's moral, social, and personal standards on the one hand, and one's egocentric and instinctional strivings -self-preservative, acquisitive, reproductive, aggressive, and destructive drives; the personal desires, needs, and strivings for possession, anger, love, and sex - on the other.
Emotional conflict may be conscious, partly conscious, or beyond conscious awareness.

EMOTIONAL FATIGUE
The fairly common type of tiredness or weariness which is out of proportion to the actual amount of physical or mental activity performed. The sources of this kind of fatigue are traceable to emotional origins.

EMOTIONAL HEALTH
A state of being which is relative rather than absolute. In general, the person who is emotionally healthy has effected a reasonably satisfactory integration of his instinctual drives. He has worked out psychologically harmonious solutions for them which are acceptable to himself, and to his social milieu. This is reflected in:
_ the satisfactory nature of his personal relationships;
_ his cheerful and willing acceptance of social responsibilities;
_ his level of satisfaction in living;
_ his flexibility in adjusting to new situations;
_ his effectiveness;
_ his actual achievements, in relation to his realistic capacities and endowment;

_ the absence of handicapping and limiting symptoms, or character defense traits;
_ his achievement of a reasonable degree of emotional equinanimity;
_ his ability to react constructively to threat or danger;
- the relative level of maturity which he has achieved.

EMOTIONAL IMMATURITY
Tendency towards emotional behavior characteristic of children or younger persons.

EMOTIONAL INDICATOR
A sign or symptom of the activity going on in an emotional state.

EMOTIONAL INSTABILITY
A pattern of overreaction emotionally in response to what appear ordinarily to be rather minor stresses. Usually the result is a decreased level of effectiveness.

EMOTIONAL MATURITY
Condition characterized by emotional development, and exhibition of emotional behavior appropriate to adults rather than to children.

EMOTIONAL PATTERN
The behavioral, psychological and peripheral responses and the set of relationships associated with a particular emotion and supposed to be characteristic of it.

EMOTIONAL SHOCK
An emotional disturbance due to an unpleasant experience. The individual becomes agitated, anxious, depressed or even hysterical.

EMOTIONAL STATE
Physical, behavioral and conscious condition of a person during emotional experiences and characteristic of emotions.

EMPATHY
The ability to recognize and relate to, and to extent share in, the emo-

tions of another. It is the power to project one's personality into someone else. The concept implies that, while a person's feelings may be engaged, he or she remains aware of his/her identity as another person. The word is necessary since sympathy is used only to refer to the sharing of unpleasant experiences and does not imply that the sympathizer necessarily retains his objectivity.

EMPHYSEMA
Abnormal condition of the lungs in which there is overinflation of the air sacs (alveoli) of the lungs leading to a breakdown of their walls, a decrease in respiratory function, and, in severe cases, increasing breathlessness.

EMPIRIC
Pertaining to treatment of disease based on observation and experience, not on knowledge of the specific causes or mechanisms of the disease.

EMPIRICAL PSYCHOLOGY
Psychology based on observation and experiment, as contrasted with rational psychology based on deduction from general philosophical principles, and sometimes also contrasting with existential psychology.

EMPIRIC RISK
The prediction of the probability that a genetic or congenital abnormality will occur in a family.

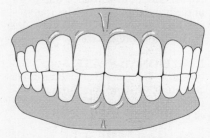

Enamel: the smooth, hard substance that covers the crown of the teeth.

EMPLASTRUM
A preparation for external application, i.e. a plaster that adheres to the skin.

EMPYEMA
Pus in the lung cavity or other body cavity, usually due to bacterial infection; treatment is by antibiotics and surgical drainage of the pus.

EMULSION
Suspension of very fine globules of oil in water, often by means of gum arabic. An emulsion is a combination of two substances that normally do not mix together properly but remain as particles of one suspended in the liquid form of the other. Many lotions are emulsions; they need to be shaken before use in case the constituent substances have separated.

ENAMEL
The smooth, hard substance that covers the crown of a tooth, overlying the dentine.

ENAMEL PULP
The jelly-like cells between the outer and inner enamel layers covering the teeth.

ENAMEL ROD
One of the elongated prismatic bodies making up the enamel of a tooth.

ENANTHEMA
A skin eruption or rash caused by specific internal diseases, such as typhoid or syphilis.

ENANTHIS
A new, tiny growth at the inner angle of the eye.

ENCAPSULATION
The process of enclosing something in a covering; the condition of being enclosed in a capsule, as the tendons or nerves are enclosed in membranous sheaths.

ENCEPHALO
Word element: association with the brain.

ENCEPHALITIS
Inflammation of the brain. It may be a specific disease due to micro-organisms such as bacteria, an insect-borne virus, or it may occur as a result of influenza, measles, German measles, chickenpox and other diseases. A very large number of living organisms invade the nervous system or its coverings, thus causing many forms of encephalitis or meningitis or a combination of both. The onset is usually that of a mild feverish illness, followed by a quiescent phase and by the disturbance in the central nervous system. Headache and drowsiness are usually present, followed in severe cases by confusion developing into stupor and coma. Convulsions may occur, particularly in young children. The pupils may be unequal and react poorly to light and accommodation. The motor functions of the cranial nerves and limbs may be little impaired. Sensory changes are variable. In the acute stage the tendon reflexes are likely to be diminished.

ENCEPHALITIS LETHARGICA
Inflammation of brain tissue characterized by the disturbances of sleep rhythm, the sufferers sleeping throughout the day and becoming wakeful and often restless and excited at night, and the damage to the upper brain stem, leading to sagging eyelids (ptosis), abnormalities in the pupils of the eyes and double vision.

ENCEPHALIZATION
The concept that the brain progressively takes more control of the functioning of the nervous system from the spinal cord, in the evolution of a species and in the development of an individual.

ENCEPHALOCELE
Congenital hernia of the brain that protrudes through an opening of the skull.

ENCEPHALOGRAPHY
The technique or act of taking X-ray photographs of the brain, usually on the basis of computerized tomography (CT scan) or after injection of a contrast medium into an artery.

ENCEPHALOID
Term used to describe a type of cancer that looks superficially like brain tissue.

ENCEPHALOMALACIA
Softening of the brain due to an inadequate supply of blood, and resulting in partial or complete deterioration.

ENCEPHALOMENINGITIS
Inflammation of the brain and its coverings.

ENCEPHALOMYELITIS
Acute inflammation of the brain and spinal cord, marked by fever, headache, neck and back pain, and vomiting. In severe cases and in weak or aged persons, seizures, coma, and death may result.

ENCEPHALON
The contents of the skull, consisting of the cerebrum, cerebellum, brain stem and membranes; the brain.

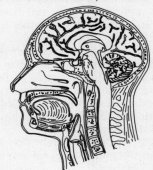

Encephalon: the brain inside the skull.

ENCEPHALOPATHY
Any malfunction or disease of the brain.

ENCHONDROMA
A benign tumor made up of cartilage. This type is especially common on fingers and toes.

ENCOPRESIS
A condition, not caused by physical illness or defect, in which the passing of feces occurs without control.

ENCOPRESIS, FUNCTIONAL
Repeated involuntary (or, much more rarely, intentional) passage of feces into places not appropriate for that purpose (e.g., clothing or floor). The stool may be of normal or near-normal consistency, or liquid, as in the case of overflow incontinence secondary to functional fecal retention.

When the passage of feces is involuntary rather than intentional, it is often related to constipation, impaction, or retention with subsequent overflow.

The constipation may develop because the child, for psychological reasons, avoids defecating, because of either anxiety about defecating in a particular place or a more general pattern of oppositional behavior.

In other children, the constipation develops for physiologic reasons, such as dehydration associated with a febrile illness or medication. Once constipation has developed, it may be complicated by an anal fissure, painful defecation, and further fecal retention.

Functional encopresis is generally referred to as primary if it has not been preceded by a period of fecal continence at least one year, and secondary if it has been preceded by a period of fecal continence lasting at least one year.

Fecal encopresis rarely becomes chronic, but, unless treated, can persist for years.

ENCOUNTER GROUP
A usually leaderless and unstructured group that seeks to develop the capacity of the individual to express feelings and to form emotional ties by unrestrained confrontation of individuals (as by physical contact, inhibited verbalization, or nudity).

END(O)
Word element: inward, within.

ENDARTERITIS
Inflammation of the inner layer of the wall of an artery, often associated with advanced syphilis and causing progressive thickening and blocking of the vessel.

ENDEMIC
Pertaining to any disease constantly present in a particular area, as opposed to epidemic, which implies a sudden explosive outburst of a disease.

ENDEMIC GOITER
Another name for euthyroid goiter.

ENDOCARDIAL FIBROELASTOSIS
A condition associated with congestive heart failure and enlargement of the heart that is characterized by the conversion of the endocardium to fibroelastic tissue.

ENDOCARDITIS
Inflammation of the endocardium (inner lining of the heart). It may involve only the membrane covering the valves or the general lining of the chambers of the heart. The condition is caused by bacterial infection or occurring as a complication of another disease (for instance, rheumatic fever). Symptoms include fever, and changes in heart rhythms; damage to heart valves may occur. Treatment consists of bedrest, antibiotics, and surgery, if necessary, to treat damaged valves.

ENDOCARDIUM
A colorless transparent membrane that lines the interior of the heart.

ENDOCERVICITIS
Inflammation of the epithelium and glands of the cervix of the uterus.

ENDOCOLPITIS
Inflammation of the lining of the vagina.

ENDOCRANIUM
Inner surface of the skull.

ENDOCRINE DISORDERS
Diseases of the pituitary, thyroid, parathyroid and adrenal glands, the islets of Langerhans in the pancreas and the endocrine parts of the ovaries and testes.

To the endocrine disorders also belong diseases of the hypothalamus-pituitary relationship (axis).

ENDOCRINE GLAND
Any ductless gland (for instance, pituitary gland) that releases its secretion - a hormone -directly into the bloodstream through which it moves to specific "target organs."

ENDOCRINE PSYCHOSYNDROME
Personality changes during the course of an endocrine disease.

ENDOCRINE SYSTEM
A number of ductless glandular structures that excrete chemical messengers called hormones and are widely distributed throughout the body. These organs and their general location are:
- pituitary gland in the brain;
- thyroid gland in the neck;
- parathyroid glands in the neck;
- adrenal glands in the abdomen;
- ovaries in the abdomen (in fe males);
- testes in the scrotum (in males).
One other organ, the pineal body, secretes hormonal products, but its function is largely unknown.

ENDOCRINOLOGIST
A physician who specializes in the diagnosis and treatment of diseases affecting the endocrine system.

ENDOCRINOLOGY
The study of the structure, function, and diseases of the endocrine system.

ENDOCRINOPATHY
Any disease caused by a disorder of an endocrine gland or glands.

ENDOCYSTITIS
Inflammation of the lining of the urinary bladder.

ENDODERM
In the embryo, the inner layer of cells from which the epithelium of the trachea, bronchi, lungs, gastrointestinal tract, and many other organs arises.

ENDOENTERITIS
Inflammation of the lining of the intestines.

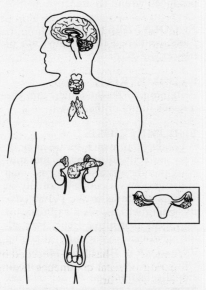

The endocrine system. From top to bottom: pituitary, thyroid and parathyroids, thymus, adrenals, and genital glands (ovaries and testicles).

ENDOGENOUS
Developed within an organism; arising within.

ENDOGENOUS DEPRESSION
A serious and persistent form of depression believed due to a complex interrelationship of biochemical, genetic and psychological factors and frequently not traceable to a specific extrinsic event.

ENDOGENOUS INFECTION
Infection caused by germs that are normally present in the body. For instance, if the bacillus Escherichia coli, which normally inhabits the large intestine, migrates to the urinary bladder, it causes cystitis (inflammation of the bladder).

ENDOGENOUS OBESITY
Obesity caused by an endocrine or metabolic disorder, not by overeating.

ENDOINTOXICATION
Poisoning of the body by a poison produced within itself.

ENDOLYMPH
Fluid contained in the labyrinth of the ear.

ENDOMETRIAL
Pertaining to the endometrium, the mucous lining of the uterus.

ENDOMETRIOSIS
A condition in which tissue more or less perfectly resembling the mucous membrane of the uterus - the endometrium -occurs abnormally in various locations in the pelvic cavity. Endometrial cells may break off into cysts that move freely through the abdomen, generally attaching themselves to the ligaments of the outer layer of the uterus, and occasionally latching on to the ovaries, Fallopian tubes, bowel or bladder. They irritate surrounding tissue, and as the infected area begins to heal, connective tissue replaces the dam-

aged tissue and a scar is formed. The scar tissue, in turn, inflames the surrounding area and the process of healing and scarring spreads outward throughout the affected area.

Although the precise cause of the disease is not known, it does seem to be linked to stress. The incidence of endometriosis has increased with the number of women entering the workforce and trying to accommodate busy lives. This stress sometimes seems to trigger abnormal tissue growth.

ENDOMETRITIS
Inflammation of the lining membrane of the uterus.

ENDOMETRIUM
Membrane lining the womb, into which the fertilized egg is embedded in order to develop. It is also responsible for menstruation.

ENDOMORPH
A person whose body tends to be more heavily developed in the torso than in the limbs, with fat accumulations giving the body a general round and soft appearance.

ENDOMORPHIC COMPONENT
The first of the three components of physique in the typology theory of Prof. W.H. Sheldon. It comprises prominence of intestines and other visceral organs, including a prominent abdomen as in the obese individual. According to this theory, such people tend to be relaxed, friendly and pleasure-loving.

ENDOMYOCARDITIS
Acute or chronic inflammation of the heart muscle (myocardium) and the inner lining (endocardium) of the heart, due to disease or infection.

ENDOMYSIUM
The supporting connective tissue surrounding a muscle fiber.

ENDONEURITIS
Inflammation of the connective tissue that forms a framework for the support of individual fibers in a nerve.

ENDONEURIUM
The fragile tissue covering the separate fibers in a nerve.

ENDONUCLEASE
An enzyme that breaks down a nucleotide chain into two or more shorter chains by attacking it at points not adjacent to the ends.

ENDOPARASITE
A parasite that lives in the internal organs or tissues of its host.

ENDOPLASM
The inner relatively fluid part of the cytoplasm.

ENDORPHIN
Any of several naturally occurring chemicals (proteins) in the brain, believed to be involved in reducing or eliminating pain and in enhancing pleasure.

END ORGAN
A structure forming the peripheral terminus of a path of nerve conduction and consisting of an effector or a receptor with its associated nerve termination.

ENDORPHIN
Any of a group of proteins with potent analgesic properties that occur naturally in the brain. Released in response to pain, endorphins bind to specialized receptors and reduce perception of pain. Narcotic analgesics such as morphine work by mimicking the action of endorphins.

ENDOSCOPY
Inspection of the body organs or cavities by the use of an endoscope. This instrument consists of a tube and optical system for observing the inside of an organ or body cavity.

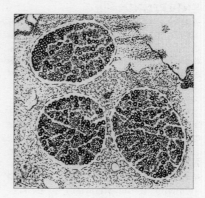

Bundles nerve fibers, each supported by endoneurium.

This may be done through a natural body opening or through a small incision.

ENDOSTEUM
The membrane lining the marrow cavity of a bone.

ENDOTHELIOMA
Tumor or growth derived from cells forming the endothelium.

ENDOTHELIUM
Membrane only one cell thick that lines the inside of the heart, blood vessels and lymph vessels, the walls of capillaries, and lymph spaces and other cavities within the body.

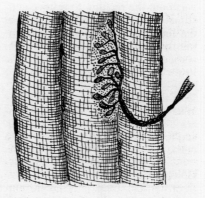

End organ: branches of a motoneuron in contact with muscle fibers.

ENDOTOXIN
A poison liberated during the destruction of a bacterial or other microbial cell. It only affects tissues in the immediate area, whereas an exotoxin is released into the blood stream and acts on distant structures.

ENDOTRACHEAL TUBE
A catheter inserted through the mouth or nose into the trachea to maintain an open airway (for instance, in severe inflammation and swelling of the pharynx), to deliver oxygen, to permit suctioning of mucus, or to prevent aspiration of stomach contents.

ENDOXANA
Brand name for a drug containing cyclophosphamide as active compound prescribed as anticancer drug for the treatment of certain types of malignant growths.

END PLATE
The ending of a motor nerve, usually embedded in a muscle fiber.

ENDURANCE
A continuing of activities while in pain or distress, without sinking or yielding.

ENEMA
Liquid introduced into the rectum to wash out the rectum, to relieve constipation, as a medical lotion to treat the lining of the bowel, or containing food products or drugs to be absorbed through the lining of the lower bowel.

ENERVATION
Weakness, loss of strength or energy. The term is also used to describe the surgical removal of a nerve.

ENGAGEMENT
In obstetrics, fixation of the presenting part of the fetus, usually the head, in the maternal pelvis. It usually occurs in late pregnancy, after which fetal movements are curtailed.

ENGORGEMENT
Congestion; the damming up of blood in a tissue or organ and indicative of obstruction to the normal flow of blood in the part.

ENGULFMENT
A form of anxiety suffered by persons who lack primary security, in which relationships with others are experienced as overwhelming threats to their identity.

ENHANCING ANTIBODY
An antibody that forms a complex with tumor-specific antigens present on the tumor surface, preventing or blocking destruction of the tumor by specific lymphocytic cells, thus favoring the growth of a tumor.

ENIGMA
A riddle, in which sometimes a specific meaning is concealed under obscure language; sometimes containing a hidden meaning that has to be guessed.

ENKEPHALIN
Any of a group of brain chemicals that influence mental activity and behavior (sometimes grouped with the endorphins as natural opiates). Evidence shows that these chemicals influence the body's immune system and help fight disease.

ENOPHTHALMUS
A condition in which the eyeball is displaced back in the eye socket, because of injury or developmental defect.

ENTELECHY
The absoluteness, or actuality, of a thing, as opposed to simple capability or potentiality. A philosophical concept of Aristotle, who styled the soul "the entelechy of the body;"

that by which it actually is, though it has the capacity of existing before.

ENTERECTOMY
Surgical removal of a portion of the intestine.

ENTERIC BACTERIA
Bacteria that live in the gastrointestinal system.

ENTERIC FEVER
Group of diseases that affect the intestines such as typhoid fever and paratyphoid fever.

ENTERITIS
Inflammation of the intestines, especially the small intestine, due to viral or bacterial infection or other disorder, usually marked by diarrhea.

ENTEROBIASIS
Infection of the large intestine with the pinworm Enterobius vermicularis, occurring especially in children. The females deposit eggs around the anus, which cause itching; if the patient scratches the area and then puts the fingers in or near the mouth, reinfection occurs. Treatment is by anthelminthics (agents that destroy worms).

ENTEROCOCCUS
Streptococcal germ found in the intestinal tract, which may cause such inflammatory conditions as appendicitis.

ENTEROCOLITIS
Inflammation of the small intestine and colon.

ENTEROCOLOSTOMY
Surgical operation to join together the small and large intestines. It usually infers that a porion of diseased intestine has been removed and the cut ends of the colon and small intestine have to be joined together.

ENTERO-ENTEROSTOMY
Surgical operation to join together two loops of the intestine. This usually means that an intermediate portion of diseased intestine has been removed and the cut ends have to be joined together.

ENTEROGASTRIC REFLEX
Reflex inhibition of the emptying of the stomach's contents through the pylorus that occurs when the duodenum is stimulated by the presence of irritants, or is obstructed.

ENTEROLITH
Stone-like body formed within the intestines.

ENTEROLITHIASIS
The presence of stone-like formations in the intestines.

ENTEROLOGY
Study of diseases of the intestines.

ENTEROLYSIS
Surgical removal of intestinal adhesions.

ENTEROMEGALY
Enlargement of the intestines.

ENTEROPEXY
Surgical fixation of part of the intestines to the abdominal wall to secure it from dropping.

ENTEROPLASTY
Surgical repair of the intestines.

ENTEROPLEGIA
Paralysis of the intestines that sometimes follows surgery within the abdomen, not necessarily on the intestines themselves. It is a form of surgical shock of the intestines.

ENTEROPTOSIS
Sagging of the intestines from their normal position down to the bottom of the abdomen.

ENTEROSPASM
Excessive, abnormal contraction of muscles of the intestine, usually causing pain.

ENTEROSTENOSIS
Narrowing or stricture of the intestinal tube.

ENTEROSTOMY
Surgical operation by which a piece of intestine is brought through the abdominal wall to the skin surface and then opened so that the contents of the intestinal tract emerge through this a bdominal opening in stead of through the back passage.

ENTEROVIRAL EXANTHEMATOUS FEVER
Viral disease of the skin characterized by: febrile, rubelliform or morbilliform rash confined to the face, neck and chest, exceptionally hemorrhagic or vascular. The course is generally benign but aseptic meningitis may occur. The disease is caused by types of coxsackie virus and echovirus. The incubation period is 3-5 days. Transmission is by direct person-to-person or fecal-oral route.

ENTEROVIRAL HEMORRHAGIC CONJUNCTIVITIS
Viral disease of the conjunctivae characterized by:
- sudden onset;
- hyperemia of conjunctivae;
- seromucous discharge;
- subconjunctival hemorrhages;
- occasionally keratitis and uveitis;
- ocular signs.
The incubation period is 1-2 days. The transmission is as follows: direct or indirect contact with eye discharges, optical instruments, possibly by droplets from the throat of infected persons.

ENTEROVIRAL LYMPHONODULAR PHARYNGITIS
Viral disease of the throat characterized by raised, direct, whitish or yellowish nodules surrounded by a narrow annular erythematic zone. The disease is caused by coxsackie virus A 10.
The transmission is as follows: droplet spread, node and throat discharges, feces of infected person. Man is the only reservoir.

ENTEROVIRAL PARALYTIC ENCEPHALOMYELITIS
Viral disease of the brain and spinal cord caused by echoviruses and coxsachieviruses. The infection may cause flaccid paralysis mainly in children, which can be severe, but may disappear after 2-3 weeks without sequelae. There is no specific treatment.

ENTEROVIRAL VESICULAR PHARYNGITIS
Viral infection of the throat characterized by:
- fever;
- malaise;
- sore throat;
- grayish papulovesicular pharyngeal lesions on erythematous base and ulcers.
The disease is caused by coxsackieviruses. The incubation time is 3-5 days. There is no specific treatment.

ENTEROVIRUS
Any of a group of picornaviruses (as the causative agent of poliomyelitis) that typically occur in the gastrointestinal tract but may be involved in respiratory ailments, meningitis, and neurological disorders.

ENTHALPY
The sum of the internal energy of a body and the product of its volume multiplied by the pressure.

ENTHELMINTH
Any intestinal worm.

ENTHUSIASM
An ecstasy of mind, as if from in-

spiration or possession by a spiritual influence.

The term is also used in the sense of complete possession of the mind by any subject.

ENTODERM
Innermost of the three germinal layers of the embryo, from which develops the lining of the digestive tract, pancreas, liver, middle ear, respiratory tract, thyroid, parathyroid and thymus glands, and other parts.

ENTOPIC
Situated in the usual place, as opposed to ectopic which means out of position.

ENTOPIC PULSE
A condition, sometimes noticed after violent exercise, in which, with every beat of the heart, the vision darkens. It is due to mechanical irritation of the retinal rods in the back of the eye by the pulsating retinal arteries. The victim often describes this sensation as threatened blackouts.

ENTROPION
Inversion of the eyelid in which the eyelashes rub against the eyeball.

ENTROPY
A measure of the unavailable energy in a closed thermodynamic system so related to the state of the system that a change in the measure varies with change in the ratio of the increment of heat taken in to the absolute temperature at which it is absorbed.

ENUCLEATION
Surgical removal of the eyeball from its socket, or the removal of a tumor or organ from its capsule.

ENURESIS
Involuntary and consistent episodic wetting during sleep by a child over the age of five or six.

ENURESIS, FUNCTIONAL
Repeated, involuntary or intentional voiding of urine during the day or at night into bed or clothes, after an age at which continence is expected.

Functional enuresis is often referred to as primary, if it has not been preceded by a period of urinary continence lasting at least one year, and secondary if it has been preceded by a period of urinary continence lasting at least one year. Either of the above types may be nocturnal (most common), defined as the passage of urine during sleep time only, diurnal, defined as the passage of urine during waking hours, or both diurnal and nocturnal.

In most cases of nocturnal functional enuresis, the child awakens with no memory of a dream and no memory of having urinated. Typically the disturbance occurs during the first third of the night. In a few cases the voiding takes place during the rapid eye movement (REM) stage of sleep, and in such cases the child may recall a dream that involved the act of urinating.

Although the great majority of children with functional enuresis do not have a coexisting mental disorder, the prevalence of coexisting mental disorders is greater in those with functional enuresis, than in the general population.

Most children with the disorder become continent by adolescence, but in approximately 1% of cases, the disorder continues into adulthood.

ENVELOPE PROTEINS
Proteins that comprise the envelope or surface of a virus. The envelope protein of the human immunodeficiency virus (HIV) is called gp 60, which splits to form two smaller molecules, gp 41 and gp 20.

ENVIRONMENT
The complex of physical, chemical,

and biotic factors that act upon an organism or an ecological community and ultimately determine its form and survival.

ENVIRONMENTALISM
A theory that views environment rather than heredity as the important factor in the development and especially the cultural and intellectual development of an individual.

ENVY
A compound of negative self-feeling and of anger. According to Sigmund Freud, penis envy occupies a central position in the psychology of women, while according to the British psychoanalyst Melanie Klein, innate envy of the mother's breast and its creativity is a primary cause of all mental illness.

Both propositions create more problems than they solve. The former raises the question of how feelings of physical completeness can arise in an intact body - in other words, it raises problems about the body-image of girls - while the latter raises questions as to how an emotion, and a complex one at that, can be innate and present from birth.

ENZYME
A protein that acts as a catalyst for the chemical reactions in the body upon which life depends. Each type of body cell produces a specific range of enzymes. Cells in the liver contain enzymes that stimulate the breakdown of nutrients and drugs; cells in the digestive tract release enzymes that help digest food.

Enzymes are themselves synthesized by other enzymes on templates derived from nucleic acids, and an average cell contains about 3,000 different enzymes. In order to function correctly, many enzymes require the assistance of metal ions or accessory substances known as co-enzymes that are produced from the diet. The action of minerals and vitamins as co-enzymes explains some of the harmful effects of a lack of such elements in the diet. Some drugs work by altering the activity of enzymes - for example, certain anticancer drugs halt tumor growth by altering enzyme function in cancer cells.

EOSIN
A red dye commonly used to stain cells, bacteria, and other materials for examination under the microscope.

EOSINOPENIA
A decrease in the number of eosinophils in the blood.

EOSINOPHIL
Granular white blood cells (leukocytes) having a nucleus with two lobes connected by a thread of chromatin, and cytoplasm containing coarse. round granules of uniform size that stains easily with the dye eosin.

EOSINOPHILIA
An increase in the number of eosinophils in the blood; it commonly occurs in allergic reactions and in some inflammatory conditions.

EOSINOPHILIC GRANULOMA
A disease of adolescents and young adults marked by the formation of granulomas in bone and the presence in them of histiocytes and eosinophilic cells with secondary deposition of cholesterol.

EOSINOPHILIC PNEUMONIAS
A group of diseases of both known and unknown cause, characterized by infiltration of the lungs and, commonly, peripheral blood by eosinophils.

EPENDYMA
Membrane lining the cavities of the brain and the central canal of the spinal cord.

EPHEDRINE
A bronchodilator; a medicine that widens the air passages of the lungs and is used to treat asthma, bronchitis, and other conditions.
Possible side effects include:
- headache;
- nervousness;
- insomnia;
- paleness;
- rapid heartbeat;
- dizziness;
- appetite loss;
- painful or difficult urination.

EPICANTHUS
Half-moon shaped skinfolds covering the inner angle of the eye commonly found in people of the Mongoloid race and being one of the signs of Down's syndrome.

EPICARDIA
That part of the esophagus between the diaphragm and the stomach.

EPICARDIUM
The innermost of the two layers of the pericardium, the membranous covering of the heart.

EPICONDYLE
Bony prominence (condyle) situated on the outer sides of the femur (thigh) and humerus (upper arm).

EPICONDYLITIS
Painful inflammation of the muscles and soft tissue around the elbow, usually caused by excessive strain, as in tennis or golf, or by carrying a heavy load.
Treatment includes rest and injection of pain-relieving medicines into the joint area, and physical therapy.

EPICRANIUM
All layers of the scalp; the coverings of the skull.

EPICRITIC
Pertaining to certain skin nerve fibers that enable us to appreciate very fine distinctions of temperature and touch.

EPICRITIC SENSITIVITY
The ability to sense fine variations in touch. Epicritic sensitivity is tested by determining the relative appreciation of light touch, temperature changes, and point-to-point distances.

EPIDEMIC
Unusual and sudden prevalence of a disease in a given area or locality, which is generally common to or affecting a great number of persons in a community at the same time, such as a contagious disease.

EPIDEMIC HEMORRHAGIC FEVER
An acute virus disease that is endemic in some Asian countries and that is characterized by acute renal failure in addition to the usual symptoms of the hemorrhagic fevers.

EPIDEMIC KERATOCONJUNCTIVITIS
A highly infectious disease of man that is often epidemic, and associated with the presence of an arbovirus, and is marked by pain, by redness and swelling of the conjunctiva, by edema of the tissues around the eye, and by tenderness of the adjacent lymph nodes.

EPIDEMIC MYALGIA
Viral infection of muscles caused by coxsackieviruses group B.
The following symptoms may occur:
- fever;
- headache;
- paroxysmal pain in the chest;
- pain in the abdomen, simulating appendicitis.
The disease has a benign course, but complications such as myocarditis or aseptic meningitis may occur. The incubation period is 3-5 days.

EPIDEMIC PLEURODYNIA

A virus disease occurring at any age, but most common in children. It is characterized by:
- sudden onset of fever;
- pain in the abdomen or chest;
- sore throat;
- malaise.

Local tenderness, muscle swelling and muscular aches may occur. The disease subsides in two to four days, but relapses may develop within a few days and symptoms may recur for several weeks.

Treatment is entirely based on the relief of symptoms.

EPIDEMIC TYPHUS

An acute, severe disease characterized by prolonged high fever, intractable headache and rash. The responsible organism is transmitted by lice.

EPIDEMIOLOGY

The study of the causes, occurrences, and control of disease. Epidemiology uses statistical and other methods to discover causative agents, determine the elements affecting the rate of incidence and the degree of severity, and establish the means of control.

EPIDERMAL NECROLYSIS

A rare but important skin condition, in which the skin becomes red and peels off all over the entire body, as though the person had been scalded. The syndrome may be caused by a variety of factors, including a

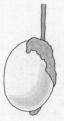 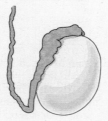

Epididymis on top of the testes.

medicine reaction; in children it is often due to staphylococcal infection.

Epidermal necrolysis calls for intensive care in a hospital.

EPIDERMIDALIZATION

Transformation of cuboidal cells derived from the stratum germinativum into flattened cells of the outer horny layer of the skin.

EPIDERMOLYSIS BULLOSA

A collective term for several uncommon, inherited conditions in which skin trauma is followed by bullae (blisters).

The dominant form gives mild symptoms, but in the recessive forms they are severe and dystrophies (developmental changes) are present.

The diagnosis will be apparent from the family history, and the clinical signs in the recessive forms are so striking that the general practitioner will promptly refer the sufferer to a dermatologist.

EPIDERMIS

The superficial, outer layers of the skin which contain numerous nerve endings but no blood vessels. Made up of squamous epithelium tissue, the epidermis is divided into an outer stratum corneum containing dead cells that are sloughed off as new cells from the inner stratum germinativum push upward; other layers are also sometimes found, especially in thick skin.

EPIDIDYMIS

Small structure lying behind and above each testicle and part of the seminal tract.

EPIDIDYMITIS

Inflammation of the epididymis.

EPIDURAL

Situated upon or over the dura, one of the coverings of the brain and spinal cord.

EPIDURAL ANESTHESIA
Local anesthesia produced by an injection of an anesthetic agent into the epidural space - that is, around but not in the spinal canal.

It effectively numbs the body from the waist down and is often used during normal childbirth and cesarean delivery.

EPIDURAL SPACE
Space between the top two membranes covering the spinal cord, containing venous sinuses.

EPIGAMIC
Term applied to characteristics such as coloring calculated to attract the other sex as a preliminary to mating.

EPIGASTRIC
Above the stomach; in the epigastrium, the region of the abdomen just below the sternum (breastbone).

EPIGASTRIC ARTERY
Any of the three arteries supplying the anterior wall of the abdomen.

EPIGASTRIC FOLD
A fold of peritoneum on the anterior abdominal wall covering the deep epigastric artery.

EPIGASTRIC REFLEX
Feeling of weakness or sinking in the stomach area frequently associated with anxiety or fear.

EPIGENESIS
Development involving gradual diversification and differentiation of an initially undifferentiated entity.

EPIGLOTTIS
A structure made of cartilage and covered with mucous membrane, situated in the throat in front of the glottis (upper windpipe). During breathing, it stands upright, but when a person swallows, it drops down to cover the glottis and pre-

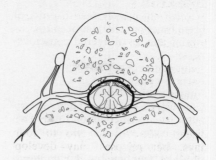

The epidural space is located between the dura and the periosteum of the vertebrae.

vents food and liquids from entering the lungs.

EPIGLOTTITIS, ACUTE
A severe, rapidly progressive infection of the epiglottis and surrounding tissues that may be quickly fatal due to sudden respiratory obstruction by the inflamed epiglottis.

Haemophilus influenzae Type B is almost exclusively the pathological agent causing the illness.

Infection, acquired through the respiratory tract, may produce initial nasopharyngitis. Subsequent downward extension produces inflammation of the epiglottis and often of the lower tracheobronchial tree.

The inflamed epiglottis mechanically obstructs the airway, increasing the work of breathing, which may result in retention of carbon dioxide and hypoxia. Clearance of inflammatory secretions is also impaired. These factors may cause fatal asphyxia.

Onset is acute and fulminating. Sore throat, hoarseness, and, usually, high fever develop abruptly in a previously well child. Dysphagia and respiratory distress characterized by drooling, dyspnea, tachypnea, and respiratory stridor develop rapidly.

As far as treatment is concerned: speed is vital. Antibiotics are important.

EPILEPSY

A recurrent paroxysmal disorder of brain function, characterized by:
- brief attacks of altered consciousness;
- altered motor activity;
- sensory phenomena;
- inappropriate behavior.

Convulsive disorders such as seizures (the most common form of attacks) begin with loss of consciousness and motor control, and jerking of all extremities, but any recurrent seizure pattern may be called epilepsy.

The cause of epilepsy is classed as either symptomatic or idiopathic: symptomatic implying that a probable cause permits a specific course of therapy, and idiopathic meaning no specific reason for the cause can be found.

No obvious cause can be found in about 50 percent of adults and in a smaller percentage of children under the age of three.

Some authorities believe that epilepsy is due to a microscopic scar in the brain resulting from birth trauma or other injury and, indeed, many patients classed during life as idiopathic epileptics show, on their deaths, evidence of such lesion at autopsy. However, it is more likely that unexplained metabolic abnormalities underlie most idiopathic cases.

EPILEPSY, TELEVISION

A form of visual reflex epilepsy in which the seizures occur regularly in light-sensitive subjects whenever they look too closely at a television screen in partial darkness.

EPILEPTOGENIC

Liable to induce an epileptic seizure, with or without convulsions.

EPILOIA

A deleterious dominant genetic trait in man marked by mental deficiency and multiple tumor formations by a high mutation rate.

EPINEPHRINE

A hormone of the adrenal medulla that acts as a powerful stimulant in times of fear or arousal and has many physiological effects, including:
- increasing breathing;
- increased heart rates;
- increased metabolic rates to provide quick energy;
- constricting blood vessels;
- strengthening muscle contraction.

EPINEURIUM

The connective tissue surrounding a nerve trunk and binding together nerve fibers.

EPINOSIC

Term used by psychoanalysts with

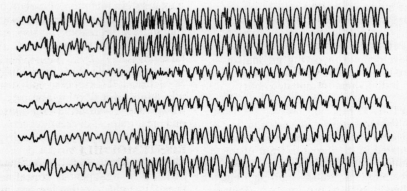

Electroencephalographic tracings of an epileptic attack.

reference to a secondary gain or advantage through illness.

EPINOSIS
An advantage or gain such as achieving social approval, and sympathy derived from neurosis.

EPIPHENOMENALISM
A philosophical theory of the relation between mental and physical, or between mind and body, which holds that mental processes have nothing that causes them that is, that the chain of cause and effect is complete on the body side, so that mental processes are merely accompanying phenomena that make no difference to the outcome.

EPIPHORA
An abnormal overflow of tears, due usually to an obstruction of the tear duct.

EPIPHYSEAL
Referring to an epiphysis.

EPIPHYSIS
The end of a long bone of the body - for example, the femur (thigh bone) or humerus (upper arm bone) - that is the growth center during growth and forms the articulating surfaces at joints. Each epiphysis remains partly cartilaginous during growth. The cartilage is eventually converted into mature bone, which is then incorporated into the main shaft. Bone-growth disorders such as rickets and some hormone disorders affect the epiphyses.

EPIPHYSIS CEREBRI
Another term for pineal body or gland.

EPIPHYSITIS
Inflammation of an epiphysis.

EPIPLOIC FORAMEN
The only opening between the omental bursa and the general peritoneal sac.

EPISCLERA
Connective tissue between the conjunctiva of the eyeball and the coat underneath.

EPISCLERITIS
Inflammation of the episcleral or subconjunctival connective tissue of the eye.

EPISIOTOMY
Surgical incision of the back part of the vaginal opening to allow the baby's head to come through at childbirth and to avoid extensive tearing. After birth, the incision is stitched up.

EPISODE
An event that is distinctive and separate although part of a larger series; especially an occurrence of a usually recurrent pathological abnormal condition.

EPISPADIAS
Congenital deformity of the penis in which the urethra (the tube that carries the urine) opens on the top surface of the penis instead of at the tip. If the urethra opens on the undersurface of the penis the condition is known as hypospadias.

EPISTASIS
Medical term used in two different meanings.
(1) Suppression of a secretion or discharge.
(2) A scum on the surface of urine.

EPISTAXIS
Nose bleeding, nasal hemorrhage. In the majority of cases, nose bleeding is due to a small ulcer in the fore part of the nasal septum and is frequently associated with nose-picking.

EPISTEMOPHILIA
Pleasure in gaining knowledge. There is a tendency to regard the thirst for knowledge as either a derivative of scopophilia - that is, as

an extension of sexual curiosity - or as a sublimation of oral drives.

EPISTERNUM
Upper part of the breast bone or sternum. Also called the manubrium.

EPITHALAMUS
A dorsal segment of the diencephalon containing the habenula and the pineal body.

EPITHELIOMA
Skin carcinoma (cancer), more common than malignant melanoma (cancer in a mole on the skin), but the mortality rate is lower.

Epithelioma is chiefly found in skin exposed to sunlight, and invades the skin in the affected areas as well as metastasizing - that is, spreading to distant parts of the body - but the rate of metastasis is relatively low. The lesion starts with a skin-colored nodule that soon ulcerates. It is treated by surgery or radiation.

EPITHELIUM
Tissue that covers external surfaces such as the skin as well as lining the tubes and cavities of the body, and consists of one or more layers of cells variously modified to serve as protection, provide sense organs or aid in excretion of waste products and the assimilation of nutrients.

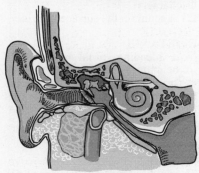

The semicircular canals (to the right of the illustration) are part of the equilibrium system.

Epithelium is also used as a general term for the various types of surface membrane.

EPITHELIZATION
The process of becoming covered with or converted to epithelium.

EPITOPE
The region on the surface of an antigen that is responsible for its specific interaction with an antibody having a matching site.

EPOGAM
Brand name of a drug containing gamolenic acid as active compound prescribed for the treatment of eczema.

EPONYM
Name for a structure, condition, or process that includes or is formed from the name of a person.

EPSOM SALT
Common name of a medicine containing magnesium sulphate as the active ingredient. Epsom salts are used as a laxative in a dose of 5-15 g per day. They should be taken with large drinks of water, and should not be used by those with congestive heart disease or impaired kidney function, or those taking diuretic medicines.

EQUANIMITY
Evenness of mind; a calm temper or firmness of mind that is not easily elated or depressed.

EQUILIBRIUM
State of balance, in which opposing forces exactly counteract each other.

EQUILIBRIUM SYSTEM
Sense organ, nerve tract and brain parts involved in maintaining the equilibrium - or, more commonly, the sense of balance - of the body. The sense organ is part of the inner ear.

The inner ear contains three semi-circular canals, containing a fluid called endolymph, that extend in three different directions from a central point, approximately at right angles to each other.

At the base of each canal are oval masses of a jelly-like substance in which all but the tips of sensitive hairs are encased. Below these are two structures: the utricle and saccule. These, too, are filled with endolymph and have pads of cells to which bristles are attached and over which is a jelly containing small granules of chalk.

When the endolymph in the semi-circular canals moves, it bends the hairs and sends messages to the brain via nerve fibers that the body is stopping or starting. When the fluid in the utricle and saccule is disturbed, the granules press against the hairs, which then send signals telling the brain in which direction the body is moving.

EQUINE ENCEPHALITIS
An infection characterized by:
– inflammation at the brain and spinal cord;
– fever;
– headache;
– vomiting ;
– neurological symptoms (for instance, visual disturbances).
The disease is caused by a virus transmitted by a mosquito from an infected horse.

EQUIPOTENTIALITY
Capacity of one part or one organ to take the place of another part or organ, with respect to the performance of a function.

ERB'S DISEASE
Condition in which there is progressive muscular dystrophy; the muscles become larger than normal, but they gradually weaken.

ERECTILE DISORDER
Persistent or recurrent partial or complete failure in a male to attain or maintain erection until completion of the sexual activity. The term may also be defined as the persistent or recurrent lack of a subjective sense of sexual excitement and pleasure in a male during sexual activity.

ERECTILE TISSUE
A type of spongy tissue (for instance, that found in the penis or clitoris) having large spaces within that can fill with blood to stiffen the structure in which it is contained.

ERECTION
Specifically refers to the alteration of the penis in which it becomes engorged with blood and erect and stiff. Erection is usually the result of sexual arousal but also occurring normally during sleep and as a result of physical stimulation.

EREMOPHOBIA
Fear of being lonely or of desolate places.

ERETHISM
Abnormally high degree of sensitivity in any part of the body.

ERGO–
Word element: association with work or exertion.

ERGOCALCIFEROL
Generic name of vitamin D.

ERGOMETER
A device for measuring the work performed by a set of muscles.

ERGONOMICS
The study and analysis of work as it relates to human physical and physiological processes.

ERGOPHOBIA
Morbid fear of work.

ERGOTISM
Ergot poisoning, resulting from pro-

longed or excessive use of ergot-containing medicines or from accidental ingestion of ergot-contaminated food.

Symptoms of ergotism include:
- excessive thirst;
- diarrhea;
- nausea and vomiting;
- cramping;
- abnormal heart rhythms;
- sometimes seizures;
- sometimes gangrene.

ERGOT PREPARATIONS
Medicines used to treat migraine and other types of throbbing headaches. Also used after delivery of babies to make the uterus clamp down and reduce excessive bleeding.

ERGONICITY
According to Sigmund Freud, the activity of a given bodily area in conveying sexually exciting stimuli to the mind.

EROGENOUS
Pertaining to stimulation of the sexual instinct, especially to the areas of the body (erogenous zones) where such stimulation leads to sexual arousal.

EROS
Greek god of sexual love. The name was used by Sigmund Freud to personify the life-force and the sexual instincts. In his later writings, Eros was contrasted with Thanatos, the god of death, the personification of the death instinct.

EROSION
Ulceration; gradually wearing down of part of the body. Commonly refers to erosion of the cervix, an ulcer of the neck of the womb, which sometimes follows childbirth.

EROTIC
Sexual, libidinal, pleasurable. According to psychoanalysis, all bodily functions accessible to consciousness may be sources of erotic pleasure, while those that involve the erotic zones habitually are - hence oral, anal, urethral, phallic, etc. erotism.

Bodily functions that are not normally sources of erotic pleasure may, by displacement, become eroticized; if this happens, the eroticized organ may become the site of a neurotic or psychosomatic symptom.

EROTOGENIC ZONE
Any area of the body from which erotic sensations may arise - typically, the sexual organs and the mucous membranes surrounding bodily openings.

EROTOMANIA
State of being excessively erotic.

ERUCTATIONS
The act of bringing up air from the stomach with a characteristic noise; belching.

ERUPTION
The act of breaking out and becoming visible, especially a rash or other skin lesion.

The term is also used to describe the emergence of a tooth as it breaks through the gums.

ERUPTION
The act of breaking out and becoming visible, especially a rash or other skin lesion. The term is also used to describe the emergence of a tooth as it breaks through the gums.

ERYSIPELAS
Also called Anthony's fire: a skin infection, usually affecting the face, caused by certain types of streptococci and common in infancy and middle age. Diffuse inflammation and swelling spread with a clear margin and cause blistering. It is a short illness with fever; if it affects the throat or brain, it may, however, cause prostration and can prove fa-

tal. It is easily and quickly treated with penicillin or one of the sulpha drugs.

ERYSIPELOID

An acute, but slowly evolving, skin infection caused by microorganism Erysipelothrix rhusiopathiae. It is an infection of the hands characterized by reddish nodules and sometimes erythema.

ERYTHEMA

Diffuse redness of the skin caused by congestion of the skin blood vessels. It is an abnormal redness of the skin resulting from dilatation of the capillaries, as occurs in sunburn.

ERYTHRASMA

Fungus disease of the skin characterized by reddish or brownish scaly patches, usually occurring on the upper, inner part of the thigh, the armpits, the folds beneath the breasts and in other moist regions.

ERYTHROBLASTOSIS FOETALIS

Also known as hemolytic disease of the newborn: severe anemia of the fetus or newborn, caused by the transmission of antibodies from the mother via the placenta, because the mother's blood is Rh negative and the baby's is Rh positive.

The antibodies break down the baby's red blood cells (a process called hemolysis), causing anemia and jaundice.

The condition is avoided by giving Rh-negative women a special injection within 72 hours of giving birth (thus preventing the formation of antibodies and protecting subsequent babies), and is treated by giving the newborn a complete transfusion.

ERYTHROCYANOSIS

Skin condition due to a disorder of the circulatory system in a particular area, found especially in young girls and young women. It is char-acterized by a bluish-red discoloration, especially in the feet and legs but more marked over the calves, and accompanied by a burning and itching sensation, sometimes with swelling of the affected areas.

ERYTHROCYTE

Another name for a red blood corpuscle. It is a mature red blood cell, which contains the pigment hemoglobin, the main function of which is to transport oxygen to the tissues.

A red blood cell is a biconcave disc with no nucleus. It is the main cellular element in the blood.

ERYTHROCYTE HEMOLYSIS TEST

A test for the susceptibility of red blood cells to hemolysis (breakdown), an indication of blood levels of vitamin A, which may be deficient in cases of anemia, infertility and malnutrition.

ERYTHROCYTE SEDIMENTATION RATE

The rate at which red blood cells settle in unclotted blood; an indication of the presence and degree of various inflammatory diseases and infections.

ERYTHROCYTOSIS

Abnormal increase in the number of red blood cells in the blood.

ERYTHRODERMA

Any skin disease characterized by an abnormal redness of the skin in which the whole thickness of the skin is involved.

ERYTHRODERMA PORPHYRIA

A genetic disorder characterized by acute skin reactions to light, no urine abnormalities and, in some sufferers, serious liver disease.

ERYTHROMID

Brand name of a drug containing

the antibiotic erythromycin as active compound prescribed for the treatment of certain types of infections.

ERYTHROPHOBIA
Fear of the color red; fear of blushing.

ERYTHROPOIESIS
The process of erythrocyte production; it normally occurs in the bone marrow.

ESCAPE LEARNING
A form of learning controlled by actual painful stimulation. Escape from the punishment brings an end to the unpleasant or painful situation and is therefore rewarding.

ESOPHAGITIS
Inflammation of the esophagus, most often caused by backflow of acid stomach contents often associated with hiatal hernia but sometimes caused by infection or irritation.

ESOPHAGOSCOPE
A special optical instrument used to examine the esophagus, to dilate the canal, or to remove a foreign object or material for biopsy.

ESOPHAGUS
The gullet; the muscular canal, about 10 inches long, that connects the pharynx and stomach; food passes through it by waves of peristalsis.

ESOPHORIA
Inward turning of the eye; squinting inwards.

ESP
Abbreviation for extra-sensory perception.

ESSENCE
That which constitutes the particular nature of a thing, and which distinguishes it from all others.

The term is also used in the sense of predominant elements or principles, or any plant or drug extracted, refined or rectified from grosser material.

ESSENTIAL HYPERTENSION
High blood pressure for which no specific cause can be found.

ESSENTIALISM
The opposite of existentialism. Freudian psychoanalysis is an essentialist theory since it explains phenomena in terms of essences.

ESTROGEN
A general term for the female hormones (including estradiol, estrone, estriol) produced by the ovaries (and in small amounts in the adrenals and testes). In women estrogen functions in the menstrual cycle and in the development of secondary sex characteristics. Synthetic estrogen medicines are used to treat menstrual irregularities, to relieve the symptoms of menopause, to treat cancer of the prostate gland, and in oral contraceptives.

ESTRUS
The periodic occurrence of sexual activity in female mammals, marked by acceptance of the male . The term is not used in reference to human sexuality.

ETHER
Colorless, highly inflammable gas used for anesthesia. It has now been largely replaced by less irritant anesthetics, as ether can cause postoperative coughing and vomiting.

ETHICAL DRUG
Prescription drug or medicine; a medicine available only by prescription.

ETHICS
The science that deals with the nature and grounds of moral obligation; moral philosophy, which

teaches people their duty and the reasons for it.

ETHMOID
Bone of the skull situated at the root of the nose and containing numerous perforations for the filaments of the olfactory nerve.

ETHMOID SINUS
A cavity in the ethmoid bone behind the bridge of the nose.

ETHMOID SINUSITIS
Inflammation of the lining of the ethmoid sinus.

ETHNOCENTRISM
Exaggerated tendency to think the characteristics of one's own group or race superior to those of other groups or races.

ETHNOGRAPHY
The branch of science that studies the distribution and characteristics of races, especially with reference to geographical conditions.

ETHNOLOGY
The branch of science that studies the culture, customs, social relationships, etc. of people and races.

ETHNOPSYCHOLOGY
Primarily, the psychology of races, and particularly primitive races, usually applied more widely to include the study of psychological interaction of races and culture contact phenomena.

ETHYL CHLORIDE
A highly flammable topical anesthetic used to treat skin irritation and in minor skin surgery. Side-effects include pain and muscle spasm.

ETIOLOGY
The study of the causes of disease.

ETOPOSIDE
Generic name of a drug prescribed for the treatment of certain cancers of the lung, lymphatic system, and testicles.

EUGENETICS
Study concerned with controlling the characteristics of future generations through selective breeding techniques.

EUNUCH
A male whose testes have been removed; an eunuch shows signs of a lack of male hormone (testosterone) such as a feminime voice and lack of facial hair.

EUNUCHOID GIGANTISM
Acromegaly (gross enlargement of the bones and other parts of the body) in which there is sexual impotence and sterility.

EUNUCHOIDISM
Condition found in the male in which most of the male characteristics are poorly developed, accompanied by obesity of the female type.

EUPHORIA
Feeling of well-being; often a pathological condition, marked by unfounded feelings of well-being, strength and optimism, characteristic of certain types of mental disorder.

EUPHRASIA
Homeopathic medicine derived from eyebright. It is prescribed for catarrh in mucous membranes (especially of eyes and nose), profuse acrid eye-watering and head cold.

EUSTACHIAN TUBE
The mucous membrane-lined tube that connects the nasopharynx and the middle ear; it allows pressure in the inner ear to be equalized with that of the atmosphere. The eustachian tubes are vital in regulation pressure within the ears, but infection in them can spread to the ears.

EUTHANASIA
Commonly called "mercy killing"; the practice of hastening or causing the death of a person suffering from a painful, debilitating and incurable disease. While frequently advocated by various groups, its practical and legal implications are so contentious that it is illegal in most countries.

EUTHYROID GOITER
An enlargement of the thyroid gland due to diminished thyroid hormone production but without symptoms of lessened function of the thyroid gland.

EVENTRATION
The protrusion of the intestine through the abdominal wall. The term is also used to describe the surgical removal of the organs in the abdomen.

EVISCERATION
The act of removing an organ or the contents of the eyeball.

EVIL EYE
A kind of influence superstitiously ascribed in former times to certain persons, their glance supposingly injuring victims.

EVOLUTION
The process by which living organisms have changed since the origin of life.

EVOKED POTENTIAL
An electrical response produced in the central nervous system by an external stimulus (e.g., a flash of light). The response can be monitored on recording equipment and used to verify the integrity of nerve connections.

EWING'S SARCOMA
A malignant tumor developing in bone marrow, usually in long bones or the pelvis; it occurs most often in adolescent boys and produces pain, swelling, and an increase in white blood cells. Treatment by radiotherapy and surgical removal.

EXACERBATION
Abnormal or disease-causing increase in the degree of functioning of an organ; subjectively, high elation.

EXAMINATION
The act of viewing and studying the body, using various procedures, techniques, and equipment to ascertain the general health of the person and the presence or absence of any disease or disorder.
The examination may include the following techniques or procedures:
- palpation;
- percussion;
- auscultation;
- blood analysis;
- urine analysis;
- radiological diagnostic procedures.

EXANTHEM
An eruption or rash on the skin. The term is also applied to an eruptive disease, especially one attended by fever, such as measles.

EXCHANGE TRANSFUSION
The repetitive removal of small amounts of blood, followed by substitution of like amounts of blood from a number of donors, until a large proportion of the body's blood has been replaced.

EXCIPIENT
A more or less inert substance, such as sugar or jelly, used as a medium or vehicle for the administration of an active medicine.

EXCISION
Cutting off or out part of an organ by surgical operation.

EXCITATORY
A term meaning having a stimulating or enhancing effect. A chemical

released from a nerve ending that causes muscle contraction is having an excitatory effect.

EXCITEMENT
A state of aroused or increased vital activity in the body or any of its tissues or organs. The term is also used in the sense of the abnormal state of the actions or sensations, or both, produced by stimulants, irritants, or the like.

EXCITING CAUSE
The stimulus that, under given conditions, produces the effect; more specially, the stimulating situation that directly produces the outbreak of a mental disorder.

EXCORIATION
A linear or hollowed-out crusted area of skin, caused by scratching, rubbing or picking.

EXCREMENT
Solid waste matter discharged from the body after digestion; feces.

EXCRETION
Waste products of the body; the act of excreting.

EXENTERATION
Surgical removal of the organs within a body cavity, as those of the pelvis.

EXERCISE
Exertion of the body that is as conductive to health; systematic exertion of the body for amusement or in order to acquire some art, dexterity, or grace.

The term is also used in the sense of activity to condition the body, maintain fitness, or correct a deformity.

EXFOLIATION
Scaling off of dead skin; this occurs naturally but may be increased in some skin diseases and severe sunburn.

EXHALATION
The process of breathing out, expelling air from the lungs.

EXHAUSTION
The state of being deprived of strength or spirits; a state of complete fatigue and physical weakness.

EXHIBITIONISM
Recurrent, intense, sexual urges and sexually arousing fantasies, of at least six months' duration, involving the exposure of one's genitals to a stranger. The person has acted on these urges, or is markedly distressed by them. Sometimes the person masturbates while exposing himself (or fantasizing exposing himself). If the person acts on these urges, there is no attempt to further sexual activity with the stranger, and therefore people with this disorder are usually not physically dangerous to the victim.

In some cases, the desire to surprise or shock the observer is consciously perceived or close to conscious awareness. In other cases, the person has the sexually based fantasy that the person observing him will become sexually aroused. The condition apparently occurs only in males, and the victims are almost entirely female (children or adults). The disorder usually occurs before age 18, although it can begin at a much later age. Few arrests are made in the older age groups, which suggests that the condition becomes less severe after age 40.

EXISTENTIAL ANALYSIS
A type of psychotherapy designed to help the individual to react spontaneously to life situations and to develop a sense of freedom and responsibility for his or her own actions.

EXISTENTIAL CRISIS
A crisis concerning the problem of finding meaning in life.

EXISTENTIAL PSYCHOLOGY
A type of psychology developed from a point of view that limits the subject matter of the science to those aspects of experience that can be observed introspectively, which means, in effect, the sensory and imagination aspects, together with feelings, all as observable mental processes.

EXOCRINE GLAND
A gland that has a duct to carry its secretions to the organ on which it will act, e.g., the pancreas whose enzymes are transported to the duodenum.

EXOGENOUS
Originating or developing from outside the body.

EXOMPHALOS
Umbilical hernia, in which some organs in the abdomen push into the umbilical cord at birth.

EXOPHTHALMUS
Protrusion of one or both eyeballs resulting from inflammation of the socket(s), edema (excess fluid), tumors, injuries or enlargement of the eyeball.

The condition may also occur during the course of increased function of the thyroid gland.

If the condition is progressive, exposure of the eyeball can lead to drying, ulceration and infection of the cornea.

EXOPHYTIC
Growing outward as a tumor that grows on the surface of an organ.

EXORCISM
The act of expelling or casting out by incantations, prayers and ceremonies or to deliver from the influence or presence of malignant spirits or demons.

EXOSTOSIS
Benign outgrowth from a bone, usually covered with cartilage.

EXOTOXIN
A poison secreted by disease-causing microorganisms into their environment, such as the host's body. This toxin will travel through the blood to act on distant organs, unlike an endotoxin, which damages tissues only in the area close to the microorganisms.

EXOTROPIA
Outward turning of one eye relative to the other.

EXPANSION
A personality characteristic, expressing itself in loquacity and lack of reserve about oneself, and grading into extreme manifestations, symptomatic of one phase of manic-depressive psychosis.

EXPECTATION
The attitude of waiting attentively for something that is usually to a certain extent defined, however vaguely; a common source of error in psychological or physical experiments, in that an examiner will often look for what he or she expects to find and perhaps not what is actually there.

EXPECTORANT
Medicine that assists in the removal of excretions from mucous membranes, either by making the secretions more watery or drying them up, causing a person to cough more effectively or soothing the lining of the airways to reduce unproductive coughs.

An expectorant is used in the treatment of a productive (sputum-producing) cough.

EXPECTORATION
The process of raising material (for instance, mucus or phlegm) from the respiratory tract by coughing and then spitting it out of the mouth.

EXPERIMENTAL PSYCHOLOGY
Employment of experimental methods to obtain psychological data or to solve psychological problems.

EXPIRATION
The act of breathing out, usually a passive mechanism.

EXPLICIT MOVEMENT
Movement easily observed and measured; overt movement.

EXPLORATORY BEHAVIOR
Movement engaged in, most frequently by children, when initially orienting themselves to new situations.

EXPLORATION
Thorough examination of an area of the body.

EXPLOSIVE DISORDER, INTERMITTENT
Discrete periods of loss of control of aggressive impulses resulting in serious assaultive acts or destruction of property.

The degree of aggressiveness expressed during the episodes is grossly out of proportion to any precipitating psychosocial stressor. There are no signs of generalized impulsivity or aggressiveness between the episodes.

The person may describe the episodes as "spells" or "attacks." The symptoms are said to appear within minutes or hours and, regardless of duration, remit almost as quickly. Genuine regret of self-reproach about the consequences of the action and the inability to control the aggressive impulse may follow each episode.

The disorder may begin at any stage of life, but more commonly begins in the second or third decade.

The disorder is believed to be more common in males than in females. The males are likely to be seen in correctional institutions, and the females in a mental health facility.

EXPRESSION
In general sense, any external sign or response indicative of a mental process; sometimes used in a restricted sense of subsidiary changes accompanying a verbal or motor response; sometimes in a comprehensive sense of the totality of motor and glandular changes, inclusive of vocal expression, taking place when an organism is faced with any situation.

EXPRESSION METHOD
The measurement of emotion or feeling through the investigation of the accompanying changes.

EXPRESSIVE LANGUAGE DEVELOPMENT
The process of acquiring the ability to use the spoken word.

EXPRESSIVITY
The extent to which a trait is manifested. The kind of degree of expression may be slight or pronounced.

EXTENDER
A substance that increases the amount of another (for instance, plasma extender, used to add to the blood volume in emergencies).

EXTENSION
Stretching; act of straightening a limb; the opposite of flexion. Also used to describe the steady pulling on a limb to treat a broken bone.

The term is also used in the sense of a mental mechanism operating outside of and beyond conscious awareness, through which the scope or boundaries of existing defenses are enlarged (that is, extended) to include areas which are adjacent or continuous; physically or through their emotional association.

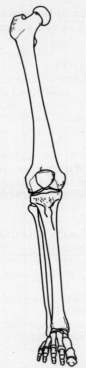

Extension (stretching) of the leg is caused by extensor muscles of the hip joint and knee joint.

EXTENSOR
A muscle that, when flexed, causes extension of a joint, or straightening of an arm or leg.

EXTERIORIZE
To place an internal organ or part of it on the outside of the body.

EXTERNALIZATION
The process by which a mental image is imagined to be outside the self, or an internal object is projected on to some figure in the external world. In this sense, it is synonymous with "projection" and the opposite of "introjection."

EXTINCTION
In psychology, the loss of a learned response because of nonreward or nonreinforcement.

EXTIRPATION
Surgical removal of an entire part, organ, or growth.

EXTRACELLULAR
Located outside of a cell.

EXTRACELLULAR FLUID
Protein and electrolyte containing fluid in blood plasma and interstitial fluid that helps control water and electrolyte movement in the body.

EXTRACTION
The act of pulling out, as a tooth.

EXTRADURAL ANESTHESIA
Anesthesia produced by injection of a local anesthetic agent on the outside of the dura mater (external membrane surrounding the spinal cord).

EXTRAPYRAMIDAL DISORDER
Motor disorder due to disturbance of certain brain systems. The pyramidal tracts are the upper pathways of nerves that connect the motor cortex (dealing with movement) with the lower motor neurons. The extrapyramidal tracts are a complex motor system that connects subcortical centers with lower motor centers in the brain stem and spinal cord.
Extrapyramidal disorders are characterized by:
(1) involuntary movements such as
- tremor;
- tics;
- athetosis;
- chorea;
- ballismus.
(2) impairment of voluntary movements:
- hypokinesia;
- akinesia.
(3) changes in muscle tone and posture:
- dystonia;
- muscle rigidity;
- disturbances of the equilibrium.
The most common disease in this

group is the Parkinson syndrome, a chronic disorder characterized by:
- slowness of movements;
- limitations of purposeful move ments;
- rigidity;
- tremor.

EXTRAPYRAMIDAL REACTIONS
Drugs that may cause abnormal reactions in the power and coordination of posture and muscular movements. Movements are not under voluntary control. Some drugs associated with extrapyramidal reactions include: amoxapionbe, antidepressants, droperidol, haloperidol, phenothiazines, rauwolfia alkaloids.

EXTRAPYRAMIDAL SYSTEM
Motor pathways from the brain to the spinal cord not running through the medullary pyramids. They regulate and control involuntary movements.

EXTRASENSORY PERCEPTION
Awareness or perception of an external event that is accomplished without using any of the known senses.

EXTRASYSTOLE
An abnormal contraction of the heart causing a brief interruption of the heartbeat. It does not usually indicate a serious condition.

EXTRAUTERINE
Situated or taking place outside the uterus, such as extra-uterine (or ectopic) pregnancy.

EXTRAVASATION
The directing of feelings and interests toward external things and the outside world rather than toward oneself; the person so inclined is an extrovert.

EXTRAVERSION
Outward-directed personality orientation characterized by sociability, activity and interest in the public environment rather than inner-directed attitudes and interests.

EXTREMITY
Any of the limbs; an arm or a leg.

EXTRUSION
The act of pushing something out by force.

EXUDATION
The slow escape (oozing) of fluids and cellular matter from blood vessels or cells through small pores or breaks in the cell membranes, sometimes the result of inflammation.

EYE
Either of two organs of sight located in a bony socket at the front of the skull. Light enters through the cornea, passes through a fluid-filled anterior chamber, passes through the opening (pupil) in the iris and then through the lens and vitreous body to strike nerve cells (rods and cones) in the retina of the eye. The impulse is then transmitted from the retina through the optic nerve to the brain.

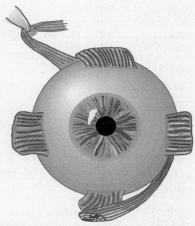

Anterior view of the eye. In the middle the lens, iris and pupil. The eye muscles are attached to the periphery of the eyeball.

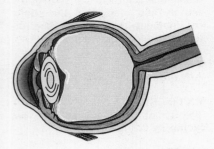

Cross section of the eye. From left to right: cornea, anterior chamber, lens, vitreous humor, retina and optic nerve. The latter contains the optic fibers transporting the visual images to the central nervous system.

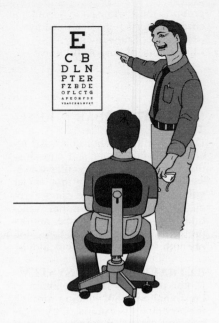

Investigation by the ophthalmologist of the eye field and characteristics of the lens.

EYEBALL
The ball or globe of the eye.

EYE BANK
A place where corneas removed from newly dead persons are stored until needed for transplantation to restore the sight of those with corneal defects.

EYEBROW
The arch or ridge forming the upper part of the socket of the eye, or the fringe of hair growing on it.

EYECUP
A device for applying lotions to the eye, consisting of a cup or glass with a rim shaped to fit snugly around the socket of the eye.

EYE DOMINANCE
Greater use of one eye that of the other in fixating on objects and greater dependence on the impressions of that eye though the other eye is functional.

EYEDROPS
Medicines used for the treatment of eye diseases.

EYE-HAND COORDINATION
The cooperative functioning of the eyes and the hand when picking up or moving objects.

EYELID
The portion of movable skin that serves as a cover for the eyeball.

EYE MOVEMENTS
The rotatory movement and positional changes of the eye as a result of the functioning of the eye muscles.

EYE SONOGRAM
A test utilizing ultrasound to detect disease of the eye.

EYESTRAIN
Discomfort or fatigue of the eyes due to excessive or incorrect use, or to uncorrected visual defects.

EYETOOTH
One of the two upper canine teeth.

EYE-VOICE SPAN
The distance, in terms of numbers or letters, by which the eye leads the voice when a person reads aloud.

F

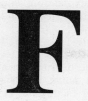

FABAHISTIN
Brand name of a drug containing the antihistamine mebhydrolin as active component.

FABLES TEST
A mental test in which the subject is required to interpret certain fables, i.e., explain the lesson taught by the fable.

FABRY'S DISEASE
A sex-linked disorder of lipid metabolism in which glycolipid accumulates in many tissues; the disease runs in families. Treatment is supportive, especially during periods of pain and fever.

FABULATION
The act of inventing or relating false or fantastic tales.

FACE
Front part of the head, bordered by hairline and chin, and consisting of the eyes, nose, mouth, forehead, cheeks and jaw. It is particularly concerned with sensibility and communication: it bears the special sense organs of vision, smell and taste, as well as especially sensitive skin.

The voice and facial expression (fine facial movements) are produced via the face, and the mobility of the neck allows these organs to be directed quickly and easily towards an object without turning the body.

FACE-BOW
A device used in dentistry to deter-

mine the positional relationships of the maxillae to the temporomandibular joints of a patient especially for the purpose of properly positioning dental casts on an articulator.

FACE LIFT
Colloquial term for the repair of sagging tissues of the cheek and eyelids by cosmetic surgery.

FACET
A smooth surface, e.g., of a bone.

FACIAL
Of or pertaining to the face.

FACIAL ANGLE
The angle that is determined by the intersection of a line connecting the nasion and prosthion with the Frankfort horizontal plane and is used as a measure of prognathism.

FACIAL ARTERY
An artery that arises from the external carotid artery just superior to the lingual artery and gives off a number of branches supplying the neck and face.

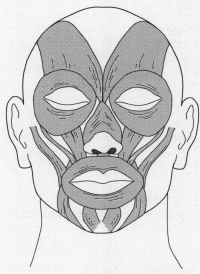

Facial muscles are important for all expressions of the face.

FACIAL BONE
Any of the bones of the facial region of the skull that do not take part in forming the braincase and that in man include 14 bones: two nasal bones, two maxillae of the upper jaw, two lacrimal bones, two zygomatic bones, two palatine bones, two nasal conchae, one vomer, and the mandible of the lower jaw.

FACIAL CANAL
A passage in the petrous part of the temporal bone that extends from the internal auditory meatus to the stylomastoid foramen and transmits various branches of the facial nerve.

FACIAL INDEX
The ratio multiplied by 100 of the breadth of the face to its length.

FACIAL MUSCLES
Group of muscles of the face innervated by the facial nerve (nervus facialis), important for facial expression, closure and opening of the eyelids, closure and opening of the mouth, blowing of the cheeks, etc.

FACIAL NERVE
The seventh cranial nerve, a mixed sensory and motor nerve that innervates much of the face, with sensory fibers extending from taste buds in the tongue and motor fi-

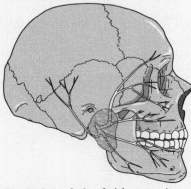

Distribution of the facial nerve (nervus facialis) that supplies the muscles of the face.

bers extending to the scalp, muscles of facial expression, and some of the lacrimal (tear) and salivary glands.

FACIAL PAIN
Pain in the distribution area of the trigeminal nerve that supplies the face. Most facial pain is related to diseases of the mouth such as caries (tooth decay) or dental abscesses, or to sinusitis. It can, however, have many causes including:
- diseases of the mouth, sinuses, nose, eyes, ears;
- diseases affecting the blood vessels, e.g., migraine;
- psychiatric disease, e.g., atypical facial pain;
- a referred condition - that is pain from a condition elsewhere in the body is felt in (or "referred" to) the face.

A chronic dull pain in the jaws characteristically affects women past middle age. Often it is a manifestation of depression and responds to anti-depressive drugs.

FACIAL VEIN
A vein that arises as the angular vein, drains the superficial structures of the face, and empties into the internal jugular vein.

FACIAL VISION
An awareness of obstacles independent of vision that is often considerably developed in blind persons and probably dependent on tactile perception of reflected sound waves.

FACIES
Facial appearance or expression indicative of a disease.

FACILITATION
Literally, making easier, promoting or fathering. In neurology, the term is used to summarize the effects of two nerve excitations, either successive in the same nerve, or simultaneous in two or more allied nerves,

though the connection may be relatively remote.

FACILITY
Ease in performance, readiness proceeding from skill or use. The term is also used in the sense of the means by which the accomplishment is rendered more easy.

FACIOPLASTY
Plastic surgery of the face.

FACTITIOUS DISORDERS
Disorders characterized by physical or psychological symptoms that are intentionally produced or feigned. The sense of intentionally producing a symptom is subjective, and can only be inferred by an outside observer.

The judgment that the symptom is intentionally produced is based, in part, on the person's ability to simulate illness in such a way that he or she is not likely to be discovered. This involves decisions as to timing and concealment that require a degree of judgment and intellectual activity suggestive of "voluntary" control. However, these acts have a compulsive quality in the sense that the person is unable to refrain from a particular behavior even if its dangers are known.

The behaviors should therefore be considered "voluntary" only in the sense that they are deliberate and purposeful (intentional), but not in the sense that the acts can be controlled. Thus, in factitious disorders, behavior that appears to be under "voluntary" control is used to pursue goals that are involuntarily adopted.

Factitious disorders are distinguished from acts of malingering. In malingering, the "patient" also produces the symptoms intentionally, but it is for a goal that is obviously recognizable when the environmental circumstances are known. For example, a claim of physical illness in order to avoid jury duty, standing trial, or conscription into the military would be classified as malingering.

Similarly, a hospitalized mental patient simulating an exacerbation of his or her illness in order to avoid transfer to another, less desirable facility would be an act of malingering.

FACTITIOUS FEVER
A fever produced artificially usually by the use of a drug.

FACTOR
A force, condition or circumstance, cooperating with others in bringing about a result; the most important technical use in psychology is in connection with mental capacity or intelligence, with respect to the factor theories of intelligence.

FACTOR I - FACTOR XIII
Factors, most of which are present in blood plasma, involved in the process of blood coagulation.

FACTOR VIII
A naturally occurring protein in blood plasma that aids in the coagulation of blood. A congenital deficiency of Factor VIII results in the bleeding disorder known as hemophilia A.

FACTOR A CONCENTRATE
A concentrated preparation of Factor VIII that is used in the treatment of individuals with hemophilia A.

FACTOR THEORY
Theory based on the nature of mental capacity, based on the statistical analysis of test results.

FACULTATIVE
Able to adjust to different environments or conditions.

FACULTATIVE ANAEROBE
A microorganism that normally lives without air (oxygen) but can survive in air.

FACULTY
The ability to do something specific (e.g., the faculty of hearing).

FACULTY PSYCHOLOGY
A pre-experimental psychology that views the mind as composed of a number of separate powers or faculties, including intellect, feeling, will and many others.

FAD
A pattern of behavior that is more expressive than useful for the individual. The individual indulges in this behavior to an excessive degree.

FAECES
See Feces.

FAIDS
Abbreviation of Feline acquired immune deficiency syndrome; AIDS in cats.

FAILURE
Cessation of supply or total defect; the act of failing or state of having failed to attain an object.

FAILURE TO THRIVE
Markedly disturbed social relatedness in most contexts that begins before the age of five and is not due to mental retardation or a pervasive developmental disorder, such as autism.

The disturbance in social relatedness is presumed to be due to grossly pathogenic care that preceded the onset of the disturbance.

The disorder may take the form of either persistent failure to initiate or respond in an age-expected manner to most social interactions or (in an older child) indiscriminate sociability, e.g., excessive familiarity with relative strangers, as shown by making requests and displaying affection. Some severe forms of this disorder, in which there is lack of weight gain and motor development, have been called hospitalism.

FAINT
A loss of consciousness or on the verge of losing consciousness.

FAINTING
Also called syncope: a state where a person nearly or totally loses consciousness. Fainting takes place when the blood supply to the brain is reduced. This can be due to minor and major problems.

True fainting lasts only a few seconds or a few minutes. Loss of consciousness that lasts for longer than this requires prompt medical evaluation in order to find out the cause. If there has been an injury to the head, even a brief period of unconsciousness should mandate a trip to a medical facility.
Fainting may occur as the result of the following causes:
- emotional shock;
- tense situation;
- exhaustion;
- hyperventilation;
- severe pain;
- drop in body temperature due to severe cold;
- blood loss;
- head injury;
- exposure to noxious fumes;
- change in heart rhythm;
- middle-ear infection;
- breath-holding;
- cardiovascular disease;
- lung problems;
- hypoxia (lack of oxygen).
Symptoms of fainting are the following:
- white or pale complexion;
- cool, moist skin;
- dizziness;
- weakness;
- sweating;
- giddiness;
- impaired vision;
- feeling of faintness;
- possible vomiting.
The severity of the condition depends on the reason for fainting.

If there are a number of attacks, medical evaluation should take place. Bodily injury may occur if a person faints while standing and/or falls over sharp or dangerous objects upon fainting. Treatment should involve the following: If a person feels faint, have him or her lie down and elevate their feet 20-25 cm, or sit down and place their head between their legs.

If a person has already fainted, make sure he or she is in a comfortable position, ensure that the nose and mouth is clear of any debris or other obstruction, and keep them lying down until they are fully alert and feeling all right again.

FAITH
Acceptance of a belief without conclusive or logical evidence, and usually accompanied, influenced or even determined by emotion.

FAITH CURE
Term that popularly covers phenomena otherwise designated mental healing, mind cure and the like.

FAITH HEALING
A method or practice of treating mental of physical illness through the patient's belief in divine intervention.

FALCIFORM LIGAMENT
Ligament attaching part of the liver to the diaphragm and abdominal wall.

FALLECTOMY
The surgical removal of part of the Fallopian tube.

FALLING
A common problem experienced among older people, due to any number of underlying causes. Evaluating people who have falls involves assessing the injuries sustained in the fall and the cause for the fall. In older people, falling frequently results in broken bones and other serious injuries which may lead to disability and sometimes death.

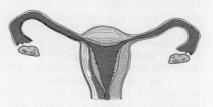

The Fallopian tube connects the ovaries to the uterus. The egg is usually being fertilized in the Fallopian tube.

FALLOPIAN TUBE
Either of a pair of slender tubes that convey the ova (eggs) from the ovaries to the cavity of the uterus.

FALLOT'S TETRALOGY
A form of congenital heart disease involving four separate but interrelated defects:
- ventricular septal defect;
- overriding aorta;
- pulmonary stenosis;
- enlargement of the right ventricle.

FALLOUT, RADIOACTIVE
(1) The descent to the earth's surface of the radioactive particles produced in a nuclear explosion.
(2) The radioactive particles themselves. It is often referred to simply as "fallout," although this term is also applied to any solid particulate matter that settles out of the air on to the surface of the earth.

FALSE LABOR
Pains resembling those of normal labor but occurring at irregular intervals and without dilation of the cervix.

FALSE-NEGATIVE
When a blood test incorrectly finds no antibodies to human immunodeficiency virus (HIV) when in reality there are some.

The term is also used for a negative test result in a subject who possesses the attribute for which the test is conducted. The labelling of a deceased person as healthy when screening in the detection of disease.

FALSE-POSITIVE
Positive test result in a subject who does not possess the attribute for which the test is conducted. The labelling of a healthy person as diseased when screening in the detection of the disease.

FALSE RIBS
The five lower ribs on each side which are not attached directly to the sternum (breastbone).

FALSE VOCAL CORDS
The upper pair of vocal cords each of which encloses a vestibular ligament, extending from one side of the thyroid cartilage in front of the arytenoid cartilage on the same side of the larynx at the back, and not directly concerned with speech production.

FALX CEREBELLI
The smaller of the two folds of dura mater separating the hemispheres of the brain that lies between the lateral lobes of the cerebellum.

FALX CEREBRI
The larger of the two folds of dura mater separating the hemispheres of the brain that lies between the cerebral hemispheres and contains the sagittal sinuses.

FAMILIAL
Running in a family; that is characteristic of several members of a family or a disease or disorder to which a family is prone.

FAMILIAL AMINOGLY-CINURIA
A benign genetic defect in the resorption of amino acids and glycine in the kidneys.

FAMILIAL MEDITERRANEAN FEVER
An inherited disorder of unknown cause, usually characterized by:
- recurrent episodes of fever;
- peritonitis;
- pleuritis;
- less commonly by arthritis and skin lesions. The disease occurs predominantly in people of American, Arabic and Sephardic Jewish ancestry, and is rare in individuals of other ethnic backgrounds. Attacks may be prevented by administering colchicine.

FAMILIAL PERIODIC PA-RALYSIS
A group of disorders, usually inherited in an autosomal dominant pattern, characterized by attacks of flaccid paralysis without alteration in consciousness.

FAMILIAL POLYPOSIS COLI
An inheritable disease of the colon in which multiple polyps carpet the colon and rectum. Malignancy develops before the age of 40 in nearly all untreated patients. Total surgery eliminates the risk of cancer.

FAMILY
The persons who live in one house and under one head. The term is also used in the sense of those who descend from one common ancestor.

FAMILY DEVELOPMENT
Changes that occur within a family over time.

FAMILY RESPONSIBILITY TASK
Growth responsibility that arises at a certain stage in the life of a family, successful achievement of which leads to satisfaction and success of later tasks; failure leads to unhappiness in the family, disapproval by society and difficulty with later developmental tasks.

FAMILY OF ORIENTATION
Unit into which one is born and

from which most basic socialization is received.

FAMILY OF PROCREATION
Family established when one gets married and reproduces.

FAMILY PLANNING
The attempt, using birth control methods, to time pregnancies in the best interests of the parents and the children. Family planning is achieved by natural restraint or by contraception. Any couple now has a number of well-established methods to consider. Factors that may play a role in their choice are:
- simplicity;
- safety to health;
- moral or religious beliefs;
- sexual satisfaction.

FAMILY PRACTICE
The physician trained in this specialty gives basic, comprehensive medical care to all members of the family on a continuing basis. Family practitioners perform the same functions as general practitioners did in earlier years.

FAMINE
Acute food shortage resulting in widespread starvation. It is usually caused by natural disasters such as drought, floods or plant diseases, causing crop failure.

FAMINE FEVER
A feverish illness caused by a spirochaetal germ transmitted to humans by mice or ticks, and characterized by:
- acute onset;
- chills;
- high temperature;
- pain in the back;
- pain in the legs;
- enlargement of the spleen;
- delirium;
- convulsions.

FAMINE PSYCHOSIS
A psychosis seen in war-torn countries when starvation is severe and widespread.

FANATICISM
Excessive and irrational enthusiasm for, or devotion to, a theory, belief or line of action, determining a highly emotional attitude and missionary zeal that shows practically no limits.

FANCONI ANEMIA
A disorder of reabsorption in the proximal convoluted tubules of the kidney that is characterized especially by the presence of glucose, amino acids, and phosphates in the urine.

FANTASTIC MELANCHOLIA
A morbid state characterized by bizarre delusions and hallucinations such as:
- evil spirits;
- death;
- ghosts;
- animals' heads;
- angels;
- floating heads.

FANTASY
Daydreaming, imagination; sometimes a consequence of frustration. It is used as a personality indicator in projective tests.

FARADISM
The application of electrical currents used in physical therapy.

FAR POINT
The point farthest of the eye at which an object is accurately focussed on the retina when the accommodation is completely relaxed, being theoretically equivalent to infinity, or, for practical purposes with respect to the normal eye, equivalent to any distance greater that 20 feet.

FAS
Abbreviation of fetal alcohol syndrome.

FASCIA
Layers of fibro-elastic tissue under the skin and between muscles, forming sheets of muscles or covering other deep structures such as nerves and blood vessels.

FASCICLE
A small cluster or bundle of nerve fibers within the central nervous system.

FASCICULATION
Muscular twitching involving the simultaneous contraction of contiguous groups of muscle fibers.

FASCIOLIASIS
Infectious disease caused by the trematode Fasciolata hepatica. The illness is characterized by:
- abdominal pain;
- eosinophilia;
- biliary colic;
- jaundice.
The incubation period is 10-60 days. The transmission is as follows: eating uncooked infested aquatic plants such as watercress.

FASCIOLOPSIASIS
Infectious disease caused by the trematode Fasciolopsis buski and characterized by:
- diarrhea;
- constipation;
- vomiting;
- anorexia;
- eosinophilia.
Massive infections may cause edemas and intestinal obstruction. The incubation period is about one month. The transmission is as follows: eating uncooked, infested, aquatic plants.

FASCIOTOMY
Surgical incision and separation or cutting of a fascia.

FASTIGIUM
The period of highest fever or greatest infection during the course of an illness.

FASTING
Abstention, wholly or in part, from food or drink, a practice common in many religions, usually linked with prayer and penance.

FATALISM
The belief that all events are predetermined, inclusive of the fate of every individual human being, and particularly the implication that no human being will or act can avert what is determined to happen.

FATALITY
The quality or state of causing death or destruction; the term is also used to designate death resulting from a disaster.

FATHER FIGURE
One often of particular power or influence who serves as an emotional substitute for a father.

FATHER IMAGE
An idealization of one's father often projected onto someone to whom one looks for guidance and protection.

FATIGUE
(1) Exhaustion, weariness, loss of strength resulting from hard or prolonged mental or physical work;
(2) temporary inability of tissues (e.g., muscle) to respond to stimuli that normally produce a response.
Fatigue, like anxiety, relative impairment, and illness or disease, is a form of human inadequacy.
All of these everyday terms lack precision and distinction, and definition is, therefore, a fundamental problem.

FATIGUABILITY
Relative rate of onset of fatigue, in an individual or in an organ.

FATIGUE FRACTURE
One occurring at the lower end of the fibula (outer bone of the lower leg) and seen in athletes, or in a

metatarsal (one of the bones extending from the ankle to the toes).

FATIGUE, PATHOLOGICAL
Kind of fatigue as a warning sign or consequence of some underlying physical disorder, perhaps the common cold or flu or something more serious, such as diabetes or cancer. In this case, other symptoms besides fatigue usually suggest the true cause.

FATIGUE, PHYSICAL
The result of overworking to the point where metabolic waste products - carbon dioxide and lactic acid - accumulate in the blood.

FATIGUE, PSYCHOLOGICAL
Fatigue resulting from emotional problems and conflicts, especially depression and anxiety. Fatigue may take the form of a defense mechanism that prevents you from having to face the true cause of your depression, such as the fact that you hate your job.

FATIGUE STATE
A neurotic reaction in which the most prominent clinical feature present is that of emotional fatigue. The emotional fatigue which is present is more or less chronic.

FAT INFILTRATION
Infiltration of tissue of an organ with excess amounts of fat.

FAT NECROSIS
Necrosis (tissue death) in the fatty tissues around the pancreas, due to acute destructive disease of the pancreas and caused by the liberation of pancreatic enzymes that attack fat.

FATTY ACID
(1) Any of numerous saturated aliphatic monocarboxylic acids including many that occur naturally in the form of esters in fats, waxes, and essential oils.

(2) Any of the saturated or unsaturated monocarboxylic acids (as palmitic acid) usually with an even number of carbon atoms that occur naturally in the form of glycerides in fats and fatty oils.

FATTY DEGENERATION
A process of tissue degeneration marked by the deposition of fat globules in the cells.

FATTY STOOLS
Stools in which fat is present due either to pancreatic disease or sprue (celiac disease).

FATUITY
Weakness or imbecility of mind; feebleness of intellect.

FAUCES
The passage that links the mouth and the throat, lying between the soft palate and the base of the tongue.

FAULT
A defect in procedure, method or apparatus, affecting the reliability of

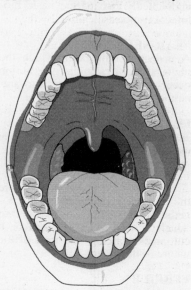

The fauces are located in the back part of the oral cavity.

the results obtained; in a special sense, failure to respond within 30 seconds in a free association test for diagnostic purposes.

FAVEOLUS
A small depression or pit, especially on the skin.

FAVERIN
Brand name of a drug containing the antidepressant fluvoxamine as active component. The drug is prescribed for certain types of depressions.

FAVISM
A severe hereditary allergic reaction caused by eating the broad bean or by inhaling its pollen that is marked by hemolytic anemia, eosinophilia, jaundice, fever and diarrhea, and is observed chiefly in southern Italy.

FEAR
Primary emotion evoked by impending danger and accompanied by the wish to flee. Despite the fact that fear is one of the elemental human experiences and that flight is undoubtedly one of the basic biological responses.

FEAR NEUROSIS
A neurotic complex in which the physical manifestations of emotion occur without any conscious awareness of such emotion.

FEATURE
The structure, form, or appearance especially of a person.

FEATURE PROFILE TEST
A type of performance test, where the subject is required to put together seven pieces of wood into which a head in profile has been cut, without being informed of the nature of the object.

FEBRILE
The state of running a temperature; having a fever.

FEBRILE CONVULSION
A seizure related to a sudden elevation of body temperature.

FEBRILE PULSE
The pulse characteristic of fever. It is full, soft and frequent, and exhibits a well-marked dicrotism (double beat).

FEBRILE REACTION
Reaction consisting of chills, fever with a rise in temperature of at least 1 degree centigrade, and sometimes headache and back pain, rarely progressing to cyanosis (bluish skin) and shock.

FECAL IMPACTION
Condition in which feces become firmly wedged in the rectum.

FECAL INCONTINENCE
Loss of involuntary control of defecation. Anal incontinence may result from injuries to or diseases of the spinal cord, congenital abnormalities, accidental injuries to the rectum and anus, extensive inflammation, tumors and deformities following dilation.

FECALITH
A concretion of dry compact feces formed in the intestine or vermiform appendix.

FECES
Bodily waste discharged through the anus. Feces consists of dietary matter that the alimentary canal has been unable to absorb together with the remnants of the mucous membranes of the alimentary tract, which are constantly being shed and renewed. (See data on feces on next page)

FECTRIM
Brand name of a drug containing the antibacterial agent co-trimoxazole as active component. The drug is prescribed for certain types of infections.

The main constituents in the feces over a 24-hour period in a healthy young man on a Western diet

Total weight	50-100 g
Water	50-75 g
Dry weight	5-30 g
Fat	3-5 g
Carbohydrate	1-5 g
Calcium	500-900 mg
Iron	10-15 mg
Ash	3-6 g

FECUNDITY
The ability to produce offspring, especially in large numbers in a short period.

FEEBLEMINDEDNESS
General term for individuals of subnormal intellectual development and deficient mental functioning, who fall into the more specific categories of moronity, imbecility and idiocy, with a range of IQ of 20-69.

FEEDBACK
The use of the output of a system to control its performance. Many examples of feedback systems can be found in the life sciences, particularly in ecology, biochemistry and physiology.

FEEDING
The taking in of food or the offering of food.

FEEDING TUBE
A rubber or plastic tube inserted into the stomach via either the mouth or the nose, for the purpose of introducing food into the stomach.

FEELING
A general term for the affective aspect of experience, i.e., the experience of pleasure and its opposite, interest and the like, usually inclusive of emotional experience; used popularly in an indefinite sense for any experience, and more particularly for touch sensations.

FEHLING'S SOLUTION
A solution of copper sulphate, potassium tartrate, and sodium hydroxide used to test for sugar (especially glucose) in the urine, which, when present, turns the solution reddish.

FEIGNING
Exhibiting behavior suggesting a condition entirely different from the real condition.

FELLATIO
A sex technique involving oral stimulation of the penis.

FELON
An acute and painful inflammation of the deeper tissues of a finger or toe, usually near the nail.

FELTY'S SYNDROME
A condition characterized by rheumatoid arthritis, neutropenia, splenomegaly and often by weight loss, anemia, lymphadenopathy, and pigment spots on the skin.

FEMALE
Pertaining to the sex that bears young (compare male).

FEMALE HORMONE
A sex hormone (as an estrogen) primarily produced and functioning in the female.

FEMALE SEXUAL AROUSAL DISORDER
Persistent or recurrent partial or complete failure to attain or maintain the lubrication-swelling response of sexual excitement until completion of the sexual activity. The term is also used in the sense of persistent or recurrent lack of a subjective sense of sexual excitement and pleasure in a female during sexual activity.

FEMININE PSYCHOLOGY
Psychology of women that stresses the cultural and social factors influ-

encing the development of a woman rather than biological ones.

FEMINISM
A social movement aiming at the advancement, politically and economically, of the female sex; in a special sense, the possession of feminine traits by the male to a marked degree.

FEMINITY
Referring to patterns of behavior, attitudes, etc., presumed by some to be psychological secondary sexual characteristics of the female.

FEMINIZATION
The development of womanlike changes (e.g., breast enlargement, loss of facial hair) in a male because of endocrine (hormonal) disorder or the administration of certain drugs.

FEMORAL
Pertaining to the femur.

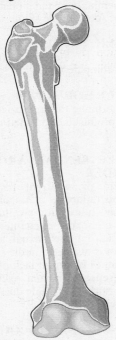

The femur or thigh bone is the longest and strongest bone of the skeleton.

FEMORAL ARTERY
The main artery of the thigh, arising from the external iliac artery in the region of the inguinal ligament and running down two-thirds of the thigh, after which it divides into several branches.

FEMORAL CANAL
The space that is situated between the femoral vein and the inner wall of the femoral sheath, measuring from a quarter to half an inch long, and extending from the femoral ring to the saphenous opening.

FEMORAL NERVE
The main nerve of the anterior (front) part of the thigh, receiving sensory impulses from the front and inner thigh and supplying the muscles of the anterior thigh.

FEMORAL PULSE
Pulse of the femoral artery, felt in the groin.

FEMORAL RING
The oval upper opening of the femoral canal; often the seat of a hernia.

FEMORAL SHEATH
The fascial sheath investing the femoral vessels.

FEMORAL VEIN
The chief vein of the thigh that is a continuation of the popliteal vein, accompanying the femoral artery in the upper part of its course, and continuing above Poupart's ligament as the external iliac vein.

FEMUR
The thigh bone, extending from the hip to the knee; the longest and strongest bone in the body.

FENBID
Brand name of a drug containing the non-steroidal anti-inflammatory preparation ibuprofen as active compound.

FENESTRA
A natural perforation, especially one in the bone between the tympanum (eardrum) and middle ear.

FENESTRATION
Any surgical procedure in which an opening is created to gain access to a cavity within an organ or bone.

FENFLURAMINE
Generic name of an appetite suppressant prescribed for obesity. Fenfluramine is related to amphetamine.

FERMENT
Any of various agents or substances, such as yeast, enzymes or certain bacteria, capable of producing chemical changes.

FERMENTATION
The decomposition of substances such as carbohydrates under the influence of ferments or enzymes.

FERRITIN
A blood protein that contains iron. It is measured to determine the amount of iron stored in the bone marrow, and to diagnose the cause of anemia or explained weakness.

FERROUS CARBONATE
A salt containing iron and occurring in nature or obtained synthetically as a white easily oxidizable precipitate and used in medicine in treating iron-deficiency anemia.

FERRUM METALLICUM
Homeopathic medicine derived from iron. The medicine is best adapted to young, weakly persons, anemic and chlorotic, when the face is habitually ashy or greenish pale.

FERTILE
Able to produce offspring.

FERTILE PERIOD
That time in the menstrual cycle in which fertilization is most likely.

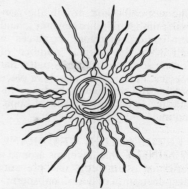

In the first phase of the fertilization process many spermatozoa surround the ovum; only one will penetrate the surrounding membrane of the egg.

FERTILITY
The ability of a woman to conceive or a man to impregnate a woman. Our social attitudes and values are undergoing profound changes at present regarding fertility and infertility. Many women now postpone childbearing until their late 20s, early 30s or even later years.

FERTILIZATION
The union of two gametes, male and female sex cells, to produce a cell from which a new individual (animal or plant) develops.

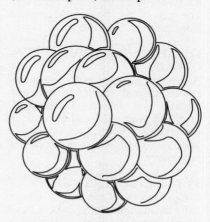

In a very short period of time, within hours, the fertilized egg starts to divide and a tiny organism of some hundred or more cells is formed.

The sex cells contain half the normal number of chromosomes, and fertilization therefore produces a cell with the normal number of chromosomes for any particular species. Fertilization may take place outside the organism's body, or inside the female as a result of copulation.

FERTILIZATION MEMBRANE
A membrane that develops around a fertilized ovum (egg) and prevents the penetration of additional sperm.

FERVOR
Intensity of feeling. The term is also used in the sense of extreme earnestness in religion, particularly in prayer.

FESTER
To become inflamed and form pus.

FESTINATION
An involuntary quickening and shortening of steps in walking, as occurs in some diseases.

FETAL
Pertaining to or having the character of a fetus.

FETAL AGE
The age of the conceptus counted from the time of fertilization.

FETAL ALCOHOL SYNDROME
A variable group of birth defects including mental retardation, deficient growth, and defects of the skull, face, and brain that tend to occur in the infants of women who consume large amounts of alcohol during pregnancy.

FETAL CIRCULATION
Circulation of blood in the unborn baby through the umbilical cord and the placenta (afterbirth).

FETAL DISTRESS
A compromised or abnormal condition of the fetus usually characterized by abnormal heart rhythm and discovered during pregnancy or labor. If possible the cause of the problem is determined and corrected.

FETAL HEART RATE
The number of heartbeats in the fetus during a given time period, normally between 100 and 160 beats per minute.

FETAL HEART SOUNDS
The sounds of the newborn baby's heart heard through the mother's abdomen.

FETAL HEMOGLOBIN
A hemoglobin variant that predominates in the blood of a newborn and persists in increased proportions in some forms of anemia.

FETAL MEMBRANES
Collectively, the amnion, chorion (sac around the amnion) and umbilical cord.

FETAL MONITOR
A device used during pregnancy, labor, and childbirth to observe the fetal heart rate and maternal uterine contractions.

FETAL MOVEMENT
Motion of the fetus itself within the uterus. The motion is usually first detected by a woman pregnant for the first time at about the 13th week of pregnancy, somewhat earlier in those who have had previous pregnancies.

FETAL POSITION
A resting position in which the body is curved, the legs and arms are bent and drawn toward the chest, and the head is bowed forward and which is assumed in some forms of psychic regression.

FETAL SOUFFLE
A murmur, heard through a stetho-

scope, that is made by the fetus's heart before birth.

FETAL SURGERY
Operative procedures on a fetus still in the womb of the mother; a newly developed branch of medicine.

FETAL UTERUS
One that has failed to develop to the size normal for the age of the woman.

FETISHISM
Recurrent, intense, sexual urges and sexually arousing fantasies, involving the use of nonliving objects (fetishes). The person has acted on these urges, or is markedly distressed by them. Among the more common fetish objects are:
- bras;
- women's underpants;
- stockings;
- shoes;
- boots;
- wearing apparel.
The person with fetishism frequently masturbates while holding, rubbing, or smelling the fetish object, or may ask his sexual partner to wear the object during their sexual encounters. Usually the fetish is required or strongly preferred for sexual excitement, and in its absence there may be erectile failure in males. Usually the disorder begins by adolescence, although the fetish may have been endowed with special significance earlier, in childhood. Once established, the disorder tends to be chronic.

FETOLOGY
The study of the fetus; that branch of medicine concerned with the fetus in the uterus, including the diagnosis and treatment of abnormalities.

FETOMETRY
The measurement of a fetus, especially the diameter of the head.

FETOPROTEINS
Proteins found in the tissues of fetuses; these can also be present in a number of malignant diseases. A greater-than-normal amount of alpha fetoprotein in the fetus often indicates an abnormality of the neural tube.

FETOSCOPE
A stethoscope placed on the mother's abdomen to detect the fetal heartbeat.

FETOSCOPY
Procedure that allows the direct observation of the fetus in the uterus through a fetoscope introduced through a small incision in the pregnant woman's abdomen.

FETUS
The life offspring while it is inside the mother (in utero), in humans, from the beginning of the third month of pregnancy until birth.

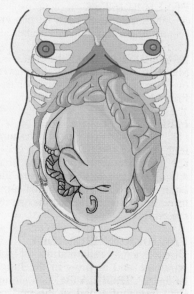

After a couple of months, when all organs have been formed, the embryo becomes a fetus. The fetus grows and develops until it has become old enough for delivery.
8-month fetus in the womb.

FEVER

Raising of the body temperature above normal. Ideal temperature is popularly thought to be exactly 37 degrees centigrade, and anything above or below that figure is suspect.

However, a normal temperature can vary between 36 and 37.2, and is usually higher in the evening than in the morning.

Fever may be due to a host of different disorders, such as:
- kidney infection;
- bowel infection;
- teeth infection;
- throat infection;
- skin infection;
- chest infection;
- cancer.

A fever without apparent cause persisting for more than two weeks is called FUO (fever of unknown origin), a favorite diagnosis of doctors when they admit people to hospital.

FEVER BLISTER

A cold sore caused by a herpes virus; a symptom of herpes simplex.

FEVERISH

Showing symptoms indicating fever (as increased heat and thirst or delirium); having a fever.

FIBER

(1) A long, threadlike structure (e.g., a nerve fiber);
(2) food content (cellulose) that adds roughage to the diet. In the latter sense fiber is a complex mixture of indigestible carbohydrate material.

FIBER-BRONCHOSCOPY

Direct visual examination of the windpipe and airways in the lungs using a flexible tube containing light-transmitting glass fibers that return a magnified image.

FIBER-OPTIC ENDOSCOPY

The use of an endoscope - a flexible tube able to bend light rays - to inspect the interior of a body cavity or organ.

FIBER OPTICS

Thin transparent fibers of glass or plastic that are enclosed by material of a lower index of refraction and that transmit light throughout their length by internal reflections.

FIBER-SCOPE

A flexible instrument containing light-carrying glass or plastic fibers used to view internal body structures.

FIBRIL

A very small fiber or a thread of a fiber.

FIBRILLATION

The twitching of certain muscle fibers without coordination or control.

FIBRILLATION, ATRIAL

Type of cardiac fibrillation involving very rapid, irregular contractions of the atria, followed irregularly by contractions of the ventricles. This may occur suddenly and for a short time or, if there is an existing heart disease, can become chronic.

FIBRILLATION, CARDIAC

A kind of heart arrhythmia (abnormal heart rhythm); uncoordinated contraction of the heart muscle occurring when the individual muscle fibers take up independent irregular contractions.

FIBRILLATION, VENTRICULAR

Type of heart fibrillation, involving contractions of the ventricles that are irregular, haphazard, and ineffective, resulting in a rapid decline of blood circulation and death. Emergency treatment may include heart massage, electrical defibrillation or drugs.

FIBRIN
A protein substance formed in blood as it coagulates and which then contracts to form a clot.

FIBRIN FILM
A pliable translucent film prepared from fibrinogen and thrombin from human blood plasma and used in the surgical repair of defects.

FIBRIN FOAM
A spongy substance prepared from fibrinogen and thrombin from human blood plasma and used especially after saturation with thrombin as an absorbable clotting agent in surgical wounds.

FIBRINOGEN
A protein present in the blood plasma and essential to the process of blood coagulation.

FIBRINOID
A homogenous acidophilic refractile material that somewhat resembles fibrin and is formed in the walls of blood vessels and in connective tissue in some pathological conditions and normally in the placenta.

FIBRINOLYSIN
A thrombolytic enzyme (enzyme that is able to dissolve a thrombus) prescribed for the breaking down of blood clots. Fibrinolysin also aids in the healing of skin ulcers.

FIBRINOLYSIS
Process in which the protein fibrin dissolves and small clots are removed.

FIBROADENOMA
A benign, nontender, hard, movable and firm tumor of the breast, most commonly found in young women and caused by high estrogen levels.

FIBROBLAST
An undifferentiated cell in connective tissue that gives rise to cells that are the precursors of bone, collagen, and other connective tissue cells.

FIBROCYSTIC
A fibrous degeneration that produces cysts.

FIBROCYSTIC BREAST DISEASE
A common condition of women characterized by the pressure of one or more cysts in the breasts. The cysts are benign. The condition is characterized by overgrowth of fibrous tissue in the breast, producing nonmalignant cysts.

FIBROELASTOSIS
A condition of the body or one of its organs (as the left ventricle of the heart) characterized by proliferation of fibroelastic tissue.

FIBROGENESIS
The development or proliferation of fibers or fibrous tissue.

FIBROID
A benign tumor made up of fibrous and muscular tissue that occurs especially in the uterine wall.

FIBROID TUMOR
A non-cancerous growth, consisting of fibrous and muscular tissue, that occurs in the womb. It can occur inside the cavity, inside the wall and on the outer surface.

FIBROMA
Benign growth composed of fibrous tissue and frequently seen as hard, pink growths in the skin.

FIBROMATOSIS
Production of many fibromas such as occurs in neurofibromatosis.

FIBROMYOSITIS
Any of a large number of disorders marked by local inflammation of muscle and connective tissue, stiffness, and joint or muscle pain. It

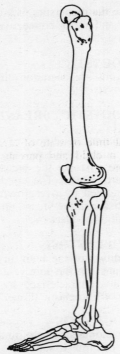

The fibula and tibia make up the lower leg, between knee joint and foot. The fibula, located on the outside, is much thinner than the tibia.

may result from infection, trauma, or other cause. Treatment includes rest, pain-relieving drugs, and sometimes massage.

FIBROSARCOMA
A sarcoma of relatively low malignancy made up chiefly of spindle-shaped cells that tend to form collagenous fibrils.

FIBROSIS
An increase in the formation of fibrous connective tissue, either normally as in scar formation, or abnormally to replace normal tissues, especially in the lungs, uterus, or heart.

FIBROSIS HEPATICA
Excess fibrous tissue in the liver, resulting (passively) from collapse and condensation of pre-existing fi-

bers or (actively) through the synthesis of new fibers by fibroblasts.

FIBROSITIS
Inflammation of fibrous tissue, such as ligaments, tendons, muscle sheets and fascia; often called muscular rheumatism.

FIBROUS
Consisting of, containing, or resembling fibers.

FIBROUS ANKYLOSIS
Immobilization or restriction of movement of a joint due to the growth of fibrous tissue.

FIBROUS JOINT
An immovable joint, such as those in the skull.

FIBULA
The outer and lesser bone of the lower leg; also called calf bone. In man it is the slenderest bone of the body in proportion to its length, articulating above with the external tuberosity of the tibia and below with the talus, and its lower end forming the external malleolus of the ankle.

FICK PRINCIPLE
A generalization in physiology which states that blood flow is proportional to the difference in concentration of a substance in the blood as it enters and leaves an organ and which is used to determine cardiac output from the difference in oxygen concentration in blood before it enters and after it leaves the lungs and from the rate at which oxygen is consumed.

FICTION
In general sense, any imaginative construction, or the product of such; used in a special sense by the Austrian psychiatrist Alfred Adler, in directive fiction, for imaginary situations created to gratify the impulse form power, and accepted as reality,

particularly, for example, the imaginary illness simulated by a neurotic in order to make others treat him or her as an invalid, or in order to avoid tasks he or she does not wish to attempt.

FIELD
(1) An area, as that seen through a microscope;
(2) the area seen (visual field);
(3) an open area during surgery (operative field);
(4) an area or expertise (e.g., field of psychiatry).

FIELD PROPERTY
In Gestalt psychology, the properties of organized wholes that influence the interpretation or action of the parts.

FIELD WORK
A method of studying social phenomena by observation under normal and natural conditions, supplementing this by enquiries and interviews.

FIGURE-GROUND PERCEPTION
Perceiving a pattern as foreground against a background. Patterns are commonly perceived this way even when the stimuli are ambiguous and the foreground-background relationships are reversible.

FIGURE PREFERENCE TEST
A psychological test consisting of 400 black and white figures for each of which the subject is asked to decide whether he or she likes or does not like it.

The test is designed to analyze some specific parameters of the personality.

FILARIA
A type of threadworm.

FILARIASIS
A disease, largely of the tropics, caused by filariae (long, threadlike worms) that enter the body through mosquito bites and infest primarily lymph glands and vessels.

Symptoms include blockage of the lymph vessels and resultant swelling and pain in the limb distal to the blockage, which, over many years, may lead to elephantiasis.

FILIAL CRISIS
Crucial time or state of affairs between a child and parents whose outcome will make a decisive difference in the relationship, for better or worse.

FILIAL MATURITY
Refers to the interdependence of an adult child's experiences with his/her parents following a healthy resolution of filial crisis.

FILIATION
The relation of a child to a father. The term is also used in the sense of the fixing of the paternity of a child.

FILTERABLE VIRUS
Any of the infectious agents that remain virulent after a fluid containing them passes through a filter of diatomite or unglazed porcelain and that include the viruses as presently understood and various other groups (as the mycoplasmas and rickettsias) which were originally considered viruses before their cellular nature was established.

FILUM TERMINALE
The slender threadlike prolongation of the spinal cord below the origin of the lumber nerves; the last portion of the pia mater.

FIMBRIA
A fringe or fringelike structure, such as the fingerlike projections around the ovarian end of the Fallopian tube.

FINAL
Usually applied to the end of a series, but may also have the sense of

purposive; in final cause the word has the sense of aim, purpose of goal of a process or series of events.

FINAL COMMON PATH
The motor neurons on which a number of motor pathways converge.

FINAL COMMON PATHWAY
A number of alternative developmental sequences converging into a single common state.

FINALISM
Philosophical interpretation or explanation of life processes in terms of their ends or purposes, and this sense is carried over into the psychology of the analytical school.

FINGER
Any of the terminal members of the hand other than the thumb.

FINGER AGNOSIA
Inability to recognize the individual fingers due to disease in the cerebral hemisphere of the brain.

FINGERNAIL
The hard protective growth at the end of each of the fingers of the hand.

FINGERPRINTS
Impressions of the loops and whorls of the papillary ridges of the fingertips.

FINGER-THUMB OPPOSITION
A significant step in muscular coordination in the development of a child, occurring on average at or

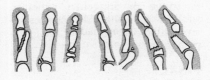

Various types of fractures of the finger.

about the age of one year and used in some test scales as a test of such development.

FINGER WRINKLE TEST
Test for certain functions of the autonomic nervous system. The functioning of the sympathetic nerves is tested by placing the person's hand in warm water for at least half an hour and noticing if the skin of the fingers wrinkled after the soaking.

The test is performed when there is suspicion of Raynaud's disease (blockage of arterial circulation, usually in extremities), diabetes or certain inflammatory conditions of peripheral nerves.

FIRE DRILL
A minor mental mechanism through which the individual concerned urgently mobilizes his emotional resources in preparing for an anticipated crisis or emergency.

FIRST AID
Emergency care or treatment given to an ill or injured person before regular medical aid can be obtained.

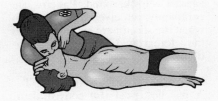

Mouth-to-mouth resuscitation is one of the most significant methods in first aid.

FIRST-DEGREE BURN
A mild burn characterized by heat, pain, and reddening of the burned surface but not exhibiting blistering or charring of tissues.

FISH PROTEIN CONCENTRATE
A protein-rich food additive obtained as a nearly colorless and

tasteless powder from ground whole fish.

FISH TAPEWORM INFECTION

An intestinal infection caused by the adult cestode Diphyllobothrium latum. Mild gastrointestinal upset may occur and, rarely, an anemia that resembles pernicious anemia.

FISSION

A splitting, as in the asexual formation of new bacterial or protozoan cells or in the splitting of an atomic nucleus, with the release of energy.

FISSURE

Any of the deep grooves of the outer covering of the brain. The term is also used in the sense of a cleft or groove in a part, whether normal of abnormal.

FISTULA

An abnormal opening or channel connecting two internal organs or leading from an internal organ to the outside.
   The following conditions may lead to the formation of a fistula:
- infection;
- inflammatory diseases;
- degeneration;
- injury;
- congenital defect;
- surgery.

FIT

(1) Popular name for an attack or manifestation of a disease characterized by loss of consciousness or by convulsions;
(2) an uncontrollable attack of any physical disturbance, such as a fit of coughing.

FIXATION

(1) The process of securing a part, as by sewing with catgut or wire (suturing);
(2) a halt in personality growth at a particular stage of psychological development;

(3) hardening and preservation of tissues for examination under a microscope.

FIXATION OF AFFECT

The establishment of a strong and relatively enduring emotional attachment.

FIXATION POINT

That phase, period or point of infantile development at which a person has become fixated, through which he or she has not completely passed and to which he or she remains liable to regress.

FIXED-ALTERNATIVE QUESTION

A question asked on a test, an examination or a survey, requiring the answer to be selected from alternatives provided by a questioner.

FIXED-COMBINATION DRUG

A preparation containing multiple ingredients in the concomitant administration of two or more drugs.

FIXED IDEA

An idea or line of thought, often emotionally entrenched, or even obsessional, that exercises or tends to exercise, a dominating influence, persistent or recurrent, on a person's attitude and mental life.

FLACCID

Limp, soft, weak, or flabby (e.g., a muscle).

FLACCID BLADDER

A type of malfunctioning bladder caused by interruption of the normal reflex arc associated with voiding.
   Important symptoms include:
- absence of bladder sensation;
- overfilling of the bladder;
- inability to urinate voluntarily.

FLACCID PARALYSIS

Abnormality characterized by weakness or loss of muscle tone due to disease or injury to the nerves affecting the involved muscles.

FLAGELLATION
The action of whipping someone else (e.g., sadism) or of being whipped (e.g., masochism) for stimulation or sexual arousal.

FLAGELLUM
A threadlike tail or other extension from an organism, as in sperm, to provide locomotion.

FLAP
A section of tissue used to cover a burn or other injury, as the pedicle flap, a tubular gathering of skin, one end of which is left attached in the original site while the other end is freed for attachment in another part of the body.

When the flap has healed at the new site, the other end is also detached and the remaining skin is sewn in place.

FLARE
(1) A reddening of the skin around a lesion produced by an allergic reaction;
(2) a reddening of the skin spreading outward from a focus of irritation or infection.

FLATFOOT
Condition in which the instep is not arched and the bottom of the foot (planta surface) is flat, sometimes causing footache and fatigue.

FLATULENCE
Real or perceived increase in the amount of intestinal gas.

The major symptoms are:
- feeling of bloating or needing to belch;
- passing much gas by the rectum;
- intestinal discomfort;
- gurgling;
- occasional cramping pain.

These may or may not be associated with an obvious cause. There are many possible causes, including:

- air swallowing;
- ulcer disease;
- inflammation of the stomach;
- small intestine disease;
- colon disorders;
- food intolerance.

The treatment depends on the cause.

FLATUS
An accumulation of intestinal gas in the stomach, intestines or other body cavity and the passing of this via the back passage.

FLAVOR
A sensory quality, or impression, primarily involving smell and, to some extent, taste (sometimes together with touch and temperature) from an object in the mouth.

FLESH WOUND
An injury involving penetration of the body musculature without damage to bones or internal organs.

FLEXIBILITAS CEREA
A symptom of some types of schizophrenia and hysteria, where the person retains a posture of body and limbs in which he or she has been placed.

FLEXIBILITY
The property of being able to be bent without breaking.

FLEXION
A bending of a joint (e.g., the elbow) that causes two adjoining bones (e.g., those in the upper and lower arm) to come closer together.

FLEXOR
A muscle that causes the bending of a limb or part.

FLEXURE
A bent or curved structure within the body.

FLIES
Members of the insect order Diptera. The housefly can carry many

harmful microorganisms (including that causing typhoid fever), and the tsetse fly carries sleeping sickness.

FLIGHT OF IDEAS
Rapid succession of superficially related, or entirely unrelated, ideas occurring in manic states of mania.

FLOATER
A spot that appears in the visual field when one stares at a blank wall. Floaters are due to bits of protein and other debris that move in front of the retina. Usually they are harmless but a sudden increase in the number of floaters may indicate a disease.

FLOATING KIDNEY
Kidney that has become detached from its normal position. Its ability to move results in the kinking of the ureter, which produces pain and, when the ureter becomes unkinked, the sudden production of a large volume of urine.

FLOATING RIB
One of the lowest pairs of ribs, not attached to the breastbone or other ribs.

FLOCCULATION
Reaction in which material that is normally invisible in a solution forms a suspension or precipitate as a result of changes in the physical or chemical conditions. This reaction is the basis of flocculation tests used to diagnose certain diseases.

FLOOD
In medicine, to have an excessive menstrual flow or a uterine hemorrhage after childbirth.

FLOXAPEN
Brand name of a penicillin antibiotic drug containing fluoloxacillin as active compound. The drug is prescribed for certain types of bacterial infections.

FLU
Short term for influenza.

FLU-AMP
Brand name for a drug containing the antibiotics ampicillin and fluoloxacillin as active compounds. The drug is prescribed for various kinds of bacterial infections.

FLUID EXTRACT
An alcohol preparation of a vegetable drug containing the active constituents of one gram of the dry drug in each millimeter.

FLUID INTELLIGENCE
Component of intelligence that is closely related to psychological and hereditary factors; ability to solve abstract problems that do not require careful monitoring of procedures to discover ways of modification.

FLUNITRAZEPAM
Generic name of a benzodiazepine preparation prescribed for insomnia (disorder in sleep mechanisms).

FLUOR
A bodily discharge.

FLUORESCENCE
A dye used in ophthalmology to detect certain defects of the cornea and other abnormalities and to determine whether the fit of a contact lens is correct.

FLUORIDATION
Addition of small quantities of fluorides to public water supplies, bringing the concentration to one part per million as in some natural water supplies. It greatly reduces the incidence of tooth decay by strengthening the teeth.

FLUORIDE
Trace element in the body. The bones and teeth contain most of the body's fluoride.

FLUORINE
A nonmetallic univalent halogen that is normally a pale yellowish flammable irritating toxic gas.

FLUOROCARBON
Any of several chemical compounds of fluorine and carbon, which, because of their ability to carry large amounts of oxygen, may become useful in artificial blood for humans who cannot have, or refuse, transfusion of human blood.

FLUOROQUINOLONES
A class of drugs used to treat bacterial infections, such as urinary tract infections and some types of bronchitis.
  These drugs include ciprofloxacin, enoxacin, lomefloxacin, norfloxacin and ofloxacin.

FLUOROSCOPY
A technique in which a special device (fluoroscope) allows the immediate projection of X-ray images of the body onto a special fluorescent screen. It eliminates the need for taking and developing X-ray photographs.

FLUOROSIS
Condition resulting from excessive intake of fluorine, usually from high concentrations in drinking water; it causes discoloration and pitting of tooth enamel in children and bone and joint changes in adults.

FLUSH
Term used in two meanings:
(1) a sudden reddening of the face;
(2) a sudden sensation of heat.

FLUTTER
Rapid movement back and forth of a part, especially of the heart chambers.

FLUTTERING HEARTS
The name given to an illusion experienced when colored fingers, on a differently colored background, are moved to and from the figures appearing to move from side to side.

FLUX
An excessive flow from an organ or cavity (e.g., diarrhea).

FLUXION
A slow or settling of blood or other fluid towards any organ with greater force than natural.

FOCAL CEREBRAL DISORDERS
Disorders of the higher (integrative) mental processes, characterized by specific signs and symptoms, and caused by injury or disease at specific sites in the cerebral cortex, either defined or presumed.

FOCAL DISTANCE
In ophthalmology, the distance between the lens and the point behind the lens at which light from a distant point is focused.

FOCAL INFECTION
Infection in which microorganisms exist in certain localized areas from where they are distributed into the bloodstream. Common sites, or foci include:
- diseased gums;
- tonsils;
- nasal passages.

FOCAL REACTION
An exacerbation or recurrence at the site of an active or healed lesion distant from the place of introduction or point of origin of the exciting agent.

FOCAL SEIZURE
A transitory disturbance, caused by abnormal electrical activity of nerve cells in a particular localized area of the brain (produced by temporary lack of oxygen, a small lesion, or trauma) and manifested by disturbance in motor or sensory function, as, e.g., profuse salivation, lip smacking, or tingling feel-

ing in a certain part of the body.

FOCAL THERAPY
Modification of psychoanalytical therapy in which one specific problem presented by the patient is chosen as the focus of interpretation.

FOCUS
(1) A point at which light, sound, or other rays, meet, as determined by positions of lenses and other devices; the point of convergence of light after passing through a convex lens is the place at which there is the clearest image;
(2) the main site of an infection or other diseased state.

FOETUS
See Fetus.

FOLD
A doubling sack or infolding (e.g., the neural fold, which leads to the development of the neural tube in the embryo).

FOLEX-350
Brand name for a drug containing folic acid (a vitamin) and iron (an important mineral for the body) as active compounds. The drug is prescribed for certain deficiency states.

FOLIC ACID
One of the B-complex vitamins, essential for cell growth and reproduction.
   Rich sources include:
- leafy vegetables;
- liver;
- kidney;
- whole grain cereals.

FOLIE
Any of several abnormal reactions; a mental disorder.

FOLIE A DEUX
The simultaneous appearance of psychoses with similar delusional content in two members of the same family.

FOLIE A TROIS
The simultaneous appearance of psychoses with similar delusional content in three members of the same family.

FOLIE DU DOUTE
The obsessional doubting mania. The original term of obsessive states.

FOLK PSYCHOLOGY
Psychology of peoples: applied to the psychological study of the beliefs, customs, conventions, etc. of peoples, especially primitive groups, inclusive of comparative study.

FOLKWAYS
Traditional forms of behavior of a particular social group, having conventional rather than moral validity in the group.

FOLLICLE
Term used in three different meanings.
(1) Pouchlike cavity, as that in the skin enclosing a hair;
(2) A saclike gland, as a sebaceous follicle that secretes sebum;
(3) Graafian follicle of the ovary, from which an ovum erupts.

FOLLICLE-STIMULATING HORMONE (FSH)
A sex hormone (gonadotropin) that is secreted by the anterior lobe of the pituitary gland and stimulates the development of egg and sperm cells.

FOLLICULITIS
Inflammation of a hair follicle.

FOMENTATION
The application of heat (usually moist) to relieve pain by causing a dilation of the blood vessels in the skin.

FOMES
Any object (as a utensil, towel,

money) that can support and transmit disease-causing organisms.

FOMITES
Inanimate objects or materials, e.g., clothing, toilet articles, dressings, bedding, on which infectious agents may be carried.

FONTANEL
One of two membrane-covered soft spots in the skull of a newborn infant, which close as the cranial bones develop. Also called soft spot.

FOOD ALLERGY
A hypersensitivity reaction to a substance - an antigen, most often a protein - ingested in food. There are two kinds of reactions to food: immediate and late.

Hypersensitivity to foods manifests itself in a variety of symptoms. One of the most common reactions is hives (urticaria). Different people may experience varying combinations of the following:
nasal symptoms, like those characteristic of allergic rhinitis;
– eye symptoms;

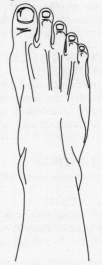

The foot consists of three major parts: the digits or toes, the metatarsus (metatarsal bones), and tarsus (tarsal bones)

– respiratory symptoms of asthma;
– gastrointestinal upset;
– nausea;
– vomiting;
– stomach ache;
– cramps (colic in infants);
– itching;
– swelling of the eyes, lips, face;
– eczema;
– migraine headache.

FOOD-CHAIN
A figure of speech for the dependence for food of organisms upon others in a series, beginning with plants or scavenging organisms and ending with the largest carnivores.

FOOD POISONING
Acute illness caused by eating food containing toxic substances or organisms and the toxins produced by them.

FOOD POISONING, STAPHYLOCOCCAL
Toxic condition of the human body characterized by the following symptoms:
- violent onset;
- severe nausea;
- vomiting;
- cramps;
- watery diarrhea;
- prostration;
- low blood pressure;
- mild or no fever.
The disease is caused by enterotoxins secreted by certain strains of Staphylococcus aureus. The incubation period is 1-6 hours, usually 2-4 hours.

FOOTDROP
Abnormal condition in which the foot is not in its normal flexion position, but rather drags; it is usually due to damage to the nerves and muscles of the foot.

FOOTLING PRESENTATION
The fetal position during childbirth when the baby is lying with the feet foremost.

FORAMEN
A hole or opening, especially in a bone or membrane.

FORAMEN OVALE
An opening between the two atria of the fetal heart that closes after birth.

FORBEARANCE
Restraint of passions: long-suffering. The term is also used in the sense of indulgence towards those who injure us.

FORCED FEEDING
The forcible administration of food (e.g., through a nasal tube) to someone who will not or cannot otherwise eat.

FORCED MOVEMENTS
Asymmetrical movements, caused by an unequal stimulation of the two sides of an organism, or by injury to one hemisphere of the brain.

FORCEPS
Any of a large variety of surgical instruments used to grasp, handle, pull or otherwise manipulate a body part of a fetus.

FORCEPS DELIVERY
An obstetrical procedure in which forceps are inserted through the vagina to grasp the head of the fetus and draw it through the birth canal; performed to shorten labor or quickly deliver a baby in distress.

FOREARM
That part of the upper extremity between the elbow and the wrist.

FOREBRAIN
The part of the brain controlling sensation, perception, emotion, learning, thinking, and other intellectual functions and including the olfactory bulb and tracts, cerebral hemispheres, and nasal ganglia as well as the thalamus, optic tracts, and hypothalamus.

FORE-EXERCISE
Preliminary practice period in an experiment or test, the object being to introduce the subject to the experimental or test situation, and any manipulation required on his or her part, and sometimes to get a base line from which to estimate variability from day to day, or the effect of the introduction of the variable condition being studied.

FOREHEAD
The part of the face which extends from the usual line of hair on the top of the head to the eyes.

FORENSIC MEDICINE
A branch of medicine concerned with the legal aspects of medical care, such as the cause of unexplained death.

FORENSIC PATHOLOGY
A branch of medicine that provides evidence used in the resolution of crimes involving the death of a person.

FOREPLAY
Stimulation of sexual arousal between partners before intercourse.

FOREPLEASURE
Term used by psychoanalysts, for sexual pleasure experienced during the excitation of an erogenous zone.

FORESKIN
The loose skin around the base of the head of the penis or clitoris; its removal constitutes circumcision.

FORMAL THOUGHT DISORDER
A disturbance in the form of thought as distinguished from the content of thought. The boundaries of the concept are not clear.

FORNIX
A part shaped like an arch, as the fornix cerebri in the hippocampus of the brain or the vaginal fornix.

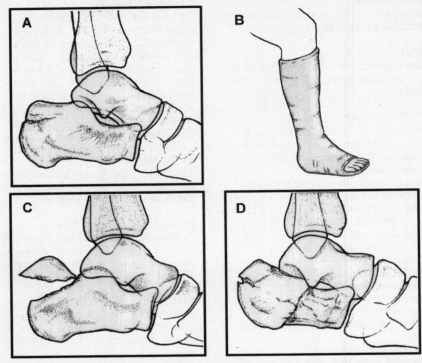

Fractures of the calcaneus (A, C and D) and the application of a plaster (B). A and D are light fractures; C is a very serious fracture.

FOSSA
A depression. The term is used in anatomy to describe various holes in the body.

FOVEA
A surface pit or small depression, especially the pit in the center of the macula of the retina.

FOVEA CENTRALIS RETINAE
The area of the retina (visual coat of the eye) that records the most distinct vision.

FRACTURE
A broken or cracked bone.

FRANK BREECH
Position of the fetus within the mother's uterus in which the buttocks present at the maternal pelvic outlet, not the head as is normal for delivery.

FRATERNAL TWINS
Twins developed from separate eggs. They are no more alike genetically than ordinary brothers and sisters, and thus may be of the same or different sexes.

FRECKLE
A small, flat brown or tan discoloration on the skin, usually resulting from exposure to the sun.

FREMITUS
A flutter than can be felt by the hand of the examiner or by listening, as the chest vibrations that occur with speech or on coughing.

FRENULUM
A band or fold of membrane that connects two organs and usually

limits the movement of one.

FRENULUM LINGUAE
The band of tissue that extends from the floor of the mouth to the under surface of the tongue.

FRONTAL
Pertaining to the front of an organ, the body or to the forehead.

FRONTAL LOBE
That part of the cerebral cortex in either hemisphere of the brain, found directly behind the forehead.

FRONTAL SINUS
One of a pair of hollow spaces (sinuses) in the frontal bone of the skull above the eye socket.

FROTTEURISM
Recurrent, intense, sexual urges and sexually arousing fantasies, involving touching and rubbing against a nonconsenting person. It is the touching, not the coercive nature of the act, that is sexually exciting.

The person with frotteurism usually commits frottage in crowded places, such as on busy sidewalks or in public transportation vehicles, from which he can more easily escape arrest. The person usually selects a victim with a body habitus very attractive to him who is wearing tight-fitting clothes.

He rubs his genitals against the victim's thighs and buttocks or fondles her genitals or breasts with his hands. While doing this he usually fantasizes an exclusive, caring relationship with his victim. However, he recognizes that in order to avoid possible prosecution, he must escape detection after touching his victim. The victim may not initially protest the frottage because she cannot image that such a provocative sexual act would be committed in such a public place.

Usually the disorder begins by adolescence. Some people with frotteurism report that they first became interested in touching others while observing others committing acts of frottage. Most acts of frottage occur when the person is 15 to 25 years of age, after which there is a gradual decline in its frequency.

FUNCTION
Term used in several senses:
(1) the activity of, or part played by, any organic structure;
(2) activity in general;
(3) mathematically, a variable quantity, whose value depends on the value assigned to the one or more parameters involved.

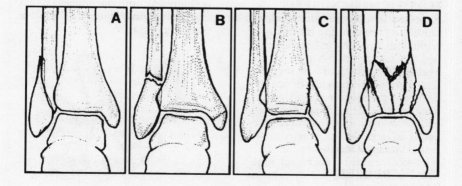

Ankle-fractures. A: fracture of the lateral ankle; B; fracture of the lateral ankle; C: fracture of the medial ankle; D: multiple fracture of the distal part of the tibia. B, C and D are serious fractures.

FUNCTIONAL DISORDER
Disorder that does not involve any change or disease affecting structure, as contrasted with organic disorder.

FUNCTIONAL ENCOPRESIS
Repeated involuntary (or, much more rarely, intentional) passage of feces into places not appropriate for that purpose (e.g., clothing or floor). The stool may be of normal or near-normal consistency, or liquid, as in the case of overflow incontinence secondary to functional fecal retention. When the passage of feces is involuntary rather than intentional, it is often related to constipation, impaction, or retention with subsequent overflow. The constipation may develop because the child, for psychological reasons, avoids defecation, because of either anxiety about defecating in a particular place or a more general pattern of oppositional behavior.

In other children, the constipation develops for physiologic reasons, such as dehydration associated with a febrile illness or medication. Once constipation has developed, it may be complicated by an anal fissure, painful defecation, and further fecal retention. The disorder usually begins by the age of four.

FUNCTIONAL ENURESIS
Repeated involuntary or intentional voiding of urine during the day or at night into bed or clothes, after an age at which continence is expected. The disorder is often referred to as primary if it has not been preceded by a period of urinary continence at least one year, and secondary if it has been preceded by a period of urinary continence lasting at least one year.

In most cases of nocturnal functional enuresis, the child awakens with no memory of a dream and no memory of having urinated. Typically the disturbance occurs during the first third of the night.

In a few cases the voiding takes place during the rapid eye movement (REM) stage of sleep, and in such cases the child may recall a dream that involved the act of urinating.

FUNDUS
The base or that part of a hollow organ farthest from its mouth.

FUNDUS UTERI
The top end of the womb. The position of the uterine fundus is used to calculate the duration of pregnancy.

FUNGUS
One of a group of simple plantlike organisms including mushrooms and yeast, some of which cause disease.

FUNNY BONE
A colloquial term for the back of the elbow, where the ulnar nerve is near the surface. A sharp blow to the site causes a most unpleasant shock or tingle.

FUSIFORM
Spindle-shaped, tapering at both ends.

FUSION
(1) Normal or abnormal joining;
(2) the combining of images from both eyes to form one image;
(3) the surgical joining of two or more vertebrae.

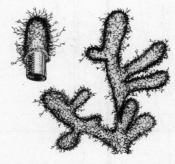

Fungal infection of the roots of a plant, which may infect humans.

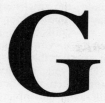

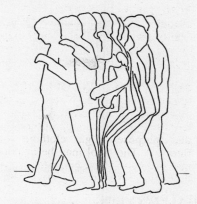

Analysis of gait in normal walking.

GAG-REFLEX
Reflex contraction of the muscles of the throat caused especially by stimulation (as by touch) of the pharynx.

GAIT
(1) A manner of walking or moving on foot;
(2) a sequence of foot movements by which an individual moves forward. A number of neurological diseases are characterized by a disorder of the gait.

GAIT-STUTTERING
A halting and hesitant gait analogous to the stammer in speech.

GALACTAGOGUE
A substance that promotes the secretion of milk.

GALACTOKINASE DEFICIENCY
An inability to metabolize galactose (the sugar derived from lactose) due to a deficiency of the enzyme galactokinase, inherited as a genetic defect.

GALACTORRHEA
Excessive production of breast milk.

GALACTOSEMIA
Increased amount of galactose in the blood. An inherited disease, the classic form is marked by enlargement of the liver, cataracts and mental retardation. Another form is marked only by cataract formation.

The diseases are due to the lack of an enzyme needed to change galactose into either glucose or some other substance. Once diagnosed, the treatment is to eliminate galactose from the diet. A blood test is performed when newborn infants show nutritional problems or gastrointestinal symptoms.

GALACTOSE
A monosaccharide (a simple sugar) found in lactose (milk sugar), sweetbreads, brains, liver, raffinose (contained in beetroot and in many gums and seaweeds).

GALACTOSTASIS
The stagnation of milk in the breast.

GALANGAL
(Alpinia galanga) Perennial plant of which the rootstock is used for medicinal purposes. The creeping rootstock is cylindrical and branched, ringed with the sheaths of former leaves, rust brown or red outside and gray-white inside. Galangal is used in the same way as ginger.

GALENICAL
A standard medicinal preparation (as an extract or tincture) containing usually one or more active constituents of a plant and made by a process that leaves the inert and other undesirable constituents of the plant undissolved.

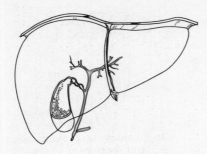

Localization of the gallbladder below the liver.

GALEN'S VEIN
Either of a pair of cerebral veins of the third ventricle that drain the interior of the brain.

GALL
A bitter fluid secreted by the liver; bile. The term is also used in the sense of bitterness of mind.

GALLBLADDER
A pear-shaped organ, about 8 centimeters (3 inches) long and located on the lower surface of the liver, that is a reservoir for bile.

Bile produced in the liver passes (through the hepatic duct) to the gallbladder, where it is stored; the presence of food, especially fats, in the duodenum and hormonal influences cause the gallbladder to contract, releasing the bile to the common bile duct for transport to the duodenum.

GALLOP RHYTHM
An extra heart sound that, when the heart rate is rapid enough, resembles the sound of a horse's gallop. It may or may not be significant.

GALLSTONE
A calculus formed in the gallbladder or common bile duct. In the early stages of formation, there are usually no symptoms. Abdominal discomfort, especially after eating a fatty meal, with occasional episodes of flatulence ("wind") associated with pain in the right side of the abdomen under the ribs, may occur. There may be one or more attacks of fever and chills, with jaundice along with these symptoms.

In most people, the cause is not known. However, gallstones are found more often in women who are middle-aged and older, in certain groups of people and in those with certain diseases (such as diabetes). As many as 10 percent of men and 20 percent of women who are between 55 and 65 years of age have gallstones, which are a common problem of aging.

For whatever reasons, the cholesterol and other substances found in the bile crystallize to form hard stones of varying sizes.

Surgery to remove the gallbladder and its stones is currently the only proven treatment. Sometimes medical treatment without surgery (diet control, certain medications) can be tried.

GALVANIC SKIN RESPONSE (GSR)
Changes in electrical conductivity of, or activity in, the skin, detected by a sensitive electronic device. The reactions are commonly used as an emotional indicator, and are also employed in lie-detector (polygraph) tests.

GALVANOCAUTERY
An instrument with a platinum-loop tip which is heated to a dull red by an electrical current and used to cut or destroy tissues.

GAMETE
The name given to the male or female reproductive cell whether it occurs in animals, humans or plants. In human beings, the female ovum and the male sperm are the gametes.

GAMETOGENESIS
Gametogeny, the production and development of gametes.

GAMMA GLOBULIN
A blood protein fraction that contains antibodies. It is given if a person is at risk of certain infectious diseases - for example, hepatitis, measles, poliomyelitis and tetanus - and to Rh-negative mothers who have given birth to Rh-positive babies, to prevent hemolytic disease of the newborn.

GAMMA RAYS
Rays emitted by radioactive substances, which have a shorter wavelength than X-rays.

GAMMOPATHY
A disorder characterized by a disturbance in the body's synthesis of immunoglobulins.

GAMONE
Any of various substances believed to be liberated by eggs or sperms and to affect germ cells of the opposite sex.

GANGLIAL, GANGLIAR
Relating to a ganglion.

GANGLIECTOMY
Surgical removal of a ganglion.

GANGLION
A small collection of nerve cells, sometimes with synapse formation, common in the autonomic and peripheral nervous systems. Also, a benign lump, often at the wrist, found close to tendons and containing a jelly-like fluid. Traditionally treated by a blow from the family Bible, they are less likely to recur after surgical removal.

The term also refers to a subsidiary nerve center in the brain or other part of the nervous system.

GANGLIONIC   BLOCKING AGENTS
Drugs that block the transmission of nerve impulses at the nerve centers (ganglia) rather than at the nerve endings (as would adrenergic blocking agents). Some of these drugs, such as hexamethonium and mecamylamine hydrochloride, may be used in the treatment of high blood pressure.

GANGLIOSIDE
Any of a group of glycolipids that are found especially in the plasma membrane of cells of the gray matter. Gangliosides have sialic acid, hexoses, and hexosamines in the carbohydrate part and ceramide as the lipid.

GANGLIOSIDOSIS
Any of several inherited metabolic diseases (as Tay Sachs disease) characterized by an enzyme deficiency which causes accumulation of gangliosides in the tissues.

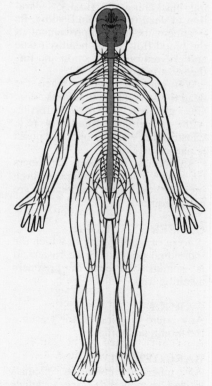

The nervous system contains numerous ganglia (plural of ganglion); most of them are located next to the spinal cord in the dorsal roots.

GANGOSA
Destructive ulcerative condition believed to be a manifestation of yaws that usually originates about the soft palate and spreads into the hard palate, nasal structures, and outward to the face, eroding intervening bone, cartilage, and soft tissues.

GANGRENE
Death of tissue following loss of blood supply, often after obstruction of arteries by injury, thrombosis (clot formation on a damaged artery wall) or embolism (blockage occurring after a portion of clot or other debris has travelled through the bloodstream until it has become stuck).

Dry gangrene is seen when arterial block is followed by slow drying, blackening and, finally, separation of dead tissue from healthy. Its treatment includes improvement of the blood flow to the healthy tissue and prevention of infection and further obstruction.

Wet gangrene occurs when the dead tissue is infected with bacteria. Gas gangrene involves infection with gasforming organisms (e.g. Clostridium welchii) and its spread is particularly rapid.

Antibiotics, hyperbaric chambers (in which oxygen is kept at high pressure) and early amputation are often required.

GANSER SYNDROME
A form of malingering in which the individual pretends to be insane. It is sometimes seen in prisoners awaiting trial.

GARGLE
Any liquid preparation for washing the mouth and throat.

GARGOYLISM
An inherited condition characterized by mental deficiency, defective vision, a very large head, a prominent abdomen and short arms and legs, and so called because the facial features resemble those of a gargoyle.

GARLIC
(Allium sativum) A plant of the onion family, rich in calcium, potassium, phosphorus and other nutrients.

It is claimed to have a beneficial effect on the digestive system and the mucous membranes, and to be helpful in treating high blood pressure, respiratory diseases and other disorders.

Garlic has antiseptic properties and has long been used to rid the body of intestinal parasites.

GAS EMBOLISM
A disorder resulting from overinflation of the lungs due to expanding pulmonary gas during reduction of surrounding pressure (e.g. during an ascent from diving), generally characterized by abrupt loss of consciousness with or without other manifestations of the central nervous system, and attributed to air bubbles in the blood vessels of the brain, which originate in the lungs.

GAS GANGRENE
That due to infection of a wound with a gas-producing microorganism. It is a progressive gangrene marked by impregnation of the dead and dying tissue with and caused by one or more toxin-producing bacteria of the genus Clostridium that enter the body through wounds and proliferate in necrotic tissue.

GASP
A labored respiration; a short painful catching of the breath.

GASSERIAN GANGLION
The large flattened sensory root ganglion of the trigeminal nerve (fifth cranial nerve) that lies within the skull and behind the orbit. Also called semilunar ganglion, trigeminal ganglion.

GASTRALGIA
Pain in the stomach; the pain is of a neuralgic type.

GASTRECTOMY
Surgical removal of part (partial or subtotal gastrectomy) or the whole (total gastrectomy) of the stomach.

GASTRIC
Pertaining to the stomach.

GASTRIC ANALYSIS
Laboratory investigation of the gastric juice. This is performed primarily to determine whether the stomach secretes hydrochloric acid, and also to show whether the stomach produces the necessary digestive enzymes and whether it contains any cancer cells.

Gastric secretions include the following:
- water;
- electrolytes;
- hydrochloric acid;
- mucin;
- pepsin;
- gastrin;
- intrinsic factor.

Gastric analysis is done by passing a tube through the nose or mouth and into the stomach. The gastric fluid is withdrawn by suction continually for one hour. Chemical analysis of the various components is then performed.

The test is done in cases of undiagnosed anemia or repeated stomach infections, when searching for stomach cancer and ulceration.

GASTRIC ARTERY
(1) A branch of the celiac artery that passes to the cardiac end of the stomach and along the lesser curvature. Also called left gastric artery.
(2) Any of several branches of the splenic artery distributed to the greater curvature of the stomach.

GASTRIC CRISIS
Paroxysms of abdominal pain with vomiting that occur in tabes dorsalis (a syphilitic disease of the nervous system).

GASTRIC GLAND
Any of various glands in the walls of the stomach that secrete gastric juice.

GASTRIC INFLUENZA
A form of gastroenteritis caused by the influenza virus.

GASTRIC JUICE
The secretions from stomach glands; the digestive juices. Gastric juice is a thin watery acid digestive fluid secreted by the glands in the mucous membrane of the stomach and containing 0.2 to 0.4 percent free hydrochloric acid and several enzymes (as pepsin).

GASTRIC NEUROSIS
A disturbance of digestion due to a psychological conflict involving dependent infantile fixations.

GASTRIC ULCER
One affecting the lining of the stomach. Has similar characteristics to a duodenal ulcer.

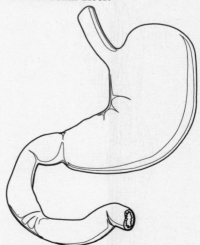

The outside of the stomach is covered with a serosal layer; the mucosal membrane of the interior is the site of numerous glands which can be investigated by chemical analysis of the gastric juice.

GASTRIN

A polypeptide hormone secreted by certain cells of the pyloric glands in the stomach. Gastrin strongly stimulates the secretion of gastric acid and pepsin and weakly stimulates secretion of pancreatic enzymes and gallbladder contraction.

Analysis of gastrin is performed when there are severe, seemingly incurable ulcers of the stomach and small intestine and in cases of suspected pernicious anemia.

GASTRITIS

Inflammation of the stomach lining, which can be either acute or chronic. The sufferer may show the following symptoms:
- sensation of dullness in the upper abdomen;
- loss of appetite;
- fever (in acute gastritis);
- nausea and vomiting (in gastritis);

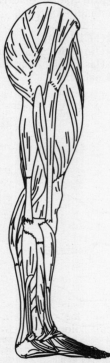

The gastrocnemius muscle occupies the dorsal or posterior part of the leg.

- diarrhea;
- general aches and pains;
- intolerance to certain foods (in chronic gastritis);
- anemia (in chronic gastritis).

The acute condition may be caused by dietary indiscretion, specific food intolerances, chemical irritants (such as alcohol and aspirin), food poisoning or many types of inflammation caused by bacteria or other microorganisms.

Chronic gastritis is a rather uncommon disease, but can be associated with gastric ulcer, cancer of the stomach wall and pernicious anemia.

Diagnosis is established with the chemical and histological analysis of gastric secretions, gastroscopy and X-rays.

The treatment depends largely on the underlying cause of the condition. For acute gastritis, removal of any irritants and resting of the stomach is usually all that is needed. Changing the diet to bland liquids and gradually increasing what is eaten are usually curative. For chronic gastritis, removal of any potential irritants (alcohol, caffeine, tobacco, spices, specific foods, etc.) and the eating of small frequent meals may be of help. If there are underlying conditions (for example, pernicious anemia), these should be treated.

GASTROCNEMIUS

The muscle that forms the bulk of the calf of the leg. It is the largest and most superficial muscle of the calf of the leg arising by two heads from the condyles of the femur and having its tendon of insertion incorporated as part of the Achilles tendon.

GASTROCOLIC

Relating to both stomach and colon.

GASTROCOLIC REFLEX

Increased contraction of the colon induced by the entrance of food into the empty stomach. This is the reason why so many people have the urge to go to the toilet after eating.

GASTROCOTE
Brand name of a drug containing the following antacids as active compounds aluminum hydroxide, sodium bicarbonate, magnesium trisilicate, and alginic acid. The drug is prescribed for certain types of gastrointestinal disorders especially excess of stomach acid.

GASTRODUODENAL
Relating to both stomach and duodenum (the first part of the small intestine).

GASTRODUODENITIS
Inflammation of both the stomach and the duodenum (the first part of the small intestine).

GASTROENTERITIS
Acute inflammation or infection of the intestinal tract, usually characterized by vomiting and/or diarrhoea. The condition shows the following symptoms:
- sudden onset of abdominal pain or discomfort, which is usually mild to crampy;
- vomiting;
- nausea;
- diarrhea.
There may or may not be fever. Symptoms are usually more severe in infants and children.

The cause is usually thought to be due to a virus infection of the small intestine, and many viruses that cause this kind of illness have been identified. However, it may be seen with infections of other parts of the body - for example, urinary tract infection, bronchitis, middle ear infection.

Gastroenteritis usually involves both vomiting and diarrhea, although every person differs in how much of each is involved. When symptoms are particularly severe or persistent, other causes (such as bacillary dysentery or parasites) must be considered.

Treatment involves replacing the liquid and the chemical elements (principally sodium and potassium) lost through vomiting and diarrhea. This is particularly vital in the very young, as babies and small children can become rapidly dehydrated; in fact, it is not uncommon for them to need medical help and possibly hospitalization to restore their fluid balance. With the replacement of liquid and bedrest, most cases of gastroenteritis eventually settle down, although antibiotics may need to be taken if a bacterial cause is suspected. Hygiene, particularly around food, must be scrupulous.

GASTROENTEROSTOMY
Surgical operation to make a connection between the stomach and small intestine when the natural passage is blocked, in cases of severe ulcers or after partial or subtotal gastrectomy (removal of part of the stomach).

GASTROINTESTINAL ALLERGY
An uncommon symptom complex due to the eating or drinking of specific food or drug allergens, manifested by nausea, vomiting, crampy abdominal pain and diarrhea.

GASTROINTESTINAL TRACT
Also called the alimentary canal, the anatomical pathway involved in the digestive system. In humans, it starts at the throat, passing into the esophagus and stomach. From this arises the small intestine, consisting of the duodenum and the great length of the jejunum and ileum. This leads into the large intestine, or bowel, consisting of the cecum (from which the vermiform appendix arises), colon and rectum. The parts from the stomach to the latter part of the colon lie suspended on a double membrane called mesentery, through which they receive their

blood supply, and lie in loops within the peritoneal cavity of the abdomen. In each part, the shape, muscle layers and epithelium are specialized for their particular functions of secretion and absorption. Movement of food in the tract occurs largely by peristalsis, the automatic contraction and relaxation of muscular tissue that pushes the food along, but is controlled at key points by sphincters, specialized rings of muscle.

In gastroenteritis, enteritis and colitis, gut segments become inflamed. Peptic ulcer affects both the duodenum and stomach, while cancer of the esophagus, stomach, colon and rectum are relatively common. Disease of the small intestine tends to cause malabsorption of various nutrients. Methods of investigating the tract include gastrointestinal X-rays as well as endoscopy, in which a viewing tube is passed in via the mouth or anus to examine the lining of the gut.

GASTRO-(O)ESOPHAGEAL REFLUX

Regurgitation or back flow of gastric juice into the lower portion of the esophagus. This will cause a burning sensation - commonly called "heartburn" - in the chest just behind the breastbone. It is thought that the muscular sphincter at the lower end of the esophagus loses the ability to stay closed under pressure from the stomach's contents; this allows the acid to enter the esophagus and irritate the lining, which is insufficiently coated to protect itself from the acid's effect. If the burning symptoms - sometimes described as cramping, sharp pain or simply as pressure - are due to gastro-esophageal reflux, they seem to be aggravated by lying down and relieved by standing up, seem to be more frequent at night, and usually occur within an hour after a heavy meal. The condition is particularly common in pregnant women, when their unborn babies grow large enough to cause pressure on the stomach.

Proper medication may relieve the symptoms. Home treatment includes allowing the stomach and intestines to rest by avoiding solid food and irritating liquids. Water, diluted fruit juices, carbonated drinks and diluted punches in small amounts, given often, are usually tolerated. Bland foods in small amounts may also work well. Sleeping in a semi-upright position can also help.

If vomiting persists, or signs of dehydration occur, prompt medical help is required. Fluid may need to be given intravenously.

GASTROPATHY
Any disease or disorder of the stomach.

GASTROPLEGIA
Paralysis of the stomach.

GASTROPTOSIS
A sagging downwards of the stomach.

GASTRORRHAGIA
Hemorrhage into the stomach.

GASTRORRHEXIS
Rupture of the stomach.

GASTROSALIVARY REFLEX
Salivation produced by the introduction of food into the mouth or stomach, especially if it contains meat or articles with a tart taste.

GASTROSCOPE
A tube-like instrument for visual examination of the inside of the stomach.

GASTROSCOPY
Examination of the inside of the stomach by means of a gastroscope.

GASTROSTENOSIS
Stricture of the stomach.

GASTROSTOMY
An operation in which a hole made in the stomach is sewn to an opening in the abdominal skin. The person can then be fed through this opening instead of swallowing food.

GATE
A mechanism or device for controlling the passage of something (as a molecule through a membrane).

GATING
The process or mechanism by which the passage of something is controlled.

GATINAR
Brand name of a drug containing lactulose as the active ingredient. The medicine is used as a laxative to treat constipation.

GAUCHER'S DISEASE
A rare disorder of lipid metabolism that can run in families, resulting in an abnormal accumulation of fats and fat-like substances (lipids) in the liver and spleen, greatly enlarging them, as well as jaundice (a yellowish pigmentation of the skin), skeletal lesions and anemia. The disease is the result of the body's inability to produce the right enzymes to break down fats, and is incurable, although surgical removal of the spleen can relieve some of the symptoms.

GELATIN
Glutinous material obtained from animal tissues by boiling; especially a colloidal protein used as food, and in medicine.

GEL FILTRATION
Chromatography in which the material to be fractionated is separated primarily according to molecular size as it moves into a column of gel and is washed with a solvent so that the fractions appear successively at the end of the column.

GELSEMIUM
Homeopathic medicine derived from the root of yellow jasmine (Gelsemium sempervirens). It is used to treat mild prostration, weakness, torpor, drowsiness with trembling of hands and body, but it is primarily employed for the relief of migraine headaches. This medicine must be used with caution, as in large doses it is extremely poisonous.

GEMELLUS (pl. GEMELLI)
Either of two small muscles of the hip that insert into the tendon of the obturator internus.

GEMINATION
A doubling, duplication, or repetition; especially a formation of two teeth from a single tooth germ.

GENDER
A sex, male or female.

GENDER IDENTITY DISORDER
Disorder due to feelings of discomfort and inappropriateness about one's physical sex. When there is confusion in sex-labelling and rearing, children will become confused about their gender identity. However, even the presence of ambiguous genitalia will not affect the child's gender identity if sex-labelling and rearing are unambiguous. Some forms of gender identity disturbance are on a continuum, whereas others may be discrete. When gender identity disturbance is mild, the person is aware that he is a male or that she is a female, but discomfort and a sense of inappropriateness about the assigned sex are experienced. When severe, as in transsexualism, the person not only is uncomfortable with the assigned sex but has the sense of belonging to the opposite sex.

Disturbance in gender identity is rare, and should not be confused with the far more common phenomena of feelings of inadequacy in fulfilling the expectations associated with one's gender role.

An example of the latter would be a person who perceives himself or herself as being sexually unattractive yet experiences himself or herself unambiguously as a man or a woman in accordance with his or her assigned sex. Although people who first present clinically with gender identity problems may be of any age, in the vast majority of cases the onset of the disorder can be traced back to childhood. In rare cases, however, an adult will present clinically for the first time with a gender identity problem and report that the first signs of the disturbance were in adult life.

GENE
The smallest particle of hereditary information that is passed from parent to offspring. Genes consist of chain-like molecules of nucleic acids: DNA in most organisms and RNA in some viruses. The genes are normally located on the chromosomes found in the nucleus of each cell. The genetic information is coded by the sequences of the four bases present in nucleic acids, with a differing three-base code for each amino acid so that each gene contains the information for the synthesis of one protein chain.

GENEALOGY
In the medical sense, the investigation in genetics of the ancestral descent of an individual.

GENE COMPLEX
A group of genes of an individual or of a potentially interbreeding group that constitute an interacting functional unit.

GENE FLOW
The passage and establishment of genes typical of one breeding population into the gene pool of another by hybridization and backcrossing.

GENE FREQUENCY
Refers to the relative proportion of each of two or more alleles of a particular gene in a given population. The gene frequency may be expressed as a percentage or as a probability.

GENE POOL
The total amount of information present at any one time in the genes of the reproductive members of a biological population. The frequency of any particular gene in the gene pool changes owing to natural selection, mutation and genetic drift. This change forms the basis of evolutionary change.

GENERAL ABILITY
Used to describe a wide range of mental capacities; or, specifically, to describe a general factor affecting all mental operations or as equivalent to general intelligence, as tested by intelligence tests.

GENERAL ADAPTATION SYNDROME
Intense physical changes in various organ systems of the body, especially the endocrine system, as a result of stress. The sequence of bodily changes consists of the alarm reaction, resistance and exhaustion.

GENERAL ANESTHESIA
Anesthesia affecting the entire body and accompanied by loss of consciousness.

GENERAL APTITUDE
The aptitude for acquiring proficiency in many activities rather than in one special set of activities. An intelligence test is designed to measure general aptitude; a typing test is designed to measure special aptitude.

GENERAL CONSCIOUSNESS
Experiences shared by all members of a group.

GENERAL INTELLIGENCE
A basic intellectual factor that functions in the solution of all intellectual problems.

GENERALIZATION
(1) In concept-formation, problem-solving and transfer of training, the detection by the learner of a characteristic or principle common to a class of objects, events or problems. (2) In conditioning, the principle that once a conditioned response has been established to a given stimulus, other similar stimuli will also evoke that response.

GENERALIZED ANXIETY DISORDER
Unrealistic or excessive anxiety and worry about two or more life circumstances, e.g., worry about possible misfortune to one's child (who is in no danger) and worry about finances (for no good reason), for a considerable period (e.g., six months or longer), during which the person has been bothered by these concerns more days than not. In children and adolescents this may take the form of anxiety and worry about academic, athletic, and social performance. When the person is anxious, there are many signs of motor tension, autonomic hyperactivity, and vigilance and scanning.
Symptoms of motor tension are:
– trembling;
– twitching;
– feeling shaky;
– muscle tension;
– aches;
– soreness;
– restlessness;
– easy fatigability.
Symptoms of autonomic hyperactivity include:
– shortness of breath;
– smothering sensations;
– palpitations;
– accelerated heart rate;
– sweating;
– cold clammy hands;
– dry mouth;
– dizziness or lightheadedness;
– nausea;
– diarrhea;
– flushes or chills;
– frequent urination;
– trouble swallowing.
Symptoms of vigilance and scanning include:
– feeling keyed up or on edge;
– exaggerated startle response;
– difficulty concentrating;
– mind going blank because of anxiety;
– trouble falling or staying asleep;
– irritability.

GENERALIZED EXFOLIATIVE DERMATITIS
A severe, widespread inflammation (erythema) and scaling of the skin.

GENERAL PARESIS
Insanity caused by syphilitic alteration of the brain that leads to dementia and paralysis; also called dementia paralytica.

GENERAL PSYCHOLOGY
A systematic discussion of general principles and laws governing the mental life in general, as distinct from peculiarities characteristic of the individual.

GENERATION
The average period between the birth of an individual of a species and the beginning of reproduction; or the offspring of two parents.

GENERATOR POTENTIAL
A stationary depolarization of a receptor that occurs in response to a stimulus and is graded according to its intensity and that results in an action potential when the appropriate threshold is reached.

GENERIC NAME
Standard name accepted for a drug. Manufacturers often use their own trade names that correspond to generic names. The generic name is the official name for a single, thera-

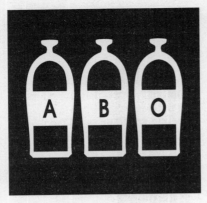

The blood groups A, B and O are genetically determined.

peutically active substance. It is distinct from a brand name or trade name, a term chosen by a manufacturer for a product containing a generic drug

GENERIC PATHWAYS
Description of general sequences that characterize multiple people or groups.

GENETIC CODE
The sequential order of the bases of DNA, which carry the genetic information.

GENETIC COUNSELOR
An advisor who is usually qualified in several medical specialties, such as internal medicine, pediatrics and genetics. The genetic counselor will compile a complete "family tree" of information about the genetic and general medical history of the patient and family. This history, together with appropriate laboratory tests, will help the genetic counselor predict the likelihood that genetic defects will occur in a family.

GENETIC DISEASE
Any disease or abnormality that results from inherited factors (genes).

GENETIC DISORDER SCREENING
Methods for the detection of heredi-

tary disorders and diseases. At the present time, nearly 3000 inherited diseases or traits (exhibited by carriers of genetic diseases who do not usually show signs of the disease) are known.

Many of these disorders reveal themselves as metabolic defects that interfere with normal body enzyme chemistry; they may also be the consequence of the lack of one or more enzymes necessary for the proper development or function of organs or tissues.

Genetic screening tests try to uncover individuals who have a greater than average risk of passing on inherited conditions.

Genetic screening may be performed on either parent-to-be prior to pregnancy; on the mother-to-be or on the fetus during pregnancy; and on the newborn infant before an inherited disorder can take effect.

In addition to genetic defects that are metabolic, abnormalities of the fetus can also come from hormonal disorders, infectious diseases, toxic drug influences and even certain kinds of malnutrition suffered by a mother during pregnancy.

GENETIC DRIFT
A process by which genetic information controlling certain features is lost from a population because it is not transmitted to the offspring. It only occurs in small isolated populations.

In large populations, any specific trait is carried by so many individuals that, unless it is unfavorable, its loss is highly unlikely. The almost total absence of blood group B in American Indians may be due to genetic drift.

GENETIC ENGINEERING
The production of new kinds of living organisms to meet human specifications. So far, only a few creatures have been manufactured in the laboratory by genetic-engineering techniques.

GENETICISM
The doctrine that behavior is inherited.

GENETIC MARKER
A readily recognizable gene that can be used to determine whether another gene is on the same chromosome.

GENETIC PSYCHOLOGY
That branch or type of psychology that studies mental phenomena and behavior by the genetic method, i.e. by investigating the origin and course of development of the various phenomena.

GENETICS
The science that studies inherited characteristics; the study of genes, their composition and function.

GENETIC SEQUENCES
The order in which structures or functions determined by genes appear in development.

GENICULATE BODY
Either of two prominences of the diencephalon that comprise the metathalamus.

GENICULATE GANGLION
A small reddish ganglion consisting of sensory and sympathetic nerve cells located at the sharp backward bend of the facial nerve.

GENICULATE HERPES
Another name for herpes zoster oticus.

GENIOGLOSSUS
A fan-shaped muscle that arises from the superior mental spine, inserting on the hyoid bone and into the tongue. The muscle serves to advance and retract and also to depress the tongue.

GENIOHYOID MUSCLE
A slender muscle that arises from the inferior mental spine on the in-

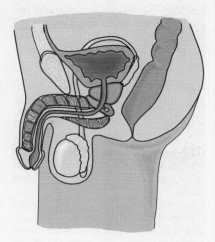

Cross section of the male genital organs. The prostate gland is located at the beginning of the penis, just below the bladder.

ner side of the symphysis of the lower jaw, inserted on the hyoid bone, and acts to raise the hyoid bone and draws it forward and to retract and depress the lower jaw.

GENITAL
Of, relating to, or being a sexual organ.

GENITAL CHARACTER
Hypothetical or ideal character displayed by a man who has been fully analyzed, who has fully resolved his Oedipus complex, who has worked through his pregenital ambivalence and achieved the post-ambivalent genital level of psychosexual development.

A genital character would, if such a person existed, be totally free of infantile dependence, and would be distinguishable by the fact that he attached equal importance to his own and his object's satisfaction - to attach more to his object's than his own would reveal him as a masochist. Although there is something absurd about the concept, which illustrates vividly the difficulties inherent in describing healthy phenomena in terms of a language rooted in psychopathology, it is a logical necessity for anyone who thinks that maturity should be definable in terms of instinct theory.

GENITAL EROTISM
Sexual excitement resulting from the stimulation of the genital organs.

GENITAL HERPES
Infection of the genital and adjacent skin area with the herpes simplex virus (type 2). It is now the commonest cause of genital ulceration. It is moderately contagious and usually spread by sexual contact. Blisters frequently develop four to seven days after contact, and the condition tends to relapse.

It is very painful, the initial attack lasting two to three weeks. Babies can be infected with the virus in the womb or during delivery, and are at high risk of congenital eye abnormalities or damage to the central nervous system. In addition, women who have contracted genital herpes are more likely to get cervical cancer.

Various vaccines and drugs have been developed to deal with genital herpes, but none of them is very effective, treatment relying mainly on the relief of symptoms. It is particularly important that those enduring an attack should abstain from sexual activity for at least a week after it is over, to prevent the spread of the disease.

GENITALITY
Term used in psychoanalytical theory to stress the importance of genital parameters in psychosexual development. While psychoanalysis has on occasion gone too far in its emphasis on genitality as a universal cure for society and thus provided a new addiction and a new commodity for many who wished to so interpret its teaching, it has not always indicated all the goals that genitality actually should and must imply.

GENITAL LEVEL
According to classical psychoanalytical theory, the last phase of libidinal development. After progressing through or up the pregenital stages of development and passing through the latency period, the individual reaches or achieves the genital level.

GENITAL ORGANS
Genitalia; the male or female reproductive organs, especially the external ones.

GENITAL PRIMACY STAGE
The final stage of psychosexual development during which the emphasis is on coition (sexual intercourse) and the pleasure is derived from the genital organs.

GENITAL STAGE
The final stage of sexual development in which a person has an affectionate relationship with a sex partner.

GENITAL WARTS
Also called venereal warts and condyloma acuminata: warts caused by a virus and usually transmitted sexually and often spread as the result of poor hygiene. They have an incubation period of from one to six months, and occur most commonly on warm, moist surfaces, such as the shaft of the penis in males, and the vulva, the vaginal wall, the cervix and the perineum (the area between the vagina and anus) in females.

Genital warts usually appear as soft, moist, minute, pink or red swellings that grow rapidly and become pedunculated (i.e., develop stalks). Several of them are usually found in the same area, often producing a cauliflower appearance. During pregnancy and in the presence of chronic discharge, they may grow more rapidly and spread.

Genital warts are treated by the careful application of a solution of podophyllum on alternate days until they disappear. A person with such warts should abstain from sex until two weeks after they have gone.

GENITOURINARY INFECTIONS

Infections of the genital and urinary systems of the body.

GENITOURINARY TRACT

The system of organ comprising those concerned with the production and excretion of urine and those concerned with reproduction.

GENIUS

The highest range of mental ability, either general, or in respect of special capacities of a creative order.

GENOCIDE

The use of calculated, systematic means to bring about the extermination of a racial or cultural group.

GENOME

All the genes found in a diploid set of chromosomes.

GENOTYPE

The total genetic make-up of a particular organism consisting of all the genes received from both parents. For any individual, the genotype determines their strengths and weaknesses during their whole life and is unique and constant for each individual. Duplication of the genotype is statistically impossible except in identical twins and in the simplest organisms.

GENTIAN VIOLET

Chemical used as an antiseptic for inflammatory skin reactions caused by bacteria, worms and fungi.

GENU VALGUM

Knock-knee; a condition in which the legs curve inward at the knees.

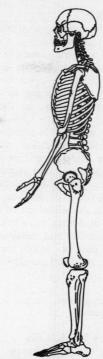

Genu varum and genu valgum are deviant position of the knee joint. The knee should be always in line with the hip joint and ankle joint.

GENU VARUM

Bow leg; a leg bowed outward at or below the knee.

GEOMEDICINE

A branch of medicine that deals with geographic factors in disease.

GEOPATHOLOGY

A science that deals with the relation of geographic factors to peculiarities of specific diseases.

GEOPHAGISM

The act or practice of eating earth, clay, chalk, etc.

GEOPHAGY

Practice of eating earthy substances (as clay) widespread among primitive and economically depressed peoples on a scanty or unbalanced diet.

GERIATRICS

The branch of medicine specializing in the care of the elderly. Although concerned with the same diseases as the rest of medicine, the different susceptibility of the aged and a tendency for these people to have a number of disorders at the same time make its scope different. In particular the psychological problems of old age differ markedly from those encountered in the rest of the population and require special management. The social and medical aspects of long-term care involve the coordination of family, voluntary and hospital services, but the individuality and freedom of the geriatric patient must be safeguarded as much as possible.

GERM

A microorganism, esp. one that causes disease.

GERMAN MEASLES

A contagious viral disease characterized by fever, mild symptoms of upper respiratory infection, and a diffuse fine red rash lasting for short period, usually three or four days.

GERMINAL CENTERS

A collection of metabolically active lymphoblasts, macrophages and plasma cells that appears within the primary follicle of lymphoid tissues following stimulation by antigens (foreign substances); part of the immune system.

GERMINATIVE LAYER

The innermost layer of the epidermis from which new tissue is constantly formed.

GERM PLASMA

(1) Germ cells and their precursors serving as the bearers of heredity and being fundamentally independent of other cells.
(2) The hereditary material of the germ cells.

GERONTOLOGY

The scientific investigation of old age or of the aging processes.

GERONTOTHERAPY

Treatment to improve the health of older persons.

GERSTMANN'S SYNDROME

Cerebral dysfunction characterized especially by finger agnosia, disorientation with respect to right and left, agraphia, and acalculia and caused by a lesion in the dominant cerebral hemisphere involving the angular gyrus and adjoining occipital gyri.

GESTALT

Form, pattern or configuration; an integrated whole, more than the sum of its parts; gives its name to the type of psychology known as Gestalt psychology.

GESTALT PSYCHOLOGY

A school of psychology concerned with the tendency of the human (or even primate) mind to organize perceptions into 'wholes' -for example, to hear a symphony rather than a large number of separate notes of different tones.

Gestalt psychology, whose main proponents were Max Wertheimer, Kurt Koffka and Wolfgang Koehler, maintained that this was due to the mind's ability to complete patterns from the available stimuli.

The school emerged as a reaction against such disciplines as behaviorism.

GESTATION

The development of young mammals in the mother's uterus from fertilization to birth.

With some exceptions, the gestation period is proportional to the adult size of the animal: thus, for human young the gestation period is about 270 days, but for those of the elephant it is closer to two years.

GESTATIONAL PSYCHOSIS
A psychosis arising during pregnancy.

GESTATION PERIOD
The length of time during which gestation takes place.

GESTOSIS
Any disorder of pregnancy, especially toxemia of pregnancy.

GESTURE
Expressive movement, usually of head or hands, for the purpose of communication, but also frequently accompanying the individual's own train of thought; it may become systematized into a gesture language, more or less conventionalized, as among deaf-mutes.

GHOST
A structure that does not stain normally because of degenerative changes; specifically a red blood cell that has lost its hemoglobin.

GHOST SURGERY
The practice of performing surgery on another physician;s patient by arrangement with the physician but unknown to the patient.

GIANT CELL ARTERITIS
Another name for temporal arteritis.

GIANT-CELL TUMOR
An osteolytic tumor affecting the metaphyses and epiphyses of long bones, composed of a stroma of spindle cells containing dispersed multinucleate giant cells, and usually benign but sometimes malignant.

GIANT HYPERTROPHIC GASTRITIS
A rare stomach disorder characterized by the lining developing huge convoluted folds and wrinkles covered in nodes and often polyps in part of or throughout the entire fundus and body of the stomach.

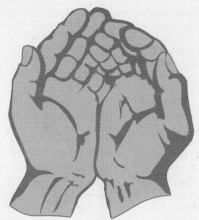

With the hand we can express a large number of gestures.

GIARDIASIS
Intestinal infection with a parasitic protozoan organism (Giardia lamblia). Although an infection may be completely without symptoms, many people with this problem (most often young children) have intestinal symptoms of abdominal pain and bloating nausea, lack of appetite, diarrhea, general listlessness and feeling poorly. Diarrhea may last for a short time or become chronic. Malabsorption of food occurs in some people and can lead to weight loss and malnutrition.

The protozoa reside and multiply in the duodenum, the first part of the small intestine. The parasite can be found either as the live protozoan stage or as the dormant cyst stage.

Although most people get this infection from contaminated water, either from a city water supply or untreated water in recreation areas, it can be passed from person to person by direct contact. It passes through households and nursery schools quickly and has been transmitted by sexual contact. The organism is found in all areas of the world and in all climates, and is one of the most common of all the intestinal parasites.

Once diagnosed, the infection can

be treated with several medications, including quinacrine.

GIBRALTAR FEVER
Another name for brucellosis.

GIDDINESS
A sensation of rolling or unsteadiness that may be due to anxiety, anemia or general debility.

GIEMSA'S STAIN
A solution for staining microorganisms, such as protozoa, rickettsiae and viral inclusion bodies, to make them detectable in laboratory samples.

GIGANTISM
A condition of abnormal size and height caused by overproduction of the growth hormone secreted by the anterior lobe of the pituitary gland.

GILBERT'S DISEASE
A metabolic disorder probably inherited as an autosomal dominant with variable penetrance and characterized by elevated levels of mostly unconjugated serum bilirubin caused by defective uptake of bilirubin by the liver.

GILLES DE LA TOURETTE SYNDROME
Single or multiple tics (facial blinking, grimaces, shoulder shrugging, arm movements) that may gradually worsen in extent and severity. Vocal tics such as grunting, sniffing, shouting and barking noises develop. The cause is unknown. Most sufferers respond to psychoactive drugs.

GINGER
(Zingiber officinale) Perennial plant of which the rootstock is used for medicinal purposes. The aromatic, knotty rootstock is thick, fibrous and whitish or buff-colored. Ginger tea, taken hot, or tincture promotes cleansing of the system through perspiration and is also said to be useful for suppressed menstruation.

GINGIVITIS
Inflammation of the gums. Major symptoms include: swelling and redness, tenderness of the gums at the base of the teeth. There may be bleeding with toothbrushing and later with chewing. Increasing swelling and inflammation lead to loosening of the teeth and periodontitis.

In most cases the gums are irritated by hard plaque that has been allowed to settle in the space between tooth and gum. Lack of good tooth cleaning allows the problem to worsen. As inflammation and swelling increase, infection settles in. Prompt care by a dentist to clean the plaque from the teeth is the best treatment. Afterwards, vigorous toothbrushing is important to keep the inflammation under control. Regular dental care is good prevention.

GINSENG
(Panax schin-seng) A small perennial plant that grows in damp woodlands in Korea. Other ginseng-varieties such as the American ginseng (Panax quinquefolius), grow elsewhere in the world, but for medicinal purposes, mostly Korean ginseng is used. As a demulcent, it is helpful for coughs, colds and various chest problems. The root is collected after flowering. Only the thoroughly dried root should be used. The best way is to make it into a tea according to one's own taste.

GLANDS
Specialized structures that secrete essential substances. They are divided into endocrine glands, which secrete hormones into the bloodstream, and exocrine glands, which are the remainder, usually secreting materials via ducts into internal organs or on to body surfaces. Lymph nodes are also sometimes termed glands.

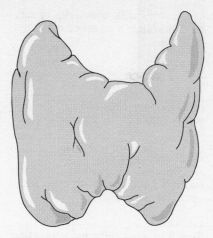

Shape of outer morphology of the thyroid gland.

In humans, there are many different exocrine glands. The skin contains two types: sweat glands, which secrete watery fluid (perspiration), and sebaceous glands, which secrete sebum. Lacrimal glands secrete tears. The cells of mucous membranes and the epithelium (lining) of internal organs secrete mucus, which serves to lubricate and protect the surface. Salivary glands (parotid, submandibular and sublingual) secrete saliva to facilitate swallowing. In the gastrointestinal tract, mucus-secreting glands are numerous, particularly in the stomach and colon, where solid food and, later, feces need lubrication. Other stomach glands secrete hydrochloric acid and pepsin as part of the digestive system. The juices of the small intestine that contain enzymes are similarly secreted by minute glandular specializations of the epithelium. The part of the pancreas secreting enzyme-rich juice into the duodenum may be regarded as an exocrine gland.

There are also a number of hormone-producing endocrine glands: the thyroid and parathyroid glands in the neck; the pituitary gland in the brain; the adrenal glands on top of each kidney; part of the pancreas; and the ovaries in females and the testes in males. The secretions of these, passed directly into the bloodstream, act on many parts of the body.

Analysis of exocrine gland secretion may be helpful in diseases of digestion, of the eyes and salivary glands and in cystic fibrosis. That of endocrine secretion is useful in a multitude of different conditions.

GLANDULAR FEVER
Common name for infectious mononucleosis.

GLANDULAR RESPONSE
One of the two classes of response of an organism to stimulation from within or without, in the change of the secretory activity of glands, the other being muscular response.

GLAUBER'S SALTS
Trade name of a drug containing sodium sulphate as the active ingredient. It is used as a saline laxative in the treatment of constipation.

GLAUCOMA
A group of eye diseases characterized by an increased pressure within the eye, causing damage to the optic disc (where the optic nerve emerges into the eye) and typical visual field defects. The acute form shows a sudden onset of increased pressure, while the chronic form is characterized by a consistent elevation of pressure inside the eyes, starting and developing gradually over a period of years. Glaucoma shows a tendency to run in families, and affects one in every 50 people over the age of 40.

In the acute condition, there is sudden and severe pain in the eye, with blurred vision. The eye is intensely red and the pupil dilated. The cause is a sudden blockage between the posterior and anterior chambers on either side of the iris, through which a watery fluid -aqueous humor - normally flows; this causes a sudden, severe increase in the pressure inside the eye. In order for acute glaucoma to occur, the anterior chamber of the eye must be narrower than normal.

The acute condition requires immediate treatment by using drugs that cause the pupil to become smaller and the pressure to go down. Surgery to remove part of the iris of the eye is done within a few days. If the pressure is reduced promptly, the risk of permanent visual damage is reduced.

In the chronic type of glaucoma, there are initially no symptoms. Then there is a gradual loss of peripheral vision (the ability to see around the sides and top), but with preservation of central vision. This condition leads gradually to what is known as tunnel vision, and this can progress to complete blindness over 10 to 30 years if not treated. The cause of this disorder is not known.

The treatment consists of eye medications to keep the pupils of the eye small and to increase the drainage of the fluid that is formed in the eye. Because of the lack of initial symptoms in chronic glaucoma, all those over the age of 40 should have their eyes checked on a regular basis.

GLEET
Chronic inflammation of the urethra, the tube carrying the urine from the bladder to the outside; a chronic form of gonorrhea.

GLENOID
Having a smooth shallow depressed form; used chiefly of skeletal articulatory sockets.

GLENOID CAVITY
The shallow cavity of the upper part of the scapula by which the humerus articulates with the pectoral girdle.

GLENOID FOSSA
The depression in each lateral wall of the skull with which the mandible articulates; also called mandibular fossa.

GLIA
Tissue that composes part of the central nervous system, consisting of supporting cells and cellular elements essential for metabolic processes.

GLIDING JOINT
A diarthrosis in which the articular surfaces glide upon each other without axial motion.

GLIOMA
Tumor of glial cells, the supporting cells of the brain and spinal cord. They never metastasize (spread), but produce signs of local damage to the brain, such as weakness, visual disturbance, personality change or epilepsy and often a characteristic type of headache. Surgery and radiation therapy may be helpful, but glial cell destruction cannot be reversed.

GLISSON'S CAPSULE
An investment of loose connective tissue entering the liver with the portal vessels and sheathing the larger vessels in their course through the organ.

GLOBULINS
Proteins insoluble in water but soluble in dilute solutions of mineral salts. They are widely distributed in plants and animals - e.g., lactoglobulin in milk and plant globulin in seeds. In humans, serum globulins are concerned in resistance to disease and in various allergies.

GLOBUS HYSTERICUS
The subjective sense of a lump in the throat occurring in absence of any palpable lump.

GLOBUS SENSATION
The subjective sensation of a lump or mass in the throat. No specific

cause or physical mechanism has been established.

GLOMERULONEPHRITIS
Acute or chronic inflammation of the glomeruli in the kidneys, caused by a streptococcal infection.

GLOMERULUS
A coil of minute blood vessels in the kidney, which passes waste fluid to the cup-shaped uriniferous tubule. A normal kidney contains about one million glomeruli.

GLOMUS
A small arteriovenous anastomosis together with its supporting structures.

GLOMUS CAROTICUM
A small body of vascular tissue that adjoins the carotid sinus. It functions as a chemoreceptor sensitive to change in the oxygen content of blood, and mediates reflex changes in respiratory activity.

GLOMUS COCCYGEUM
A small mass of vascular tissue situated near the tip of the coccyx.

GLOMUS JUGULARE
A small mass of chemoreceptors in the adventitia of the dilation in the internal jugular vein where it arises from the transverse sinus in the jugular foramen.

GLOMUS TUMOR
A painful benign tumor that develops by hypertrophy of a glomus.

GLOSSA
The tongue; *glossal*: relating to the tongue.

GLOSSECTOMY
Removal of the tongue.

GLOSSITIS
Inflammation of the tongue, usually a complication of anemia and malnutrition.

GLOSSOLALIA
"Speaking in tongues": speech in an unknown or fabricated language uttered by individuals under hypnosis, suffering from certain mental illnesses or in trance, or by groups undergoing religious ecstasy.

GLOSSOPHARYNGEAL NERVE
A mixed nerve that is either of the 9th pair of cranial nerves, that has sensory fibers arising from the superior and petrosal ganglia and motor fibers arising with those of the vagus nerve from the lateral wall of the medulla, and that supplies chiefly the pharynx, posterior tongue, and parotid gland with motor and sensory fibers including gustatory and autonomic secretory and vasodilator fibers.

GLOSSOSPASM
A spasm of the tongue consisting of an inward-outward movement, lasting several minutes.

GLOTTIS
Narrow opening at the upper end of the larynx; the gap between the vocal cords.

GLUCAGON
Hormone produced by the pancreas. It converts protein and fat molecules into blood sugars to be used as energy, and also causes insulin to be released into the body. Glucagon is sometimes injected to help diagnose excess glycogen (glucose stored mainly in the liver). Glucagon values are greatly increased with tumor of the pancreas, uncontrolled diabetes and inadequate amounts of insulin. On occasion, glucagon is decreased with certain forms of hypoglycemia (low blood sugar).

GLUCOCORTICOID
Any of a group of corticoids (as hydrocortisone or dexamethasone) that are involved especially in car-

bohydrate, protein, and fat metabolism, and that tend to increase liver glycogen and blood sugar by increasing glyconeogenesis, and that are anti-inflammatory. The glucocorticoids are used widely in medicine (as in the alleviation of the symptoms of rheumatoid arthritis).

GLUCONEOGENESIS
Formation of glucose within the body especially by the liver from substances (as fats and proteins) other than carbohydrates.

GLUCOSE
A monosaccharide (simple sugar), also known as dextrose (a grape sugar), found in certain foodstuffs, especially fruits. It is the end product of carbohydrate metabolism, and is the chief source of energy for living organisms, its utilization being controlled by insulin. Excess glucose is converted into glycogen and stored in the liver and muscles for use as needed; beyond that, it is converted to fat and stored in the fat cells of adipose tissue.

The level of glucose can be measured as the amount of glucose floating in the blood or excreted by the kidneys. Such a test is really a measure of how well the body handles carbohydrate metabolism, the breakdown of starches such as vegetables as well as all the various sugar products in the foods we eat.

A uniform blood glucose level is generally maintained in the body through insulin secretion (which decreases it), despite variations due to dietary increase in sugar and energy expenditure.

For the test, blood is taken from a vein to assess the level of glucose in the serum; glucose in whole blood, plasma, urine or spinal fluid may also be tested.

GLUCOSE-GALACTOSE MALABSORPTION
Another name for carbohydrate intolerance.

GLUCOSE 6-PHOSPHATE DEHYDROGENASE
An enzyme normally found in red blood cells. In people with a deficiency of this enzyme (an inherited condition), red blood cells are no longer protected from oxidation, causing hemolysis (destruction of red blood cells and subsequent separation of hemoglobin), which can lead to severe anemia.

Deficiency in this enzyme, while not usually serious or chronic, can at times be fatal. It does not show itself until the person takes drugs or food that precipitate the hemolytic anemia.

GLUCOSE TOLERANCE TEST
Method to investigate how well a person's body uses glucose as well as the working mechanism of insulin; it is particularly used for those who have, or are suspected of having, diabetes. In preparing for this test, the person eats his or her usual amount of carbohydrate for several days. Then he/she fasts for 8 to 12 hours prior to the test. First, a fasting blood glucose and urine glucose are measured. Then the person is given 100 g (3½ oz) of glucose in water or squash to drink. Thirty minutes afterwards both the blood and urine are again examined for sugar levels. (Glucose testing after eating is called postprandial.) Every hour thereafter for the next five hours, urine and blood samples are taken to determine how long it takes the body to metabolize the 100 g of glucose. Fasting blood glucose levels normally range from 80 to 120 mg per 200 ml of blood serum, 60 to 100 mg per 100 ml of whole blood. Postprandial levels should not exceed 180 mg per 100 ml of whole blood.

During the entire five to six hours of the glucose tolerance test, the peak should remain below 180 mg per 100 ml, and after two hours, the levels should return to the same as for fasting.

GLUE-SNIFFING
Common name for inhalant abuse. Glue-sniffing is the deliberate inhalation of volatile organic solvents from plastic glues that may result in symptoms ranging from mild euphoria to disorientation and coma.

GLUTAMIC ACID
An amino acid, one of the group that the body manufactures. The richest natural sources are wholegrain wheat and milk. Glutamic acid is also available in tablets but only as a digestive aid. It is sometimes used in the treatment of epilepsy.

GLUTAMIC OXALACETIC TRANSAMINASE
Enzyme, primarily present in heart and liver, involved in amino acid metabolism. The enzyme is unique in that it is released into the blood when there is heart muscle damage and liver cell destruction. The level of this enzyme is elevated following a heart attack.

GLUTAMINASE
An enzyme that hydrolyzes glutamine to glutamic acid and ammonia.

GLUTATHIONE
An enzyme, a deficiency of which may lead to hemolytic anemia. Glutathione is a peptide that contains one amino acid residue each of glutamic acid, cysteine, and glycine, that occurs widely in plant and animal tissues, and that plays an important role in biological oxidation-reduction processes and as a coenzyme.

GLUTEAL
Relating to the buttocks.

GLUTEAL ARTERY
Either of two branches of the internal iliac artery that supply the gluteal region. The largest branch of the internal iliac artery that sends branches to the gluteal muscles is called superior gluteal artery. A branch that is distributed to the buttocks and backs of the thighs is called the inferior gluteal artery.

GLUTEAL NERVE
Either of two nerves arising from the sacral plexus and supplying the gluteal muscles and adjacent parts. One nerve arising from the first sacral nerve and distributed to the gluteus muscles and to the tensor fasciae latae is called superior gluteal nerve. Another nerve arising from the posterior part of the fifth lumbar nerve and from the first and second sacral nerves and distributed to the gluteus maximus is called inferior gluteal nerve.

GLUTEAL TUBEROSITY
The lateral ridge of the linea aspera of the femur that gives attachment to the gluteus maximus.

GLUTEI
The large muscles that form the buttocks.

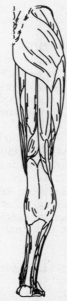

The gluteal muscles are part of the buttocks.

GLUTEN

A mixture of two proteins (gliadin and glutenin) found in wheat, rye and other cereal flours. In the rising of bread, gluten forms an elastic network that traps carbon dioxide, giving a desirable crumb structure on baking. The proportion of gluten in wheat flour varies from 8 to 15 percent, the level determining the suitability of the flour for different uses. The high gluten content of hard wheat is right for bread and pasta, while soft wheat (low gluten) is used for biscuits and cakes.

An intolerance to gluten is likely to be the cause of celiac disease, a condition in which chronic diarrhea can lead to malnutrition. A gluten-free diet is required.

GLUTEN ENTEROPATHY

Another name for celiac disease.

GLUTEUS MAXIMUS

The outermost muscle of three muscles found in each of the buttocks that arises from the sacrum, coccyx, back part of the ilium and adjacent structures that is inserted into the fascia lata of the thigh and the gluteal tuberosity of the femur.

GLUTEUS MEDIUS

The middle muscle of the three muscles found in each of the human buttocks that arises from the outer surface of the ilium and that is inserted into the greater trochanter of the femur.

GLUTEUS MINIMUS

The innermost muscle of the three muscles found in each of the buttocks that arises from the outer surface of the ilium and that is inserted into the greater trochanter of the femur.

GLYCERIN

Another name for glycerol.

GLYCEROL

Also called glycerin: a colorless, viscous liquid with a sweet taste; a trihydric alcohol.

Its fatty-acid esters constitute natural fats and oils, from which glycerol is obtained as a byproduct of soap manufacture; it is also synthesized from propylene, a petroleum product. It is used to reduce inflammation, as a mouthwash and throat spray and to prevent skin chapping.

GLYCOGEN

Animal starch made up of glucose molecules. Glycogen is the form in which glucose is stored in the body, primarily in the liver and muscles, and is called into use to replenish the glucose levels in the body as the glucose is burned to provide energy. This replenishing process is controlled in the main by the hormones secreted by part of the pancreas: glucagon inhibits its use and insulin increases it.

GLYCOGENESIS

Any of several metabolic disorders that are characterized by hypoglycemia and abnormal deposits of glycogen and are caused by enzyme deficiencies in glycogen metabolism.

GLYCOGEN STORAGE DISEASES

A group of hereditary disorders caused by lack of a specific enzyme involved in glycogen synthesis or breakdown, and characterized by the deposition of abnormal amounts or types of glycogen in the tissues.

GLYCOHEMOGLOBIN

Hemoglobin in combination with glucose molecules. The greater the amount of glucose in the blood, the greater the percentage of glycosylated hemoglobin.

The amount of glycohemoglobin in the blood is determined in those with diabetes to ascertain that their blood sugar level is properly controlled.

GLYCOL SALICYLATE
A counter-irritant drug that is applied to the skin to produce dilatation of blood vessels, causing redness and warmth. This reaction is used to bring relief from deep--seated pain in cases of rheumatic diseases.

GLYCOLYSIS
The enzymatic breakdown of a carbohydrate (as glucose of glycogen) by way of phosphate derivatives with the production of pyruvic or lactic acid and energy stored in high-energy phosphate bonds of ATP.

GLYCOSIDE
Any of numerous sugar derivatives that contain a nonsugar group attached through an oxygen or nitrogen bond and that on hydrolysis yield a sugar (as glucose).

GNOTOBIOTICS
Term used to describe laboratory organisms that are either free of all known contaminating organisms (e.g. bacteria, fungi, yeasts) - and thus are "germ-free" - or germ-free organisms specifically contaminated with a known organism. Animals that are not contaminated with specific organisms (but otherwise normal), the so-called "specific pathogen free" (SPF) animals, are not gnotobiotic. SPF and gnotobiotic animals are widely used in medical research.

GOITER
Enlargement of the thyroid gland that is commonly visible as a swelling of the anterior part of the neck, and that often results from insufficient intake of iodine and then is usually accompanied by hypothyroidism and that in other cases is associated with hyperthyroidism usually together with toxic symptoms and exophthalmos.

GOITRE
See Goiter

GOLD
Chemical element, atomic number 79, symbol Au. Gold compounds (all of which are poisonous) are used in medicine, chiefly in the treatment of rheumatoid arthritis. Possible side effects include:
- skin rashes;
- blood disorders;
- intestinal disorders;
- stomach discomfort;
- sensitivity of the skin to sunlight.
It should be used with caution by pregnant women, and not at all by those with impaired liver or kidney function or blood or skin disorders.

GOLD COMPOUNDS
Medicines which use gold as their base and are usually used to treat joint or arthritic disorders. These medicines include aurothioglucose, gold sodium thiomalate, auranofin.

GOLGI APPARATUS
A cytoplasmic organelle that appears in electron microscopy as a series of parallel, sometimes vesicular, membranes without ribosomes and is probably active in cellular secretion.

GOLGI TENDON ORGAN
A spindle-shaped sensory end organ within a tendon that provides information about muscle tension.

GONADOTRAPHON
Brand name for chorionic gonadotrophin prescribed for certain cases of infertility.

GONADOTROPIC
Stimulating the function of the sex organs.

GONADOTROPIC HORMONE (GONADOTROPIN)
A hormone secreted by the pituitary gland that stimulates the growth and development of the sperm and eggs

in the gonads and causes the secretion of the hormones androgen and estrogen.

GONADOTROPIN- RELEAS-ING HORMONE

Hormone produced by the hypothalamus that stimulates secretion of gonadotropins by the anterior part of the pituitary gland.

GONADS

The reproductive organs of animals, which produce gametes (reproductive cells). The female gonad is the ovary, producing eggs (ova), and the male gonad the testis, producing spermatozoa.

GONIOPUNCTURE

A surgical operation for congenital glaucoma that involves making a puncture into the sclera with a knife at the site of discharge of aqueous fluid at the periphery of the anterior chamber of the eye.

GONIOSCOPE

An instrument consisting of a contact lens to be fitted over the cornea and an optical system with which the interior of the eye can be viewed.

GONIOTOMY

Surgical relief of glaucoma used in some congenital types and achieved by opening the canal of Schlemm.

GONOCOCCAL

Relating to the gonococcus.

GONOCOCCUS

Also called Neisseria gonorrhea: the bacterium responsible for gonorrhea.

GONORRHEA

Common venereal disease caused by the bacterium Neisseria gonorrhoea and transmitted through contact with an infected person or with secretions containing the bacteria.

Symptoms include:
- painful urination and burning;
- itching and pain around the urethra;
- greenish-yellow and pus-containing discharge.

If untreated the infection spreads, especially in women, infecting the reproductive organs, causing inflammation of the liver, and, if widespread, leading to septicemia and polyarthritis, with painful lesions in joints and tendons and infection of the conjunctiva of the eye that can lead to blindness. Treatment is by antibiotics.

GOODPASTURE'S SYNDROME

An uncommon hypersensitivity disorder of unknown cause manifested by hemorrhage in the lungs with associated severe and progressive glomerulonephritis, and characterized by circulating antibodies and by the depositing of immunoglobulin in the kidneys.

GOOSEFLESH

Skin marked by the prominent appearance of the hair follicles, which stand up as the result of a stimulus to a minute muscle called the erector pilli. Spasm of this muscle is usually a sequel to cold, but sometimes to fright.

GOUT

Disease in which a defect in uric acid metabolism causes the acid and its salts to accumulate in the blood and joints, causing pain and swelling of the joints (especially the big toe area), accompanied by fever and chills. The disease is more common among men than women and usually has a genetic basis. Treatment includes a diet And the use of drugs.

GRAAFIAN FOLLICLE

A liquid-filled cavity in an ovary containing a mature egg before ovulation.

GRACILIS
The most superficial muscle of the inside of the thigh arising from the lower part of the pubic symphysis and the anterior half of the pubic arch and having its tendon inserted into the inner surface of the shaft of the tibia below the tuberosity.

GRAFT
Skin, muscle, bone, nerve or other tissue taken from a living organism and employed to replace a defect in a corresponding structure.

GRAFT REACTION
The immunological reaction between the graft recipient and antigens present in the graft which results in the destruction of the tissue of the graft.

GRAFT-VERSUS-HOST REACTION
Reaction of a graft containing immunologically competent lymphocytic cells against antigens in the tissues of a graft recipient whose immune system is defective or has been reduced by radiation treatment or immunosuppressive drugs.

GRAINS
Edible grasses, including wheat, rice, oats, millet, maize, buckwheat and rye.

All grains are rich sources of carbohydrates and most are high in protein as well, if their nutritious elements have not been refined away.

Whole-grain cereals have not had their husks removed by milling and are excellent sources of protein, B vitamins and other nutrients. All whole-grain products must be treated as perishables.

GRAM-NEGATIVE MICROORGANISMS
Those that do not retain the violet dye used in the Gram stain method, and take the color of the counterstain.

GRAM-POSITIVE MICROORGANISMS
Those that retain the violet dye used in the Gram stain method, and do not accept the counterstain.

GRAM'S STAIN
Test for the distinguishing of various types of bacteria, developed by Dr H. C. J. Gram in 1884. Gram-negative means that when a microorganism is stained with a dye such as gentian violet that is then fixed with iodine, it loses the stain or becomes decolorized by alcohol, a primary characteristic of bacteria having a cell-wall surface more complex in chemical composition than the Gram-positive bacteria. The latter types of bacteria retain the stain or resist decolorization by alcohol. Sputum, joint fluid, urine, sinus discharge, urethral discharge, vaginal fluid and exudates from infections can all be examined in this manner under the microscope.

The test is used primarily to evaluate and distinguish infectious microorganisms in various body fluids and to aid in the precise choice of therapy. Certain antibiotics are effective only against Gram-positive microorganisms, while other antibiotics are effective only against Gram-negative ones.

GRANDIOSE
Characterized by affection of grandeur or splendor or by absurd exaggeration.

GRAND MAL
Major form of epileptic seizure; the person usually cries out and then falls to the ground unconscious.

GRAND MULTIPARA
A woman who has given birth seven or more times.

GRANULAR LAYER
The deeper layer of the cortex of the cerebellum containing numerous small closely packed cells.

GRANULATION TISSUE
The bright red, granular tissue that develops during the healing of a wound. The tissue consists initially of fine blood vessels and therefore bleeds easily. Later, fibrous tissue is laid down and a scar replaces the granulation tissue.

GRANULE CELL
One of the small neurons of the cortex of the cerebellum and cerebrum.

GRANULOCYTE
Also called polymorphonuclear leukocyte or polymorph: 70 percent of all white blood cells comprise the granulocytes, which have small granules scattered throughout them and segmented nuclei.

There are three different types, all of which become stained when dyed:
(1) neutrophils, the most common and the most faintly staining;
(2) eosinophils, the granules of which become red when exposed to the acidic dye eosin;
(3) basophils, with granules that become blue when stained with methylene blue dye.

Granulocytes destroy bacteria and other invaders such as parasites and allergens.

They respond quickly to any infection, and because they are easily counted, an increase in their number usually points to the diagnosis of an acute infection.

GRANULOCYTOPENIA
An acute or chronic reduction in the granulocytes found in the blood, resulting in increased susceptibility to bacterial infection in proportion to the severity and duration of the condition.

GRANULOMA
Tumor formed of granulation tissue. One form of granuloma is the so-called "proud flesh" that develops in a surface ulcer. They are caused by chronic infection, and can occur in tuberculosis and syphilis.

GRANULOMA INGUINALE
Venereal disease characterized by large areas of swollen, red, meaty skin around the genitals.

The disease is diagnosed by the discovery of bacteria, called Donovan bodies, in tissue scrapings from the infected area, and is more common in tropical areas. The treatment is the giving of tetracycline, four times a day for 10 to 15 days.

GRANULOMATOSIS ILEITIS
Another name for regional enteritis.

GRANULOMATOUS ARTERITIS
Another name for temporal arteritis.

GRAPHOKINESTHETIC
Relating to the motor sensations involved in writing.

GRAPHOLOGY
The study of handwriting, particularly the deduction, from its form, of information about the character of the writer.

GRAPHOMANIA
An obsessive urge to write, indicative of some abnormality or some mental disorder and, in the latter case, usually resulting in confused, irrational and rambling statements or, in extreme cases, in a mere meaningless succession of written, sometimes nonsense words.

GRAPHOPATHOLOGY
The scientific investigation of changes in, and other characteristics of, handwriting, indicative of physical or mental abnormality or disorder.

GRASPING REFLEX
Response by fingers or toes to an object brought into contact with them by which the object is held, characteristic of human infants at an early stage.

GRAVES' DISEASE

Another name for toxic goiter, a disease of the thyroid gland.

GRAVIDA

A pregnant woman.

GRAY COMMISSURE

A transverse band of gray matter in the spinal cord appearing in sections as the transverse bar of the H-shaped mass of gray matter.

GRAY MATTER

Neural tissue especially of the brain and spinal cord that contains cell bodies as well as nerve fibers, having a brownish gray color, and forming most of the cortex and nuclei of the brain, the columns of the spinal cord, and the bodies of ganglia.

GRAY SYNDROME

A potentially fatal toxic reaction to chloramphenicol especially in premature infants that is characterized by:
- abdominal distension;
- cyanosis;
- vasomotor collapse;
- irregular respiration.

GREATER CEREBRAL VEIN

A broad unpaired vein formed by the junction of Galen's veins and uniting with the inferior sagittal sinus to form the straight sinus.

GREATER CURVATURE

The boundary of the stomach that in man forms a long convex curve on the left from the opening for the esophagus to the opening into the duodenum.

GREATER OMENTUM

A part of the peritoneum attached to the greater curvature of the stomach and to the colon and hanging down over the small intestine.

GREATER TUBERCLE

A prominence on the upper lateral

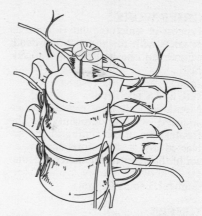

In the gray matter the spinal motoneurons are located from which the peripheral motor nerves originate.

part of the end of the humerus that serves as the insertion for the supraspinatus, infraspinatus, and teres minor muscles.

GREENSTICK FRACTURE

Common name for an incomplete fracture where the bone is not completely broken. These are common in children, whose bones are still made up of a proportion of cartilage and therefore are not as hard and brittle as those of adults.

GREEN STOOLS

Stools seen in babies when the contents of the intestine are rushed through before the bile has been digested, so that they emerge as green instead of the normal yellow-brown. However, unless the baby has lost its appetite, has a fever and seems to be failing to thrive, green stools are not a cause for concern.

GREW INDURATION

Diffuse fibrosis of the lung found in chronic pneumonia.

GRIEF

An emotional attitude or a complex emotion, more or less synonymous with sorrow, as generally used, but usually implying greater intensity and more specific reference.

GRIEF WORK
Process in which the individual tries to cope with reactions to the death of a loved one and attempts to adjust.

GRIEG'S DISEASE
Mental and physical retardation associated with a deformity of the frontal area of the skull and characterized by a low forehead, wide bridge of the nose, increased distance between the eyes and divergent strabismus (squint).

GRIPPE
Another name for influenza.

GROSS ANATOMY
A branch of anatomy that deals with the macroscopic structure of tissues and organs.

GROUP
(1) A number of individuals assembled together or having some unifying relationship.
(2) an assemblage of related organisms.

GROUP ANALYSIS
Group psychotherapy in which the therapist restricts his/her activities to interpretation of the dynamics of the group.

GROUP BEHAVIOR
Behavior characteristics of a social group as such, or of an individual as a member of a social group.

GROUP DYNAMICS
The interacting force within a small human group. The term is also used to designate the sociological study of these forces.

GROUP FALLACY
The assumption of a collective mind.

GROUP PSYCHOANALYSIS
Psychoanalytic technique applied to the group treatment of mental disorders; a particular version of group psychotherapy based on psychoanalytic principles.

GROUP PSYCHOLOGY
That branch of psychology concerned with the behavior of groups and with the psychology of membership of groups. It is probably not distinguishable from social psychology. Psychoanalytical formulations stress identification between members, identification of members with a leader and the relationship with the common enemy, all three factors playing an important role in diminishing the disruptive effects of rivalry between members.

GROUP PSYCHOTHERAPY
Any form of psychotherapy in which more than two clients are present. In most forms of group psychotherapy, the group is initially created by the therapist selecting the members, but it is assumed that the common relationship to the therapist will lead to the formation of a genuine group situation.

GROUP THERAPY
A group discussion or other group activity with a therapeutic purpose participated in by more than one client at a time.

GROWING PAIN
Pains occurring in the legs of growing children having no demonstrable relation to growth.

GROWTH
An increase in size of an organism or any of its parts, as occurs normally in a child, and abnormally in a tumor.

GROWTH CURVE
A curve on a graph representing the growth of a part, organism, or population as a function of time.

GROWTH FACTOR
A substance (as a vitamin) that pro-

motes the growth of an organism.

GROWTH HORMONE
One of the pituitary hormones, also called somatotropin, which controls the height an individual attains. Testing for growth hormone offers the earliest indication of generalized pituitary problems. Today drugs are available to stop excessive growth hormone secretion (preventing gigantism or abnormally tall individuals) as well as drugs to allow normal growth hormone secretion .

GROWTH PLATE
The region in a long bone between the epiphysis and diaphysis where growth in length occurs.

GUANASE
An enzyme found in the blood that is sometimes markedly elevated in those with hepatitis and other types of liver disease and in infectious mononucleosis (glandular fever).

GUIDANCE
Employed in a technical sense in two connections:
(1) Child guidance, meaning the organization and cooperation of medical, psychological, educational and psychiatric advice and treatment, through special clinics, in dealing with difficult or retarded children presenting either behavior or educational problems.
(2) Educational guidance, meaning the employment of standardized tests, mental and educational. Together with progress records, school reports, etc., it acts as a basis of advice to children and parents regarding educational courses that should be followed after the child has passed through the elementary school.

GUILLAIN-BARRÉ SYNDROME
An acute, rapidly progressive form of degeneration of peripheral nerves and characterized by muscular weakness and numbness that starts in the feet and spreads upwards, and usually begins shortly after a mild infectious disorder, surgery or an immunization. The paralysis may progress until it involves the muscles used in breathing. Corticosteroids have been advocated, but the best present evidence is that their usage improves the acute symptoms, but not the eventual outcome.

Recovery over a period of months is usual if the person survives the acute episode. Residual defects may require retraining, orthopedic appliances or corrective surgery.

GUM ARABIC
Mucilaginous excretion of the acacia tree, mainly used as soothing agent in skin applications.

GUM DISEASES
Disorders and ailments of the gums,

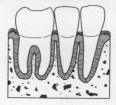

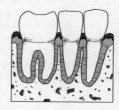

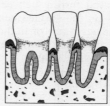

The development of gum diseases is mainly due to improper flossing and brushing of teeth.

the tissue that surrounds the necks of teeth and covers the alveolar parts of the jaws; broadly: the alveolar portion of a jaw with its enveloping soft tissues. Inflammatory processes and degeneration may occur.

GUMMATOUS OSTEITIS
Inflammation of the substance of bone characterized by the formation of syphilitic growths in or on bones.

GUMMA
Hard swelling of a consistency resembling India rubber, with a tendency to necrosis (tissue death) and caseation (cheese-like dead tissue). It is one of the features of syphilis.

GUSTATION
The sense of taste.

GUSTATORY
Relating to the sense of taste.

GUT
The intestines; the alimentary canal or part of it (as the intestine or stomach).

GUTHRIE TEST
Also called the Guthrie bacterial inhibition assay: a blood or urine test for phenylalanine, an amino acid. Elevated levels in babies may indicate phenylketonuria (PKU), an inherited enzyme deficiency disease that causes mental retardation if not diagnosed and treated soon after birth.

GUTTER
A depressed furrow between body parts (as on the surface between a pair of adjacent ribs or in the dorsal walls of the body cavity on either side of the spinal column).

GYMNASTICS
A system of exercise designed not only to maintain and improve the physique, but also as a sport. In ancient Greece, gymnastics -including track and field athletics and training for boxing and wrestling - were important in education. Competitive gymnastics are a series of exercises on set pieces of apparatus: parallel bars, horizontal bar, side and vaulting horses, beam and asymmetric bars. The US system, derived from the German, is designed to assist physical growth; the Swedish system aims at rectifying posture and weak muscles; and the Danish system seeks general fitness and endurance.

GYNANDROMORPH
An abnormal individual exhibiting characters of both sexes in various parts of the body.

GYNECOGENIC
Tending to induce female characteristics; for example a gynecogenic hormone.

GYNECOLOGY
The medical specialty concerned with the health care of women, including function and diseases of the reproductive organs. It combines both medical and surgical and is usually practiced in combination with obstetrics.

GYNECOMASTIA
Enlargement of the male breasts. This usually occurs if a man is given female sex hormones or one of a small number of drugs.

GYNOGENESIS
Development in which the embryo contains only maternal chromosomes due to activation of an egg by a sperm that degenerates without fusing with the egg nucleus.

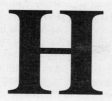

HABENULA
Either of two nuclei one which lies on each side of the pineal gland under the corresponding trigonum habenulae, composed of two groups of nerve cells. It forms a correlation center for olfactory stimuli.

HABIT
A learned stimulus-response sequence. The term is also used in the sense of an automatic response to specific situations, acquired normally as a result of repetition and learning; strictly applicable only to motor responses, but often applied more widely to habits of thought perhaps more correctly called attitudes.

HABITAT
The place or type of site where a plant or animal naturally or normally lives and grows. The term is also used to designate a housing for a controlled physical environment in which people can live surrounded by inhospitable conditions.

HABITUAL
Having the nature of a habit.

HABITUAL ABORTION
Spontaneous abortion occurring in three or more successive pregnancies.

HABITUATION
(1) The process of becoming accustomed to something;
(2) in pharmacology, the dependence on a drug resulting from repeated use but without severe physiological signs of addiction or need to increase dosage;
(3) in psychology, the decrease or loss of response to a particular stimulus after repeated exposure to that stimulus.

HABITUS
Term with two different meanings.
(1) The general physical build of a person (e.g., an athletic habitus);
(2) a person's tendency to require or be affected by something, as a disease.

HAEMOGLOBIN
See Hemoglobin.

HAEMORRHAGE
See Hemorrhage

HAEMORRHOID
See Hemorrhoid.

HAIR
Threadlike, keratin-containing appendage of the outer layer of the skin present over most of the body surface except the palms, soles, lips, and a few other small areas. A hair develops inside a tubular hair follicle beneath the skin with the root of the hair expanded into a bulb. The part above the skin consists of an outer cuticle that covers the cortex, which contains pigment and gives the hair its color, and an inner medulla.

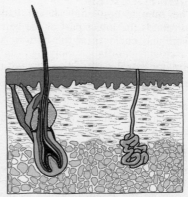

Localization of the root and shaft of a hair in a cross section of the skin.

HAIR, BEADED
Hair marked with alternate swellings and constrictions, as in monilethrix.

HAIR, BURROWING
Hair that grows horizontally beneath the surface of the skin.

HAIR, CLUB
Hair whose root is surrounded by a bulbous enlargement composed of keratinized cells, preliminary to normal loss of hair from the follicle.

HAIR, TERMINAL
The coarse hair on various areas of the body during adult years.

HAIR, TWISTED
Hair which at spaced intervals is twisted through an axis of 180 degrees, being abnormally flattened at the side of the twisting.

HAIR BULB
The bulbous expansion at the base of a hair from which the hair shaft develops.

HAIR CELL
Cell with hairlike processes; for example, one of the sensory cells in the auditory epithelium of the organ of Corti.

HAIR FOLLICLE
The tubular epithelial sheath that surrounds the lower part of the hair shaft and encloses at the bottom a vascular papilla supplying the growing basal part of the hair with nourishment.

HAIR SHAFT
The part of a hair projecting beyond the skin.

HALATION
Indistinctness of the visual image caused by strong illumination coming from the same direction as the object being viewed.

HALF-LIFE
The time in which the radioactivity originally associated with a particular isotope is reduced by half through radioactive decay. In pharmacology, the term is used for the time the body takes to reduce the blood level of a drug by half. Knowledge of the half-life of drugs helps to determine frequency of dosage.

HALF-LIFE, ANTIBODY
A measure of the mean survival time of antibody molecules following their formation, usually expressed as the time required to eliminate 50 percent of a known quantity of immunoglobulin from the animal body.

HALF-LIFE, BIOLOGICAL
The time required for a living tissue, organ, or organism to eliminate one-half of a radioactive substance which has been introduced into it.

HALIBUT LIVER OIL
Oil rich in vitamins A and D.

HALITOSIS
Commonly called bad breath: an unpleasant odor to the breath. This may be produced by ingesting or inhaling substances that are partially excreted by the lungs, by gum disease, by fermentation of food particles in the mouth or in association with diseases of other organ systems. Oral hygiene will eliminate most cases of halitosis, but when gum or other disease is the cause, this must be treated before the unpleasant odor will disappear.

HALITUS
The breath or moisture of the breath. The term is also used in the sense of vapor exhaled from the body.

HALLUCINATION
An experience similar to a normal perception but with the difference

that sensory stimulus is either absent or too minor to explain the experience satisfactorily. Certain abnormal mental conditions produce hallucinations, as does the taking of hallucinogenic drugs.

They may also result from exhaustion, fever or alcoholism (delirium tremens), or may be experienced while falling asleep (hypnogogic) or waking (hypnopompic), and also by individuals under hypnosis.

A negative hallucination is lack of perception despite adequate stimulus. Mass hallucination is hallucination shared by the members of a group; it may particularly result from mass hypnosis.

HALLUCINOGEN
A drug that causes hallucinations, characterized by unreal perceptions of surroundings and objects. Alcohol taken in large amount may also have an hallucinogenic effect.

HALLUCINOGENIC DRUGS
Drugs that cause hallucinations or illusions, usually visual, together with personality and behavior changes. The last may arise as a result of therapy, but more usually follow deliberate exposure to certain drugs for their psychological effects, commonly called "tripping."

LSD (lysergic acid diethylamide), heroin, morphine and other opium narcotics, mescaline (peyote) and psilocybin ("magic mushrooms") are commonly hallucinogenic and cannabis sometimes so.

The type of hallucination is not predictable and many are unpleasant ("bad trip"). Recurrent hallucinations may follow use of these drugs; another danger is that altered behavior may inadvertently cause death or injury.

Although psychosis may be a result of their use, it may be that recourse to drugs represents an early symptom of schizophrenia.

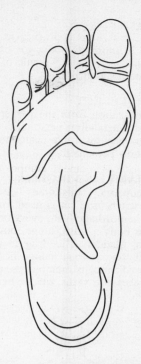

Plantar view of the toes; the big toe or hallux should not deviate laterally or medially.

HALLUCINOSIS
A mental disorder in which hallucinations are the main symptom.

HALLUX
The big toe; the innermost digit of the lower limb.

HALLUX RIGIDUS
Restricted mobility of the big toe due to stiffness of the metatarsophalangeal joint, especially when due to arthritic changes in the joint.

HALLUX VALGUS
Deviation of the big toe towards the other toes, forming a bunion. Hallux valgus is an abnormal deviation of the big toe away from the midline of the body or toward the other toes of the foot.

HALLUX VARUS
Deviation of the big toe away from the other toes.

HALO

A circle of light appearing to surround a luminous body; for example one seen as the result of the presence of glaucoma.

HALO EFFECT

Generalization from the perception of one outstanding personality trait to an overly favorable evaluation of the whole personality.

HAMAMELIS VIRGINIA

Homeopathic medicine derived from witch hazel. It is used for venous hemorrhage from every orifice of the body - nose, lungs, bowels, uterus, bladder. The drug is prescribed for venous congestion of skin and mucous membranes, phlebitis, varicose veins, ulcers, hemorrhoids.

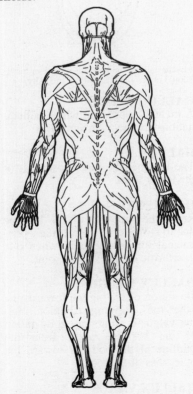

The hamstring occupies most of the posterior part of the thigh.

HAMARTOMA

A tumor-like mass of cells that arises from faulty development in the embryo; a typical example is the vascular birthmarks called nevi.

HAMARTOPHOBIA

Fear of making a mistake.

HAMMER

The malleus, a small bone in the middle ear.

HAMMER TOE

A deformity of one of the toe joints nearest the foot, in which the soft tissues have contracted and prevent the toe from being straightened. This condition usually affects only one toe, often the second, which is frequently overly long and has been under pressure from footwear. A painful bunion may form on top of it, which can be relieved by protecting it with pads; however, surgery is often necessary.

HAMSTRING MUSCLE

Any of three muscles at the back of the thigh that function to flex and rotate the leg and extend the thigh.

HAMSTRINGS

The tendons of the hamstring muscles, located at the back of the knee. They serve to bend the knee and turn the foot.

HAM TEST

A test for paroxysmal nocturnal hemoglobinuria.

HAND

The part of the upper limb distal to the forearm and extending from the wrist to include the fingers. It contains 27 bones, including 8 in the wrist, 5 in the metatarsal region, and 14 in the fingers.

HANDEDNESS

Refers to the side of the body, and in particular to the hand, that is most used in motor tasks. Most peo-

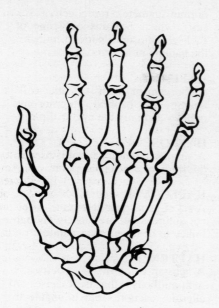

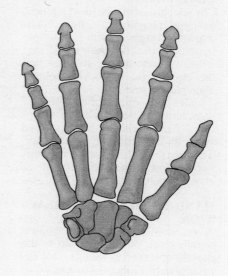

Dorsal view of the skeleton of the hand consists of the carpus, metacarpus and phalanges. The carpus, or wrist consists of eight small bones united to each other by ligaments. The bones are arranged in two transverse rows, with four bones in each row.

Palmar view of the skeleton of the hand consists of the carpus, metacarpus and phalanges. The carpus, or wrist consists of eight small bones united to each other by ligaments. The bones are arranged in two transverse rows, with four bones in each row.

ple are right-handed and few are truly ambidextrous - that is, equally skilled with either hand.

In the brain, the paths for sensory and motor information are crossed, so that the right side of the body is controlled by the left cerebral hemisphere and vice versa. The left hemisphere is usually dominant and also contains centers for speech and calculation. The non-dominant side deals with aspects of visual and spatial relationships, while other functions are represented on both sides. In some left-handed people, the right hemisphere is dominant. Suppression of left-handedness may lead to speech disorders.

HANDICAP
Any physical or mental defect or characteristic, congenital or acquired, preventing or restricting a person from participating in normal life or limiting his/her capacity to work.

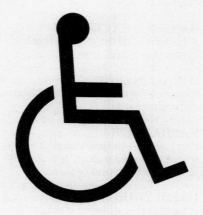

International symbol used, for instance, for a parking place for an individual with a handicap.

HAND-SCHUELLER-CHRISTIAN DISEASE

Chronic histiocytosis (development to large phagocytic cells) of unknown origin with multiple lipogranuloma (nodules of lipid material) of bone and of the skin and the viscera; the histiocytes contain abundant cholesterol.

Males are more often affected than females. As a rule the symptoms begin within the first five years of life, but can appear later. The course of this disease is relatively benign, with a mortality rate of about 10 percent.

HAND-TO-MOUTH REACTION

A reaction of bringing all objects within reach of the hand up to the mouth, observed in infants until approximately 12 months of age.

HANGNAIL

A small strip of skin, partly detached from the fold of the nail.

HANGOVER EFFECT

The same feelings as a "hangover" after too much alcohol consumption. Symptoms include:
- headache;
- irritability;
- nausea.

HANSEN'S BACILLUS

A bacterium of the genus Mycobacterium that causes leprosy.

HAPALONYCHIA

Abnormal softness of the fingernails or toenails.

HAPHALGESIA

Pain upon physical contact with something which does not usually induce the sensation of pain.

HAPHEPHOBIA

A morbid fear of being touched.

HAPLOID

The number of chromosomes in a normal gamete (reproductive sex cell), which contains only one of each chromosome pair; in humans, the haploid number is 23.

HAPLONT

An organism with somatic cells having the haploid chromosome number and only the zygote diploid.

HAPLOSCOPE

A simple stereoscope that is used in the study of depth perception.

HAPLOTYPE

A set of genes that determine different antigens but are closely enough linked to be inherited as a unit.

HAPTEN

A substance that reacts specifically with antibody - that is, it causes an allergic reaction - but is unable to induce antibody formation unless attached to other carrier molecules, usually proteins.

HAPTICS

The branch of science that studies the sense of touch.

HAPTOGLOBULIN

A blood protein that combines with hemoglobulin. A low level of haptoglobulin indicates a breakdown of red blood cells, as may occur in certain diseases, snakebite or drug ingestion. Levels are increased in some inflammatory conditions.

HAPTOPHORE

Having an ability to enter into combination with specific receptors of a cell.

HARELIP

Congenital deformity of the upper lip and often associated with cleft palate. The human embryo commences as a flat plate that folds in upon itself to form a tube, and it is the incomplete closure of this tube that causes such a developmental abnormality. It is more common in boys than girls, and tends to run in families and to be associated with other physical and mental abnormalities. It can be repaired by cosmetic surgery.

HARMALINE
A hallucinogenic alkaloid found in several plants (e.g., Pergamum harmala) and used in medicine as a stimulant of the central nervous system.

HARRIS'S OPERATION
Removal of the prostate gland by the suprapubic route (i.e. over the pubic bone).

HARTMANN'S SOLUTION
Solution containing sodium lactate and chloride, potassium chloride and calcium chloride. It is used to replace fluid in those who are dehydrated.

HARTNUP DISEASE
A rare disease due to abnormal absorption and excretion of tryptophan and other amino acids, characterized by rash and abnormalities in the central nervous system.

HASHIMOTO'S DISEASE
Chronic inflammation and enlargement of the thyroid gland. This form of goiter is produced by an abnormality in the auto-immune system, and is most common in middle-aged women.

HASHISH
Drug produced from a resin obtained from the hemp plant (Cannabis sativa), particularly from its flowers and fruits. It is a non-addictive drug whose effects range from feelings of euphoria to fear. Hashish is mainly produced in the Middle East and India, and has been in use for many centuries, although it is still illegal in many countries.

HAUSTRATION
The formation of sac-like depressions in the wall of the large intestine.

HAVERSIAN CANAL
Any of the small canals through which the blood vessels ramify in bone.

HAVERSIAN SYSTEM
Haversian canal with the concentrically arranged laminae of bone that surround it.

HAY FEVER
An acute allergic nasal catarrh and conjunctivitis that is sometimes accompanied by asthmatic symptoms.

HCG
Abbreviation of human chorionic gonadotrophin, used as a drug for certain types of infertility.

HEAD
(1) The upper part of the body, especially that which contains the brain and organs of sight, hearing, taste, and smell.

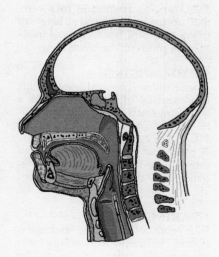

Cross section through the head and the skull (without brain) to show the relationship of the facial structures, tongue, pharynx and larynx and the transitional area of the skull and spine.

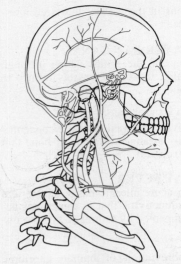

Lateral view of the skeleton of the head and upper part of the spine.

(2) the rounded portion of a bone, which fits into a groove in another to form a joint;
(3) that part of a muscle that is away from the bone that it moves.

HEADACHE
Pain, ranging from mild to severe, that occurs in the head. There are many causes of headache and treatment depends on the cause.

HEAD-BANGING
Uncontrolled physical movements characteristic of a young child in a temper tantrum.

HEALING
A process of cure; the restoration of integrity to injured tissues and organs; also the natural process of cure.

HEARING
The sense of receiving and interpreting sounds. Sound waves enter the outer ear, cause vibrations of the eardrum and bones of the middle ear and are transmitted to the inner ear from which they are transmitted along the auditory nerve to the brain for interpretation.

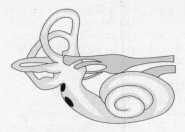

The cochlea (in the left part of the illustration) is the organ of hearing. It is located in the inner ear in close relationship with the organ of equilibrium, consisting of the semicircular canals.

HEARING LOSS
Loss of hearing can be sudden or gradual, and can range from mild and almost unnoticed to very severe. There are two types: nerve deafness and conductive deafness. With nerve deafness the acoustic nerve is unable to receive the signals of sound and transmit them to the brain. This kind of deafness usually affects only certain pitches, and a person is able to hear in some of the ranges of noise or sound. Nerve deafness can be either sudden or gradual in onset and congenital or acquired.

Conductive deafness or hearing loss, on the other hand, is caused by something that interferes with the transmission of sound from the outside, across the eardrum and the small bones of the middle ear to the nerve. This can be a deformity, a collection of fluid or pus or a problem with the bones of the middle ear. This type of deafness can usually be helped by hearing aids, while nerve deafness cannot, and it is also often preventable.

HEART
The muscular, roughly cone-shaped organ that pumps blood throughout the body. Lying behind the breastbone between the lungs, it is about the size of a closed fist, about 12 cm (5 inches) long, 8 cm (3 inches) wide at its broadest upper part, and about 6 cm (2.3 inches) thick and

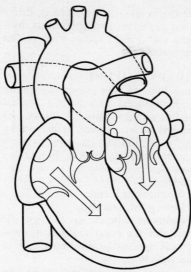

Cross section through the heart showing the direction of the blood flow. To the left are the right atrium and right ventricle, to the right the left atrium and left ventricle. The arc of the aorta is shown above the heart.

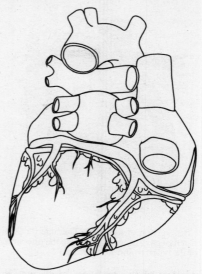

Posterior view of the heart. The various incoming and outgoing vessels are shown at the top.

weighs about 275-345 g (10-12 ounces). Under outer epicardium membranes, the heart wall - myocardium - consists of cardiac muscle; the innermost layer – endocardium – is continuous with the lining of the blood vessels.

The heart is divided into left and right sides by a septum; each side has an upper atrium (auricle) and lower ventricle. Through coordinated nerve impulses and muscular contractions, initiated in the sinoatrial node of the right atrium, the heart pumps blood throughout the body.

HEART ATTACK
Technically called myocardial infarction: the death of a portion of heart muscle which may result in disability or death of the individual, depending on how much of the heart is damaged.

A heart attack occurs when an obstruction in one of the coronary arteries prevents an adequate oxygen supply to part of the heart. Symptoms may be none, mild or se-

vere and may include chest pain (sometimes radiating to the shoulder, arm, neck or jaw), nausea, cold sweat and shortness of breath.

Doctors often refer to a heart attack in terms of the type of obstruction (i.e., coronary occlusion, coronary thrombosis or simply "coronary") or the heart muscle damage (myocardial infarction). In common usage, the term "heart attack" is often incorrectly used to describe irregular heartbeats or attacks of angina pectoris.

HEART BLOCK
Conditions in which the spread of the electrical impulses across the heart is slowed or interrupted in a portion of the normal conduction pathway of the heart. The normal impulse conduction pattern is from the upper chambers (the atria) to the lower chambers (the ventricles) along specialized conducting tissue. The impulse causes contraction of the heart muscle and, thus, pumping of blood either to the next chamber or out of the heart to the lungs or

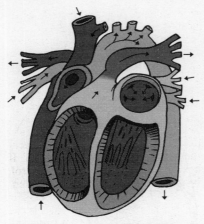

Cross section of the heart. The anterior part is removed. The arrows indicate the direction of the blood to and from the heart.

the rest of the body. A blockage in this conducting system can occur with age or infection or can result from certain drugs.

HEARTBURN

Esophagitis, a burning sensation of "indigestion" located in the upper abdomen or lower chest. It is frequently worse after large meals or on lying flat, especially with hiatus hernia (when part of the stomach bulges up into the esophagus). Acid stomach contents irritate the lining of the esophagus and may lead to the formation of an ulcer; relief is obtained with antacids. Heartburn is also loosely applied to other pains in the same situation.

HEART CATHETERIZATION

A diagnostic procedure that involves inserting a narrow tube called a catheter into a vein or artery and advancing it, under fluoroscopic guidance, into the blood vessels or chambers of the heart. Contrast medium is injected to aid in visualization, and blood samples and pressure readings may be taken at different stages.

HEART DRUGS

Medicines that have a direct effect on the heart such as digitalis, drugs used to correct abnormal heart rhythms and drugs used to treat angina pectoris.

HEART FAILURE

Inability of the heart to pump enough blood to maintain normal body requirements. It may be caused by congenital defects or by any condition that damages or overloads the heart muscle. Symptoms include:
- edema;
- shortness of breath;
- feelings of faintness.
Treatment depends on the specific cause of the heart malfunction and on the age and general condition of the patient.

HEART MASSAGE

Also called cardiac massage: an emergency technique using compression of the heart to keep the blood pumping through the body in the event of the heart not pumping effectively. External heart massage involves pressing on the chest to compress the heart between the breastbone and the spine. Internal cardiac massage is usually done in the operating theater where the heart is directly compressed by the surgeon's hand through an incision in the chest.

HEART MURMUR

Abnormal sound heard on listening to the chest over the heart with a stethoscope. Normally there are two major heart sounds due to valve closure, separated by silence. Murmurs can arise in heart valve disease, with narrowing (stenosis) or leakage (incompetence). Holes between the heart's chambers, valve roughening and high flow of blood also cause murmurs. Most murmurs are completely harmless.

HEART RATE CHANGES

The sensation of a changing or irregular heartbeat is very bothersome for people, especially if they have or think they have heart disease. Palpitations are the sensations of the heart skipping a beat, beating irregularly or pounding in the chest.

Most people have changes in the heart rate and rhythm as part of a normal day, and palpitations may signal no disease at all. Others have this as a sign of heart disease. When palpitations are pronounced or frequent, or if they are associated with symptoms of light-headedness or difficult breathing, it is important that a person seek prompt medical care.

HEART SCAN
A scan of the heart after injection of a harmless radioactive substance into a vein, to determine size, shape and location; to diagnose pericarditis (inflammation and fluid accumulation around the heart); or to view the heart's chambers. A blood pool scan can measure damage sustained after a heart attack.

HEART SURGERY
Any surgical procedure involving the heart. In closed heart surgery, a small incision is made into the heart; the heart-lung machine is not used. In open-heart surgery, the heart is opened, the chambers of the heart made visible, and blood detoured from the operating field through the heart-lung machine.

HEAT CRAMPS
Severe cramps of skeletal muscle resulting from excessive sweating due to exertion and/or high ambient temperature. In most instances, heat cramp is prevented and also rapidly relieved by drinking fluids or eating foods containing salt.

HEAT EXHAUSTION
Excessive fluid and salt loss during particularly hot weather. The symptoms include: excessive sweating; cool, clammy skin; and sudden weakness and fatigue. Blurred vision, nausea, headache and dizziness may also be experienced. Extreme thirst and salt loss may occur. Exercise in hot weather makes a person even more susceptible to heat exhaustion.

Extreme heat coupled with excessive water and salt loss (through profuse sweating) will eventually lead to dehydration, further complicated by inadequate fluid replacement and an inability to cool off. If heat exhaustion gets out of control, heatstroke (a serious, life-threatening emergency) may occur. It is therefore imperative that steps be taken to avoid heat exhaustion and to treat it immediately so a more serious problem does not arise.

HEAT RASH
Also called prickly heat: rash occurring in hot, moist weather, in which the sweat ducts become plugged, balloon up and form red blisters. This heat rash usually occurs in folds of the skin or in areas covered by tight clothing.

It often occurs beneath the breasts in women or under the scrotum in men. The primary treatment is to discard restrictive clothing in order to let the skin breathe.

Keep the skin as dry as possible; antiseptic dusting powder and calamine lotion can reduce itching. Cortisone cream helps clear up the rash at first; then proper skin care is required.

HEAT STROKE
Mild to grave reactions to high temperature due to inadequate or inappropriate responses of the heat-regulating mechanisms of the body. Prolonged exposure to high ambient temperatures may lead either to severe muscle cramp, excessive blood fluid loss and shock, or the failure of the body's heat-loss mechanisms and dangerous and possibly fatal high body temperatures.

Common sense is the best preventive; strenuous exertion in a very

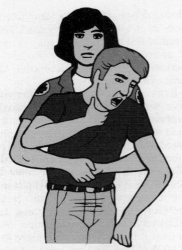

Method of the Heimlich maneuver is case of choking.

hot environment, inadequately ventilated rooms and heavy, insulating clothing should be avoided. Loss of fluid and electrolytes (salt and potassium) should be replaced by the continuous drinking of fluids that are slightly salty to taste.

If someone collapses from heat stroke, this is an emergency: remove the person to a cool place; if he or she is conscious, give slightly salty water to drink; if possible, apply ice packs or cold wet sheets to the body until the temperature falls; call for medical help urgently.

HEBEPHRENIC SCHIZOPHRENIA

A form of schizophrenia, characterized by extremely silly, seemingly childlike "happy" behavior. The victim often laughs hilariously over nothing, wets the bed and behaves in other inappropriately infantile ways. Although hebephrenics may seem almost blissful in their own mad way, this is actually the most extreme of all forms of schizophrenia as well as the least amenable to treatment.

The stricken individual is in grave danger of complete withdrawal from contact with the real world.

HEDONISM

The theory that people seek pleasure and avoid pain; an extreme form of the theory is that pleasure or happiness is the highest good.

HEGAR'S SIGN

Soft consistency of a compressible area between the cervix and the body of the uterus, indicating pregnancy.

HEIMLICH MANEUVER

The manual application of sudden upward pressure on the upper abdomen of a choking victim to force a foreign body from the windpipe.

HELIOTHERAPY

Treatment by exposure to sunlight or ultra-violet light.

HELIX

The rounded edge of the external ear.

HELLEBORE

Term for various varieties of poisonous perennial plants - black hellebore (Helleborus niger), stinking hellebore (Helleborus foetidus) and green hellebore (Helleborus viridis) - of which the rootstock is used for medicinal purposes.

Black hellebore is used variously to stimulate the heart and to treat depression, mania, epilepsy and skin problems.

The leaves and rootstock contain a variety of glycosides similar in activity to the heart drug digitalis. Hellebore is not for use without medical direction under any circumstances.

HELLER'S OPERATION

Surgical procedure (cutting) of the muscular layer at the junction between the esophagus and the stomach; performed to relieve the difficulties in the passage of food and swallowing in cases of spasm of the muscular cardiac sphincter in that area.

HELMINTAGOGUE
Substance or medicine that destroys worms.

HELMINTH
A general term covering several varieties of intestinal and parasitic worms.

HELMINTHIASIS
The condition of having worms in the intestines or other parts of the body.

HELOMA
Commonly called a corn: a cone-shaped overgrowth and hardening of the epidermis of the skin, with the point of the cone in the deeper layers. It is produced by friction or pressure.

HEM
The pigment-carrying portion of hemoglobin.

HEMADSORPTION
Adherence of red blood cells to the surface of something.

HEMAGGLUTINATION
Agglutination of red blood cells (erythrocytes).

HEMAL
Term with two different meanings.
(1) Of or relating to the blood or blood vessels.
(2) Relating to or situated on the side of the spinal cord where the heart and chief blood vessels are placed.

HEMANALYSIS
Chemical and microscopic analysis of a blood sample.

HEMANGIOBLAST
A mesodermal cell which gives rise to both vascular endothelium and hemocytoblasts.

HEMANGIOMA
A benign tumor made up of newly formed blood cells; this malformation of blood cells may occur in any part of the body.

HEMANGIOMA, CAVERNOUS
A red-blue spongy lesion made up of a connective tissue framework enclosing large, cavernous, vascular spaces containing blood.

HEMANGIOMA, SCLEROSING
A solidly cellular lesion purportedly developing from a hemangioma by proliferation of endothelial cells and connective tissue stroma.

HEMANGIOMATOSIS
The presence of multiple malformations of blood vessels, such as multiple birthmarks.

HEMAPHERESIS
Any procedure in which blood is withdrawn, a portion (plasma, leukocytes, platelets, etc.) is separated and retained, and the remainder is retransfused into the donor.

HEMARTHROSIS
Accumulation of blood into a joint or its synovial cavity. In the long term, the irritant effect of hemoglobin may destroy the joint.

HEMATEMESIS
The vomiting of blood.

HEMATIN
Any of the iron-containing constituents of blood.

HEMATINEMIA
The presence of hematin (hem) in the peripheral blood.

HEMATINURIA
The presence of hematin (hem) in the urine.

HEMATITE-MINER'S LUNG
A form of severe silicosis; a lung disorder caused by the inhalation of stone dust or sand, occurring in the iron (hematite) industry.

HEMATOCRIT

The percentage of blood cells (mostly red blood cells) comprising the total blood volume. A blood sample from a vein is centrifuged, the solid matter being forced to the bottom of a specially marked tube, leaving the clear plasma in the upper section. In a sense, the test measures the viscosity of blood as well as the amount of fluid in the blood. Many doctors feel the hematocrit test is a better measure of anemia than the hemoglobin test, especially if the person's diet includes normal amounts of iron.

HEMATOCYST

Effusion of blood into the bladder or a cyst.

HEMATOCYTE

Rarely used term for a blood cell or blood corpuscle.

HEMATOGENOUS

Produced by or derived from the blood; disseminated through the blood stream.

HEMATOIDIN

A substance apparently chemically identical with bilirubin but formed in the tissues from hemoglobin, particularly under conditions of reduced oxygen tension.

HEMATOLOGY

The medical and chemical science dealing with the structure and chemistry of blood and blood-forming tissues, and with their physiology and pathology.

HEMATOLYSIS

The breaking-down of hemoglobin, when the hemoglobin separated from the red blood cells and appears in the plasma of the blood.

HEMATOMA

A localized collection of blood outside the vessels, usually clotted, in an organ, space or tissue; a swelling filled with blood. This sometimes accompanies a bruise (contusion).

HEMATOMA, SUBDURAL

A massive blood clot beneath the dura mater that causes neurologic symptoms by pressure on the brain.

HEMATOMETRA

An accumulation of blood in the uterus; usually of menstrual origin.

HEMATOPOIESIS

The formation and development of the various types of blood cells.

HEMATOPOIESIS, EXTRA-MEDULLARY

Formation and development of blood cells occurring outside the bone marrow, as in the spleen, liver, and lymph nodes.

HEMATORRHEA

Hemorrhoids (piles) characterized by a copious loss of blood.

HEMATOSALPINX

An accumulation of blood in the Fallopian, or uterine, tube.

HEMATOSTEON

Hemorrhage (bleeding) into the medullary cavity of a bone.

HEMATURIA

The presence of blood in the urine; when no cause for this can be determined, the condition is called essential hematuria.

HEMATURIA, ESSENTIAL

The presence of blood in the urine for which no cause has been determined.

HEMATURIA, FALSE

Redness of the urine due to ingestion of food or drugs containing pigment and not due to the presence of red blood cells.

HEMATURIA, RENAL

The presence of red blood cells in

the urine due to a disorder of the kidney; the blood in the urine comes from the kidney.

HEMATURIA, URETHRAL
The presence of blood in the urine, which comes from the urethra.

HEMATURIA, VESICAL
The presence of blood in the urine in which the blood comes from the bladder.

HEMERALOPIA
Day blindness; defective vision in bright light.

HEMIANACUSIS
Loss of hearing in one ear.

HEMIANESTHESIA
Anesthesia (loss of sensation) of one side of the body.

HEMIANALGESIA
Insensibility to pain down one side of the body.

HEMIANOPIA
Blindness in one half of the field.

HEMIATROPHY
Diminution in size of cells, tissues and organs on one side of the body or one half of an organ or part.

HEMIBALLISM
Violent, flinging limb movements caused by injury in the area of the subthalamic nucleus of the mid-brain, usually a small infarct. The disorder is confined to the side opposite the injury. The head is sometimes also affected. The repeated violent movements incapacitate and may exhaust the sufferer.

HEMICHOREA
Irregular and spasmodic movements, out of control of the person, limited to one side of the body.

HEMICOLECTOMY
Surgical procedure (mostly for severe cancer of the large intestine) in which approximately half of the colon is removed.

HEMICRANIA
Commonly called migraine: headache affecting one side of the head, associated with nausea, vomiting or both and sometimes preceded by disturbances of vision, such as seeing flashing or colored lights.

HEMIDIAPHORESIS
Hyperhidrosis (excessive perspiration) in one half of the body.

HEMIPLEGIA
Paralysis affecting only one side of the body.

HEMISPHERICAL DOMINANCE
The tendency of one side of the brain to control bodily movements resulting in laterality. In most people the left hemisphere is dominant.

HEMIZYGOUS
Since males have only one X chromosome, they are said to be hemizygous with respect to X-linked genes.

HEMOCHROMATOSIS
Also called bronzed diabetes: a disorder of iron metabolism with excess deposition of iron in the tissues resulting in brown pigmentation of the skin and cirrhosis of the liver. The person has often diabetes.

HEMOCONCENTRATION
Decrease in the fluid content of the blood, with a resulting increase in the concentration of the various types of blood cells.

HEMOCYTOBLAST
The free stem cell, from which the blood cells are formed.

HEMOCYTOMETER
An instrument used in the counting of blood cells.

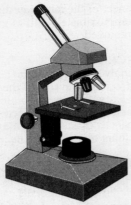

The morphological properties of blood can be investigated by a microscope.

HEMODIALYSIS
Removal of certain elements from the blood (usually the waste products from the metabolism of cells and tissues) by virtue of the difference in their rates of diffusion through a semi-permeable membrane; such a technique is used in the artificial kidney.

HOMOGENTISIC ACID
An acid present in urine in alkaptonuria, a rare metabolic disease.

HEMOGLOBIN (Hb)
The oxygen-carrying pigment of the red blood cells (erythrocytes), formed by the developing cell in the bone marrow, and made up of four different globin polypeptide chains, each composed of several hundred amino acids.

There are many different forms of hemoglobin in the blood; these forms are usually measured together as the total hemoglobin.

Hemoglobin is made up of an iron compound hem and a protein substance globin, which are manufactured inside the newly forming red blood cells and stored there for the life of the cells. Because of hemoglobin's unique affinity for oxygen, its task is to pick up oxygen as the red blood cells pass through the lungs and deliver that oxygen to tissue cells throughout the body. The amount of oxygen that the blood can carry depends not only on the amount of hemoglobin present but also on its effectiveness.

Exposure to toxic substances can alter the hemoglobin molecule: for example, carbon monoxide gas will easily replace the oxygen attached to hemoglobin to form carboxyhemoglobin; this will prevent vital oxygen from reaching tissue cells.

HEMOGLOBIN C DISEASE
A moderately severe anemia due to an inherited abnormality of hemoglobin formation.

HEMOGLOBIN F
Fetal hemoglobin; in adults or children, abnormally elevated levels may indicate various blood diseases and conditions, including aplastic anemia, leukemia and thalassemia, a type of hemolytic anemia.

HEMOGLOBINOMETER
An instrument used to determine the hemoglobin content of the blood by measuring the intensity of its red color.

HEMOGLOBINOPATHY
Genetic abnormality of the hemoglobin molecule shown by changes in chemical characteristics or physical properties.

HEMOGLOBINURIA
Presence of blood pigment (hemoglobin) in the urine. Paroxysmal nocturnal hemoglobinuria is a disease that occurs in certain people after middle age. Symptoms may include:
- attacks of anemia;
- generalized aches and pains;
- chills;
- fever;
- excessive amounts of hemoglobin in the urine as a consequence of hemolysis (destruction of defective red blood cells), and these usually occur during sleep.

The disorder is believed to be caused by a defect in the membranes surrounding red blood cells, which, it seems, are unusually sensitive to the blood's complement (a constituent of serum that plays a major role in the immune system), and this causes them to self-destruct.

Because the condition is so insidious, it can take years before a diagnosis is made. One way this is done is by the HAM test: blood is taken from a vein and the serum is tested in an acid solution.

HEMOGRAM
A laboratory record, either written or graphic, of a differential blood count, with special emphasis on the size, shape, special characteristics and numbers of the solid constituents of the blood.

HEMOLYSIN
A substance that releases hemoglobin from red blood cells so that it appears in the blood plasma; the agent causes disintegration of red blood cells.

HEMOLYSIS
The dissolving or destruction of red blood cells by a chemical substance or disease.

HEMOLYTIC DISEASE OF THE NEWBORN
Another name for erythroblastosis fetalis.

HEMOLYTIC REACTION
Reaction accompanied by hemolysis (breakdown) of the recipient's or the donor's red blood cells (usually the latter) during of following a transfusion of solutions, plasma, blood or blood components.

HEMOLYTICS
Drugs that separate hemoglobin from the blood cells.

HEMOPERICARDIUM
An effusion of blood within the pericardium (outer covering of the heart).

HEMOPERITONEUM
An effusion of blood in the peritoneal cavity.

HEMOPHILIA
A hereditary disease in which the blood clots only very slowly, so that a minor cut or bruise can cause prolonged bleeding, and there is a tendency to bleed internally without any obvious cause. It affects only males, but is transmitted in the genes of females. The genetic defect is the inability to synthesize a protein - called Factor VIII - needed for normal clotting of the blood. The severity of the disease depends on how much Factor VIII is produced by the body. In severe cases, where no Factor VIII is made, internal bleeding can lead to massive hemorrhages and can erode the joints of arms and legs. The disease can now be controlled by giving the hemophiliac transfusions or intravenous injections of Factor VIII that has been collected from donated blood.

HEMOPHILUS
A genus of Gram-negative bacteria, including Haemophilus influenzae, a species once thought to cause epidemic influenza.

HEMOPHILUS VAGINITIS
An inflammation of the vagina caused by the bacterium Haemophilus vaginalis. The uncontrolled reproduction of this bacteria, triggered perhaps by a change in vaginal acidity, produces the infection. In the earliest stage, the woman notices a scant vaginal discharge associated with mild burning and itching. As the infection spreads, the discharge becomes more profuse, either white or gray, and carries a foul small. Vaginal itching and irri-

tation increases, intercourse may become painful, and there may be a sensation of burning during urination.

HEMOPHOBIA
Fear of the sight of blood.

HEMOPHTHALMIA
Bleeding into the eyeball.

HEMOPNEUMOTHORAX
A collection of blood and air within the pleural cavity, the space between the lungs and the chest wall.

HEMOPOIESIS
The formation and development of blood.

HEMOPTYSIS
Splitting up of blood. This may occur in conditions such as bronchitis or a catarrhal cold, or it may be the first sign of a growth in the lung or of active tuberculosis.

HEMORRHAGE
Acute loss of blood from any site. Injury to major arteries, veins or the heart may lead to massive hemorrhage.

Gastrointestinal tract hemorrhage is usually accompanied by the loss of blood in vomit or feces and mat lead to shock; ulcers and cancer of the bowels are important causes.

HEMORRHEOLOGIC AGENTS
Medicines to help control bleeding.

HEMORRHOID
Commonly called a pile. Piles are varicose veins of the back passage that may either be internal and bleed frequently, thus producing anemia, or become large and protrude from the anus, causing pain and discomfort.

There is no known cause, although they are more common in pregnant women and in those with cirrhosis of the liver. The pain and discomfort can be relieved by the application of suppositories, and they can be treated by the injection of an irritant fluid that will cause scarring around the hemorrhoid and so obstruct it. Surgery can also be employed to close them off. All hemorrhoids should be treated by a doctor; they mimic the early signs of cancer of the rectum, making a proper diagnosis vital.

HEMORRHOIDAL
Pertaining to hemorrhoids (piles).

HEMORRHOIDECTOMY
Surgical removal of hemorrhoids.

HEMOSIDEROSIS
Increase of iron deposits in body tissues without tissue damage.

HEMOSTASIS
The arrest of bleeding, either naturally (by physical properties such as vasoconstriction and coagulation) or artificially by surgical means.

HEMOTHORAX
Collection of blood in the pleural cavity.

HENOCH-SCHOENLEIN DISEASE
Another name for allergic purpura.

HEPAR
The liver.

HEPATALGIA
Pain in the liver or capsule surrounding the liver.

HEPATECTOMY
Surgical procedure (mostly for liver cancer), in which all or part of the liver is removed.

HEPATICA
Another name for liverwort.

HEPATIC COMA
Another name for portal-systemic encephalopathy.

HEPATIC ENCEPHALO-PATHY

Another name for portal-systemic encephalopathy.

HEPATITIS

An inflammation of the liver, characterized by:
- jaundice;
- loss of appetite;
- abdominal discomfort;
- enlarged liver;
- abnormally functioning liver.

It may be caused by bacterial or viral infection, infestation with parasites, alcohol, drugs, toxins, transfusions of incompatible blood, or as a complication of another disease and may be mild and brief or prolonged and severe, even life-threatening.

HEPATITIS ASSOCIATED ANTIGEN

An antigen often found in the blood serum of people who have had hepatitis; the blood test for this antigen is used to detect type B (serum) hepatitis, and to differentiate it from type A (infectious) hepatitis.

HEPATIZATION

Transformation of an organ into a liver-like mass, especially the solid state of the lung in certain types of pneumonia.

HEPATOCIRRHOSIS

Hardening and other degenerative changes (fibrosis) in the liver.

HEPATOMA

A tumor of the liver that is usually malignant.

HEPATOMEGALY

Enlargement of the liver, due to some disease or disorder of the liver.

HEPATORENAL SYNDROME

A disease or disorder affecting both the liver and kidneys.

HEPATOTOXIC

Medicine or agent having an injurious effect on liver cells.

HEPATOTOXICS

Medications that can possibly cause toxicity or decreased normal function of the liver.

HEREDITARY ANGIO-EDEMA

A form of angio-edema (swelling of the loose tissues of the body) transmitted as an autosomal dominant trait and associated with a deficiency in the blood.

HEREDITARY ATAXIAS

A group of hereditary diseases characterized by degenerative changes in the spinal cord, the cerebellum and, often, the brainstem, peripheral nerves and other portions of the nervous system, resulting in impaired coordination of body movements.

HEREDITY

(1) The process by which specific traits or characteristics are transmitted, through genes, from parents to offspring;
(2) the total genetic makeup of an individual.

HEREDITARY HEMOR-RHAGIC TELANGIECTASIA

An abnormal widening of arterioles (tiny arteries) and capillaries, resulting in tumors of the skin and mucosa, inherited as an autosomal dominant trait.

HEREDITARY LEPTOCY-TOSIS

Another name for thalassemia.

HEREDITARY NEPHRITIS

A disorder that runs in families and is characterized by hematuria (blood in the urine), functional impairment of the kidneys, deafness due to a damaged acoustic nerve and, on occasion, abnormalities in vision.

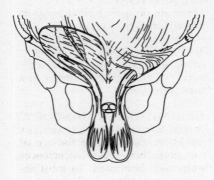

Frontal view of the inguinal region of the male individual.

HERMAPHRODITIC DREAM

Dream that is bisexual in character, and evidence, in the opinion of some psychoanalysts, of the bipolarity of the sexual impulse itself.

HERMAPHRODITISM

Presence of both male and female reproductive organs in the same organism.

HERNIA

Protrusion of abdominal contents through the abdominal wall in the inguinal or femoral part of the groin, into the navel (umbilicus, infants only) or through the diaphragm (hiatus hernia).

Hernia may occur because of a congenital defect or because there is an area of muscle weakness. Parts of the intestines and omentum (a fold of membrane that hangs down in the abdominal cavity) are commonly found in hernial sacs, and if there is a tight constriction at the neck of the sac (i.e., the hernia is strangulated), the intestines may be obstructed or suffer gangrene. In hiatus hernia, part of the stomach protrudes into the esophagus.

Inguinal, femoral and umbilical hernias may need surgery to reposition the intestines and close the defect, but this is rare in hiatus hernia.

HERNIA, HIATUS

Protrusion of abdominal contents, usually a portion of the stomach, through the muscular ring - the cardiac sphincter - that separates the stomach and the esophagus, or through another gap in the diaphragm. Symptoms include a sensation of fullness or pain behind the breastbone, especially after eating, and heartburn and chest or upper abdominal pain are common.

Symptoms commonly occur after a large meal or when there is pressure on the abdomen. Problems may be accentuated by lying down.

Hiatus hernia often appears in middle or old age; the potential gap may have always been present but did not cause symptoms. Anything that increases the pressure inside the abdomen will tend to push the abdominal contents into the chest, and this is why the condition is especially common in pregnant women. The condition can lead to severe pain or discomfort, as well as to esophagitis (inflammation of the esophagus) if stomach acid repeatedly spills up into the esophagus. Severe chest pain can also cause justified worry about heart disease. Some people with this problem repeatedly regurgitate food and liquid, especially at night, and have chronic aspiration and pneumonia.

Treatment involves dieting if the person is overweight, avoiding bending down and drinking before bedtime, sleeping propped up on two or three pillows and regularly taking antacids to neutralize stomach acid. If all this fails, there is a surgical operation that can be performed to repair the weakness in the diaphragm, but today this is rarely needed.

HERNIA, INGUINAL

Protrusion of intestines or other abdominal contents through a gap in the muscles and tissues of the groin. More common in men than in women, the protruding mass can usually be felt in the groin or in the scrotum and may be large or small. The hernia is usually first noted as a swelling in the groin and/or scrotum, usually without discomfort if small, but as it becomes larger, it may cause a feeling of dragging in the groin or scrotum. Swelling may come and go or change in size. The cause is failure of the normal gap between tissues in the groin to close. The opening is normal in fetal life, especially in males because the testicles need to descend down through it. With increased pressure inside the abdomen, the intestine is pushed down through the gap, leading to swelling of the testicles. This may result from injury or straining.

The condition is a nagging problem that can be relieved by the wearing of a truss -a special belt that holds in the hernia - but it really requires surgical correction, in which the defect is "darned." In infancy there is a significant risk for the hernia to incarcerate (get stuck in the gap), leading to probable damage to the bowel itself.

HERNIOPLASTY
Surgical procedure for the repair of a hernia in order to prevent recurrence.

HERNIORRHAPHY
Surgical procedure for the repair of a hernia in which the weak area is reinforced by some of the person's own tissues.

HERNIOTOMY
A cutting operation for the repair of a hernia.

HEROIN
A strongly addictive drug made from morphine; it has no specific medical use but is widely abused.

HERPES
A virus with several forms, capable of causing painful infection of lips, trunk, nerves or genital organs.

There are several different but related herpes viruses. The first, and probably the best known, is herpes simplex I (or herpes virus hominus type I). It is the cause of the common cold sore (fever blister) that frequently appears on the lips, in and around the mouth, and sometimes in the throat. Most often, those who acquire a herpes simplex I infection do so before the age of five and then have recurrences throughout their lives. In most instances, the sores heal within a week or two.

Herpes simplex II (herpes virus hominus type II) causes sores similar to cold sores but they are almost always in, on and around the genital organs and urinary passageways. Today, genital herpes, as herpes simplex II is also known, is considered one of the most potentially dangerous sexually transmitted diseases (formerly called venereal diseases). Not only can it cause miscarriage, especially in the first months of pregnancy, but it can also damage an unborn baby's central nervous system, if it is affected while still in the womb, or its eyes if it becomes infected during delivery. It is also believed that herpes simplex II slightly increases the risk of cancer of the cervix. The third herpes virus is herpes zoster, or varicella-zoster virus, and is the cause of chickenpox as well as shingles, so-called because of the narrow layers of blister-like skin eruptions that appear around the trunk or extremities of the body when the virus travels down the nerves to the skin surface. While chickenpox is commonly a disease of childhood, herpes zoster is largely a disease of late middle and old age. Other herpes viruses are: herpes virus simiai, primarily the cause of a disease in monkeys in captivity, but a condition that can bring on encephalitis and herpes zoster-like symptoms in humans if they are bitten by infected monkeys; cytomegalovirus; and the Epstein-Barr virus that causes glandular fever (infectious mononucleosis).

HERPES GENITALIS
Another name for genital herpes.

HERPES LABIALIS
The sores or blisters that sometimes occur around the mouth in association with the common cold.

HERPES SIMPLEX
Also called cold sores: a recurrent viral infection characterized by the appearance on the skin or mucous membranes of single or multiple clusters of small blisters, filled with clear fluid, on slightly raised inflammatory bases. There is no medicine, either taken by mouth or placed directly on the cold sores, that will do anything to eliminate them. Treatment is based on the relief of symptoms.

HERPES SIMPLEX KERATITIS
A herpes simplex virus infection in which the cornea of the eye becomes inflamed, commonly leading to chronic inflammation, blood shot eyes, scarring and loss of vision.

HERPES ZOSTER
Commonly called shingles: an acute infection of the central nervous system involving primarily the dorsal root ganglia, and characterized by the eruption of blisters and acute neuralgic pain in the areas of the skin supplied by peripheral sensory nerves arising in the affected root ganglia.

Shingles last from ten days to five weeks and can be very painful. If all of the blisters appear within 24 hours, the length of the disease is shortened.

It can be set off by exposure to someone with chickenpox (which is caused by the same virus). There is no specific treatment. However, a corticosteroid, may relieve pain in severe cases.

HERPES ZOSTER OTICUS
Inflammation of the sensory nerve cell bodies of the eighth cranial nerve caused by the herpes zoster virus, producing severe ear pain, hearing loss, dizziness and paralysis of the facial nerve. Corticosteroid therapy is the treatment of choice.

HETEROEROTISM
Sexual interest in persons other than oneself, especially of the opposite sex.

HETEROMORPHOSIS
Development of an organ or structure in a position other than that in which it is normally found.

HETEROPHIL ANTIBODY TEST
A test using the red blood cells of sheep to diagnose glandular fever (infectious mononucleosis).

HETEROPLASTY
Transplantation of tissues or cells from one individual to another of a different species.

HETEROSEXUAL
Attracted towards the opposite sex; pertaining to, characteristic of the opposite sex.

HETEROTOPIC
Situated in an abnormal location; said of grafts placed in an abnormal site in the recipient, e.g., a kidney transplant placed in one of the iliac fossae (a depression at each lower corner of the abdomen).

HETEROTROPIA
Another name for strabismus.

HETEROZYGOTE
An individual possessing different alleles (alternative forms of the same gene) at a given locus on a pair of homologous chromosomes.

HEXACHLOROPHENE
Generic name of an antiseptic substance used to prevent skin infections.

HEXOSE
A monosaccharide (simple sugar) containing six carbon atoms in each molecule.

HGH
Abbreviation of human growth hormone, secreted by certain types of cells in the anterior part of the pituitary gland. A deficiency of this may lead to restricted growth.

HIATAL HERNIA
Section of stomach that protrudes into the chest cavity.

HIATUS
An empty space or opening.

HIATUS HERNIA
Protrusion of the stomach above the diaphragm (see Hernia, hiatus).

HICCUP
Repeated involuntary spasmodic contractions of the diaphragm, followed by sudden closure of the glottis (small space between the vocal cords), which checks the inflow of air and produces the characteristic sounds. A sudden onset of forceful hiccups may persist for hours or days. They can cause exhaustion and soreness of the muscles of the abdomen.

Many things have been tried with varying success: breath-holding, distraction, sudden scares, drinking water. Most often, the hiccups go away in a short time, regardless of what is done. For severe, long-lasting hiccups, medical evaluation and treatment is needed. Sedative drugs, antacids and medications that reduce intestinal movement are most often tried.

On rare occasions surgery to cut the nerve that supplies the diaphragm is needed.

HIDRADENITIS SUPPURATIVA
An inflammation of the apocrine sweat glands resulting in obstruction and rupture of the ducts with painful local inflammation. Most lesions occur in the armpits or groin, but they may also be found around the nipples or anus. Susceptible people should avoid antiperspirants and other irritants. Early simple cases are treated with rest, moist heat and prolonged systemic antibiotic therapy.

HIGH BLOOD PRESSURE
Common name for hypertension.

HILUM
A depression or pit on an organ, giving entrance and exit to vessels and nerves - for example, hilum pulmonis, the depression on the medial surface of the lung.

HINTON TEST
A blood test for syphilis.

HIP
Area of the body formed by the lower part of the torso (pelvis) and the upper part of the thigh.

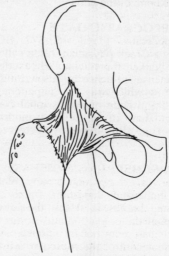

Anterior view of the hip joint. The capsule and its ligaments are shown.

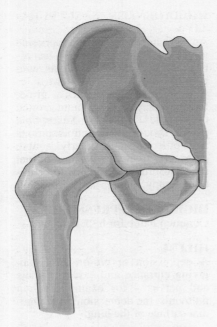

Anterior view of the hip joint. The head or caput of the femur fits into the acetabulum of the pelvis.

HIP JOINT
A ball-and-socket joint in which the head of the femur (thigh bone) fits into the acetabulum of the innominate bone of the pelvis.

HIPPOCRATIC OATH
Hippocrates (circa 460-377 BC) was a Greek physician, often called the "father of medicine." He exerted immense influence by his writings, among which was the "Hippocratic Oath," a code of professional conduct that, in its revised modern form, is still followed by doctors today.

HIRSCHSPRUNG'S DISEASE
Also called congenital megacolon: an inherited condition found in young babies in which the lower part of the colon contains no nerve cells, is enormously dilated and cannot control the muscular movements that normally push the feces out.

The baby will have severe abdominal pain, swelling, constipation and, occasionally, vomiting. Surgery is needed to remove the ineffective part of the colon and to attach the remaining healthy intestine to the anus.

HIRSUTE
Shaggy, hairy.

HIRUDOID CREAM
Nongreasy cream containing heparin in an absorbable base; useful for inflammation of the skin and hemorrhoids (piles).

HIS BUNDLE ARRHYTHMIA
An arrhythmia (abnormal heart rhythm) that results from sustained enhanced automaticity within the bundle of His, the major impulse conduction system of the heart.

HISTAMINE
Substance produced by the body as part of an allergic reaction; it causes dilation of blood vessels, lowered blood pressure and stimulation of secretions from the stomach and other organs.

HISTIDINE
An amino acid obtainable from many proteins by the action of sulphuric acid and water; it is essential for optimal growth in infants. Histamine is derived from the decomposition of this.

HISTIOCYTE
A large phagocytic cell of tissue origin.

HISTIOCYTOSIS
A condition marked by the abnormal appearance of histiocytes in the body - for example, as in Hand-Schueller-Christian disease.

HISTOLOGY
Medical and biological science dealing with the microscopic study of tissues.

HISTONE
A simple protein found combined as salts with acidic substances - for instance, the protein combined with the globin of hemoglobin.

HISTOPLASMA AGGLUTININS
Agglutinins - that is, antibodies in the blood involved in the agglutination (sticking together) of foreign antigens - associated with fungal lung infection.

HISTOPLASMOSIS
An infectious disease that is endemic in parts of Africa, South America and the United States and is caused by the fungus Histoplasma capsulatum. It is characterized by damage to the lungs and occasional anemia, with ulcerations of the mouth and the gastrointestinal tract, enlargement of the liver and spleen, disorder of the lymph glands and necrosis (tissue death) of the adrenal glands. If not treated early with an antifungal agent, a severe attack can be fatal. It is particularly common in infants and older men.

HISTRIONIC PERSONALITY DISORDER
A pervasive pattern of excessive emotionality and attention-seeking, beginning by early adulthood and present in a variety of contexts.

People with this disorder constantly seek or demand reassurance, approval, or praise from others and are uncomfortable in situations in which they are not the center of attention. They characteristically display rapidly shifting and shallow expression of emotions.

Their behavior is overly reactive and intensely expressed; minor stimuli give rise to emotional excitability.

Emotions are often expressed with inappropriate exaggeration, for example, the person may appear much more sad, angry, or delighted then would seem to be warranted. People with this disorder tend to be very self-centered, with little or no tolerance for the frustration of delayed gratification. Their actions are directed to obtaining immediate satisfaction.

These people are typically attractive and seductive, often to the point of looking flamboyant and acting inappropriately. They are typically overly concerned with physical attractiveness. In addition, their style of speech tends to be expressionistic and lacking in detail. For example, a person may describe his vacation as "Just fantastic!" without being able to be more specific.

The disorder is apparently common, and is diagnosed much more frequently in females than in males.

HIVES
Another name for urticaria.

HLA SYSTEM
A group of tissue antigens - human leukocyte antigens - that appear on the surfaces of cells throughout the body; their positions and types are inherited. They are responsible for rejection reactions in organ transplants: the HLA antigens on the transplant are recognized by the body as "foreign.". More than 50 such antigens have been identified, each of us having four of them. They are what is looked for in "tissue typing."

HOARSENESS
The state or quality of having a harsh, rough, grating voice, as when affected with a cold.

Hoarseness, roughness or harshness of the voice arises when there is interference with the vibrations of the vocal cords. This is most often caused by inflammation of the vocal cords and surrounding areas, due either to infection or to irritation. Inflammation causes swelling of the lining tissues, so the vibrations are distorted.

Hoarseness can also be caused by growths on the vocal cords, which also interfere with their usual vibrations because of distortion. More unusual causes of hoarseness are paralysis of a vocal cord and a few congenital abnormalities of the vocal cords and windpipe.

Hoarseness as a symptom can occur with abuse of the voice (e.g., screaming). With this and other sudden causes, the symptoms are usually temporary. If hoarseness or another change in the voice persists over several weeks, be sure to obtain a medical evaluation.

HOBNAIL LIVER
Popular term for severe cirrhosis of the liver, usually due to alcohol abuse or a parasitic disease.

HODGKIN'S DISEASE
A malignant disorder in which there is painless, progressive enlargement of lymph tissue. Symptoms include:
- generalized itching;
- weight loss;
- loss of appetite;
- low-grade fever;
- night sweats.

It occurs more often among males and usually manifests itself between the ages of 15 and 35.

Treatment with radiotherapy and/or chemotherapy effects long-term remissions in more than half of cases and cures in a larger percentage those with localized disease.

HOLISM
The principle that an organism comprises more than the sum of its parts and must be studied as a whole. The term holistic medicine is used to describe the treatment of the whole person - his/her body, emotions, mind and spirit - not just a symptom or a disease.

HOLISTIC-DYNAMIC PSYCHOLOGY
Theory based on the innate goodness of human nature. In this, the fundamental human needs are good or neutral rather than evil.

HOMAN'S SIGN
Passive dorsal flexion (bending of the foot towards the calf) that causes pain in the calf muscles. It is indicative of established venous thrombosis (inflammation of a vein usually associated with a clot) of the leg.

HOMEOPATHY
A medical system, based on the idea that "like cures like," which uses drugs or other substances that would produce in healthy persons the symptoms shown by the sick person, e.g., treating a fever by giving small doses of a drug that raises body temperature.

HOMEOSTASIS
The self-regulating mechanisms whereby biological systems attempt to maintain a stable internal condition in the face of changes in the external environment. It was the 19th-century French physiologist Claude Bernard who first realized that the internal environment of any free living organism is maintained constant within certain limits.

Homeostasis is generally achieved through two types of regulating systems: on-off control and feedback control. Hormones often play a vital role in maintaining homeostatic stability.

HOMO-EROTISM
Erotic or libidinal feeling directed towards a person of the same sex.

HOMOGRAFT
A tissue or organ that is transplanted from one individual to another of the same species, such as in kidney or heart transplants.

HOMOSEXUALITY
Sexual preference for persons of the same sex.

HOMOVANILLIC ACID
A product of normal metabolism; elevated urine levels may indicate various tumors of the adrenal gland.

HOMOZYGOTE
An individual possessing a pair of identical alleles (variations of the same gene) at a given position on a pair of homologous chromosomes.

HONEYMOON CYSTITIS
Common bladder condition, usually the result of very frequent intercourse. The symptoms are bladder cramps, burning during urination and blood in the urine. The disease need not be the result of a bladder infection; it may be caused by an inflammation of the wall of the bladder. Excessive stimulation of the cervix during sexual intercourse can lead to a low-grade cervicitis (erosion of the cervix), and the inflammation can spread via the lymphatic pathways to part of the bladder wall, resulting in honeymoon cystitis. If the condition is of bacterial origin, appropriate antibiotics will be given. Otherwise, treatment is for the relief of symptoms. Sometimes a change in position during sexual intercourse or using alternative forms of love-making can help.

HOOKWORM DISEASE
Also called ancylostomiasis: a symptomatic infection caused by the worms Ancylostoma duodenale or Necator americanus and characterized by abdominal pain and iron-deficiency anaemia. The 12 mm (1/2 in) worms live in the small intestine and produce enormous numbers of eggs. These are passed out in the faeces, when they can pollute soil and drinking water.

Preventing soil pollution and avoiding direct skin contact with the soil are effective but impractical measures in most endemic areas. Periodic mass treatment with anthelmintics (drugs that kill parasitic worms) and dietary iron supplements may be effective.

HORDEOLUM
Stye on the eyelid that looks like a barley grain.

HORIZONTAL DECALAGE
Ability to transfer what is learned in one area to another.

HORMONES
Substances produced in living organisms to affect growth, differentiation, metabolism, digestive function, mineral and fluid balance, and usually acting at a distance from their site of origin.

Hormones are secreted by endocrine glands (or analogous structures) into the bloodstream, which then carries them to their point of action. The rate of secretion, efficacy on target organs and rate of removal are all affected by numerous factors including feedback from their metabolic effects, mineral or sugar concentration in the blood and the action of controlling hormones. The latter usually originate in the pituitary gland, and those controlling the pituitary come from the hypothalamus. Important hormones include: insulin; thyroid hormone; adrenaline; steroids; parahormone (parathyroid gland hormone); glucagon; gonadotrophins; estrogen; progesterone; androgens; oxytocin; antidiuretic hormone (ADH); growth hormone; prolactin; vasopressin; thyroxine; thyroid-stimulating hormone (TSH); adrenocorticotrophic hormone (ACTH); gastrin; secretin.

HORMONOTHERAPY
Treatment by hormones; usually as substitution therapy in cases of a deficiency in the body of particular hormones.

HORN
A substance mainly composed of keratin, of which hair and nails are composed.

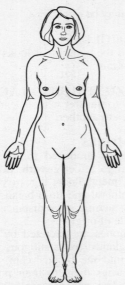

The contours of the female human body differ from the contours of the male.

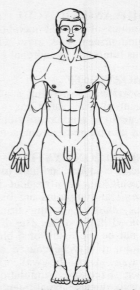

The contours of the male human body differ from the contours of the female.

HORNER'S SYNDROME
A collection of symptoms characterized by
- sinking in of the eyeball;
- ptosis (drooping) of the upper eye lid;
- slight elevation of the lower lid;
- miosis (contraction) of the pupil;
- anidrosis (abnormal reduction of sweat) of the affected side of the face.
 The syndrome is due to paralysis of the cervical part of the sympathetic nervous system (in the neck).

HORSESHOE KIDNEY
A congenital defect in which the kidneys, instead of being separate, are joined at their lower ends, forming a horseshoe shape. It is more common in males than in females.

HORTON'S SYNDROME
A condition characterized by bouts of severe headache due to the release of excessive amounts of histamine in the body.

HOSPITALISM
A syndrome resulting from institutionalization in infancy after early separation from the mother, and characterized by a lag in mental and physical development, apathy, immobility, withdrawal reactions in the presence of strangers, frequent infections and sometimes death.

HOST
The organic structure upon which parasites thrive; the recipient of a transplanted organ or tissue.

HOUSEMAID'S KNEE
Popular term for an inflammation of the bursa in the front of the knee.

HUMAN BODY
The physical substrate of humans, Homo sapiens. In terms of anatomy, it consists of the head and neck; a trunk divided into the chest, abdomen and pelvis; and four limbs -two arms and two legs.
  The head contains (within the bony structure of the skull) the brain, which is connected by cranial nerves to the special sense organs for vision (eyes), hearing and balance (ears), smell (nose) and taste

(tongue and nose). On the front of the head is the face, specialized for communication (including the special senses), and through which the voice emanates.

The head sits at the top of the spinal column of vertebrae, which continue through the neck and the thorax and lumbar regions of the back to the sacrum and coccyx in the pelvis.

The spinal column is the central structural pillar of the musculoskeletal system, and it is on to this that the ribs and pelvic bones are jointed. Within the bony spinal canal is the spinal cord - the downward extension of the brain concerned with relaying information to and from the body and with segmental reflex behavior. It is linked with the various parts of the body by the peripheral and autonomic nervous systems. The chest, abdomen and pelvis contain many vital organs comprising the various functional systems.

HUMANISTIC PSYCHOLOGY
An offshoot of existentialism and tectorium. This branch of psychology stresses the holistic approach, creativity and self-actualization, intentionalism, free choice and spontaneity.

HUMANIZED MILK
Cow's milk that has been reduced in fat and increased in sugar so that it closely resembles human milk.

HUMAN PLACENTAL LACTOGEN
A hormone secreted by the placenta during pregnancy; levels may be decreased in certain abnormalities of pregnancy.

HUMATROPE
Brand name of a drug containing as active compound somatropin, a synthetic pituitary hormone, used for the treatment of certain deficiency states.

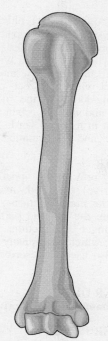

Anterior view of the right humerus.

HUMERUS
The bone of the upper arm.

HUMORAL
Pertaining to bodily fluids, as opposed to cellular elements; hence, those aspects of the immune response that are associated with circulating antibody.

HUMORAL IMMUNE SYSTEM
That portion of the immune system mediated by antibodies produced by B cells. B cells comprise 30 percent of blood lymphocytes.

HUMORS
In ancient and medieval medicine, the four bodily fluids whose balance was required for the individual's health. They correspond to the four elements: blood (fire); phlegm (water); choler, or yellow bile (air); and melancholy, or black bile (earth).

Excess of blood (hot and dry), for example, made one sanguine;

phlegm (cold and wet), phlegmatic, etc. Cure was by enantiopathy -that is, treatment with opposites - so that a fever would be treated with cold and so forth. The idea may have originated with the Greek philosopher Empedocles in the fifth century BC, and we still retain some-thing of it in modern words such as "choleric" and "phlegmatic."

HUNGER
Normally referring to appetite (impulse, drive) for food; may refer also to the mass of uneasy sensations from the gut and particularly from hunger contractions in the stomach, which accompany the appetite; also used to describe sexual appetite.

HUNGER DRIVE
A drive based on food deprivation.

HUNGER PANGS
The twinges of pain experienced during stomach contractions.

HUNTERIAN CHANCRE
The hard sore of primary syphilis.

HUNTINGTON'S CHOREA
A hereditary disease beginning in adulthood, characterized by involuntary movements and mental deterioration. Symptoms usually begin between the ages of 30 and 50, but personality changes and inappropriate behavior may precede the involuntary jerky, irregular movements. The chorea responds to some drugs. There is no treatment for the mental decline. Children of a parent with this disease have a 50/50 chance of developing it.

HURLER'S SYNDROME
An inherited metabolic disease (a mucopolysaccharidosis) due to deficiency of the enzyme l-iduronidase, characterized by the following symptoms:
- gargoyle facial expression;
- dwarfism;
- severe physical and skeletal changes;
- cloudy corneas and deafness;
- enlargement of the spleen and liver;
- contractures of some joints.

HUTCHINSON'S PUPIL
A diagnostic sign of hemorrhage into the brain. The pupil on the side of the hemorrhage is dilated, that on the other side is contracted.

HUTCHINSON'S TEETH
Peg-shaped incisor teeth, notched at the cutting edge, seen in those suffering from hereditary syphilis.

HUTCHINSON'S TRIAD
Three conditions diagnostic of hereditary syphilis. They are:
(1) diffuse inflammation of the eye, especially of the cornea.
(2) disease of the labyrinth of the ear.
(3) Hutchinson's teeth.

HYALINE
A clear, homogenous, glassy-looking material occurring normally in cartilage and the vitreous body of the eye, in the colloid contained in the thyroid gland, and in the umbilical cord, but also seen in tissue degeneration.

HYALINE MEMBRANE DISEASE
Another term for respiratory distress syndrome.

HYALURONIDASE
An enzyme preparation used to facilitate the diffusion of injected drugs. It is also found in snake venom.

HYDATID
The cyst formed by larvae of the tapeworm, Echinococcus.

HYDATIFORM MOLE
Another term for trophoblastic disease.

HYDRADENITIS
Inflammation of the sweat glands in the armpit.

HYDRAMNIOS
Accumulation of fluid in the amniotic sac in which the unborn baby lies.

HYDRARGAPHEN
Generic name of a drug containing mercury as the active compound. It is used in skin applications for the treatment of skin infections, both by bacteria and fungi.

HYDRARTHROSIS
An accumulation of effused watery fluid in a joint cavity, due to allergic conditions or injury.

HYDROA
General term for any skin disease characterized by the formation of little blisters.

HYDROCELE
Collection of fluid in the tunica vaginalis of the testis or along the spermatic cord.

HYDROCEPHALIC
Relating to hydrocephalus.

HYDROCEPHALUS
Enlargement of the brain ventricles due to increased cerebrospinal fluid (CSF) within the skull. In children, it causes a characteristic enlargement of the head. Brain tissue is attenuated (stretched) and damaged by long-standing hydrocephalus.

It may be caused by a block to CSF drainage in the lower ventricles or brainstem aqueduct (e.g. by tumor and malformation, including those seen with spina bifida) or by prevention of its reabsorption over the brain surface (e.g., following meningitis).

Apart from attention to the cause, treatment may include draining the CSF, using either the Spitz-Holter or Pudenz-Heyer shunt in which a tube runs between the ventricle in the brain and, respectively, the right atrium of the heart or the abdomen.

HYDROCORTISONE
Naturally occurring corticosteroid isolated from the adrenal glands of animals and humans. It is given by mouth and injection, and it is also applied externally in ointments, creams and lotions.

Hydrocortisone is readily and quickly absorbed from the gut, even in malabsorption syndromes or after total or partial removal of the stomach.

High corticosteroid levels are reached within one hour and persist (though falling) for six to eight hours. Taking the drug by mouth is preferred for long-term therapy.

HYDRO-ENCEPHALOCELE
An aberration of brain development in which the brain cavity protruding from the skull connects with the cerebral ventricles.

HYDROGEN
Chemical element, atomic number 1, symbol H. It is a colorless, odorless gas. The hydrogen ion concentration is a measure of the acidity or alkalinity of body fluids, ranging from pH 1 to 14, 7 being approximately neutral.

HYDROGEN PEROXIDE
Oxidizing agent, which may cause poisoning. Hydrogen peroxide is an oxidizing liquid marketed as aqueous solutions ranging from the common concentration of 3 percent as a topical antiseptic, 6 percent in hair preparations (bleaches, neutralizers and so forth), to 30 percent for industrial and laboratory use and 90 percent for use in rocket propulsion.

HYDROLYSIS
The chemical splitting of large molecules into simpler substances by the addition of water.

HYDROMA
Accumulation of watery fluid in a sac, cyst or bursa. A congenital hydroma, situated in the neck, may be present at birth.

HYDROMYELIA
A dilation of the central canal of the spinal cord associated with an increase of fluid in this canal due to a tumor or injury.

HYDRONEPHROSIS
Distention of a kidney because of the retention of an abnormal amount of urine. This is a result of the blockage of the ureter, interrupting the flow of urine out of the kidney, and leads to progressive loss of kidney function.

HYDROPERICARDIUM
Fluid in the pericardial sac covering the heart, usually in the absence of inflammation. This condition can occur in heart failure, but also in severe kidney failure.

HYDROPERITONEUM
The presence of fluid within the abdominal cavity.

HYDROPHOBIA
Dread of water, one of the defining symptoms of rabies, in which the sufferer is unable to face swallowing fluids.

HYDROPNEUMOTHORAX
A collection of fluid and gas in the pleural cavity (containing the lungs), impeding normal breathing movements. The condition is mostly due to a severe inflammation such as tuberculosis.

HYDROPS FETALIS
Another name for erythroblastosis foetalis.

HYDROSALPINX
Accumulation of watery fluid in the Fallopian tube; the condition is usually due to severe inflammation, such as pelvic inflammatory disease.

HYDROTHERAPY
The use of water to treat disorders, mostly limited to exercises in special pools for rehabilitation of paralyzed patients.

HYDROTHORAX
The accumulation of fluid in the pleural cavity (the cavity between the lungs and the wall of the chest).

HYDRO-URETER
Distention of the ureter, the tube leading from the kidney to the bladder, due to an obstruction at its lower end.

HYDROXYPROLINE
An amino acid (one of the basic building blocks of proteins). Hydroxyproline is unique in that it exists mostly in collagen, a substance found in bone and in slightly smaller amounts in the skin. While hydroxyproline levels in the blood are primarily an indication of a bone condition or bone disease, a test to discover them is also used to search for certain inherited conditions. Although hydroxyproline can be found in the blood, the test is most often performed on urine.

5-HYDROXYTRYPTAMINE
A substance in blood and tissues that constricts blood vessels and transmits nerve impulses. The level of it is elevated in the urine in carcinoid syndrome -a condition produced by a type of tumor found in the appendix or lower intestinal tract, and sometimes in the lungs.

HYGIENE
The principles of maintaining health. In common usage, hygiene has become almost synonymous with "cleanliness," but it covers many other areas, such as baths, clothing, diet, exercise, sanitation, ventilation, water supplies and, in

particular, the cooking, storing and preserving of food.

HYMEN
Also called the maidenhead: a fold of mucous membrane that partially blocks the external opening of the vagina. The hymen is located beyond the labia minora, about 1 cm (½ in) inside the vaginal opening. A small membrane or rudiment of a membrane, it is usually broken after the first sexual intercourse, but fragments will remain in place throughout a woman's life. When it is broken, the hymen looks like small pieces of flesh around the circumference of the vaginal wall. Occasionally, the hymen lingers as a long piece of flesh, and this can be surgically removed if it is bothersome. Some women are born with extremely small hymens. These women will have little problem or pain during first intercourse; sometimes the hymen does not even rip.

HYMENECTOMY
Surgical operation to remove the hymen in a case of imperforated hymen. If the hymen is completely closed, a problem would develop when a girl starts menstruation - the blood will collect behind the hymen period after period, and cause severe pain, eventually requiring surgical intervention.

HYMENOTOMY
Surgical incision or division of the hymen.

HYOID
U-shaped bone at the base of the tongue, which can be felt in front of the neck, just above the Adam's apple.

HYPERACIDITY
Abnormally large amounts of acid in the stomach.

HYPERACTIVITY
Abnormal and excessive activity.

HYPERACUITY
Abnormal perception of sound. Hyperactivity is also the most characteristic symptom of the Attention deficit disorder with Hyperactivity (ADHD).

HYPERALGESIA
Increased sensibility to pain.

HYPERBILIRUBINEMIA
Excessive bilirubin (a by-product of the liver) in the blood, classified as conjugated or non-conjugated, according to the predominant form of bilirubin present. A characteristic form is the jaundice of the newborn.

HYPERCALCEMIA
An excess of calcium in the blood - for instance, conditions associated with overdosages of vitamin B or severe kidney disease. Infantile hypercalcaemia is a rare condition found in children.

HYPERCALCEMIA-CAUSING MEDICATIONS
Medicines that cause too much calcium in the blood.

HYPERCALCIURIA
An excess of calcium in the blood, such as in the overfunctioning of the parathyroid glands; the condition may lead to the occurrence of kidney stones.

HYPERCAPNIA
An excess of carbon dioxide in the blood.

HYPERCHOLESTEROLEMIA
Excessive amount of cholesterol in the blood. A person with this condition is generally predisposed to atherosclerosis and resulting artery and heart disorders.

HYPEREMESIS
Excessive vomiting; sometimes a complication of pregnancy that may become serious.

HYPEREMESIS GRAVIDARUM

Severe nausea and vomiting to the extent that the pregnant woman becomes dehydrated and her blood becomes too acid. Those with this disorder do not gain weight and usually lose weight.

It differs from "morning sickness" in that many pregnant women with morning sickness feel as though they are vomiting everything that is ingested, but they continue to gain weight and do not become dehydrated.

Psychological factors are prominent in this syndrome but do not lessen the danger. Antihistamines or tranquillizers may halt the vomiting, and pyridoxine (vitamin B6) may stop it completely; however, many sufferers have to enter hospital where their diet and fluid intake can be carefully controlled. The cause for this is not known.

HYPEREXTENSION

Extreme or excessive extension of a limb or part; overextension is, to some degree, a physical phenomenon in the elbow joint.

HYPERFLEXION

Extreme or excessive bending of a limb or part.

HYPERGLYCEMIA

Excessive amount of sugar in the blood; if untreated, it can lead to a diabetic coma.

HYPERGLYCINEMIA

Excessive amount of the amino acid glycine in the blood. This is an inherited metabolic disorder, usually characterized by:
- episodic vomiting;
- lethargy;
- dehydration;
- ketosis (poisoning by various by-products of the partial metabolism of fats).
- increased susceptibility to infection.

HYPERHIDROSIS

Also spelled hyperidrosis: excessive perspiration, sometimes due to a disorder of the autonomic nervous system.

HYPERINSULINISM

Also called a "hypo" reaction: a deficiency of sugar in the blood, due to an excess of insulin. This can be a life-threatening condition for diabetics, and emergency medical help is required.

HYPERKERATOSIS

Excessive formation of the horny layer of the skin, or enlargement of the cornea.

HYPERKINESIS

Abnormally increased muscular function or activity; usually due to a disturbance of the basal ganglia of the brain.

HYPERLIPEMIA

High blood level of cholesterol and/or triglycerides.

HYPERLIPOPROTEINEMIA TYPE I

A relatively rare disorder due to either a congenital deficiency of lipoprotein lipase activity or the congenital absence of the lipase-activating protein apolipoprotein.

HYPERLIPOPROTEINEMIA TYPE II

A genetic disorder of lipid metabolism characterized by an elevated level of cholesterol in the blood in association with xanthelasma (a skin disease), tendon and tuberous xanthomas (soft, yellow cholesterol deposits), accelerated atherosclerosis and early death from heart attack.

HYPERLIPOPROTEINEMIA TYPE III

A less common disorder that runs in families and is characterized by the accumulation in blood serum of a low-density lipoprotein, associated with the presence of xanthomas and a marked predisposition to severe premature atherosclerosis.

HYPERLIPOPROTEINEMIA TYPE IV
A common disorder, often running in families, characterized by variable elevations of triglycerides in the blood and a possible predisposition to atherosclerosis.

HYPERLIPOPROTEINEMIA TYPE V
An uncommon disorder, sometimes running in families and associated with defective clearance of triglycerides (both those taken into the body and those produced by the body itself) and the risk of life-threatening pancreatitis (inflammation of the pancreas).

HYPERMANIA
An extreme manic state characterized by excessive activity and excitement.

HYPERMETABOLISM
Increased metabolism; a high metabolic rate, characteristic of increased function of the thyroid gland (thyrotoxicosis).

HYPERMETROPIA
Long-sightedness: a condition of the eye in which incoming parallel light rays focus behind the retina due to an abnormal shortness of the eyeball or to subnormal refraction.

HYPERMOBILITY
Excessive mobility in a joint, usually due to laxity of fibrous bands.

HYPERPARATHYROIDISM
Overactivity of the parathyroid glands, usually due to a small tumor.

HYPERPERISTALSIS
Excessive activity of the involuntary muscles of the gastrointestinal tract that push food through the system.

HYPERPHAGIA
Uncontrolled excessive eating. This may be caused by diabetes mellitus or by disease of or injury to the hypothalamus in the brain.

HYPERPHORIA
A condition in which the visual axis of one eye is above or below that of the other.

HYPERPIGMENTATION
Abnormally increased pigmentation of the skin, usually due to an endocrine disorder.

HYPERPITUITARISM
Overfunction of the pituitary gland, resulting in acromegaly or gigantism.

HYPERPLASIA
Abnormal increase in the number of normal cells in normal arrangement in an organ or tissue, which increases its volume.

HYPERPNEA
Abnormal increase in the rate and depth of breathing. This can occur normally as part of exertion, or it can be caused by a blood or brain disorder.

HYPERPOTASSEMIA
Excessive amount of potassium in the blood. This may cause a disturbance in the function of excitable cells, particularly the muscle fibers of the heart.

HYPERPYREXIA
Another name for heat stroke.

HYPERSECRETION
Excessive secretion of endocrine or exocrine cells.

HYPERSENSITIVITY
Excessive sensitivity of tissues to substances or other stimuli inside or

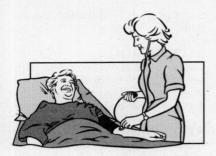

Regular measurement of the blood pressure is the only way to detect hypertension.

outside the body. Hypersensitivity may be a serious reaction to many medications.

HYPERSPLENISM
Various disorders in which blood cytopenia is associated with enlargement of the spleen. The cardinal features of the syndrome are: a reduction of one or more blood cell elements and enlargement of the spleen. This blood disorder is corrected by surgical removal of the spleen.

HYPERTELORISM
Abnormally increased distance between two organs or parts; in the case of orbital hypertelorism (increased distance between the orbits, or eye sockets) it is often a sign of mental deficiency.

HYPERTENSION
A common disorder, often with no symptoms, in which the blood pressure is persistently above 140/90 mm Hg. Causes of hypertension include:
- adrenal disorders;
- kidney disorders;
- toxemia of pregnancy.
In most cases - called essential hypertension -the cause is unknown although there are a number of predisposing factors such as:
- stress;
- obesity;
- hypercholesterolemia;
- high blood sodium level.

Symptoms, when present, include:
- headache;
- palpitations;
- fatiguability.
Treatment is by diuretics, vasodilators, central nervous system depressants and inhibitors and ganglionic blocking agents.

HYPERTENSIVE ENCEPHALOPATHY
An acute or subacute condition occurring in those with severe hypertension (high blood pressure), and marked by headache, obtundation, confusion or stupor and convulsions. Treatment consists of deliberate but progressive reduction of the blood pressure to more nearly normal ranges, by the taking of certain drugs.

HYPERTHERMIA
Greatly increased body temperature, usually due to a disturbance in the temperature regulating center in the hypothalamus of the brain.

HYPERTHYROIDISM
A condition in which the thyroid gland is overly active. This may eventually result in an increased rate of heartbeat. Symptoms are:
- weakness;
- tremors;
- sweating;
- weight loss;
- nervousness;
- heat intolerance can be profound;
- rapid and irregular heartbeat;
- diarrhea;
- a warm, moist skin.
All are indicators that the body metabolism has speeded up. The eyes may protrude (exophthalmos), and the person may tend to stare. There may be blurred or double vision. The thyroid gland is usually enlarged (goiter).

Most often the cause is unknown and associated with Graves' disease (also called toxic goiter and thyrotoxicosis), a condition involving the enlargement of the thyroid gland

and exophthalmus. Other causes include tumors that secrete thyroid hormone, tumors of other endocrine glands and inflammation of the thyroid gland.

HYPERTONIA
Increased tone of muscle or increased blood pressure.

HYPERTONIC
Pertaining to hypertonia.

HYPERTONIC SALINE
Salt solution with a greater osmotic pressure than normal physiological (body) pressure.

HYPERTONIC SOLUTION
One that has a higher osmotic pressure than a standard (reference) solution.

HYPERTRICHOSIS
Excessive hair growth in areas usually not hairy. An inherited or racial tendency is common. An endocrine disorder may be implicated in women and children. The underlying disorder should be treated.

HYPERTROPHIC CARDIAC DISEASE
Primary disease of the heart muscle characterized by hypertrophy of the heart muscle with no significant cardiac dilation or inflammation.

HYPERTROPHY
Increase in the size of the constituting cells of tissues or organs, independent of natural growth; sometimes due to excessive function such as heart hypertrophy in athletes.

HYPERVENTILATION
Overbreathing: increased inspiration and expiration of air as a result of an increase in the rate or depth of respiration or both.

HYPERVITAMINOSIS
A condition due to the ingestion of an excess of one or more vitamins.

HYPERVOLEMIA
Increase in the volume of circulating blood.

HYPHEMIA
Hemorrhage within the anterior chamber of the eye.

HYPNO-ANALYSIS
Form of psychotherapy in which the patients are made drowsy by sedation prior to their therapeutic session. The rationale of such treatment is based on the idea that the patients' sleepiness will reduce resistance and make them more receptive to the therapist's interpretations and suggestions.

HYPNOLOGY
Scientific investigation of sleep and waking.

HYPNOPOMPIC
Used to describe the state between sleep and waking, before one is fully awake.

HYPNOSIS
An artificially induced mental state characterized by an individual's loss of critical powers and his/her consequent openness to suggestion. It may be induced by an external agency or by the individual him/herself (autohypnosis).

Hypnotism has been widely used in medicine (usually to induce analgesia) and especially in psychiatry and psychotherapy.

Here, the particular value of hypnosis is that, while in trance, the individual may be encouraged to recall deeply repressed memories that may be at the heart of, for example, a complex; once such causes have been elucidated, therapy may proceed.

HYPNOTHERAPY
The use of hypnosis as an adjunct to psychotherapy.

HYPNOTICS
Measures, particularly the taking of certain drugs, designed to induce sleep.

HYPNOTIC TRANCE
The dream-like state of heightened suggestibility induced in a subject by a hypnotist.

HYPNOTISM
The process of inducing a hypnotic trance.

HYPOCAPNIA
Decreased amount of carbon dioxide in the blood.

HYPOCHLOREMIA
Reduced amount of chlorides in the blood; a form of alkalosis.

HYPOCHLORHYDRIA
Diminished amount of hydrochloric acid in the gastric juices.

HYPOCHONDRIA
Also called hypochondriasis: a mental condition involving undue anxiety about real or supposed ailments, usually in the belief that these are incurable. The source of hypochondria was once thought to be the hypochondrium, that part of the abdomen containing the spleen and liver.

HYPOCHONDRIACAL NEUROSIS
Preoccupation with the fear of having, or the belief that one has, a serious disease, based on the person's interpretation of physical signs or sensations as evidence of physical illness. A thorough physical evaluation does not support the diagnosis of any physical disorder that can account for the physical signs or sensations or for the person's unwarranted interpretation of them, although coexisting physical disorder may be present. The unwarranted fear or belief of having a disease persists despite medical reassurance, but is not of delusional intensity, in that the person can acknowledge the possibility that he or she may be exaggerating the extent of the feared disease or that there may be no disease at all.

HYPOCHONDRIUM
The upper regions of the abdomen beneath the ribs. The right hypochondrium contains the liver and gallbladder and the left hypochondrium the stomach and the spleen.

HYPODERMIC
Beneath the skin. Commonly refers to an injection beneath the skin.

HYPOFUNCTION
Diminished function.

HYPOGASTRIUM
The middle region of the abdomen below the navel and above the pubic bone.

HYPOGLOSSAL
Beneath the tongue, or pertaining to the 12th cranial nerve (hypoglossal nerve), which supplies the muscles of the tongue.

HYPOGLYCEMIA
An abnormally low level of glucose in the blood. Symptoms are:
- tremulousness;
- sweating;
- irritability;
- restlessness;
- feeling of extreme hunger;
- headache;
- nausea;
- chronic fatigue;
- weakness.
With severe hypoglycemia, the person may lose consciousness.

There are many possible causes. Hypoglycemia that occurs several hours after a person has eaten may be related to: too much insulin in the blood because the pancreas is secreting too much, because a tumor is secreting insulin or, in the case of diabetics, too much insulin has been injected (a "hypo" reaction); certain liver diseases and certain endocrine conditions. Low blood sugar that occurs after meals can have multiple causes.

HYPOMANIA
Psychiatric term for the condition of persons who display a mild form of the elation and psychomotor acceleration of mania. Differentiation of hypomania from exuberant and indefatigable vitality depends on demonstrating that the person uses manic defences against depression.

HYPOMANIC EPISODE
A distinct period in which the predominant mood is either elevated, or irritable and there are associated symptoms of the manic syndrome. By definition, the disturbance is not severe enough to cause marked impairment in social or occupational functioning or to require hospitalization.

HYPOMENORRHEA
A condition in which the menstrual cycle is prolonged and often irregular due to malfunction of the ovaries. There is scanty loss of blood and the intervals between periods may be measured in months.

HYPOMETABOLISM
Decreased metabolic rate; characteristic for a reduced function of the thyroid gland.

HYPON
Brand name of a medicine containing codeine, aspirin, phenolphthalein and caffeine as active ingredients. It is used as a pain reliever.

HYPONATREMIA
A decrease in the sodium concentration in the blood below the normal range; salt depletion.

HYPOPARATHYROIDISM
Diminished activity of the parathyroid glands. These are situated behind the thyroid gland in the neck and control calcium metabolism.

HYPOPHORIA
Eye disorder characterized by a downward deviation of the visual axis of one eye in the absence of visual functional stimuli.

HYPOPHOSPHATEMIC RICKETS
An inherited disorder characterized by impaired resorption of phosphate in the proximal renal tubules of the kidneys, with consequent lower content of phosphate in the blood, defective intestinal absorption of calcium and rickets (osteomalacia) that is unresponsive to vitamin D.

HYPOPHYSECTOMY
Removal of the pituitary gland at the base of the skull.

HYPOPHYSIS CEREBRI
Pituitary gland; a small oval reddish gray very vascular endocrine organ that is attached to the infundibulum of the brain, and consists of an epithelial anterior lobe and a posterior lobe of nervous origin. The various hormones synthesized and excreted by the hypophysis exert a controlling and regulating influence on other endocrine organs and bodily functions.

HYPOPIESIS
Abnormally low blood pressure.

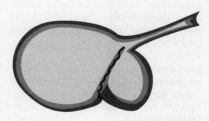

Gross anatomy of the pituitary gland. The gland consists of three part: anterior and posterior lobe and a small intermediary part.

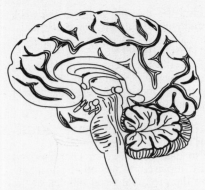

The hypothalamus is located between the telencephalon (hemispheres and basal ganglia) and the brain stem.

HYPOPIGMENTATION
A congenital or acquired decrease in melanin (pigment) production in the skin.

HYPOPITUITARISM
Diminished function of the pituitary gland.

HYPOPLASIA
Defective development of a tissue or organ.

HYPOPROTEINEMIA
Deficiency of protein in the blood. This may lead to edema (swelling) because of low osmotic value of the blood - that is, the fluid in the blood more readily passes through vessel walls into tissue.

HYPOSENSITIZATION
A treatment involving the administration of increasingly large doses of an allergen to gradually build tolerance to the allergen in a sensitive individual.

HYPOSMIA
Decrease in the normal sensitivity to smell.

HYPOSPADIA
A birth deformity in which the opening of the urethra (the tube carrying urine from the bladder to the outside) is situated on the undersurface of the penis instead of at the tip.

HYPOSTASIS
The collection of blood in the parts of a body or an organ closest to the ground immediately after death. It is one way by which a pathologist can tell whether a body has been moved after death.

HYPOTENSION
Low blood pressure. Symptoms may include:
- weakness;
- lightheadedness;
- dizziness.
Some medications that might cause hypotension include alcohol, enzyme inhibitors, antidepressants, lidocaine, opioid anesthetics, phenothiazines, etc. If you take any of these medications, be sure to tell a dentist, anesthesiologist or anyone else who intends to give you an anesthetic to put you to sleep.

HYPOTHALAMUS
Central part of the base of the brain, closely related to the pituitary gland. It contains vital centers for controlling the autonomic nervous system, body temperature and water and food intake, and is the center for primitive physical and emotional behavior. It also produces hormones for regulating pituitary secretion and two systemic hormones (e.g., vasopressin).

HYPOTHENAR
The pad of soft tissue on the palm of the hand at the base of the little finger.

HYPOTHERMIA
Subnormal temperature of the body. Initial symptoms are:
- weakness;
- slurred speech;
- confusion;
- shivering;
- clumsiness.
If the condition progresses, the

weakness is replaced by stiff muscles, the person feels unable to move and drowsiness and sleepiness occur. The body is no longer able to conserve heat, and the body temperature falls rapidly.

HYPOTHYROIDISM
A condition in which the thyroid gland is underactive, resulting in the slowing down of many of the body processes, including the heart rate.

HYPOTONIA
Diminished tone or activity, usually of muscles.

HYPOTONIC SOLUTION
One that has a lower osmotic pressure than a standard (reference) solution.

HYPOVENTILATION
Reduced rate and depth of breathing.

HYPOVOLEMIA
Abnormally decreased volume of circulating blood in the body.

HYPOXIA
Lack of an adequate amount of oxygen in air that is breathed in; reduced oxygen content or tension.

HYSTERECTOMY
Surgical removal of the uterus, with or without the ovaries and Fallopian tubes. It may be performed via either the abdomen or the vagina, and is most often used for fibroids, benign tumors of the womb or for diseases causing heavy menstruation. If the ovaries are preserved, hormone secretion remains intact, though periods cease and infertility is inevitable.

HYSTERIA
Medical diagnostic term for:
(1) Illnesses characterized by the lack of physical symptoms.
(2) The absence of physical signs, or any evidence of physical disease.

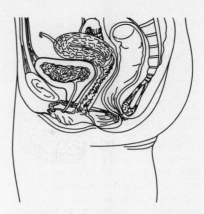

In hysterectomy the uterus or womb will be removed either through an abdominal incision or through the vagina.

(3) Behavior suggesting that the symptoms fulfil some psychological function.

HYSTEROGRAM
X-ray record of the uterus after injection of contrast medium into the uterine cavity.

HYSTEROSALPINGOGRAPHY
X-ray investigation of the uterus and the Fallopian tubes.

HYSTEROSALPINGOSTOMY
Surgical operation in which an anastomosis (link) is made between a Fallopian tube and the uterus. This is used to try to correct infertility, caused by blockage of the Fallopian tube as a result of inflammation.

HYSTEROSCOPY
A procedure that allows direct visual examination of the uterus with a tubular instrument (endoscope) for diagnostic or treatment purposes.

HYSTEROTOMY
A form of abortion in which the fetus is removed via a surgical incision in the uterus. This is very uncommon today, and should not be undertaken unless other methods are impossible.

IATROGENIC DISEASE
Disease produced by medical treatment. For example, in order to correct an overactive thyroid gland, part of it is removed. If, too much is cut out, the gland becomes underactive and this condition is then referred to as an iatrogenic disease.

IATROGENIC PSYCHOSIS
A severe behavior disorder induced by a doctor's diagnosis, attitudes and/or behavior and not the result of the treatment for the complaint.

ICHOR
A thin watery fluid, such as serum or whey. The term is also used in the sense of a thin, watery, acrid discharge from a sore or a wound.

ICHTHAMMOL
Thick black substance derived from coal. It is incorporated in ointments as a treatment of eczema and to relieve pruritus (itching).

ICHTHYOSIS
Congenital condition of the skin which is deficient in grease glands and so is dry and scaly for the whole of the sufferer's life.

ICTERUS
Jaundice. The word icterus derives from the Greek for a yellow bird, the color of the jaundiced patient being comparable to that of the bird.

ICTERUS GRAVIS NEONATORUM
Another name for erythroblastosis foetalis.

ICTERUS INDEX
Measurement of concentration of bilirubin (causing jaundice) in the blood plasma.

ICTUS
Sudden onset of illness, such as a convulsion ("fit") or stroke.

ID
Term introduced by Sigmund Freud; the mass of unbound energies, both libidinal and aggressive, that constitute part of the unconscious and influence conscious action by seeking discharge and immediate gratification in accordance with its governing influence; the instinctive part of behavior.

IDEA
The most common word for any mental process on the cognitive side.

It is usually employed, in contrast to "impressions," for processes on the ideational and conceptual levels, i.e., as inclusive of images and thoughts, but exclusive of percepts.

IDEAL
Emotionally colored thought about a personality, type of character or line of conduct, as representing a goal to be striven after, though possibly not to be attained, by the individual.

IDEALISM
Any one of a variety of systems of philosophical thought, which would make the ultimate reality of the universe expressible or intelligible only in terms of ideas, rather than in terms of matter or space.

IDEAS OF REFERENCE
An idea, held less firmly than a delusion, that events, objects, or other people in the person's immediate environment have a particular and unusual meaning specifically for him or her.

IDENTICAL TWINS
Twins developed from a single egg. They are always of the same sex, and commonly very much alike in appearance, although some characteristics may be in mirror image, e.g., one right-handed, the other left-handed.

IDENTIFICATION
The process by which a person either:
- extends his/her identity into someone else;
- borrows his/her identity from someone else;
- fuses or confuses his/her identity with someone else.

IDENTIFICATION FIGURE
Adult model copied, partly unconsciously, by the child; especially the child's parents.

IDENTITY
The condition of sameness in essential character. The sense of self, providing a unity of personality over time. Prominent disturbances in identity or the sense of self are seen in schizophrenia, borderline personality disorders, and identity disorders.

IDENTITY CRISIS
Emotional disturbance seen particularly in young people. The individual has difficulty in experiencing or establishing a consistent personality irregardless of changes in time, circumstances or roles.

IDENTITY DISORDER
Severe subjective stress, regarding inability to integrate aspects of the self into a relatively coherent and acceptable sense of self.

There is uncertainty about a variety of issues relating to identity, including:
- long-term goals;
- career choice;
- friendship patterns;
- sexual orientation and behavior;
- religious identification;
- moral value systems;
- group loyalties.

These symptoms last at least three months and result in impairment in social or occupational (including academic) functioning.

IDENTITY FORMATION
The process of achieving adult personality integration, as an outgrowth of earlier identifications and other influences.

IDEOMOTOR
Psychological term for mental energy; also, producing jerky automatic movements of muscles (for instance, arm or leg muscles) to indicate mental agitation.

IDIOCY
Congenital condition of mental deficiency; a mental age of two years or less.

IDIOGAMY
Term used in psychoanalysis for the restriction of male potency to cohabitation with one woman.

IDIOLALIA
Also called idioglossia: private or invented language of individuals of low mentality.

IDIOPATHIC
Term descriptive of a disease that arises spontaneously and is not due to or associated with any other disease, as far is known to medical knowledge. Sometimes a cause is discovered for such diseases, which, of course, then removes them from the idiopathic category.

IDIOSYNCRASY
Peculiar characteristic of body, mind or temperament. In a medical sense, a peculiarity or constitution that makes an individual react differently from most persons to drugs or treatments, such as the person who cannot take aspirin without be-

coming giddy and developing a skin rash.

IDIOT
The lowest grade of feeblemindedness, attaining, when adult, a mental age of no more than two years or an IQ not above 25.

Ig
Abbreviation of immunoglobulin.

ILEAC
Relating to the ileum, the lower part of the small intestine.

ILEECTOMY
Surgical removal of the ileum.

ILEITIS
Also called regional enteritis and Crohn's disease: inflammation of the ileum.

ILEO-CECAL VALVE
The muscular ring at the junction of the terminal ileum (last part of the small intestine) and the cecum (first part of the large intestine). It prevents a reflux of the contents of the cecum back into the ileum.

ILEOCOLIC
Relating both to the ileum (lowest part of the small intestine) and the colon (the large intestine).

ILEOCOLITIS
Inflammation of the intestines, located in the ileum and large intestine.

ILEOCOLOSTOMY
Surgical formation of a passage between the ileum (last part of the small intestine) and the colon to bypass a diseased cecum (first part of the bowel).

ILEOCYSTOPLASTY
Operation for a severe disturbance of the urinary bladder, in which tissues of the small intestine (ileum) are used.

ILEOILEOSTOMY
Surgical operation in which a diseased piece of the ileum (last part of the small intestine) is removed and the cut ends rejoined.

ILEOSIGMOIDOSTOMY
Operation in which the ileum (last part of the small intestine) is joined to the sigmoid colon to bypass a diseased portion of the cecum and the ascending or transverse colon.

ILEOSTOMY
Surgical operation by which the ileum is brought to the surface of the abdominal wall to form an opening for the discharge of its contents.

ILEUM
Lower part of the small intestine between the jejunum and the cecum.

ILEUS
Paralysis of the intestine. This causes an obstruction, and can sometimes follow surgery on the intestines.

ILIOCOCCYGEAL
Pertaining to the ilium (haunch bone) and the coccyx (lowest part of the vertebral column).

ILIOFEMORAL
Pertaining to the ilium (haunch bone) and the femur (thighbone).

ILIOINGUINAL
Relating to the ilium (haunch bone) and the groin.

ILIOPSOAS
Two muscles that lie together low down in the rear of the abdomen. (See illustration on next page)

ILIUM
Also called the haunch bone: upper broad wing-shaped bone that sticks out from the true pelvis and forms the ridge of bone popularly referred to as the hip. (See illustration on next page)

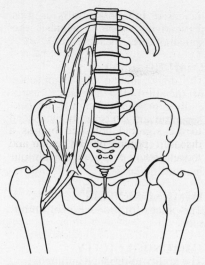

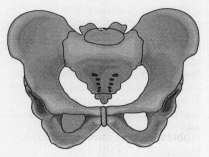

The ilium or iliac bone is part of the pelvis. The internal surface of the ilium seen from the medial side is the iliac fossa. Its superior border, the iliac crest ends anteriorly in the anterior superior iliac spine. The anterior inferior iliac spine is located inferior to the anterior superior spine.

Iliopsoas muscle; important for movement of lower part of the spine and pelvis. The muscle is attached to part of the spine, iliac bone and minor trochanter of the femur.

ILLOGICAL THINKING
Thinking that contains obvious internal contradictions or in which conclusions are reached that are clearly erroneous, given the initial premises. It may be seen in people without mental disorder, particularly in situations in which they are distracted or fatigued. Illogical thinking has psychopathological significance only when it is marked, and when it is not due to cultural or religious values or to an intellectual deficit.

ILLUSION
An erroneous perception of reality, often the result of misinterpretation by the brain of information received by the senses. Most commonly, the sense involved is sight: one of the exploitations of optical illusion is the use by artists of perspective. Optical illusions may also have external causes, such as refraction, as in the observation of a stick held in water. Examples of auditory illusion include the apparent change in pitch of a train's whistle as it passes. Rather different classes of illusion are hallucinations and eidetic images. The unconscious falsification of the memory of a past experience is also termed an illusion.

ILLUSION OF ORIENTATION
Misidentification of environmental stimuli due to impaired senses. It occurs in typhoid fever, malaria, pneumonia and scarlet fever.

IMAGE
A revived sense experience, in the absence of sensory stimulation, e.g., seeing with the mind's eye.

IMAGINARY AUDIENCE
Mental configuration characterizing adolescent egocentrism in which the individual imagines that everyone is watching him/her.

IMAGO
Psychoanalytic term for the unconscious, idealized representation of an important figure from childhood, usually a parent, often markedly influencing later life in the form of control and standards.

IMBALANCE
Out of balance, term commonly used to describe certain muscular activity, as well as the upset of the

acid-base relationship and the electrolytes in the body fluid.

IMBECILE
Individual with a degree of mental defect intermediate between the idiot and the feebleminded, or having a mental age between two and seven years, or an IQ between 25 and 50.

IMMUNE GLOBULIN
Also spelled immunoglobulin; any of a group of structurally related blood proteins responsible for a number of immunological properties and responses. The name is also used for a preparation injected to prevent infectious diseases.

IMMUNE RESPONSE
The reaction of the body to the introduction into it of an antigen.

IMMUNITY
A state of relative resistance to an infection. Active immunity is acquired naturally during an infectious disease or artificially by vaccination (immunization) with dead or living microorganisms. Passive immunity is also acquired naturally when antibodies of the mother pass to the unborn child via the placenta, but it too can be acquired artificially by administering immune blood serum containing antibodies.

IMMUNITY, ACTIVE
Immunity that is acquired by vaccination against a disease or by recovery from a previous infection.

IMMUNITY, PASSIVE
Immunity that is acquired from antibodies obtained either from the mother (such as through breastfeeding) or by injection (such as from an immune person or animal who has active immunity).

IMMUNIZATION
The process by which resistance to an infectious disease is induced or increased. Immunization is used as preventive measure against the spread of infectious diseases.

IMMUNOASSAY
The determination of the presence or quantity of a substance, especially a protein, through its properties as an antigen or antibody.

IMMUNODEFICIENCY
A reduction of a person's normal immune defenses.

IMMUNOGENESIS
The process of production of immunity.

IMMUNOGENICITY
The ability to produce immunity.

IMMUNOGLOBULIN (Ig)
A protein of animal origin with known antibody activity, synthesized by lymphocytes and plasma cells and found in blood serum and other body fluids and tissues. There are five distinct classes based on structural and antigenic properties: IgA, IgD, IgE, IgG and IgM.

IMMUNOHEMATOLOGY
The study of antigen-antibody reactions and similar phenomena as they relate to blood disorders.

IMMUNOHETEROGENOUS
Occurring in two or more immunoreactive forms.

IMMUNOLOGY
The study of the body's response to foreign invasion (e.g., bacteria, virus, fungus, transplanted tissue).

IMMUNOMODULATION
Adjustment of the immune response to a desired level, as in immunopotentiation, immunosuppression or induction of immunological tolerance.

IMMUNOPARESIS
An inadequate immunological re-

sponse to an infectious agent.

IMMUNOPATHOGENESIS
The process of development of a disease in which an immune response or the products of an immune reaction are involved.

IMMUNOPATHOLOGY
That branch of biological and medical science concerned with immune reactions associated with disease.

IMMUNOPOTENCY
The immunogenic capacity of an antigen molecule or one of its parts to initiate a synthesis of antibodies.

IMMUNOPOTENTIATION
Accentuation of the immune response by administration of another substance.

IMMUNOSUPPRESSANTS
Powerful drugs that suppress the immune system. Immunosuppressants are used in patients who have had organ transplants or severe disease associated with the immune system.

IMMUNOSUPPRESSION
The artificial prevention or diminution of the immune response, such as by the use of radiation, anti-metabolites, etc. Immunosuppressive drugs are used in the treatment of cancer and rheumatoid arthritis, and after transplant operations.

IMMUNOTHERAPY
Passive immunization of an individual by the administration of antibodies that have been actively produced by another individual.

IMMUNOTRANSFUSION
Transfusion of blood from a donor previously rendered immune to the disease affecting the person.

IMPETIGO
An infectious skin disease that generally affects children. The outer

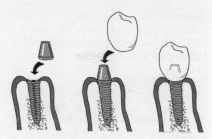

Examples of an implant in the lower jaw.

layers of the skin - most often the scalp and face - become infected with the bacterium Staphylococcus aureus, which produces clusters of small abscesses that dry up, leaving infectious yellowish-brown scabs. Contact with these - either by other parts of the person's body or by someone else - spreads the disease.

Antibiotic cream applied to the affected areas usually clears up the condition, but in severe cases, an antibiotic may have to be taken by mouth or injection.

IMPLANT
(1) To set permanently in the consciousness or habit patterns.
(2) To insert artificial teeth in the bony structure of the lower or upper jaw.

IMPLANTATION
The insertion of living cells or solid materials into the tissues, or the insertion or grafting into the body of biological, living, inert or radioactive material.

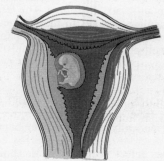

Implantation of an embryo in the internal lining (mucosa) of the uterus.

The term is also used for the embedding of the six-day-old embryo (called a blastocyst) in the epithelial lining of the uterus.

IMPOTENCE
The inability of the male to achieve erection of the penis or, less commonly, to ejaculate. The term is also used in the sense of weakness.

IMPULSE
Push or communicated force; a sudden mental urge to do an action. The term is also used in the sense of a tendency to action without deliberation.

IMPULSIVE
Term referring to the character of an act as immediate, and without deliberation or volition, on the mere presentation of a situation, either in perception or idea.

INACTIVE COLON
Another term for colonic inertia.

INADEQUACY
Inability to cope with a situation in which an individual is placed, either because of a lack of the necessary personal qualities, or the requisite mental ability or special skill.

INANITION
Exhaustion as the result of starvation.

INARTICULATE
Without joints, disjointed. The term particularly applies to the utterance of vocal sounds that are not capable of being understood. It popularly means speechless or indistinct pronunciation.

INBORN ERROR OF METABOLISM
A genetically determined biochemical disorder in which a specific enzyme defect produces a metabolic block that may produce a disease.

INCEST
Sexual intercourse between persons to whom marriage is forbidden on grounds of kinship. These grounds vary with culture and epoch. First-cousin marriage, for example, once prohibited under the tenets of Roman Catholicism and, later, Protestantism, is now generally permissible.

Almost universally forbidden are marriages between parents and children, or between siblings, but the ancient Egyptians and the Incas of Peru both allowed brother-sister marriages in the ruling family.

INCEST BARRIER
Term employed in psychoanalysis for the barrier placed upon the development of the libido by social law regarding incest, at the same time stressing the feelings of guilt - evoked by thoughts, or fantasies or dreams - involving the breaking down of the barrier.

INCEST TABOO
Social norm that prevents a person from marrying within the family group; system that forbids marriage between certain relatives, including to one's mother, father, siblings, grandparents, uncles, aunts, nieces and nephews.

INCIDENCE
The number of cases of a disease (or other event) that occur during a prescribed period of time; this is often expressed as a rate.

INCIDENCE RATE
Number of cases of a disease appearing per unit of population within a defined time interval.

INCIPIENT MOVEMENT
The imperceptible or barely perceptible beginning of movement that is then overtly carried out, such as occurs in the speech organs during speech.

INCISION
Surgical cut. Incisions are named after their location, shape and direction, after the organ or structure in which they are made, and frequently after the surgeon who first used them.

INCISOR TOOTH
One of the eight cutting teeth at the front of the mouth.

INCISURA PULSE
One showing a sharp fall in pulse pressure.

INCLUSION BODY
Object found within the body's cells during virus diseases, sometimes representing the virus itself.

INCOHERENCE
Quality of being incoherent; absence of connection of ideas or of language. Incoherence is speech that, for the most part, is not understandable, owing to any of the following:
- a lack of logical or meaningful connection between words, phrases, or sentences;
- excessive use of incomplete sentences;
- excessive irrelevancies or abrupt changes in subject matter;
- idiosyncratic word usage;
- distorted grammar.

Incoherence may be seen in some organic mental disorders, schizophrenia, and other psychotic disorders.

INCOMPATIBLE
Usually refers to substances such as drugs that are incapable of being used or put together because they interact wrongly chemically or have opposing qualities.

INCOMPETENCE
Insufficiency or inability to perform its function, as in an incompetent (or leaky) heart valve.

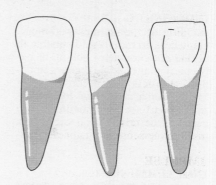

From left to right: anterior, lateral and posterior view of an incisor.

INCONTINENCE
The inability to control urination and/or defecation.

INCOORDINATION
Term used generally to describe movements in which muscles or muscle groups do not cooperate smoothly or adequately in a complex movement. The term may also be used by extension to describe certain faulty mental functions.

INCREMENT
An increase, such as the increase in the tone of a muscle as a contraction is building in strength.

INCUBATION PERIOD
The time between exposure to infection and the first symptoms of illness.

INCUBATOR
A cabinet heated to a constant temperature to allow cultures of bacteria to grow; or a temperature-regulated apparatus for premature babies.

INCUS
Also called the anvil: central of the three tiny bones situated in the middle ear that receive vibrations from the eardrum and transmit them to the organ of hearing where they are interpreted as sound.

INDECISION
An attitude, sometimes pathological, where an individual is unable to decide on a course of action, or between two alternative courses of action, and action is accordingly inhibited for a shorter or longer period. The term is sometimes also used to describe a characteristic, more or less enduring, of an individual.

INDETERMINISM
A theory of the will, to the effect that it is possible for an individual to act, or to choose a course of action, independently of the stimuli affecting him/her, or the motives prompting him/her at the time.

INDEX
Formula expressing the ratio of one dimension of an object to another dimension. The term is also used generally for a sign directing to a particular statement, fact or point; a sign indicative of some phenomenal change.

INDEX FINGER
Forefinger, the finger next to the thumb.

INDIAN HEMP
Common name for Cannabis indica.

INDICAN
Potassium indoxyl sulphate, a product of the decomposition of the amino acid tryptophan in the intestines that is excreted in urine. Elevated levels may indicate that the person is on a high protein diet or suffering from gastrointestinal disease.

INDICANURIA
Excessive amount of indican in the urine.

INDICATION
Sign; any symptom, cause or occurrence in a disease that indicates its course of treatment. The term is also used to designate a disorder, symptom, or condition for which a drug or treatment may be prescribed.

INDIGESTION
Also called dyspepsia: any upset of the normal digestive process, resulting in symptoms of discomfort; lack of digestion; imperfect digestion. The symptoms may be pain, flatulence ("wind") or a feeling of distension.

INDIGOCARMINE
Dye used for testing the function of the kidney.

INDISPOSITION
Slight ailment or health disorder.

INDIVIDUALITY
The sum total of the characteristics of an individual, which distinguish him/her from other individuals; sometimes wrongly used as a synonym for personality, which has, or may have, dynamic and also normative implications, absent in the case of individuality, which is necessarily descriptive.

INDOLE
With skatole, the chemicals that give odor and color to feces.

INDOLENT
Literally, slothful, lazy; medically, it means causing no pain, such as a painless ulcer that is slow to heal.

INDUCED LABOR
Labor started artificially, either by the midwife or obstetrician rupturing the membranes, or by giving intravenous drugs that stimulate the womb to contract.

INDUCED PSYCHOTIC DISORDER
A delusional system that develops in a second person as a result of a close relationship with another person (the primary case) who already

has a psychotic disorder with prominent delusions. The same delusions are at least partly shared by both persons.

INDUCTION

Term used in a special physical or psychological sense to describe the production of an effect elsewhere than at the original locus of activity. Also used in the sense of induction of labor.

INDUCTIVE TECHNIQUE

Style of parental discipline consisting of a cognitive component that helps a child to learn specific rules or limits for behavior, understand the reasons for such rules and anticipate the consequences of breaking them.

It is sometimes accompanied by a love-oriented technique, but not necessarily.

INDURATION

The hardening of tissue as in hyperemia (congestion of a part with blood); infiltration by a malignant tumor.

INDUSTRIAL DISEASE

Also called occupational disease: a disease contracted by occupational exposure to an industrial agent known to be hazardous - for instance, dust, fumes, chemicals, irradiation - the notification of, safety precautions against and compensation for which are usuallycontrolled by law.

INDUSTRIAL PSYCHOLOGY

The branch of applied psychology that concerns itself with the application of psychological methods and results to problems arising in the industrial or economic field, inclusive of the selection and training of workers and methods and conditions of work.

INERTIA

The tendency of a body to persist in

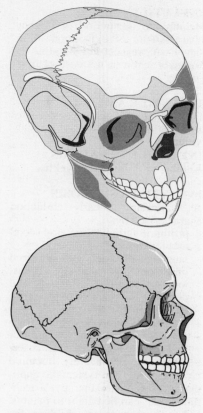

The skull of an infant (above) consists of loosely connected cranial bones, while the cranium of an adult (below) is fully ossified.

its state of rest or motion. The term is sometimes used figuratively in psychology to describe perseverations or latent time.

IN EXTREMIS

At the point of death.

INFANCY

The period of helplessness and dependency in humans or other organisms. In humans, it roughly comprises the first two years.

INFANT DEBILITY

A condition of retarded development found among some institutionalized infants, and attributed to the lack of affectionate care.

INFANTILE
Relating to the period of infancy; characteristic of the period of infancy with respect to mentality and behavior, even in the case of older people.

INFANTILE AMNESIA
Forgetfulness of the experiences of early childhood.

INFANTILE PARALYSIS
Another term for poliomyelitis.

INFANTILE PSYCHOSIS
A syndrome of early childhood characterized by:
- profound failure to develop social relationships;
- language disorder with impaired understanding, echolalia (meaningless repetition of words and phrases) and reversal of pronouns (e.g. "you" for "I").
- rituals and compulsive behavior;
- general retardation in intellectual development, in most cases.

For the most severely impaired children, only the systematic application of behavior therapy, a technique that can be taught to parents, helps to manage the child in the home and at school. Treatment may take a considerable time.

INFANTILE SEXUALITY
General term embracing those aspects of sexuality exhibited by most children less than about five years old.

They do not in general persist into adulthood, though the adult may suffer from a complex caused by guilt concerning them.

INFANTILE SPINAL MUSCULAR ATROPHY
Also called motor neuron disease: disorder beginning in infancy or childhood, characterized by skeletal muscle wasting due to progressive degeneration the anterior horn cells in the gray matter of the spinal cord and of the brainstem.

INFANTILISM
Persistence of child-like characteristics into adult life. Organs that fail to mature and produce an adult function are also described as infantile.

INFANT MORTALITY
The death of live-born children who have not reached their first birthday. This is usually expressed as a rate - that is, the number of infant deaths during a reporting period per 1000 live births reported in the same period.

INFARCT
The area of tissue that is damaged or dies as a result of receiving an insufficient blood supply. Frequently used in the phrase myocardial infarct (commonly called "heart attack"), referring to the area of heart muscle injury due to the interrupted flow of blood through the coronary artery that normally supplies it.

INFECTION
The invasion of disease-producing microorganisms into a body where they may multiply, causing a disease.

INFECTIOUS ARTHRITIS
Arthritis resulting from infection of the synovial tissues with pyogenic (pus-producing) bacteria or other infectious agents.

INFECTIOUS DISEASE
Disease cause by pathogenic microorganisms.

INFECTIOUS MONONUCLEOSIS
Commonly called glandular fever: an acute disease that is thought to be caused by the Epstein-Barr virus, and spread by close contact, including kissing. It is characterized by:
- high fever;
- sore throat;
- generalized disorder of the lymphatic system

(resulting in swollen glands);
- and by an increase in white blood cells. In 15 percent of cases, a rash develops and, in severe cases, some vital organs can become involved.

Treatment aims to relieve symptoms. Bedrest is very important during the acute phase of fever and malaise, and can be prolonged (up to six months) if the liver has become inflamed. Aspirin or other pain relievers usually control headache. Isolation of sufferers is unnecessary. Antibiotics are of no value unless secondary bacterial infection is present.

INFERIORITY COMPLEX
Term used by the Austrian psychoanalyst Alfred Adler to describe the complex of fears and emotions arising out of feelings of inferiority or inadequacy, particularly those concerned with (usually imagined) inferiority of the sexual organs.

INFERIORITY FEELING
The normal feeling of weakness and comparative helplessness or inefficiency experienced by all children. This is sometimes strongly reinforced by special inferiorities, such as in illness, health, deformity or defect.

Children's attempts to overcome this always stimulates them to efforts to secure recognition by others, and even to secure superiority over others, and this often leads to neurotic symptoms of various kinds, including inferiority complexes.

INFERTILITY
The condition of being unable to bear young - in a woman the inability to conceive, in a male, an inability to impregnate.

INFLAMMATION
Reaction of the tissues to injury or infection and characterized by local heat, swelling, redness and pain. The causes are innumerable.

INFLUENZA
An acute, contagious, virus-caused infection of the respiratory tract. Treatment is symptomatic.

INFORMATION TEST
A type of mental test devised with the object of throwing light upon a person's knowledge of facts in a variety of fields, general and special, and frequently forming one of a battery of intelligence tests.

INFORMED CONSENT
Practice whereby participants involved in any experimental procedure, from research to therapy, must give free consent to participate after having been informed about all essential aspects of the procedure, including possible side effects.

INFRACLAVICULAR
Below the clavicle (collarbone).

INFRARED
Electromagnetic radiation of a wave length greater than that of the red end of the spectrum. Used therapeutically for the production of heat in the tissues.

INFRATEMPORAL
Below the temporal bone, the bone forming the front of the skull.

INFUNDIBULUM
Any funnel-shaped passage or part, such as the stalk of the pituitary gland or the wide funnel-shaped region of the Fallopian tube at its fimbriated (fringed) end near the ovary.

INFUSION
Extract made by adding boiling water to some vegetable substance - tea, for instance.

INFUSION PUMP
An apparatus or machine for administering a continuous, controlled amount of a drug or other fluid through a needle inserted into a vein

or under the skin. It consists of a small battery powered pump that controls the flow of fluid from a syringe into the attached needle.

The pump may be strapped to the patient and preprogrammed to deliver the fluid at a constant rate.

INGUINAL
Relating to the groin.

INGUINAL CANAL
A passage about one and a half inches long that lies parallel to and half inch above the inguinal ligament.

INGUINAL LIGAMENT
The thickened lower border of the aponeurosis of the external oblique muscle of the abdomen extending from the anterior superior iliac spine to the pubic tubercle continuous below with the fascia lata, and forming the external pillar of the superficial inguinal ring and a part of the anterior boundary of the femoral ring.

INGUINAL RING
The hole in the abdominal muscles of males through which the testicles pass before birth from the region near the kidney to the scrotum (testicle bag).

The ring is normally closed at birth but occasionally closure is incomplete and portions of the abdominal contents, such as intestine, protrude to form an inguinal hernia - commonly called a rupture.

INHALATION
Breathing of steam or medicated vapors into the nose or lungs.

INHALATION ANESTHESIA
That induced by the inhalation of an anesthetic vapor.

INHALER
A device used for administering a drug in powder or vapor form. In-

halers are used principally in the treatment of respiratory disorders such as asthma and chronic bronchitis.

Among the medications administered in this way are corticosteroids and bronchodilator drugs.

INHERITANCE
Acquisition of characteristics transmitted from parents to their children.

INHIBITED ORGASM
A relatively rare phenomenon in which intravaginal ejaculation does not occur or there is an inability to masturbate to ejaculate.

INHIBITION
The action of a mental process or function in restraining the expression of another mental process or function; for example, fear of social condemnation inhibiting fulfillment of sexual desire.

Most often the ego or superego inhibits instinctual behavior. Inhibition may play a role in neuroses.

INHIBITORY
Showing restraint; showing a blocking effect. The term is, for example, used for a chemical released from a nerve ending that prevents muscle contraction.

INITIAL REFLEX
The first reflex evoked by a series of stimuli, gradually increasing in strength from a first stimulus, below threshold strength.

INITIATION
The process of beginning an activity or movement; in a special sense, used to describe the preparation for becoming a member of some society, or the enjoyment of certain privileges, e.g., as a full or adult member of a social group or community.

This is often marked by a special ritual or ceremony.

INJECTION
The act of introducing a fluid (under pressure) into the tissues, a vessel, cavity or hollow organ.

INK-BLOT TEST
Also called the Rorschach test: test, sometimes described as a test of fertility of imagination, where a series of irregular figures, such as ink blots, is presented to subjects, and they are required to say what objects they see, or can imagine, in the figures.

The result depends generally on the number of objects they can report in a given time, though the kind of objects they may report may also be significant.

INNATE
Inborn, belonging to the body and mind by nature. The term is also used in the sense of something derived from the constitution of the mind, as opposed to being derived from experience.

INNERVATION
Stimulation of a part through the action of nerves; the distribution and function of the nervous system; nerve supply of a part.

INNOMINATE ARTERY
Also called the brachiocephalic artery: largest branch of the arch of the aorta, the main artery from the heart.

INNOMINATE BONE
Bone forming the front wall and sides of the pelvic cavity.

INNOMINATE VEINS
Two veins that join to form the superior vena cava, the main vein bringing blood back to the heart from the head and neck.

INOCULATION
Introduction of a germ, a poison produced by a germ or serum into the body to set up the production of

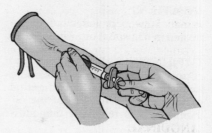

Injection of a drug in the vein of the arm of a patient.

antibodies that will subsequently protect the individual from an attack of the disease. This is called preventive inoculation.

INOPERABLE
Any condition that cannot or should not be operated upon. It commonly refers to a cancerous condition that has spread far beyond the original site, making it pointless to operate on the original growth because of growth deposits in all the surrounding organs, or an operation may be impossible because of the damage that would occur to surrounding tissues and organs.

INOSITOL
A cyclic sugar alcohol, one of the components of the vitamin B complex. It is not an essential nutrient.

INOSUTURIA
The presence of inositol in urine.

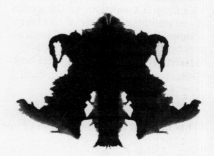

Ink blot test (Rorschach test), used to gain more insight into the characteristics of the personality of a client or patient.

INPATIENT
A patient who is lodged, fed and treated in a hospital or infirmary.

IMPRINTING
A species-specific type of learning that occurs within a limited period of time early in the life of the organism and is relatively unmodifiable thereafter.

INQUEST
Enquiry held by a coroner into the cause of violent or sudden death or to determine the ownership of treasure trove.

INSANITY
Legal term for severe mental disorder involving irresponsibility and incompetence in the conduct of the individual's affairs.

INSEMINATION
Deposit of seminal fluid within the vagina. Also called semination.

INSERTION
The attachment of a muscle to the bone it moves.

INSIDIOUS
Having an imperceptible commencement, such as a disease with a late manifestation of definite symptoms.

INSIGHT
As a technical term in psychology, this means an awareness of one's own mental condition, or the grasp of a principle behind a problem without the apparent use of logical process. Insight learning is direct, bypassing the process of trial and error.

IN SITU
In its normal place; confined to the site of origin.

INSOMNIA
A condition characterized by difficulty falling asleep or staying asleep or by seriously disturbed sleep. The essential feature of these disorders is a predominant complaint of difficulty in initiating or maintaining sleep, or of not feeling rested after sleep that is apparently adequate in amount (nonrestorative sleep).

There is great variability in the normal length of time it takes a person to fall asleep or in the amount of sleep normally required for a person to feel alert and rested. For the vast majority of people, sleep begins within 30 minutes of creating an environment that encourages sleep and lasts from four to ten hours. Typically, a young person with an insomnia disorder complains that it takes too long to fall asleep. An older person complains that he or she awakens too frequently, or is unable to stay asleep long enough to feel rested the next day. In some cases a person with insomnia complains only of nonrestorative sleep, despite apparently having no difficulty falling asleep or staying asleep.

INSPIRATION
The drawing of air into the lungs.

INSTABILITY
(1) Lack of steadiness of aim, steadiness of control, effectiveness in action, due to what is popularly termed "nervousness."
(2) More importantly used in the sense of emotional instability, a definite defect characterized by excessive and variable manifestations of emotional excitement.

INSTEP
The arch of the foot on the dorsal surface.

INSTILLATION
Administration of a liquid drop by drop.

INSTINCT
A phenomenon whose effects can be observed in animals and humans,

but whose precise nature is little understood. In general, one can say that instinctive behavior comprises those fixed reactions to external stimuli that have not been consciously learned. In fact, such behavior seems to stem from a complex of hereditary and environmental factors, since animals placed from birth in artificial environments display some, but not all, instinctive reactions characteristic of their species. It has been further suggested that embryos may have some learning ability - that is, that some learning before birth is possible. Numbered among the instincts are the sex drive, aggression, territoriality and the food urge, but much debate surrounds such classification.

INSTRUMENTAL LEARNING
Behavior changes that occur as a result of the consequences of a given behavior; also referred to as operant conditioning.

INSUFFLATION
Blowing of a powder, vapor or gas into a body cavity.

INSULIN
Hormone manufactured in the pancreas by little areas of tissue called the islets of Langerhans, and then secreted into the blood where it controls the digestion of carbohydrates. A lack of insulin or a disturbance of its use by the cells is the cause of diabetes.

INSULINASE
Enzyme that inactivates insulin.

INTAKE CASEWORKER
Individual (usually in a health service clinic) who compiles a developmental history and preliminary statement regarding the problem of the individual or family.

INTEGRATION
The organization of parts into harmoniously operating whole, as in the expression "integrated personality."

In psychoanalysis, two types of psychological integration are marked by the terms primary integration and secondary integration, the first being the development, in young children, of the recognition of their bodies as distinct from objects in the environment, and the second, the organization into the complete psychosexual unit of its pregenital components, in earlier stages of development.

INTEGRITY
Behavior in accordance with a strict code of values - moral, artistic, etc. The term is also used in the sense of the quality of wholeness, something without mark or stain.

INTEGUMENT
A covering, especially the skin.

INTELLECT
Mind in its cognitive aspect, and particularly with reference to the higher thought processes.

INTELLECTUALISM
The tendency in psychology to emphasize the intellectual or cognitive aspect, and to neglect the emotional and volitional, or the attempt to explain them in terms of the intellectual psychology.

INTELLECTUALIZATION
A defense mechanism employing intellectual functions in the attempt to understand or explain a personal problem rather than the acknowledgement of the emotion evoked by the problem.

INTELLIGENCE
The ability to learn, to understand, to apply experience, and to make judgments.

INTELLIGENCE SCALE
Any series of intelligence tests, normally arranged in order of diffi-

culty, by means of which an individual's mental level, or mental development, can be determined.

INTENSITY
One of the dimensions of sensory experience; a quantitative measure of strength or degree, e.g., a bright light has a high intensity, a soft tone a low intensity. A change in intensity is distinguished from a change in quality, which is a change in kind.

INTENTIONALISM
A type of psychological theory, sometimes referred to as "act of psychology," that emphasizes the act of intending or referring to an object as the most fundamental characteristic of the psychological process or of the mental life.

INTERACTION
Change in the body's response to one drug when another is taken. Interaction may decrease the effect of one or both drugs, increase the effect of one or both drugs or cause toxicity.

INTERACTIONAL PSYCHO-THERAPY
A psychotherapeutic technique based on manipulation of transference phenomena and adjustment of the technique to the type of sociogenic disorder.

INTERACTIONISM
A theory of the relation between mind and body, which assumes interaction or reciprocal causation between the two - that mind acts on body and body on mind -as the solution of the psycho-physical problem. This involves a philosophical dualism, which need not prevent the psychologist adopting it as the simplest working hypothesis.

INTERCOSTAL
Between the ribs. This is usually used to describe the nerves, muscles and blood vessels that lie between each pair of ribs, and the diseases affecting them.

INTERCOSTAL NEURALGIA
Neuralgia (nerve pain) occurring in the nerves running round the chest. Often associated with a herpes zoster infection such as shingles.

INTERCOURSE
Communication, coitus.

INTERCURRENT DISEASE
Illness occurring in someone already suffering from another disease. For instance, if a person suffering from chronic heart disease then contracts pneumonia, the pneumonia is the intercurrent disease.

INTERFERON
A class of small soluble proteins produced and released by cells invaded by a virus, which induce in non-infected cells the formation of an anti-viral protein that inhibits viral multiplication. Interferon production may also be induced by certain bacteria and specifically sensitized lymphocytes. There are indications that interferon may be useful in the treatment of certain types of cancer.

INTERMENSTRUAL PAIN
Also called mittelschmerz: pain occurring at the time of ovulation. Normally, ovulation causes no pain, or sometimes just a dull cramping, but occasionally it is combined with such severe pain that a woman cannot walk and is confined to bed. The pain can also sometimes be associated with vaginal bleeding. The pain may be due to spasms of one of the Fallopian tubes, or to intra-abdominal bleeding from the ovulation site. This last causes a reaction from the peritoneum that lines the abdomen, which results in pain from the nerve endings. The vaginal bleeding that occurs is usually due to spillage of a hormone, mostly es-

trogen hormone, which can alter the contraction pattern of the uterus. Some of the endothelial lining of the uterus is then shed, resulting in bleeding. The pain usually disappears in a few days. There is no treatment save bedrest with a heating pad and the taking of a pain-reliever such as aspirin or paracetamol.

INTERMITTENT
Occurring at intervals.

INTERMITTENT CLAUDICATION
Pain in the muscles of a limb (usually the leg), similar to angina pectoris, that occurs intermittently - during stress but not at rest.

This condition frequently accompanies diseases of the peripheral blood vessels, such as athero-sclerosis and thromboangiitis obliterans.

The resting muscle has an adequate blood supply, but when the need for blood increases (as during exercise), the disease impairs the circulation.

An inadequate blood supply and the build-up of waste products of metabolism in the tissues cause pain.

INTEROCEPTIVE SYSTEM
The system of nerve receptors located within the body as distinguished from the exteroceptive system, situated near the surface of the body, and the proprioceptive system, sited within the locomotor system.

INTEROCEPTOR
A sense organ or nerve receptor located inside the body, e.g., the walls of the blood vessels.

INTEROCULAR DISTANCE
The distance between the central points of the pupils of the two eyes when they are in the normal position of fixation.

INTERPERSONAL AWARENESS
Knowledge of one's self who is separate and distinct from other human beings.

INTERPERSONAL PSYCHOTHERAPY
A treatment technique that emphasizes the interpersonal nature of the events occurring in the treatment as well as in the patient's life in an attempt to help the patient become conscious of those parts of himself that he has a stake in keeping out of awareness.

INTERSEX
Term employed of an individual intermediate between a male and a female, in a normally bisexual species.

INTERSEX STATES
Conditions in which the appearance of the external genital organs is either ambiguous or at variance with the chromosomal, gonadal or genetic sex of the individual.

INTERSEXUALITY
The possession of both male and female characteristics.

INTERSTITIAL
Situated between two important parts; occupying the interspaces or interstices of a part; or pertaining to the finest connective tissue of an organ.

INTERTRIGO
Form of moist eczema that occurs where two folds of skin rub against each other. It is due to the chafed skin being constantly moist with perspiration, which causes it to break down and become inflamed. The commonest sites for intertrigo are beneath a pendulous breast and in a groin or armpit.

INTERVENTRICULAR
Between two ventricles, particularly

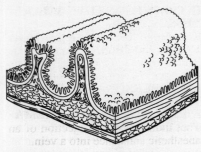

Schematic drawing of the microscopic structure of part of an intestinal wall showing some villi.

the cardiac ventricles, the two lower chambers of the heart. The term also refers to the ventricles in the brain, the spaces containing cerebrospinal fluid.

INTERVERTEBRAL DISC
Cartilaginous plate between each pair of spinal vertebrae that acts as a natural shock absorber.

INTESTINES
That part of the alimentary canal or digestive system extending from the pyloric opening of the stomach to the anus.

INTIMA
An innermost structure, such as the inner lining of a blood vessel.

INTOLERANCE
Inability to withstand or consume; inability to absorb or metabolize nutrients.

INTOXICATION
State in which a person is overtly affected by an excess of a drug or poison. It is often used to describe the psychological effects of drugs and, particularly, alcohol, in which behavior may become disinhibited, morose or aggressive and in which judgement is impaired.

Late stages of intoxication affecting the brain include stupor and coma. Ingestion of very large amounts of water causes water in-

toxication and may lead to coma and death. Poisoning with toxins and drugs may cause intoxication of other organs (e.g. heart with digitalis overdosage).

INTRA-ABDOMINAL
Within the abdomen.

INTRA-AMNIOTIC INSTILLA-TION
Use of saline (salt water) or prostaglandin to cause abortion by stimulating the uterus to contractions similar to those of labor. The products of conception are then expelled, mimicking a natural miscarriage.

Abortions of this type are considered major procedures and should only be performed in hospitals on an in-patient basis so that the woman can be carefully watched throughout the entire procedure.

INTRA-ARTERIAL
Within an artery.

INTRA-ARTICULAR
Within a joint.

INTRA-ATRIAL BLOCK
Slowed conduction through the muscle of the atria of the electrical impulse produced by the atrioventricular node in the heart.

INTRACARDIAC
Within the heart.

INTRACELLULAR
Within a cell or cells.

INTRACEREBRAL
Within the cerebrum or cerebral hemispheres of the brain.

INTRACUTANEOUS
Within the skin tissues; within the substance of the skin.

INTRAMURAL
Within the layers of the wall of a hollow tube or organ.

INTRAMUSCULAR
Within the muscular substance, within a muscle.

INTRAMUSCULAR INJECTION
Injection of a drug into a muscle, usually in the upper arm or buttock. The drug is absorbed from the muscle into the bloodstream.

INTRA-OCULAR TENSION
The pressure produced by the fluid within the eyeball. It may be estimated by a tonometer, or by palpation (pressing) with the fingers.

INTRA-ORAL
Within the mouth.

INTRAPERITONEAL
Within the peritoneal cavity of the abdomen. Since the whole abdomen is lined with peritoneum, the term literally means "intra-abdominal."

INTRAPLEURAL
Within the pleural cavity of the chest. The pleural membrane lines the chest wall and covers the lungs, and the pleural cavity is the space between the two layers of membrane.

INTRAPULMONARY
Within the substance of the lung.

INTRASPINAL
Within the spinal canal.

INTRATHECAL SPACE
The space between the arachnoid and pia mater covering the brain and spinal cord, which contains cerebrospinal fluid.

INTRATHORACIC PRESSURE
Pressure within the chest cavity.

INTRATRACHEAL
Within or through the windpipe.

INTRA-UTERINE
Within the uterus or womb.

INTRA-UTERINE DEVICE
Full name of IUD.

INTRAVENOUS
Within a vein, such as intravenous injection - the injection of a fluid into a vein.

INTRAVENOUS ANESTHESIA
That induced by the injection of an anesthetic substance into a vein.

INTRAVENOUS FEEDING
Method of supplying nutrients for growth or maintenance of body mass when the gastrointestinal tract is unable to provide adequate nutrition because of certain diseases of the gut or following surgery.

INTRAVENOUS INFUSION
Prolonged, slow injection of fluid (often a solution of a drug) into a vein. The fluid flows at a controlled rate from a bag or bottle through a fine tube inserted into an opening into a vein. An intravenous infusion may also be administered via an infusion pump.

INTRAVENOUS INJECTION
Direct injection of a drug into a vein, which puts the drug immediately into the circulation. Because it has a rapid effect, intravenous injection is useful in an emergency.

INTRAVENOUS PYELOGRAM
X-ray of the kidneys and urinary tract after intravenous injection of a contrast medium to aid visualization.

INTRAVENTRICULAR
Within a ventricle, one of two lower chambers of the heart. The term may also refer to the ventricles of the brain, the spaces containing cerebrospinal fluid.

INTRINSIC
Situated within; the inherent characteristics of an object occurring within itself.

INTRINSIC FACTOR
Also known as Castle's factor: substance normally contained in gastric juice and absent in pernicious anemia. It is vital for the absorption of vitamin B12, which in turn is vital for the formation of red blood cells.

INTROITUS
Any opening in the body; an entrance to a cavity, particularly the vagina.

INTROJECTION
Psychologically, the ascribing to inanimate objects of characteristics of living creatures. In psychoanalytical literature, the term is used for absorbing into oneself environmental influences and characteristics, but more particularly, the personal characteristics of other persons, and reacting to external events accordingly.

INTROSPECTION
Observation by an individual of his own mental processes; systemic self-observation.

INTROVERSION
Inner-directed personality orientation characterized by interest in personal thoughts and feelings rather than in social concerns of external matters.

INTROVERSION-EXTRAVERSION TEST
A type of test, usually of the questionnaire type, designed to bring out an individual's general direction of interest, inwards or outwards.

INTROVERT
Individual who tends to live with his own thoughts and avoids socializing.

INTUBATION
Passing a tube into a part, especially the introduction of a tube into an opening made into the trachea (windpipe) at the front of the neck to relieve obstructed breathing in certain conditions.

INTUSSUSCEPTION
The descent or doubling in of a higher portion of intestine into a lower one, thus creating an obstruction. Also, the act of taking foreign matter into the substance of a living body. In addition, the term is used in the sense of the process by which nutriment is absorbed into and goes to form part of the system.

INULIN CLEARANCE
The rate at which the kidneys excrete inulin; tested to evaluate kidney function and diagnose muscle or liver diseases.

INVAGINATED
Process of becoming ensheathed; the state of burrowing or infolding to form a hollow space within a solid structure. Typical examples are the invagination of the lining membrane of the nose into the skull bone during embryological development in order to form a nasal sinus, and the invagination by one piece of intestine into another, producing an intussusception.

INVASION
In a medical sense, the entry of bacteria into the body.

INVERSION
A turning inward, inside out, or other reversal of the normal relation of a part. Inversion of the uterus is a turning of the uterus whereby the fundus is forced through the cervix, protruding into or completely outside the vagina.

IN VITRO
Literally, "in glass." It refers to actions taking place in laboratories as opposed to those that take place in the body (in vivo). In many cases, in vitro tests prove successful but when applied to the body the same result is not obtained. The most

common use of the term is in vitro fertilization, where conception takes place while both egg and sperm are outside the woman's body; the conceptus is placed in the woman's uterus a few days after fertilization.

IN VIVO
Occurring within the body.

INVOLUCRUM
Sheath of new bone that is formed over a dead bone in, say, osteomyelitis.

INVOLUNTARY
Something that occurs independently of the will.

INVOLUNTARY MUSCLES
Those muscles not under the control of the will and which act without the individual making any conscious effort. They include those in the heart, intestines, the bladder and the respiratory apparatus.

INVOLUTION
Turning inwards; shrinkage. Also refers to the return of the womb to normal size and shape following childbirth or its regression after the change of life.

INVULNERABILITY
The quality or state of being incapable of being wounded or of receiving injury.

IODINE
An essential mineral necessary for the thyroid gland to function properly. Ocean foods are rich natural sources; seaweed is extremely rich in iodine, while fish, especially cod, are also a good source. The most readily available source is iodized table salt, which provides all the iodine normally needed. A lack of iodine can lead to enlargement of the thyroid gland (goiter).

IODISM
Chronic poisoning by iodine or io-

dides (salts of iodine), with head cold, excessive production of saliva, frontal headache, weakness and skin eruptions.

IODOFORM
A mild antiseptic made of iodine, alcohol and potash. It is sometimes used on wounds and skin ulcers.

ION
An atom or molecule that has gained or lost one or more electrons and acquired a positive charge (a cation) or negative charge (an anion). In electrolysis, an ion passes to one or another pole.

IPPB
Abbreviation of "intermittent positive pressure breathing" another term for artificial respiration.

IQ
Abbreviation of "intelligence quotient".

IRIDECTOMY
Surgical removal of part of the iris, the colored part of the eye. This is sometimes performed to relieve the pressure inside the eye in glaucoma.

IRIDOCHOROIDITIS
Inflammation of the iris of the eye and the choroid, the middle membrane covering the eyeball.

IRIDOCYCLITIS
Inflammation of the iris and the ciliary body of the eye.

IRIDOLOGY
Also known as iris diagnosis, iridology, iriscopy, iris science and diagnosis from the eye: this is based on the findings of Ignatz von Peczely of Hungary, a physician and surgeon, and N. Liljequist of Sweden.
The basic premise of iridology is that each organ of the body is represented by an area of the iris. Iridology charts show the pupil area as corresponding to the navel, and the

organs occupy areas in the iris in relation to the position they occupy with regard to the navel and the medial and lateral aspects of the body.

IRIDOTOMY
Surgical cutting of the iris of the eye without the removal of any part.

IRIS
Colored circular part of the eye made of muscle and fiber and surrounding the black pupil. Responsible for regulating the amount of light entering the eye, it separates the front and back chambers of the eyeball and rests against the front of the crystalline lens. Its color is determined by the location of pigment bodies known as melanophores: if these are at the back of the iris, it appears blue or gray; if in the middle, it appears brown.

IRITIS
Inflammation of the iris. Symptoms include pain in or just above the eye, watering of the eye, pain on exposure to light (photophobia), redness around the edges of the iris, dimness of vision. It can be caused by an allergic reaction, as a secondary reaction to syphilis, gonorrhea, tuberculosis, diabetes, ankylosing, rheumatoid arthritis and ulcerative colitis, or is a result of a direct injury to the iris. Treatment involves the wearing of dark glasses, and resting the eye by the application of atropine eye drops, which will paralyze the muscles in the iris. Steroid eye drops or ointment may also be given to reduce the inflammation.

IRON
Metallic element essential for hemoglobin synthesis in the body and used in various drugs.

IRON-BINDING CAPACITY
A measure of the iron uptake and return in blood, in relation to the synthesis and breakdown of hemoglobin.

IRON-DEFICIENCY ANEMIA
Chronic anemia characterized by small, pale red blood corpuscles and depletion of iron stores.

IRON SUPPLEMENTS
Products that contain iron in a form that can be absorbed from the intestinal tract. Supplements include ferrous fumarate, ferrous gluconate, ferrous sulfate, iron dextran, iron-polysaccharide.

IRREDUCIBLE
Not capable of being restored to a normal position. It usually refers to a hernia which cannot be returned to within the abdomen by non-surgical means (i.e. a truss) and becomes a fixed, painful swelling and may produce the signs of intestinal obstruction that can only be relieved by surgery.

IRREGULARITY
A part exhibiting or causing something to be irregular or impairing uniformity. The term is also used in the sense of defecation or menstruation that does not follow a previous pattern, or an action or behavior constituting a breach of morality.

IRREGULAR PULSE
A pulse in which the beats occur at irregular intervals or in which the force, or rhythm and force, varies.

IRRITABILITY
In biology and psychology, the ability to be affected by external stimuli.

IRRITABLE BOWEL SYNDROME
Also called irritable colon or spastic colon: a motility disorder involving the small intestine and large bowel and associated with variable degrees of abdominal pain, constipation or diarrhea, apparently as a reaction to stress in a susceptible individual. No physical cause can be found. The sympathetic under-

standing and guidance of the doctor is of over-riding importance, and the sufferer must be reassured that no organic disease is present. Since psychological stress, particularly depression may be a significant factor in this illness, it should be diagnosed, evaluated and treated.

IRRITANT
That which excites or irritates; a medical application that causes pain or heat; an irritant poison.

IRRITATION
Angry feeling, or a feeling of heat or pain in a part of the body. The term is also used in the sense of the change or action that takes place in muscles or organs when a nerve or nerves are affected by the application of external bodies.

ISCHEMIA
A local, usually temporary, deficiency of oxygen in some part of the body, often caused by a constriction or an obstruction in the blood vessel supplying that part.

ISCHEMIC HEART DISEASE
Also called coronary thrombosis, coronary artery disease and coronary heart disease: heart ailments caused by narrowing of the coronary arteries and therefore a decreased blood supply to the heart .

ISCHEMIC SYNDROME
Disorder of the system of blood vessels in the brain caused by insufficient circulation.

ISCHIAL SPINES
Small points on the posterior border of the hip bones.

ISCHIUM
The lower part of the innominate bone of the pelvis; the bone on which the body rests when sitting.

ISCHURIA
Insufficient passage of urine either because of a suppression of the urge to urinate or bladder retention.

ISLETS OF LANGERHANS
Clusters of special cells scattered throughout the pancreas. They comprise two types of cells: alpha cells produce the hormone glucagon, which acts to increase the amount of glucose in the blood; and beta cells produce the hormone insulin, which is vital for the ability of body cells to use this glucose.

ISO-ANTIBODY
An antibody produced by one individual that reacts with iso-antigens of another individual of the same species.

ISO-ANTIGEN
An antigen existing in alternative forms in a species, thus inducing an immune response when one form is transferred to members of the species who lack it.

ISOCHROMOSOME
A chromosome in which the arms on either side of the centromere are identical.

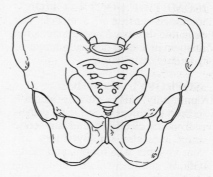

Anterior view of the human pelvis. The two coxal bones of a newborn consist of three components: a superior ilium, an inferior anterior pubis, and an inferior and posterior ischium. Eventually, the three separate bones fuse into one. The ischium contains a prominent ischial spine, a lesser sciatic notch below the spine. The rest of the ischium, the ramus, joins with the pubis and together they surround the obturator foramen.

ISO-ENZYME
Variation of an enzyme, with a slightly different chemical structure, but producing the same effects as the enzyme itself.

ISOGRAFT
Transfer of tissue between identical twins.

ISO-IMMUNIZATION
Development of antibodies in response to iso-antigens. An example of this is the immunization of an Rh-negative mother by an Rh-positive foetus; the woman then develops antibodies against Rh-positive blood and these can damage any future Rh-positive babies she may have.

ISOLATION MECHANISMS
Psychoanalytical term for a symptom characteristic of compulsion neuroses, which are marked by blank pauses after a highly unpleasant or personally significant experience.

ISOLEUCINE
One of the essential amino acids.

ISOMETRIC CONTRACTION
Increased tension in a muscle that does not shorten. Muscle tone is the maintenance of a normal amount of isometric contraction.

ISOPROPYL ALCOHOL
Commonly called rubbing alcohol: a clear, colorless liquid used principally as a cleansing and antiseptic agent. It is also employed as a solvent in some skin lotions and medications, and in cosmetics and perfume. Isopropyl alcohol is approximately twice as toxic as ethyl alcohol and the probable lethal dose is 2 to 4 fl. oz in children. Poisoning may also occur from inhalation of high concentrations. Deep coma has resulted from sponging a feverish child with a concentrated isopropyl alcohol solution.

ISOTONIC CONTRACTION
The shortening of a muscle under constant load.

ISOTONIC SOLUTION
One that has the same power of diffusion as another. Such a solution can be added to body fluid without causing any disturbance. An example is an isotonic saline (salt water) solution that is injected into the bloodstream.

ISOTOPE
One of a variety of forms in which a chemical element can appear. Isotopes of an element are identical in number of protons and electrons in each atom, but differ in atomic weight, and therefore have different properties. Isotopes are used to trace movements of chemical substances in the body, as are radioactive isotopes. The latter can also be used to treat certain types of cancer.

ITCH
An uneasy sensation of irritation, or light prick pain, on the skin accompanied by an impulse to scratch the area.

IUD
Abbreviation of "intra-uterine device".

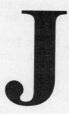

J

JABORANDI
South American plant (Pilocarpus microphyllus), which belongs to the rue family. Its leaves contain the alkaloid pilocarpine, which causes an increase in saliva and profuse perspiration; it is used to decrease the pressure inside the eyeball in glaucoma.

JACKET CROWN
An artificial crown that is placed over the remains of a natural tooth.

JACKSONIAN EPILEPSY
Also called focal epilepsy: form of epilepsy that is characterized by convulsive movements starting in a single muscle or a group of muscles, and in which consciousness is generally retained. The aura is often the most prominent part of the attack.

JACKSON'S LAW
The name sometimes given to the principle that, in the impairment or loss of mental acquisition, the more recent memories are the first to be affected or to disappear, that the order of degeneration is the
reverse of the order of development or acquisition.

JACKSCREW
A device operated by means of a screw to expand the dental arch and move individual teeth.

JACOBSON'S ORGAN
A slender horizontal canal in the nasal mucosa than ends in a blind pouch and that has an olfactory function. It is rudimentary in human beings but highly developed in most reptiles.

JACQUEMIER'S SIGN
Blueness of the mucosa of the vagina seen in early pregnancy.

JACTITATION
Severe restlessness that appears at times in gravely ill persons.

JAIL FEVER
Another name for epidemic typhus.

JAMAIS VU
A disorder of memory characterized by the illusion that familiar is being encountered for the first time.

JAMES-LANGE THEORY
A classical theory of emotion, named for the two men who independently proposed it. The theory states that a stimulus first leads to motor responses, and then the awareness of these responses constitutes the experience of emotion.

JAPANESE B ENCEPHALITIS
An encephalitis that occurs epidemically in Japan in the summer, and is caused by an arbovirus. The virus usually produces a subclinical infection.

JARGON
Gibberish or babbling speech associated with aphasia, idiocy, or a severe mental illness.

JARISH-HERXHEIMER REACTION
An increase in the symptoms of a spirochetal disease (as syphilis, Lyme disease, or relapsing fever) occurring in some persons when treatment with spirocheticidal drugs is started.

JAUNDICE
Yellow color of the skin and whites of the eyes caused by excess bilirubin pigment in the blood. The hemoglobin in the blood is broken

down to form bilirubin which is excreted by the liver in the bile. If blood is broken down more rapidly than normal (hemolysis), the liver may not be able to remove the abnormal amount of bilirubin fast enough. Jaundice occurs with liver damage (hepatitis, late stages of cirrhosis) and when the bile ducts leading from the liver to the duodenum (first part of the small intestine) are obstructed by stones from the gallbladder or by cancer of the pancreas or bile ducts.

It is not uncommon for newborn babies to have a trace of jaundice during the first days of life; this is treated by exposing the baby to sunlight or to a powerful artificial ultraviolet light. Severe cases do occur and these can be dangerous, as bilirubin may be deposited in various parts of the brain, causing permanent damage. If exposure to ultraviolet light does not work, a complete change of blood (exchange transfer) may be needed.

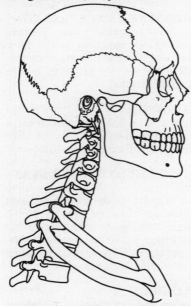

Side view of the skull and upper part of the spine. The upper jaw is a fixed part of the skull, the lower jaw can move in the temporomandibular joint.

JAUNDICE, CHOLESTATIC
Jaundice that results from abnormality of bile flow in the liver.

JAUNDICE, HEPATOGENOUS
Jaundice associated with hemolytic anemia.

JAUNDICE, NEWBORN
Icterus neonatorum; abnormally high amounts of the bile pigment bilirubin in the blood, usually characterized by jaundice. It is a common disorder, usually due to immaturity of the liver, deficiency of enzymes, and normal destruction of fetal red blood cells. In many cases is subsides spontaneously, it other cases the condition is treated by phototherapy.

Severe cases, more often due to an abnormal condition (e.g., erythroblastosis fetalis), produce signs of spleen and liver enlargement, anemia, kernicterus (sometimes leading to mental retardation), and other complications, sometimes leading to death.

JAUNDICE, OBSTRUCTIVE
Jaundice that is due to blocking of bile flow.

JAUNDICE, PHYSIOLOGIC
Mild icterus neonatorum (newborn jaundice) lasting the first few days of life.

JAUNDICE, RETENTION
Jaundice that is due to the inability of the liver to dispose of the bilirubin provided by the circulating blood.

JAW
Either of two complex cartilaginous or bony structures that border the mouth, support the soft parts enclosing it, and bear teeth on their oral margin.

JAW BONE
Either the maxilla (upper jaw) or mandible (lower jaw).

JAW-JERK REFLEX
Short spasmodic contraction of the jaw muscles elicited by striking the relaxed and open jaw with a percussion hammer.

J CHAIN
A relatively short polypeptide chain with a molecular weight of about 35,000 daltons and a high number of cysteine residues that is found in immunoglobin of the IgM and IgA classes.

J-CURVE
A distribution curve of the behavior of individuals, in the form of an inverted J. It appears when social controls are placed upon behavior, e.g. at an intersection when traffic is regulated by a stop sign.

JEALOUS TYPE DELUSIONAL DISORDER
Presence of a persistent, nonbizarre delusion that is not due to any other mental disorder, such as schizophrenia. When delusions of jealousy are present, a person is convinced, without due cause, that his or her spouse or partner is unfaithful.

Small bits of "evidence," such as disarrayed clothing or spots on the sheets, may be collected and used to justify the delusion. Almost invariably the person with the delusion confronts his or her spouse or partner and may make extraordinary steps to intervene in the imagined infidelity.

These attempts may include restricting the autonomy of the spouse or partner by insisting that he or she never leave the house unaccompanied, secretly following the spouse or partner, or investigating the other "lover."

The person with the delusion may physically attack the spouse or partner and, more rarely, the other "lover."

The age of onset of a delusional disorder is generally middle or late

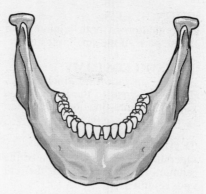

Superior view of the lower jaw or mandible. The rounded structures in the upper part of the illustration are part of the temporomandibular joint.

adult life, but can be a younger age. In most studies average age at onset has been found to be between 40 and 55.

JEALOUSY
A special form of anxiety resulting from fear of loss of a loved one's affection to a rival, with both emotional and motivational consequences.

JEJUNAL
Pertaining to the jejunum, part of the small intestine.

JEJUNECTOMY
Surgical removal of all or a portion of the jejunum.

JEJUNITIS
Inflammation of the jejunum.

JEJUNOCOLOSTOMY
Surgical operation by which the jejunum is joined to the colon (large intestine).

JEJUNOILEAL BYPASS
A surgical bypass operation performed especially to reduce absorption in the small intestine that involves joining the first part of the jejunum with the more distal segment of the ileum.

JEJUNOILEITIS
Inflammation of both jejunum and ileum, parts of the small intestine.

JEJUNOILEOSTOMY
Surgical operation in which the jejunum is joined to the ileum and a part of the intestine between them is removed.

JEJUNOJEJUNOSTOMY
Operation in which a portion of the jejunum is removed and the cut ends rejoined.

JEJUNOTOMY
Surgical opening of the jejunum, usually performed to remove a foreign body such as a small object swallowed by a child.

JEJUNUM
Part of the small intestine between the duodenum and the ileum. It is about 2.5 m (8 ft) long.

JELLY
A soft, resilient substance; generally, a colloidal semisolid mass.

JELLY, CARDIAC
A gelatinous substance present between the endothelium and myocardium of the embryonic heart that transforms into the connective tissue of the endocardium.

JELLY, WHARTON
The soft, jelly-like intracellular substance of the umbilical cord.

JERK
Sudden involuntary movement of a muscle.

JERK, ACHILLES
Plantar flexion of the foot elicited by a tap on the Achilles tendon, preferably while the patient kneels on a bed or chair, the feet hanging free over the edge.

JERK, ELBOW
Involuntary flexion of the elbow on striking the tendon of the biceps or triceps muscle.

JERK, KNEE
A kick reflex produced by sharply tapping the patellar ligament.

JERK, TRICEPS SURAE
Plantar flexion of the foot elicited by a tap on the Achilles tendon, preferably while the patient kneels on a bed or chair, the feet hanging free over the edge.

JERKY PULSE
A pulse in which the artery is suddenly and markedly distended as occurs in aortic regurgitation (backflow of blood into the heart).

JET LAG
A condition that is characterized by various psychological and physiological effects (as fatigue and irritability), occurring following long flight through several time zones, and probably resulting from disruption of circadian rhythms in the human body.

JOINT
The point where two or more bones meet. A joint may be immovable, as those of the skull; slightly movable (cartilaginous), as those connecting the vertebrae; or freely movable, as those of the elbow and knee.

JOINT, BALL-AND-SOCKET
A synovial joint in which a spheroidal surface on one bone ("ball") moves within a concavity ("socket") on the other bone.

JOINT, BIAXIAL
A joint with two chief axes or more bones.

JOINT, CONDYLOID
A joint in which an ovoid head of one bone moves in an elliptical cavity of another, permitting all movements except axial rotation.

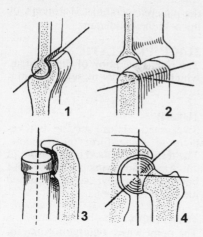

Various types of joints.
1. hinge joint with one axis;
2. saddle-shaped joint with two axes;
3. rotating joint with one axis;
4. ball-shaped joint with three axes.

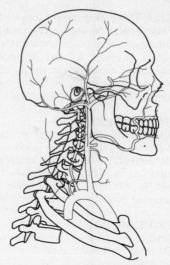

Side view of the skull and upper part of the spine. Between the vertebrae numerous small joints are located.

JOINT, ELBOW
The articulation between the humerus, ulna, and radius.

JOINT, ELLIPSOIDAL
A joint representing a spheroidal joint, but having an ellipsoidal articular surface.

JOINT, FIBROUS
A joint in which the bones are united by fibrous tissue.

JOINT, SADDLE
A joint having two saddle-shaped surfaces at right angles to each other.

JOINT, SPHEROIDAL
A synovial joint in which a spheroidal surface on one bone moves within a spheroidal cavity on the other bone.

JOINT, UNIAXIAL
A joint which permits movement in one axis only.

JOY-RIDES
Brand name of a drug containing as active compound hyoscine used for the prevention of motion sickness.

JUGULAR
Refers to any structure in the neck but particularly three large veins - the internal, anterior and external jugular veins -which carry blood from the head and neck to the subclavian vein and then to the heart.

JUGULAR FORAMEN
A large irregular opening from the posterior cranial fossa that is bounded anteriorly by the petrous part of the temporal bone and posteriorly by the jugular notch of the occipital bone and that transmits the inferior petrosal sinus, the glossopharyngeal, vagus, and accessory nerves, and the internal jugular vein.

JUGULAR FOSSA
Depression on the basilar surface of the petrous portion of the temporal bone that contains a dilation of the internal jugular vein.

JUGULAR NOTCH
A notch in the inferior border of the occipital bone behind the jugular

process that forms the posterior part of the jugular foramen. The term is also used to designate a notch in the petrous portion of the temporal bone that corresponds to the jugular notch of the occipital bone and with it makes up the jugular foramen.

JUGULAR PROCESS
Quadrilateral or triangular process of the occipital bone on each side that articulates with the temporal bone and is situated lateral to the condyle of the occipital bone on each side articulating with the atlas.

JUGULAR TRUNK
Either of two major lymph vessels that drain the head and neck.

JUGULAR VEIN
Any of several veins of each side of the neck.
(1) A vein that collects the blood from the interior of the cranium, the superficial part of the face, and the neck, running down the neck on the outside of the internal and common carotid arteries, and uniting with the subclavian vein to form the innominate vein. This vein is called the internal jugular vein.
(2) The external jugular vein is a smaller and more superficial vein that collects most of the blood from the exterior of the cranium and deep parts of the face and opens in the subclavian vein.
(3) The anterior jugular vein is a vein that commences near the hyoid bone and joins the terminal part of the external jugular vein or the subclavian vein.

JUICE
Any fluid from animal, plant of human tissue.

JUICE, GASTRIC
The liquid secretion of the glands in the wall of the stomach.

JUICE, PANCREATIC
The enzyme-containing secretion of the pancreas, conducted through its ducts to the duodenum.

JUICE, PROSTATIC
The liquid secretion of the prostate, which contributes to semen formation.

JULEP
Sweetened mixture serving as a vehicle to some form of medicine. The term is also used in the sense of an American drink composed of bourbon whiskey, sugar, crushed ice and mint leaves.

JUNCTION
The point where two parts come together (e.g., neuromuscular junction, the point where a nerve and muscle come together).

JUNCTIONAL NEVUS
A nevus that develops at the junction of the dermis and epidermis and is potentially cancerous.

JUNCTIONALLY RHYTHM
A cardiac rhythm resulting from impulses coming from a locus of tissue in the area of the atrioventricular node.

JUNCTIONAL TACHYCARDIA
Tachycardia (rapid heartbeat) associated with the generation of impulses in a locus in the region of the atrioventricular node.

JUNCTION, GAP
A narrowed portion of the intercellular space in such tissues as that of the myocardium (muscle layer of the heart), containing channels linking adjacent cells and through which pass ions, most sugars, amino acids, nucleotides, vitamins, hormones, and cyclic AMP.

JUNCTION, ILEOCECAL
The junction of the ileum and cecum, located at the lower right side of the abdomen and fixed to the posterior abdominal wall.

JUNCTION, MUCOGINGIVAL
The histologically distinct line marking the separation of the gingival tissue from the oral mucosa.

JUNCTION, MYONEURAL
The site of apposition between a nerve fiber and the motor endplate of the skeletal muscle which it innervates.

JUNCTURE
The line or point at which two bodies are joined; particularly, a point rendered critical or important by a concurrence of circumstances.

JUNGLE FEVER
A severe form of malaria or yellow fever.

JUNGLE YELLOW FEVER
Yellow fever endemic in or near forest or jungle areas in Africa and South America and transmitted by mosquitoes other than members of the genus Aedes.

JUVANTIA
Drugs or devices that ease pain or discomfort.

JUVENILE
Referring or relating to a young person, usually below the age at which compulsory attendance at school ceases.

JUVENILE-ONSET DIABETES
A form of diabetes mellitus which usually starts before the age of 20 and is less common and usually more severe that maturity-onset diabetes.

JUVENILE RHEUMATOID ARTHRITIS
A form of rheumatoid arthritis in children involving the larger joints, resulting in interference with growth and development.

JUXTAGLOMERULAR APPARATUS
Functional unit near a kidney glomerulus that controls renin release and is composed of juxtaglomerular cells and a macula densa.

JUXTAGLOMERULAR CELL
Any of a group of cells that are situated in the wall of each afferent arteriole of a kidney glomerulus near its point of entry adjacent to a macula densa and that produce and secrete renin.

JUXTAPOSITION
Side by side, adjacent.

JUXTARESTIFORM BODY
A part of the inferior cerebellar peduncle containing nerve fibers that reciprocally connect the cerebellum and the vestibular nuclei of the medulla oblongata.

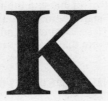

KAHN SYMBOL TEST
A structured play test used in diagnostic evaluation of children and sometimes adults. The test involves the arrangement of small plastic objects.

KAHN TEST
A serum-precipitation reaction for the diagnosis of syphilis.

KAINOPHOBIA
A pathological fear of new situations and things. If this condition develops into a severe neurosis, some form of psychotherapy should be applied.

KALA-AZAR
Also called dumdum fever and visceral leishmaniasis: disease of tropical and subtropical countries caused by a protozoan (a microorganism) and transmitted by sandflies. The incubation period is from one to four months but cases have occurred as long as two years after exposure. It is associated with enlargement of the spleen and liver, great wasting of the body and an irregular fever of long duration.

KANNER'S SYNDROME
Infantile autism characterized by:
- profound failure to develop social relationships;
- language disorder with impaired understanding;
- echolalia (automatic repetition of words and phrases);
- reversal of pronouns;
- rituals and compulsive phenomena;
- general retardation in intellectual development, in most cases.

KANTREX
Brand name of kanamycin.

KAOLIN
A mineral clay that remains white after firing, used internally in diarrhea to absorb fluid and irritants, and externally in poultices.

KAPOSI'S HEMORRHAGIC SARCOMA
Multiple vascular tumors that commonly appear on the toes or legs as purple or dark brown plaques or nodules. The lesions do not at first produce symptoms, but lymphedema (swelling) of the legs may develop later. Death may result from the bleeding of such tumors into the gastrointestinal tract, or from an associated lymphoma. The sarcoma is probably related to AIDS (acquired immune deficiency syndrome).

KAPOSI'S VARICELLIFORM ERUPTION
Skin eruption occurring in children with eczema. It is a severe generalized bullous (blister-producing) eczema that, if untreated, will cause death.

KARYOGENESIS
Formation and development of a cell nucleus.

KARYOPLASM
The substance of the nucleus of a cell, containing chromosomes, nucleolus and deoxyribonucleic acid (DNA).

KARYOPYKNOSIS
Shrinkage of the cell nuclei of epithelial cells (as of the vagina) with breakup of the chromatin into unstructured granules.

KARYOPYKNOTIC INDEX
An index that is calculated as the

percentage of epithelial cells with karyopyknotic nuclei exfoliated from the vagina, being used in the hormonal evaluation of a patient.

KARYOSOMA
A chromatin mass in the nucleus of a cell.

KARYOTYPE
The full complement of chromosomes; the term covers the number, relative sizes and structure of the chromosomes.

KARYOTYPING
Analysis of chromosomes that is performed on fetal cells obtained by amniocentesis to detect the sex and various genetic factors or diseases of an unborn child.

Karyotyping is also performed on children and young adults to detect genetic abnormalities and diseases.

KATZENJAMMER
A feeling of worry, uneasiness or nervousness, usually on the basis of the development of a mild neurosis.

KAWASAKI DISEASE
An acute febrile disease affecting young children that was first described in Japan and is characterized by:
- erythema of the conjunctiva;
- erythema of the mucous membranes of the upper respiratory tract;
- erythema and edema of the hands and feet;
- rash following by desquamation;
- cervical lymphadenopathy.

KAYSER-FLEISCHER RING
A brown or greenish brown ring of copper deposits around the cornea that is characteristic of Wilson's disease.

KELLER'S OPERATION
Surgical procedure for the correction of a hallux valgus (outward displacement of the big toe) or hallux rigidus (stiffness of the joint between the big toe and the foot). The operation consists of cutting away the half of the proximal phalanx (middle bone of the big toe) nearest the inner side of the foot, plus any osteophytes and exostoses (respectively, bone spurs and overgrowths) on the head of the metatarsal bone. The toe is fixed in the correct position; after healing, a fibrous, flexible joint results.

KELLY-PATTERSON SYNDROME
Combination of severe glossitis (inflammation of the tongue) with difficulty in swallowing and secondary anemia.

KELOIDS
Ugly scars produced by a healing abnormality after surgery. The development of keloids has nothing to do with the surgical technique of a doctor; it is probably genetic. Although there is no known cure for keloids, plastic surgery techniques are being developed to remove them. One technique for dealing with keloids involves a steroid injection combined with the removal of the scars. This has been found to decrease the re-formation of the keloids in many cases.

KELP
An edible seaweed, extremely rich in iodine, as well as calcium, potassium and the trace minerals. Kelp is available as a mineral supplement and as a salt substitute. It comes dehydrated, in tablets, powder and granules.

KENNY METHOD
A procedure for the treatment of poliomyelitis involving both hot applications and physical exercises.

KENOPHOBIA
Fear of large empty spaces. Sometimes behavioral therapy is necessarily.

KERATALGIA
Pain in the cornea of the eye.

KERATECTOMY
Removal of a portion of the cornea.

KERATIASIS
Occurrence of multiple warts on the skin.

KERATIN
An insoluble protein, containing sulphur, present in skin, hair and nails.

KERATINOUS CYST
A slow-growing benign cystic tumor of the skin containing follicular, keratinous and sebaceous material and frequently found on the scalp, ears, face, back or scrotum. Surgical treatment is most effective.

KERATITIS
Inflammation of the cornea. Superficial punctate keratitis is a scattered, fine loss of epithelium from the corneal surface of one or both eyes. It is often associated with trachoma, blepharitis (inflammation of the eye lids), conjunctivitis or an inflammation of the respiratory system. It may be due to a viral infection or may be a reaction to local medication and is commonly the cause of intense pain after exposure to ultraviolet light (for instance, from welding arcs, sun lamps).
Symptoms include:
– photophobia (intolerance to light);
– pain;
– watery eyes;
– conjunctival infection;
– diminution of vision.
The application of an antibiotic to the cornea will be given promptly, usually with good success.

KERATOCANTHOMA
A round, firm, usually flesh-colored lesion with a characteristic central crater containing keratinous material.

KERATOCONJUNCTIVITIS SICCA
A chronic dryness of the conjunctiva and sclera of both eyes, leading to the drying up of the surface of the eye.
Frequent use of artificial tears containing methylcellulose or polyvinyl alcohol can be effective. Most cases are treated adequately throughout the sufferer's lives with such supplementation.

KERATOCONUS
A slowly progressive ectasia (dilatation) of the corneas of (usually) both eyes, beginning between the ages of 10 and 20. Surgery may be necessary if the cornea becomes thin.

KERATODERMA
The horny layer of the skin, consisting of dead cells and keratin.

KERATODERMATOSIS
Any skin disease characterized by thickening of the skin and accumulation of keratin.

KERATODERMIA
A thickening of the horny layer of the outer layer of the skin (epidermis), especially on the palms of the hand.

KERATOHYALIN
A colorless translucent protein that occurs in granules of the stratum granulosum of the epidermis and stains deeply with hematoxylin.

KERATO-IRITIS
Inflammation of the cornea and iris.

KERATOLALACIA
A condition associated with vitamin A deficiency and protein-calorie malnutrition, characterized by a hazy, dry cornea that becomes denuded.
Corneal ulceration with secondary infection is common. Vitamins and antibiotics are beneficial.

KERATOLYSIS
Loosening or separation of the layer of the epidermis of the skin.

KERATOMA
Any horny growth, such as a wart or callus.

KERATOPATHY
Any disease of the cornea; non-inflammatory disease of the cornea.

KERATOPHAKIA
Surgical treatment for correction of hypermetropia (long-sightedness). A slice of a donor's cornea is shaped to the desired curvature and then inserted between layers of a recipient's cornea to change its curvature.

KERATOPLASTY
The operation by which damaged corneal tissue is replaced by healthy tissue.

KERATOSIS
Disease in which horny overgrowths develop, primarily on the skin, in this area, these are a number of different conditions (see below). When these horny overgrowths appear on the larynx (voice box), this is considered a preliminary to the development of laryngeal cancer.

KERATOSIS SENILIS
Skin disease appearing in elderly people and characterized by brownish warty growths, occurring chiefly on the face, backs of the hands and feet and other surfaces exposed to the wind and sun.

KERION
Inflammatory ringworm of the hair follicle of the beard and scalp accompanied by secondary bacterial infection and marked by spongy swelling and the exudation of sticky pus from the hair follicles.

KERNICTERUS
A disease occurring in infancy manifested by jaundice two or three days after birth, which, if untreated, produces convulsions, rigidity, coma and death in 75 percent of cases. Mental deficiency, epilepsy, chorea (involuntary jerky movements) or athetosis (slow writing movements of hands and feet) often result in those who survive.

The disease is caused by the incompatibility of the blood of the fetus with the mother's blood, such as occurs in erythroblastosis foetalis. The liver is unable to cope with the massive increase in the number of red blood cells that it is supposed to break down, and yellow bile pigments spill over into the blood, producing jaundice. When these settle in the brain, major damage results in the basal ganglia.

KERNIG'S SIGN
Test performed in the diagnosis of meningitis (inflammation of the meninges, the membranes covering the brain and spinal cord). When the thigh is flexed upon the abdomen and pain is produced by extending the lower leg or there is marked resistance, the sign is positive.

KETOGENIC DIET
A high-fat diet that produces ketosis. It is sometimes prescribed in the treatment of epilepsy and infections of the urinary tract.

KETONE BODIES
A group of compounds, similar to acetone, produced by fatty acid metabolism, found only when a metabolic disturbance is present.

KETONEMIA
A high content of ketone bodies in the blood.

KETONURIA
The presence of ketone bodies in the urine. This condition may be present in diabetes or as a result of an unbalanced high-protein diet.

KETOSIS
Condition in which ketone bodies are present in the blood, as occurs in states of acidosis. It is a symptom of severe diabetes and starvation.

KETOSTEROIDS
A group of compounds that chemically resemble cholesterol, in which ketone groups are attached to carbon atoms. When the ketone is in the number 17 position of the nucleus, it is known as a 17-ketosteroid. The substances are normally present in the urine, 10-25 mg being excreted in the urine in 24 hours by a male and 4-15 mg by a female. Below average values occur in hypopituitarism, Addison's disease and hypogonadism, and the value may be doubled in Cushing's disease and tumors of the adrenal gland.

Testosterone and other androgens (sex hormones), which have male sex hormone characteristics, are 17-ketosteroids.

KETY METHOD
A method of determining coronary blood flow by measurement of nitrous oxide levels in the blood of a patient breathing nitrous oxide.

KHAT
A shrub cultivated by the Arabs for its leaves and buds that are the source of a habituating stimulant when chewed or used as a tea.

KIDNEY
Either of two bean-shaped excretory organs that filter wastes from the blood and excrete them and water in urine and help to regulate the water, electrolyte, and pH balance of the body.

KILLER CELL
T cell that functions in cell mediated immunity by destroying a cell (as a tumor cell) having a specific IgG antigenic molecule on its surface by causing lysis of the cell or by releasing a nonspecific toxin.

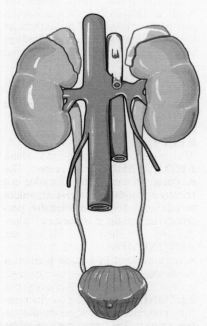

Urinary apparatus; From top to bottom: kidneys and blood supply, ureters, urinary bladder.

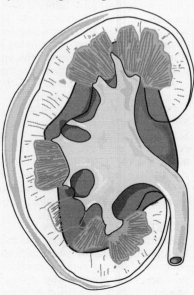

Cross section of the right kidney. From left to right: cortex, medulla (with renal pyramids and papillae, renal pelvis (where the urine is collected) and the first part of the ureter.

KILLIAN'S OPERATION
Curetting of the frontal sinus of the skull, leaving the supra-orbital ridge (eyebrow) intact to reduce deformity.

KIMMELSTEIN-WILSON SYNDROME
Also called intercapillary glomerulosclerosis: severe kidney disease, present in diabetics, with high blood pressure, edema (swelling) and a high concentration of albumin in the urine.

KINESIOLOGY
The study of the principles of mechanics and anatomy in relation to human movement.

KINESITHERAPY
The therapeutic and corrective application of passive and active movements (as by massage) and of exercise.

KINESTHESIS
General term covering sensations of movement of any part of the body, arising from stimulation of nerve receptors in joints, muscles and tendons, and sometimes inclusive of sensations from the organ of balance in the ear.

KINESTHETIC MEMORY
Memory in terms of ideal representation of movement sensations.

KINEPHANTOM
An illusion of direction of movement, or its pattern, when a movement is seen in silhouette shadows.

KINEPLASTIC SURGERY
Surgical operation whereby certain muscle groups are isolated and utilized to work certain modified prostheses such as an artificial hand.

KINESIA
Motion sickness, such as seasickness, car sickness, etc.

KINESALGIA
Discomfort or pain caused by muscular movement, usually on the basis of a tear or bruise in the muscle.

KINESIONEUROSIS
A functional disorder characterized by nervous tics and muscular spasms. If a severe neurosis develops, some form of psychotherapy should be applied.

KININ
Any of a group of peptides having the ability to produce vasodilatation (widening of blood vessels) and smooth muscle contraction, and formed from kininogens in the plasma by the action of some esterases. They can induce pain and probably are instrumental in migraine headache, as well as in allergic reactions.

KINOGEN
An inactive precursor of a kinin.

KIRCHNER WIRE
A metal wire inserted through bone and used to achieve internal traction or immobilization of bone fractures.

KISS OF LIFE
Method of artificial respiration. Exhaled breath of rescuer inflates the victim's lungs.

KLEPTOMANIA
The persistent impulse to steal, which may have a sexual cause. The essential feature of this disorder is a recurrent failure to resist impulses to steal objects not needed for personal use or their monetary value; the objects taken are either given away, discarded, returned surreptitiously, or kept and hidden. Almost invariably the person has enough money to pay for the stolen objects. The person experiences an increasing sense of tension immediately before committing the act and when immediate arrest is probable (e.g., in full view of a policeman), it is

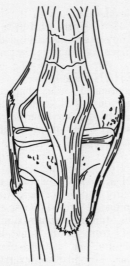

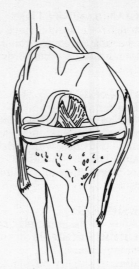

Cross section of the right kidney. From left to right: cortex, medulla (with renal pyramids and papillae), renal pelvis (where the urine is collected) and the first part of the ureter.

Anterior view of the knee with part of the femur (above) and below the fibula (left) and tibia (right). The various ligaments are shown. The patella and the patellar ligament is located in front of the knee.

not planned, and the chances of apprehension are not fully taken into account. The stealing is done without long-term planning and without assistance from others.

KLIEG EYES
Watering and inflammation of the eyes caused by immoderate exposure to very bright lights.

KLINEFELTER'S SYNDROME
Relatively common chromosome anomaly occurring in about one in every 700 live male births. There is an extra X-chromosome, thus making 47 in total. Most affected males are normal in appearance and intellect, although many are sterile.

KLUMPKE'S PARALYSIS
Paralysis and atrophy (wasting) of muscles of the forearm and hand, with sensory and pupillary disturbances due to injury to sympathetic nerves arising in the neck.

KNEE
The joint complex formed, fronted

by the kneecap, at which the thighbone and lower leg connect. It includes joints at which the femur and tibia meet, a joint where the femur and patella meet, and numerous ligaments and bursae.

KNEECAP
The movable bone covering the knee joint in front.

KNEE JERK
Reflex that is an involuntary jerk forward of the lower leg produced by tapping of the ligament below the kneecap when the leg hangs loosely bent at the right angles. The knee jerk is normally present, but when it is absent, it is indicative of a disorder of the central nervous system. It may be difficult to elicit in some nervous people because they hold the leg rigid and refuse to allow it to kick out.

KNOCK-KNEE
Inward curvature of the legs, causing the knees to knock together in walking. This is very common in

young children, who tend to outgrow it by the age of seven. It can also be caused by rickets, and by rheumatoid and osteoarthritis, when the knee joints collapse inward.

KNUCKLEBONE
A bone forming the knuckle of the finger, the rounded end of the fingerbone at a joint.

KNUCKLES
Joints of the fingers, especially the joints at the roots of the fingers; the rounded prominences of such joints when the fingers are bent.

KOCHER'S FORCEPS
A strong forceps for controlling bleeding in surgery having serrated blades with interlocking teeth at the lips.

KOCH'S BACILLUS
Older term used for the tuberculosis bacillus.

KOCH'S PHENOMENON
The response of a tuberculous animal to reinfection with tubercle bacilli marked by necrotic lesions that develop rapidly and heal quickly and caused by hypersensitivity to products of the tubercle bacillus.

KOEHLER'S DISEASE
Inflammation of both the bone and cartilage (osteochondritis) of the navicular bone in the foot; confined to children three to five years old.

KOILONYCHIA
Spoon-shaped (concave) nails, characteristic of iron-deficiency anemia.

KOLMER'S TEST
A blood test for syphilis.

KOPLIK'S SPOTS
Small white spots inside the mouth, during the first days of measles.

KOROTKOFF SOUNDS
Arterial sounds heard through a stethoscope applied to the brachial artery distal to the cuff of a sphygmomanometer that change with varying cuff pressure and that are used to determine systolic and diastolic blood pressure.

KORSAKOFF'S SYNDROME
Also called alcoholic dementia: an amnesic state in which the inability to record new memory traces may lead to the invention of stories to make up for the lost memory and a paradoxic situation in which the person can carry out complex tasks learned before his/her illness but cannot learn the simplest new skills.

The course of the syndrome reflects its cause. It is often transient and has a good prognosis in head injury.

In alcoholism (where the syndrome is caused by a lack of thiamine, a B vitamin that is destroyed by alcohol), and other conditions where destruction is irreversible, the prognosis is poor and prolonged institutional care may be required.

KRABBE'S DISEASE
Genetically determined degenerative disease associated with mental subnormality.

KRAUROSIS
A dry, atrophied (wasted) condition of the skin and mucous membranes.

KRAUROSIS VULVAE
A dry condition of the membranes of the vulva.

KRAUSE'S CORPUSCLE
Any of various rounded sensory end organs occurring in mucous membranes (as of the conjunctiva or genitals).

KRAUSE'S MEMBRANE
One of the isotropic cross bands in a striated muscle fiber that consists of disks or sarcoplasm linking the individual fibrils.

KREBS CYCLE
A sequence of reactions in the living organism in which oxidation of acetic acid or acetyl equivalent provides energy for storage of phosphate bonds,

KRUKENBERG TUMOR
A secondary malignant tumor of the ovary. The primary growth is usually in the stomach.

KUDER REFERENCE RECORD
A self-report inventory designed to reveal relative interest in ten broadly defined vocational areas by the administration of items dealing with the interests.

KUENTGER NAIL
Used to fix fractures of long bones, especially the femur. The nail has a clover-leaf cross-section.

KUPFER CELL
A fixed histiocyte of the walls of the liver sinusoids that is stellate with large oval nucleus and the cytoplasm commonly packed with fragments resulting from phagocytic action.

KURU
A progressive fatal disorder due to degeneration of the central nervous system, transmitted during cannibalistic rites and occurring only in natives of the New Guinea highlands. Discovery of this disease led to great progress in research into slow viruses.

KUSSMAUL BREATHING
Abnormally slow deep respiration characteristic of air hunger and occurring especially in acidotic states.

KVEIM TEST
Test for the diagnosis of sarcoidosis, a condition in which the lymph glands enlarge and fibrous nodules appear in the chest and other body areas.

KWASHIORKOR
A condition common in children of some areas of the Third World, where there is protein malnutrition even though there is a relatively adequate calorie intake. In affected children, the following symptoms are seen:
– excess body fluid;
– distended abdomen;
– skin and hair changes;
– loss of appetite;
– diarrhea;
– liver disturbance;
– apathy.
   Its name derives from the Ghanaian for "deposed one," from its occurrence in children who are removed from breastfeeding at an early date, often because of the birth of another baby. There also seems to be an element of emotional deprivation involved. Therapy involves rehydration, treatment of infection and a balanced diet with adequate protein, as well as attention and affection given to the child.

KWINT PSYCHOMOTOR TEST
An inventory of psychomotor activities based on age, and designed for use with brain-damaged children.

KYMOGRAPHY
A technique used to record graphically motions of the body, such as the heart and the large blood vessels.

KYPHOSCOLIOSIS
A curvature of the spine sideways and backwards.

KYPHOSIS
An abnormal backward curving of the upper part of the spine, so that a hump appears in the shoulder area and the lower back is abnormally arched. In its severe form, it is known as "hunchback."

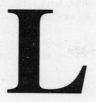

L

LABIA
The lip or lip-like structure.

LABIAL
Pertaining to a lip, or labium.

LABIAL ARTERY
Either of two branches of the facial artery of which one is distributed to the upper and one to the lower lip.

LABIAL GLAND
One of the small tubular mucous and serous glands lying beneath the mucous membrane of the lips.

LABIALISM
Defective speech with the use of labial sounds.

LABILE
Gliding, moving from point to point over the surface; unstable, fluctuating.

LABILITY
The quality of being labile; in psychiatry, emotional instability.

LABIOCHOREA
A choreic affection of the lips in speech, with stammering.

LABIOCLINATION
Outward inclination of a front tooth toward the lips.

LABIODENTAL
Pertaining to the lips and teeth.

LABIOGINGIVAL
Pertaining to or formed by the labial and gingival walls of a tooth cavity.

LABIOPLACEMENT
Displacement of a tooth toward the lip.

LABIUM
A fleshy border or edge; a lip-like edge or lip-like structure. The term is mostly used for any of the folds at the margin of the vulva.

LABIUM MAJUS
An elongated fold of skin in the female, on either side of the vaginal opening.

LABIUM MINUS
A small skin fold on either side, between the labium majus on either side of the vaginal opening.

LABIUM ORIS
Lip of the mouth.

LABOR
The function of the female organism by which the product of conception is expelled through the vagina to the outside world; the first stage begins with the onset of regular uterine contractions and ends when the cervix is completely dilated and flush with the vagina; the second extends from the end of the first stage until the expulsion of the infant is completed; the third extends from expulsion of the infant until the placenta and membranes are expelled and contraction of the uterus is completed.

LABOR COACH
A person who assist a woman in labor by providing emotional support and encouragement to use breathing, concentration, and exercise techniques learned in childbirth-preparation classes.

LABOR, DRY
Labor in which the amniotic fluid escapes before the onset of contractions of the uterus.

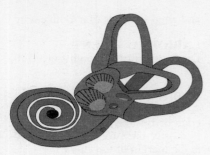

Structure of the labyrinth with the cochlea (left) and the semicircular canals (right).

LABOR, INDUCED
Expulsion of the fetus from the womb, brought on by artificial means.

LABOR PAIN
The discomfort and pain caused by contractions of the uterus during labor; pain sensation accompanying the rhythmic contractions of the womb that result in the birth of an infant.

LABOR, POSTPONED
Labor occurring two weeks or more after the expected date of confinement.

LABOR, PRECIPITATE
Labor occurring with undue rapidity.

LABOR, PREMATURE
Expulsion of a viable infant before the normal end of gestation; usually applied to interruption of pregnancy between the 28th and 37th week.

LABOR ROOM
A hospital room where a woman in labor is kept before being taken to the delivery room.

LABORATORY
A place equipped for making tests or doing experimental work.

LABORATORY, CLINICAL
One for examination of materials derived from the human body for the purpose of providing information on diagnosis, prevention, or treatment of disease.

LABRUM
An edge, rim, or lip; a lip-like structure.

LABRUM GLENOIDALE
The cartilage of the glenoid cavity in the shoulder joint.

LABYRINTH
The internal ear, made up of the vestibule, cochlea, and semicircular canals.

LABYRINTHECTOMY
Surgical removal of the labyrinth.

LABYRINTH, ETHMOID
Either of the paired lateral masses of the ethmoid bone, consisting of many thin-walled cellular cavities, the ethmoidal cells.

LABYRINTH, MEMBRANOUS
A system of communicating epithelial sacs and ducts within the bony labyrinth, containing the endolymph.

LABYRINTHINE NYSTAGMUS
Regular movements of the eyeball (nystagmus) associated with disorders of the labyrinth.

LABYRINTHINE SENSE
A complex sense concerned with the perception of bodily position and motion, mediated by end organs in the vestibular apparatus and the semicircular canals, and stimulated by alterations in the pull of gravity and by head movements.

LABYRINTHINE VERTIGO
Vertigo (an extreme form of giddiness) associated with disorders of the labyrinth.

LABYRINTHITIS
Inflammation of the labyrinth of the inner ear.

LABYRINTHITIS, CIRCUMSCRIBED

Inflammation of the labyrinth due to erosion of the bony wall of a semicircular canal with exposure of the membranous labyrinth.

LACERATION

Tear or irregular wound produced by tearing or crushing of a part, particularly the skin.

LACERTUS FIBROSUS

An aponeurosis extending from the medial border of the biceps tendon to the fascia of the ulnar side of the forearm.

LACRIMA

Tear.

LACRIMAL ABSCESS

An abscess in a tear duct or gland.

LACRIMAL APPARATUS

The structures that secrete and drain tears from the eye. Tears produced in the lacrimal gland drain through small openings at the corner of the eye into special ducts that pass into the nasal cavity.

LACRIMAL ARTERY

A large branch of the ophthalmic artery that arises near the optic foramen, and that passes along the superior border of the lateral rectus muscle, supplying the lacrimal gland.

LACRIMAL BONE

A small fragile facial bone located at the inner part of the orbital cavity. The lacrimal bone makes up part of the front inner wall of each orbit and provides a groove for the passage of the lacrimal ducts.

LACRIMAL DUCT

A short canal leading from a minute orifice on a small elevation at the medial angle of each eyelid to the lacrimal sac. The term is also applied to any of several small ducts that carry tears from the lacrimal gland to the fornix of the conjunctiva.

LACRIMAL GLAND

A gland under the upper eyelid that secretes and produces tears. The gland is located laterally and superiorly to the bulb of the eye in a shallow depression on the inner surface of the frontal bone.

LACRIMAL NERVE

Branch of the trigeminal nerve supplying the accessory structures of the eye.

The lacrimal nerve enters the lacrimal gland with the lacrimal artery and supplies the lacrimal gland and the adjacent conjunctiva and the skin of the upper eyelid.

LACRIMAL SAC

Either of two oval-shaped dilated ends of the nasolacrimal duct that fill with tears secreted by the lacrimal glands.

LACRIMATION

Secretion and discharge of tears.

LACRIMATOR

An irritant that causes the secretion of tears.

LACTAGOGUE

A substance that stimulates the secretion of milk from the breasts.

LACTALBUMIN

A protein belonging to the albumin class, found in milk. It is a protein fraction from whey that includes lactoglobulin and is used in foods and in preparing protein hydrolases.

LACTASE

An enzyme found in the small intestine, liver, and kidney that catalyzes (speeds up) the breakdown of lactose (milk sugar) into the simple sugars glucose and galactose. Lactase is particular abundant during infancy.

LACTASE DEFICIENCY
Another name for carbohydrate intolerance.

LACTATE
Any salt or ester of lactic acid.

LACTATE DEHYDROGENASE
Any of a group of isoenzymes that catalyze reversibly the conversion of pyruvic acid to lactic acid. They are found in the liver, kidneys, striated muscle, and the myocardium, and tend to accumulate in the body when these organs or tissues are deceased or injured.

LACTATION
The production of breast milk; also the time during which milk is produced. The term is also used in the sense of the act of nursing or suckling young.

LACTEAL
(1) Pertaining to milk;
(2) any of the intestinal lymphatics that transport chyle.

LACTEAN
One of the numerous minute lymphatic vessels that absorb or take up lymph from the alimentary canal and convey it to the thoracic duct.

LACTESCENCE
Resemblance to milk.

LACTIC ACID
The end product of the metabolism of sugar, the formation of which causes milk to sour. Lactic acid is produced in muscles after their cells have broken down glycogen for energy, and it is this accumulation of lactic acid that causes muscle fatigue. Blood levels of lactic acid are also elevated in persons with lactic acidosis, diabetes, anemia, leukemia and in other abnormal conditions.

Lactic acid is also an ingredient in preparations for warts and emollients.

LACTIC ACIDOSIS
A condition characterized by a marked "anion gap." Normally the amount of sodium and potassium in the blood (the anion group) equals the total amount of chloride and bicarbonate in the blood (cation group). When the difference between the two groups is greater than 30 (that is, when the cation group is decreased), an anion gap exists and is an ominous sign of lactic acidosis. Blood is taken from a vein and the whole blood is tested.

LACTIFEROUS DUCT
The ducts of the mammary glands (i.e. breasts) that lead to the tip of the nipple.

LACTIFEROUS SINUS
An expansion in a lactiferous duct at the base of the nipple in which milk accumulates.

LACTIFUGE
Any agent used to stop milk secretion in the mammary glands.

LACTOBACILLUS
Any of the rod-shaped bacteria that produces lactic acid in the fermentation of milk and carbohydrates. These bacteria require little or no oxygen; they require carbohydrates for growth and ferment them chiefly to lactic acid.

LACTOFERRIN
A red iron-binding protein synthesized by neutrophils (a type of white blood cells) and glandular epithelial cells, found in many human secretions (as tears and milk), and retarding bacterial and fungal growth.

LACTOGEN
Any substance that enhances the secretion of milk.

LACTOGEN, HUMAN PLACENTAL
A hormone secreted by the pla-

centa; it has lactogenic and growth-promoting activity, and inhibits insulin activity of the mother.

LACTOGENIC
Stimulating milk production.

LACTOGENIC HORMONE
Prolactin, a hormone produced in and secreted by the anterior lobe of the pituitary gland that stimulates growth and development of mammary glands in females and the production of milk after parturition.

LACTOGLOBULIN
A crystalline protein fraction that is obtained from the whey of milk.

LACTO-OVO-VEGETARIAN
One who follows a diet of milk, eggs, vegetables, fruits, grains, and nuts.

LACTOSE
Milk sugar that is broken down into galactose and glucose in the intestines. Its levels in the urine are elevated in late pregnancy, during lactation and in certain rare metabolic diseases.

LACTOSE INTOLERANCE
Also called carbohydrate intolerance; the inability of the body to digest milk sugar.

LACTOSE TOLERANCE
The capacity of the body to handle lactose/glucose metabolism.

LACTOSURIA
The presence of milk sugar in the urine.

LACTOTHERAPY
Treatment by milk diet.

LACTOVEGETARIAN
(1) A person who subsists on a diet of milk (or milk products) and vegetables;
(2) pertaining to such a diet.

LACTULOSE
A laxative drug. It is a synthetic disaccharide, able to alter the bacterial contents of the bowel and increase the fluid bulk of the motions, and leads to stimulation of bowel movement.

LACUNA
A small pit or hollow cavity.

LACUNA, ABSORPTION
A pit or groove in developing bone that is undergoing resorption; frequently found to contain osteoclasts.

LACUNA, BONE
A small cavity within the bone matrix, containing an osteocyte from which slender small canals radiate and penetrate the adjacent lamellae to anastomose with neighboring small canals, thus forming a system of cavities interconnected by minute canals.

LACUNA, CARTILAGE
Any of the small cavities within the matrix of cartilage, containing a chondrocyte.

LAENNEC'S CIRRHOSIS
Alcoholic cirrhosis in the liver. It is a hepatic cirrhosis in which increased connective tissue spreads out from the portal spaces comprising and distorting the lobules, causing impairment of liver function, and ultimately producing the typical hobnail liver.

LAENNEC'S PEARL
Small gelatinous bodies found in the sputum of asthmatic patients.

LAFORA BODY
Any of the cytoplasmic inclusion bodies found in neurons of parts of the central nervous system in myoclonic epilepsy and consisting of a complex of glycoprotein and mucopolysaccharides.

LAG
The interval between the cessation of a stimulus and the cessation of its effect.

LAG INFANT
Abbreviation for "large-for-gestational-age" infant.

LAGOPHTHALMOS
Inability to close the eyelids completely.

LAG PHASE
The period of time between the introduction of a microorganism into a culture medium and the time it begins to increase exponentially.

LALIATRY
The study and treatment of disorders of speech.

LALLATION
A babbling, infantile form of speech; unintelligible speech-like utterances. The term is also used for a speech disorder in which the sound "l" is used in place of other sounds, especially "r" sounds, or the sound "l" is mispronounced.

LALOGNOSIS
The understanding of speech.

LALLOPATHOLOGY
The branch of medicine dealing with disorders of speech.

LALOPLEGIA
Paralysis of the organs of speech.

LALORRHEA
Excessive flow of words.

LAMAZE METHOD OF CHILDBIRTH
A method of psychophysical preparation for childbirth, developed by the French obstetrician Ferdinand Lamaze in the 1960s; that is now the most widely used method of natural childbirth. In classes during pregnancy and in practice sessions at home, the pregnant woman, usually with the help of a coach learns the physiology of pregnancy and childbirth, techniques of relaxation, concentration, breathing, and exercises certain muscles to promote control during labor and childbirth.

LAMBDA
The point of meeting of the sagittal and coronal sutures (immovable unions of two bones) of the skull.

LAMBDA CHAIN
Polypeptide chain of one of the two types of light chain that are found in antibodies and can be distinguished antigenetically and by the sequence of amino acids in the chain.

LAMBDACISM
Speech disorder marked by incorrect or excessive pronunciation of the sound "l" or substitution of the sound "r" for "l".

LAME
Incapable of normal locomotion; deviation from normal gait.

LAMELLA
Medicated disc or tiny tablet that is inserted inside the lower eyelid in the treatment of eye infections. Also, a lamina or layer; a basement membrane in an organ.

LAMELLA, CIRCUMFERENTIAL
One of the layers of bone that underlie the periosteum and endosteum.

LAMELLA, ENDOSTEAL
One of the bony plates lying beneath the endosteum.

LAMELLA, HAVERSIAN
One of the concentric bony plates surrounding a Haversian canal.

LAMELLA, INTERSTITIAL
One of the bony plates that fill in between the Haversian systems.

LAMINA
A thin, flat plate or layer, used in anatomic nomenclature to designate such a structure, or a layer of a composite structure.

LAMINA BASALIS
One of a pair of longitudinal zones of the embryonic neural tube, from which develop the ventral gray columns of the spinal cord and the motor centers of the brain.

LAMINA CRIBROSA
The horizontal plate of ethmoid bone forming the roof of the nasal cavity, and perforated by many foramina of olfactory nerves.

LAMINA, DENTAL
A thickened epithelial band along the margin of the gum in the embryo, from which the enamel organs are developed.

LAMINA DURA
The thin hard layer of bone that lines the socket of a tooth and that appears as a dark line in radiography.

LAMINA FUSCA
The pigmentary layer of the sclera.

LAMINA PROPRIA
A vascular layer of connective tissue under the basement membrane lining a layer of epithelium.

LAMINA SPIRALIS
A double plate or bone winding spirally around the modiolus, dividing the spiral canal of the cochlea into the scala tympani and scala vestibuli.

LAMINA TERMINALIS
A thin layer of gray matter in the telencephalon that extends backward from the corpus callosum above the optic chiasm and forming the median portion of the rostral wall of the third ventricle of the cerebrum.

LAMINA, VERTEBRAL ARC
Either of the pair of broad plates of bone flaring out from the pedicles of the vertebral arches and fusing together at the midline to complete the dorsal part of the arch and provide a base for the spinous process.

LAMINECTOMY
A surgical procedure in which the bony arches of one or more vertebrae are chipped or removed to relieve pressure on the spinal cord, to remove tumors, or to treat disorders involving the vertebral column.

LAMPAS
A congestion of the mucous membrane of the hard palate just posterior of the incisor teeth.

LANATOSIDE
Any of three poisonous crystalline cardiac steroids occurring in the leaves of a foxglove (Digitalis lanata).

LANCEFIELD GROUP
One of the serologically distinguishable groups into which streptococci can be divided.

LANCET
A small, pointed, two-edged surgical knife.

LANDMARK
An anatomical structure used as a point of orientation in locating other structures (as in surgical procedures). The term is also used to designate a point on the body or skeleton from which anthropological measurements are taken.

LANDOLT RING
One of a series of incomplete rings or circles used in some eye chart to determine visual discrimination or acuity.

LANGERHANS CELL
A dendritic cell of the interstitial

spaces of the epidermis that resembles a melanocyte but lacks tyrosinase.

LANGHANS GIANT CELL
Any of the large cells found in the lesions of some granulomatous conditions (as leprosy and tuberculosis) and containing a number of peripheral nuclei arranged in a circle or in the shape of a horseshoe.

LANGUAGE
Means of communication. The psychological definition is: a conventional system of expressive signs functioning, psychologically, in the individual as an instrument of conceptual analysis and synthesis and, socially, as a means of intercommunication, from which it follows that the unit of language is a sentence or statement.

LANGUAGE ACQUISITION DEVICE
Preprogramming of the central nervous system providing for a propensity of thought and feeling.

LANGUAGE CENTER
Areas in the cerebral cortex whose functions are involved in different aspects of spoken and written language.

LANGUAGE DYSFUNCTION
Disorders of various nature. Defects in language function (aphasia) may be of an expressive nature (difficulty in planning, coordinating and using speech), a receptive nature (unable to understand what is said), or amnesic (unable to remember sounds), and testing for the type of aphasia helps locate the exact area of brain disease.

LANGUAGE LEARNING
The process of acquiring the techniques of symbolic communication, including the identification of the meanings that have been assigned to series of sounds or other symbols, the recognition and reproduction of the symbols used in the customary linguistic orders and structures, and the acquisition of the motor skills necessary to use the symbols learned.

LANGUOR
A complex of mental and neuromuscular conditions, with, on the one hand, physical and general sensation akin to those of fatigue, with disinclination for active employment; and, on the other, a state of relaxation.

LANOLIN
A purified, fat-like substance from the wool of sheep, mixed with 25 to 30 percent water; used in a water-in-oil ointment base.

Lanolin easily penetrates the skin, and because it is capable of taking up water, it makes an ideal base for medicinal products intended to be absorbed through the skin.

LANUGO
Fine hair on the body of the fetus; it is normally shed during the ninth month of gestation but may be present on newborns, especially premature newborns.

LAPARO–
Word element: loin, flank, abdomen.

LAPARO-ENTEROSTOMY
Surgical creation of an opening into the intestine through the abdominal wall.

LAPARORRHAGY
Suture of the abdominal wall.

LAPAROSCOPE
A long slender optical instrument for insertion through the abdominal wall that is used to visualize the interior of the peritoneal cavity.

LAPAROSCOPY
Examination by means of a laparo-

scope: an endoscope for examining the peritoneal cavity. The laparoscope is inserted through a small incision in the abdominal wall. The procedure is also used in women as a sterilization method in which the Fallopian tubes are ligated.

LAPAROTOMY
Incision through the flank or, more generally, through any part of the abdominal wall. The method is often done for exploration, as, for instance, to examine abdominal organs.

LARGE INTESTINE
That portion of the digestive tract containing the cecum, appendix, ascending, transverse and descending colons, and the rectum.

LARGE MUSCLE SKILLS
Ability to perform movements - such as sitting, crawling, climbing, jumping, and walking - that require coordination of the large muscles. Also called gross motor skills.

LARSEN'S SYNDROME
A syndrome characterized by cleft palate, flattened facies, multiple congenital joint dislocations and deformities of the foot.

LARVA
An independent, immature stage in the life cycle of an animal in which it is unlike the parent and must undergo changes in form and size to reach the adult stage.

LARVA MIGRANS
Creeping eruption; a convoluted threadlike skin eruption that appears to migrate, caused by the burrowing beneath the skin of roundworm larvae, particularly Ancylostoma larvae.

LARVA MIGRANS, VISCERAL
A condition due to prolonged migration of nematode larvae in human tissue other than skin; commonly caused by the larvae of Toxocara canis, which do not complete their life cycle in humans.

LARVICIDE
An agent that kills insect larvae.

LARYNG–
Pertaining to the larynx: the organ of voice.

LARYNGALGIA
Pain in the voice box or region of the voice box.

LARYNGEAL ARTERY
Either of two arteries supplying blood to the larynx. The inferior laryngeal artery is a branch of the inferior thyroid artery that supplies the muscles and mucous membranes of the dorsal part of the larynx. The superior laryngeal artery is a branch of the superior thyroid artery or sometimes of the external carotid artery that supplies the muscles, mucous membranes, and glands of the larynx and anastomoses with the branch of the opposite side.

LARYNGEAL CANCER
A malignant tumor of the larynx or voice box. While not a common disease, it does account for 2 to 5 percent of all cancer cases. The outcome of this form of cancer is almost entirely dependent on how early it is discovered and treatment begun. If diagnosed early, when the cancer is commonly limited to one vocal cord, the disease can be cured. In the great majority of such cases, a normal voice will still be possible. In the disease's later stages, however, when the cancer has spread to other areas of the larynx and throat, treatment often involves laryngectomy, the surgical removal of the larynx.

Cancer of the larynx is primarily a disease of men in the 50s and 60s; it is rarely seen before the age of 40 and the frequency with which it occurs levels off after the age of 65. The ratio of male to female sufferers is about 7 to 1.

Several environmental or occupational factors have been linked with laryngeal cancer, and habitual smoking and heavy drinking are among the most important of these.

LARYNGEAL NERVE

Either of two branches of the vagus nerve supplying the larynx. The superior laryngeal nerve arises from the ganglion of the vagus situated below the jugular foramen in front of the transverse processes of the first two cervical vertebrae and that passes down the neck to supply the cricothyroid muscles.

The inferior laryngeal nerve or recurrent laryngeal nerve arises below the larynx, loops under the subclavian artery on the right side and under the arch of the aorta on the left, and returns upward to the larynx to supply all the muscles of the thyroid except the cricothyroid.

LARYNGISMUS STRIDULUS

A sudden spasm of the larynx that occurs in children especially in rickets and is marked by difficult breathing with prolonged noisy inspiration.

LARYNGITIS

Inflammation of the larynx; may be acute or chronic in character, and catarrhal, suppurative, diphtheric, tuberculous or syphilitic in type.

The acute catarrhal type that accompanies a heavy cold is most common, and is characterized by hoarseness and sometimes by complete loss of voice.

The larynx becomes inflamed as a result of:
- inhaling smoke;
- chemical fumes;
- gases;
- vapors or dust;
- overuse or abuse of voice;
- excessive use of alcohol;
- diseases such a sinusitis, tonsillitis, bronchitis, flu;
- the common cold;
- pneumonia and pharyngitis;
- polyps in the throat;
- cancer.

Hoarseness is most often a temporary, minor problem. However, chronic or persistent hoarseness may signal a minor to serious underlying problem. If hoarseness continues for two weeks, it is best to have the problem evaluated by a doctor.

Treatment of mild laryngitis is by steam inhalation, which has the added benefit of opening the airways in the nose, the blockage of which may be greatly contribute to the condition.

LARYNGOSCOPE

Surgical instrument consisting of a long-handled mirror that is placed at the back of the throat to inspect the inside of the larynx.

LARYNGOSPASM

Spasm of the interior of the larynx and vocal cords.

LARYNGOTRACHEITIS

Inflammation of both the larynx (voice box) and the trachea (windpipe).

LARYNGOTRACHEOBRON- CHITIS

Inflammation of the larynx, trachea, and bronchi. It is an acute severe infection of these parts marked by swelling of the tissues and excessive secretion of mucus leading to more or less complete obstruction of the respiratory passages.

LARYNGOTRACHEOTOMY

Surgical operation to make an artificial airway by cutting through the cartilaginous rings of the upper portion of the trachea (windpipe) and inserting a small tube so that the person will breathe through the tube instead of through the mouth.

LARYNX

The enlarged upper end of the trachea (windpipe); the organ of voice, a specialized structure capable of utilizing air expired from the lungs to produce "voice" or sounds, but not (on its own) speech. It also serves as an essential part of the air passageway of the respiratory tract, conveying air into and out of the lungs.

The larynx is located in the midline of the front part of the neck. Above, the larynx is continuous with the pharynx (throat), and below with the trachea.

It consists of a framework of cartilage held together by ligaments, membranes and muscles, and lined by a mucous membrane. Its most important structural feature is a pair of vocal cords that are essential in the production of the voice.

Nine pieces of cartilage form the framework of the larynx. There are three large single pieces - the thyroid and cricoid cartilages and the epiglottis - and three smaller paired pieces - the arytenoid, corniculate and cuneiform cartilages. Two groups of ligaments are found in the larynx. The extrinsic ligaments serve to connect the cricoid cartilage and the trachea at the lower border, and the thyroid cartilage and epiglottis with the hyoid bone (at the base of the tongue) at the upper border.

A number of intrinsic ligaments serve to join the cartilages of the larynx to each other. True joints are formed between the thyroid and cricoid cartilages, and between the arytenoid cartilages and the cricoid cartilages, allowing rotation and gliding movements.

Two bands of elastic fibers covered by mucous membrane pass around the whole of the interior of the larynx, forming shelf-like folds. The upper folds, called the false vocal cords, are stationary, and to a degree they protect the lower pair of folds, the true vocal cords. These vocal cords are sharp, prominent folds capable of being moved. The space between the two vocal cords is called the glottis, and the width of the glottis is modified by the action of the ligaments that move the arytenoid cartilages.

The larynx serves primarily as part of the passageway for conduction of air to and from the lungs, and as an organ of voice. Voice or sound is produced by vibration of the vocal cords as expired air is forced out between them. The width of the glottis opening and the tension of the cords are controlled primarily by the intrinsic ligaments of the larynx.

LASER

Abbreviation for light amplification by the stimulated emission of radiation; a device for amplifying light radiation, in which a beam of light is shot through a crystal, causing it to emit an intense, direct light beam; the heat from this acts as a cutting tool that is particularly useful in certain types of microsurgery (eye complications; ear surgery; skin surgery; cutting calcium deposits from the inner wall of atherosclerotic arteries).

The laser is also used to repair a detached retina in the eye, and to coagulate bleeding blood vessels in the retinas of diabetics. Other uses include coagulating bleeding ulcers in the stomach and duodenum, vaporizing cervical cancer cells, brain surgery and removal of tattoos, birthmarks and moles.

LASSA FEVER

A frequently fatal, contagious virus infection carried by a species of rat found in West Africa. The disease involves most organs of the body but spares the central nervous system. The incubation period is about ten days. The onset of severe symptoms - the major one being a very high temperature - is gradual; most persons have symptoms for four to five days before hospitalization is needed. Severe lower abdominal pain and intractable vomiting are common.

Because this is a virus, there is no specific drug treatment, the relief of symptoms being the primary concern.

LASSITUDE
A feeling of weariness or weakness; listlessness of body and mind.

LATE LUTEAL PHASE DYSPHORIC DISORDER
Variety of physical and emotional changes associated with specific phases of the menstrual cycle. Generally, these changes are not severe, cause little distress, and have no effect on social or occupational functioning. In some women, the disorder is characterized by a pattern of clinically significant emotional and behavioral symptoms that occur during the last week of the luteal phase and remit within a few days after the onset of the follicular phase. These symptoms occur in the week before, and remit within a few days after, the onset of menses.

LATENCY PERIOD
In psychoanalytic theory, a period of sexual development between the age of four or five and the beginning of adolescence, separating infantile from normal sexuality.

LATENT CONTENT
The real or unconscious meaning of a dream.

LATENT PERIOD
Delay between exposure to a disease-causing agent and the appearance of manifestations of the disease. After exposure to ionizing radiation, for instance, there is a latent period of five years, before development of leukemia, and more than twenty years before development of

certain other malignant conditions.

The term latent period is often used synonymously with induction period, that is, the period between exposure to a disease-causing agent and the appearance of manifestations of the disease. It has also been defined as the period from disease initiation to disease detection.

LATERAL
Of or pertaining to the side, situated at, preceding from or directed towards a side (of the body).

LATERAL GENICULATE BODY
A sensory relay nucleus that is part of the visual system. It is a part of the thalamus in the brain where the optic tract synapse joins with visual fibers that run to the visual region of the cerebral cortex.

LATERAL HUMERAL EPICONDYLITIS
Another name for tennis elbow.

LATEROPULSION
The tendency to fall involuntarily to one side, found in certain diseases of the cerebellum of the brain and the labyrinth of the ear.

LATEROVERSION
A tendency to or a turning towards one side.

LATEX FIXATION TEST
A blood test to detect various antibodies and factors indicative of such conditions as rheumatoid arthritis, systemic lupus erythematosus, dermatomyositis and chronic infections.

LATISSIMUS DORSI
A broad flat superficial muscle of thwe lowwr part of the back that originates mostly in a broad aponeurosis attached to the spinous processes of the vertebrae of the lower back, the supraspinal ligament, and the crest of the ilium. The

muscle is inserted into the bicipital groove of the humerus.

LAUDANUM
Popular name for tincture of opium.

LAV (lymphadenopathy-associated virus)
A retrovirus recovered from a person with lymphadenopathy (enlarged lymph nodes) who was also in a group at high risk for AIDS, and now believed to be the same virus as HIV-III.

LAXATIVE
Drug or food taken to promote bowel action and to treat constipation. They may act as irritants (cascara, senna, phenolphthalein, castor oil), softeners (mineral oil), or bulk agents (bran, methylcellulose and magnesium sulphate). Laxative abuse may cause gastrointestinal tract disorders, potassium deficiency and lung disease.

LAXATIVE, BULK-FORMING
Any of a group of medicines taken by mouth to encourage bowel movements to relieve constipation and to prevent straining. This type of laxative is not digested but absorbs liquid in the intestines and swells to form a soft, bulky stool. The bowel is than stimulated normally by the presence of the bulky mass.

Some bulk-forming laxatives, like psyllium and polycarbophil, may be prescribed to treat diarrhea. Laxatives should not be given to young children (up to 6 years of age) unless prescribed by their doctor.

LAXATIVE, EMOLLIENT
Any of a group of medicines taken by mouth to encourage bowel movements by helping liquids mix into the stool and prevent dry, hard stool masses. This type of laxative has been said not to cause a bowel movement but instead allows the patient to have a bowel movement

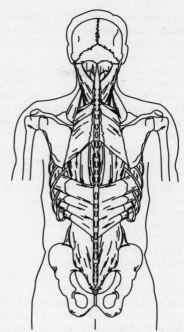

The latissimus dorsi is one of the major muscles of the back, running from the arm to the spine.

without straining. Emollient laxatives are available without a prescription; however, your doctor may have special instructions for the proper use and dose for your medical condition.

LAXATIVE, STIMULANT
Any of a group of laxatives, taken to encourage movements by acting on the intestinal wall. They increase the muscle contractions that move along the stool mass. Stimulant laxatives are available in many brand names, and dosage forms. They are a popular type of laxative for self-treatment.

LDH
Abbreviation for lactate dehydrogenase. It is a measurement of cardiac enzymes used to confirm some heart conditions.

LEAD POISONING
Medically called plumbism; result-

ing most commonly from repetitive absorption of increased amounts of lead through the gastrointestinal tract.

Acute poisoning from a single, massive dose of lead salts taken by mouth is exceptionally rare. The chronic course of poisoning may be punctuated by episodes of acute symptoms.

In the young child, increased lead absorption results most commonly from repetitive ingestion of old paint, old putty and lead-contaminated dirt and dust, and symptoms are most common during summer and are generally found in children with "pica" (a craving for an unusual food such as paint or dirt). In older children and adolescents in whom pica (except in retarded children) can be excluded, alternative sources should be checked, for example, lead objects retained in the stomach, making toy soldiers, illicit whiskey, part-time jobs in battery and other lead manufacturing plants, home repair involving burning and scraping off old paint surfaces.

Treatment
Identification of the source of overexposure and separation of the child from it, are the most important aspects of treatment. Medical treatment involves chelation therapy, drugs that promote the excretion of metals and serve to reduce dangerous levels of lead in the tissues quickly. It is most efficacious if it is given before acute symptoms appear, on the basis of clearly abnormal metabolic tests.

LEARNING
Any process that modifies experience and behavior. Thus, life itself is a continual learning situation, as we constantly modify our attitudes, opinions and behavior in the light of each new experience. As we grow older, we tend to become less receptive to new learning, more rigidly set in ways determined by previous learning responses that have now become habitual. This resistance to change is one of the most prominent features of aging. This is not due entirely to a natural reluctance to change established patterns of behavior, since aging also brings a falling off in the brain's capacity to utilize new information.

LEARNING DISABILITY (DISORDER)
Any of several abnormal conditions of children who, although having at least average intelligence, have difficulty in learning specific skills, or have other problems with normal learning procedures.

Hyperactivity, impulsiveness, emotional instability, muscle incoordination and certain perceptual difficulties may be observed before the child starts school. Some mothers state that, as an infant, their child was irritable and disliked being picked up or held; some even stiffened and pushed away.

Most children with learning disorders are identified during the early school years because of academic failure. Behavioral signs usually exist that suggest a general inability to control impulses and to integrate various cognitive and sensory-processing functions. Many of these children are hyperactive (constantly moving), touching, handling or otherwise unwittingly drawing critical attention to themselves.

Their behavior appears disordered, they lack a clear focus or sense of direction, and their efforts appear unrelated to assigned tasks. Many have a short attention span for auditory and visual stimuli, and because they cannot screen out even weak, irrelevant stimuli, they are easily distracted; yet at other times, persevere with whatever they are doing despite outside attempts to intervene. Their conduct is unpredictable, immature and impulsive, and when overstimulated, some become aggressive and destructive.

LEARNING, IDEATIONAL
Learning involving the use of ideational material, as in learning through the connection of ideas or memorization, in contrast to motor learning.

LEARNING, INCIDENTAL
The occurrence of learning in the absence of formal instruction, intent to learn as ascertainable motive.

LEARNING, MOTOR
Any form of learning that is described in terms of the activities of muscles and glands which it involves.

LEARNING, PERCEPTUAL
Learning of a new perceptual response, or learning that consists of modifying an already existing perceptual response.

LEARNING, PROGRAMMED
A learning method consisting of materials that are presented in a predetermined order with provisions enabling the student to check his/her answers and to proceed at his/her own pace.

LEARNING RESPONSE
Learning to make a specific set of responses to reach a goal.

LEARNING SET
A generalized approach to problem situations, which includes the assumption by the subject that a specific method can be discovered to solve the problem.

LEARNING, SUBLIMINAL
The acquisition of a habit which cannot be remembered because the learning of it was not on a conscious level or because it has not progressed far enough.

LECITHIN
A fatty substance (one of the phospholipids) found in blood, bile, brain, nerves and other tissues, as well as in egg yolk. It may be measured in ratio with sphingomyelin to determine fetal lung maturity.

LECITHIN/SPHINGOMYELIN RATIO
The ratio between the two components of amniotic fluid, which surrounds the fetus in the womb; found to be a predictor of fetal lung maturity.

LEEUWENHOEK, ANTONIE VAN (1632-1723)
Microscopist, the first scientist who observed bacteria.

His researches on lower animals refuted the doctrine of spontaneous generation. He grounded over 350 lenses.

LEFT-HANDEDNESS
Condition of being more adept in the use of the left hand. If you are born left-handed you tend to go through life with the feeling that the world is a place for other people. Ink smears when you write, doors open against you, screws turn the wrong way and even chewing gum wrappers seems to have been carefully and intentionally designed to thwart you.

Left-handers tend to be more creative and imaginative than their right-handed counterparts, to have better hearing, to be better athletes and musicians and artists.

Some of these anomalies are easily explained: left-handers are better typists, for instance, simply because the typewriter or keyboard was designed with a built-in bias that greatly favors the left hand.

LEG
One of the two lower extremities, including the femur (thighbone), tibia (shinbone), fibula and patella (kneecap); specifically the part between the hip and ankle. The length and direction of the long bones determine the basic form of the limb, which may be long, short, straight,

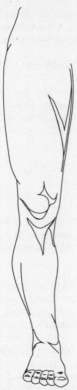

Anterior view of the thigh, knee joint, leg and foot. The ankle joints form the transition of the leg to the foot.

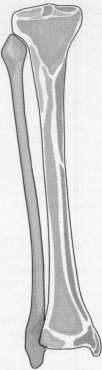

The two major bones of the leg: tibia (right) and fibula (left). The tibia, or shinbone, is the larger, medial bone of the leg. It bears the major portion of the weight on the leg. The fibula is parallel, and lateral, of the tibia. It is considerable smaller than the tibia.

knock-kneed or bowed. The femur, or thighbone, slants inward from the acetabulum, the cup-shaped depression of the hip joint, to the knee, and in the adult female, this angle is usually more marked than in the male because of the shorter length of the femur and the greater width of the pelvis.

The general shape of the limb is given by the muscles (within their envelopes of fibrous fascia) that surround the bones. The rather stark outline that this produces is smoothed out by the layer of subcutaneous fat. In females, the layer is thicker than in males, particularly in the thighs and buttocks, giving a more rounded appearance to the female limb.

The fullness of the buttock is due to the gluteus maximus muscle, and the size of the gluteal fat pad determines its final shape. The gluteal fold or buttock crease, does not represent the lower border of the gluteus maximus muscle, which extends well below the gluteal fold on its way to its insertion into the gluteal tuberosity of the femur and the iliotibial tract.

LEGIONNAIRES' DISEASE
Severe lung infection caused by a small Gram-negative, non-acid-fast bacillus Legionella pneumophila. After an incubation period of two to ten days, the illness begins with the non-specific symptoms of malaise, headache and muscular aches and

pains, succeeded in a few hours by high fever and shivering. A dry cough, or a cough producing a small amount of bloodstained sputum, is present in the beginning. Watery diarrhea with abdominal distention, occurring in about 50 percent of sufferers, may precede the onset of fever.

The main pathological changes are found in the lungs which on X-ray show patchy areas of consolidated tissue. Samples of this tissue reveal large numbers of the bacilli. Treatment is by specific antibiotics such as chloramphenicol and erythromycin.

LEIOMYOMA
A tumor made up of smooth (involuntary) muscle tissue.

LEIOMYOSARCOMA
A malignant tumor containing smooth muscle tissue.

LEISHMANIASIS
A group of conditions caused by a species of Leishmania and transmitted by several types of sandflies. The manifestations of the disease may be seen in the internal organs (kala-azar, and dum-dum fever) or on the skin (the Oriental sore, Dehli boil, Baghdad boil, American leishmaniasis) and the strain of infecting organisms and the host's immunologic status apparently can greatly modify the clinical manifestations.

LEPROSY
Chronic infectious disease caused by Mycobacterium leprae, an organism that is highly infectious but does not produce disease in the majority of those infected. It has a predilection for cooler regions - skin, mucous membranes and the nerves on the outer parts of the body (e.g., hands and feet).

Symptoms include the gradual development of flat skin sores which may eventually thicken and form ulcers. The sores may be numb or have unusual sensations in them. Small tumors under the skin may occur, and the infection progresses gradually, destroying skin, underlying tissue and even the ends of fingers and toes.

Drug treatment with specific anti-leprosy medicines is effective, but treatment takes years in order to be effective. Deformities will persist after treatment. Care of the sores and nodules as well as surgical treatment of the ulcers are important.

LEPTOMENINGES
The two soft membranes that envelop the brain and spinal cord.

LEPTOSPIRA
Any of the thin-coiled, aerobic bacteria normally found on rodents and other small mammals, some of which can infect humans.

LEPTOSPIRA AGGLUTININS
Agglutinins (a certain type of antibody) found in blood of persons with Weil's disease, an infectious type of jaundice caused by the Leptospira organisms.

LEPTOSPIROSIS
A condition resulting from a Leptospira infection.

LESBIANISM
Female homosexuality.

LESION
An abnormal, localized change in the structure of an organ or tissue, resulting from disease or injury.

LETHAL
Causing, or able to cause, death.

LETHARGY
Generally taken to mean "morbid drowsiness;" used technically for the earliest stage of hypnosis with some anesthesia and muscular limpness.

LEUCINE
A white crystalline amino acid, formed in various ways, especially by pancreatic digestion of proteins in the body; one of the essential amino acids, which cannot be manufactured by the body.

LEUCOCYTE
Alternative spelling of leukocyte.

LEUKAPHERESIS
A process in which blood is withdrawn from a vein, white blood cells are selectively removed in a cell separating machine, and the remaining fluid of the blood is reinfused in the donor. The white blood cells may be used for treatment, research, or other purposes.

LEUKEMIA
One of the major types of cancer; a malignant neoplasm of blood-forming tissues, characterized by abnormalities of the bone marrow, spleen, lymph nodes, and liver and by rapid and uncontrolled proliferation of abnormal numbers and forms of leukocytes (white blood cells).

Leukemia may be acute, rapidly progressing from signs of fatigue and weight loss to extreme weakness, repeated infections, and fever, or it may be chronic, progressing slowly over a period of years.

Leukemia is usually classified according to the type of white blood cell that is proliferating abnormally. Treatment involves chemotherapy, blood transfusions, antibiotics to control infections, and sometimes bone marrow transplants.

LEUKOCYTE
A white blood cell or corpuscle; a colorless blood cell active in the defense against infection and bacteria and occasionally found in body tissues. There are five different types of leukocytes:
- neutrophils;
- eosinophils;
- basophils;
- lymphocytes;
- monocytes.

LEUKOCYTE ALKALINE PHOSPHATASE TEST
A blood test employed to detect various diseases that stimulate the secretion of this enzyme, such as cirrhosis, polycythemia and certain infections. It is also used to differentiate chronic myelocytic leukemia from leukemia-like reactions.

LEUKOCYTOGENESIS
The formation of leukocytes in the tissues of the body.

LEUKOCYTOLYSIS
Destruction of leukocytes, usually by invading bacteria or viruses.

LEUKOCYTOSIS
A temporary increase in the number of leukocytes in the blood, usually caused by an infection and not indicative of leukemia.

LEUKODERMA
A deficiency of pigment in the skin, usually occurring in patches.

LEUKOPENIA
An acute decrease of leukocytes in the blood.

LEUKOPLAKIA
Formation of white, smooth spots or patches, irregular in size and shape, usually on the mucous membrane lining the inside of the cheek, but can occur on the male and female genital organs. The lesions are usually benign, but may become malignant.

LEUKORRHEA
Also called whites: a condition in which vaginal secretion increases to an abnormal amount. Leukorrhea is a white vaginal discharge containing white blood cells and excreted dead or damaged vaginal cells. It can be caused by a vaginal infection

such as trichomonas or candidiasis (thrush), or irritation by a foreign body such as an IUD, a forgotten tampon or even a vaginal tumor.

When leukorrhea becomes a source of vaginal pain or irritation, a woman should go to see her doctor.

LEUKOTOMY
Surgical operation involving the cutting of white nerve fibers in the frontal lobes of the brain, and formerly used to relieve severe depression and other psychotic states. It has now largely been abandoned in favor of safer (and reversible) drug therapy.

LEVATOR
A muscle that raises a part of the body. It is also the name of a surgical instrument used to raise a depressed part of the skull.

LEVITATION
Rising in the air without material support; a term employed in psychical research to describe alleged movement of heavy objects against gravity, due to an observable or known physical agency.

LEVULOSE
Fructose, a natural sugar found in honey and many fruits, used in foods, medicines, and preservatives.

LIBERTINE
Sexually unrestrained and promiscuous individual.

LIBERTINISM
Unrestrained sexual activity especially with reference to the male.

LIBIDO
Originally and still popularly, the sexuality or general sex drive of the individual. In Freudian psychoanalysis, the libido, with its source in the ID, is a type of mental energy (through it may, as in sexuality, generate physiological energy or activity) that is responsible for all human constructive action.

LIBIDO DAMMING
Frustration of psychosexual development.

LIBMAN-SACKS ENDO-CARDITIS
A noninfectious form of verrucous endocarditis associated with systemic lupus erythematosus.

LICE
There are three types of lice that live on humans:
- Pediculus corporis, the body louse;
- Phthirius pubis, the pubic louse, commonly called crabs;
- Pediculus capitis, the head louse.
In general, infestation with any of these has nothing to do with cleanliness or the absence of it.

LICHEN
Any of several skin diseases characterized by the eruption of flat papules.

LICHENIFICATION
Thickening of the skin with accentuation of the skin margins.

LICHEN PLANUS
A recurrent skin inflammation characterized by itchy, flat-topped, reddish-brown pimples that may coalesce into rough scaly patches, often found on the wrists and frequently accompanied by lesions in the mouth. The cause is unknown.

LICHEN SIMPLEX CHRONICUS
Dermatitis marked by one or more clearly defined patches produced by chronic rubbing of the skin.

LICHEN SPIRULOSUS
A skin disease characterized by the eruption of follicular papules from which keratotic spines protrude.

LIDOCAINE
A local anesthetic agent, used topically on the skin and mucous membranes and parenterally to treat heart rhythm disorders. Adverse effects from systemic use include heart arrest and central nervous system disturbances; from topical use, hypersensitivity reactions may occur.

LIE DETECTOR
Common name for polygraph, an apparatus that measures changes in pulse, breathing, blood pressure and the electrical conductivity of the skin of persons to whom questions are posed that must be answered. The assumption is that the emotional disturbance associated with telling a lie will exhibit itself in these physical changes.

LIENORENAL LIGAMENT
A mesenteric fold passing from the spleen to the left kidney and affording support to the splenic artery and vein.

LIFE
The property whereby things live. Despite the vast knowledge that has been gained about life and the different forms of life, the term still lacks any generally accepted definition. Physiologists regard as living any system capable of eating, metabolizing, excreting, breathing, moving, growing, reproducing and able to respond to external stimuli. In terms of thermodynamics, it has been said that life is exhibited by localized regions where net order is increasing.

LIFE CYCLE
The series of stages in form and functional activity through which an organism passed between successive recurrences of a specific primary stage.

LIFE EXPECTANCY
An expected number of years of life based on statistical probability.

LIFE HISTORY
A history of the changes through which an organism passes in its development from the primary stage to its natural death. The term is also apply to designate the history of an individual's development in his social environment.

LIFESAVING
The skill or practice of saving or protecting the lives especially of drowning persons.

LIFE SPAN
The physical and psychological environment of an individual or group.

LIFE STYLE
An individual's typical way of life, including diet, kinds of recreation, job, home environment, location, temperament and smoking, drinking and sleeping habits.

LIFE-SUPPORT SYSTEM
A system that provides all or some of the items (as oxygen, food, water, control of temperature and pressure, disposition of carbon dioxide and body water) necessary for maintaining life or health. A life-support system may be used to maintain the health of a person in outer space, underwater, or in a mine. The term is also applied to a system used to maintain the life of an injured or ill person unable to maintain certain physiological processes without artificial support.

LIFE TABLE
A summarizing technique used to describe the pattern of mortality and survival in populations. The survival data are time-specific and cumulative probabilities of survival of a group of individuals subject (throughout life) to the age-specific death rates in question. The life table method can be applied to the

study not only of death, but also of any defined endpoint such as the onset of disease or the occurrence of specific complications of disease.

LIGAMENT

A band, sheet or cord of fibrous connective tissue that supports bodily organs or links bones together. Tough, strong ligaments hold the two bones in either side of a joint firmly together, while allowing movement. The tearing or twisting of such a ligament is called a sprain.

The ligaments supporting the soft internal organs of the abdomen are, in fact, thickened or folded parts of the peritoneum, the membrane that lines the abdominal cavity. Other ligaments attach soft or muscular tissues (such as the penis) to a nearby bone, while the lens of the eye is also held in place by tiny ligaments.

LIGATION

The surgical process of tying up an anatomical channel.

LIGATURE

A thread, wire or the like for tying blood vessels to
prevent hemorrhage, or for removing tumors by strangulation.

LIGHT ADAPTATION

The adjustments including narrowing of the pupillary opening, decrease in rhodopsin, and dispersion of melanophores by which the retina of the eye is made efficient as a visual receptor under strong conditions of illumination.

LIMB

One of the jointed appendages of the body, such as an arm or leg.

LIMBO

A suspended state of mind, usually between alternatives.

LIMEN

The threshold, as of consciousness.

LIMINAL SENSITIVITY

Sensory acuity as measured by the lowest value of a stimulus giving rise to sensation.

LINCTUS

Any thick, syrupy medicine, but usually referring to cough medicaments.

LINEA ALBA

A median vertical tendinous line on the abdomen formed of fibers from the aponeuroses of the two rectus abdominis muscles and extending from the xiphoid process to the pubic symphysis.

LINEA ASPERA

A longitudinal ridge on the posterior surface of the middle third of the femur.

LINEA NIGRA

Dark line sometimes seen on the skin of pregnant women, running from above the navel to the pubic bone.

LINE OF SIGHT

A line from an observer's eye to a distant point toward which he is looking.

LINE OF VISION

A straight line joining the fovea of the eye with the fixation point.

LINGUA

The tongue or a part that resembles the tongue.

LINGUAL ARTERY

An artery arising from the external carotid artery between the superior thyroid and facial arteries and supplying the tongue.

LINGUAL GLAND

Any of the mucous, serous, or mixed glands that empty their secretions onto the surface of the tongue.

LINGUAL NERVE
A branch of the mandibular division of the trigeminal nerve supplying the anterior two thirds of the tongue and responding to stimuli of pressure, touch, and temperature.

LINGUAL TONSIL
A variable mass or group of small nodules of lymphoid tissue lying at the base of the tongue just anterior to the epiglottis.

LINGULA
A tongue-shaped process or part; a ridge of bone in the angle between the body and the greater wing of the sphenoid bone.

LINIMENT
A liquid preparation, usually oily, for rubbing on or applying to the skin to relieve stiff muscles or aching joints. It creates heat by mildly irritating the skin (a process known as counterirritation).

LININ
The substance forming the net-like structure that connects the chromatin granules in the nucleus of a cell.

LINKAGE
The tendency for characters to be linked together in hereditary transmission. The term is applied in a specific sense for the relationship between genes on the same chromosomes that causes them to be inherited together.

LINKAGE GROUP
A set of genes at different loci on the same chromosome that except for crossing-over tend to act as a single pair of genes in meiosis instead of undergoing independent assortment.

LINOLEIC ACID
An essential nutrient and found in all fats, plant oils being a rich source. They are vital for the proper structure and functioning of cells; particularly nervous tissue.

LINOMYCINS
A family of antibiotics used to treat certain infections. These antibiotics include erythromycin, erythromycin estolate etc.

LINSEED OIL
A yellowish drying oil obtained from flaxseed and used in liniments, pastes, and green soap and as a laxative.

LIP
Either of two fleshy parts or folds forming the margins of the mouth and performing an important function in speech.

LIPASE
An enzyme that accelerates the hydrolysis or synthesis of fats or the breakdown of lipoproteins.

LIPECTOMY
The excision of subcutaneous fatty tissue especially as a cosmetic procedure.

LIPEMIA
The presence of lipids in the blood.

LIPIDOSIS
A disorder of fat metabolism involving the deposition of fat in an organ, as the liver or spleen.

LIPIDS
A diverse group of organic compounds found in plants, animals and microorganisms and characterized by their solubility in fat solvents such as ether, chloroform and alcohol. When discussing food, lipids are referred to as "fat". Lipids include many heterogenous substances and, unlike proteins and carbohydrates, have no characteristic type of building block. They are classified into fats, phospholipids, waxes, steroids, terpenes and other types, according to their products on hydrolysis. Most commonly, these are

fatty acids, particularly those having an even number of carbon atoms. Other components found in many lipids include glycerol, choline and derivatives of isoprene.

LIPO-ATROPHY
An allergic reaction to insulin medication that is manifested as a loss of subcutaneous fat tissue.

LIPODYSTROPHY
A disorder of fat metabolism involving loss of fat from or deposition of fat in tissue.

LIPOPOLYSACCHARIDE
A large molecule consisting of lipids and sugars joined by chemical bonds.

LIPOPROTEIN
Any of a large class of conjugated proteins composed of a complex of protein and lipid and separable on the basis of solubility and mobility properties.

LIPOSARCOMA
A sarcoma arising from immature fat cells of the bone marrow.

LIPOSOME
One of the fatty droplets in the cytoplasm of a cell. The term is also used to designate an artificial vesicle composed of one or more concentric phospholipid bilayers and used to enclose a drug and in the study of biological membranes.

LIPOTROPIC
Tending to promote the utilization of fat and thus prevent excessive fat deposits in the liver.

LIPREADING
The interpreting of a speaker's words by watching his lip and facial movements without hearing his voice.

LIQUEFACIENT
A liquefying agent, such as a drug

that causes the liquefaction of solid deposits.

LIQUID PARAFFIN
A lubricating agent used as a laxative for the treatment of certain types of constipation.

LISTERIOSIS
A serious commonly fatal disease caused by a bacterium of the genus Listeria monocytogenes and taking the form of a severe encephalitis accompanied by disordered movements ending in paralysis, fever, monocytosis.

LITHIASIS
The formation of stony concretions in the body, as in the urine tract or gallbladder.

LITHIUM
A metallic element; lithium compounds are used to treat certain types of mental illness. There is only one treatment in psychiatry generally accepted with only a minimum of controversy: the treatment of manic depressive illness with lithium.

It is not used to treat all types of depression.

LITHOTOMY
The surgical operation of removing stones from the bladder.

LITHOTRITY
The surgical operation in which stones in the bladder are crushed into particles that can then be washed out.

LITHURESIS
Passage of crushed calculi (stones) by urination.

LITHURIA
An excess of uric acid or of its salts in the urine.

LITTLE FINGER
The fourth and smallest finger of

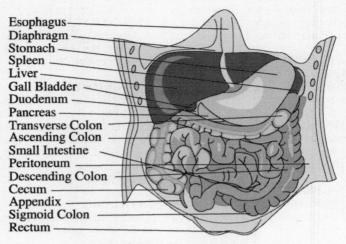

Esophagus
Diaphragm
Stomach
Spleen
Liver
Gall Bladder
Duodenum
Pancreas
Transverse Colon
Ascending Colon
Small Intestine
Peritoneum
Descending Colon
Cecum
Appendix
Sigmoid Colon
Rectum

Localization of organs in the abdominal cavity.

the hand counting the forefinger as the first.

LITTLE LEAGUE ELBOW
Inflammation of the medial epicondyle and adjacent tissues of the elbow especially in preteen and teenage baseball players who make too strenuous use of the muscles of the forearm.

LITTLE'S DISEASE
Another name for congenital cerebral palsy; a congenital form of spastic paralysis affecting all four limbs and held to be caused by impaired development of the pyramidal tracts.

LITTLE STROKE
A transient blockage of one or more arteries in the cerebrum causing temporary numbness or impaired function of a part, slowed mentation, speech defects, dizziness, and nausea.

LIVE BIRTH
The complete expulsion or extraction from its mother of a product of conception (irrespective of the duration of the pregnancy) that, after such separation, breathes or shows any other evidence of life such as heartbeat, umbilical cord pulsation or definite movement of voluntary muscles, whether or not the umbilical cord has been cut or the placenta is attached. Each product of such a birth is considered live born.

LIVER
The largest organ in the body; approximately 21-22 cm across at its widest point, 15-18 cm at its greatest height, and 10-13 from front to back and weighing 1200-1600 g.

The reddish-brown liver is the largest gland. Its primary secretion, the bile, is poured into the duodenum (the first part of the small intestine) through the common bile duct. In addition, it has important functions as a "ductless" gland in connection with the metabolism of carbohydrates and nitrogenous waste products.

The liver has an intricate and complex system of blood vessels. It receives its arterial supply from the hepatic artery. There is a much larger supply of blood vessels from the portal vein, which conveys blood from the stomach, intestines,

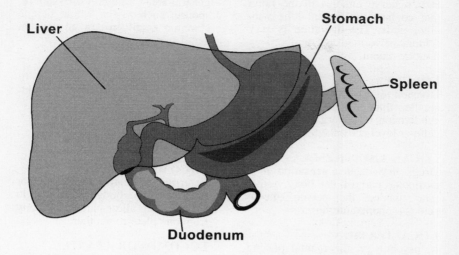

Liver

Stomach

Spleen

Duodenum

The liver in relation to the stomach, spleen and duodenum.

pancreas and spleen to the liver. The hepatic veins, by which the blood of the liver passes into the inferior vena cava, usually pass from the liver through two large and several small openings on the back surface of the organ.

Liver functions

The liver receives blood, via the portal vein, that has come from the intestines; this blood contains the final products of digestion as well as decomposition products. From this, the liver removes glucose, which it turns into glycogen and then stores. When the body needs energy, the liver converts the glycogen back into glucose, which then travels through the bloodstream to the cells where it is needed.

The liver incorporates amino acids into proteins; it probably makes such proteins as albumin, prothrombin components, fibrinogen, transferrin, and glycoprotein.

The liver is important in the transformation (sometimes called detoxification) of such substances as indole and skatole, which may be absorbed into the blood from the in-

testine. It is also instrumental in the clearing out of harmful drugs and other chemicals from the body.

The liver excretes the bile pigments -bilirubin and biliverdin - formed in the cells of the reticuloendothelial system from hemoglobin.

LIVER FLUKE

Common name for Fasciolata hepatica, a parasite that can infect the liver. It is spread by sheep, who act as hosts during the later stages of the fluke's life, but humans in our country mainly catch the infection by eating contaminated wild watercress. Once the flukes become established in the liver, there is pain in the upper abdomen, liver enlargement and fever; jaundice then sets in and eventually the liver is destroyed, a process that can take months or years.

Specific medicines are helpful, but sometimes surgery is needed to cut away abscesses in the liver.

LOBOTOMY

A treatment for some psychotic disorders involving the severing of certain nerve bundles in the brain that connect the frontal lobe with other parts. The operation is very seldom performed and replaced by drug treatment.

LOBULE
Division of an organ (e.g., liver) smaller than a lobe; the smallest subdivision of an organ before the cellular level is reached.

LOCAL ANESTHESIA
Drugs that deaden sensation in a particular part of the body, rather than making the person unconscious (general anesthesia).

LOCALIZATION
In psychology, the mental placing of a source of a particular stimulus, or particular experience at a particular point in space or time. In medicine, the term is used to describe the restriction of symptoms, etc. to a particular place in or area of the body.

LOCALIZED NEURODERMA-TITIS
Another name for localized scratch dermatitis.

LOCALIZED SCRATCH DERMATITIS
Also called localized neurodermatitis; a chronic, superficial itching inflammation of the skin, characterized by dry, scaling, well-demarcated, highly pigmented, lichenified plaques of oval, irregular or angular shape.

The disease has a strong psychological component, and it is important for doctors to help their patients realize that scratching and rubbing produce the skin changes. The itching may be controlled with medication.

LOCATION SCORE
One of the major components in the scoring or coding of Rorschach (or inkblot) tests, which denotes the general area of the blot used in a response, such as the whole blot, a common detail area or an unusual detail area.

LOCHIA
The discharge from the uterus of blood, mucus and tissue after childbirth, late miscarriage or abortion.

LOCKJAW
Another name for tetanus.

LOCOMOTOR
Referring or relating to any part or function of the body that has to do with moving all or part of the body from one place to another.

LOCOMOTOR ATAXIA
Also called tabes dorsalis; a disease of the spinal cord, marked by intense pain, difficulty in coordination and walking and, eventually, paralysis. The type caused by syphilis can be successfully treated in all but the later stages by penicillin.

LOCUS
The precise location of a gene on a chromosome. Different forms of the genes are always found at the same locus on the chromosome.

LOCUS CERULEUS
A blue area of the brain stem with many norepinephrine-containing neurons.

LOEFFLER'S SYNDROME
A mild pneumonitis marked by transitory pulmonary infiltration and eosinophilia and usually considered to be basically an allergic reaction.

LOGAGNOSIA
Disorder of the brain producing the inability to recognize words; word-blindness.

LOGOCLONIA
Inability to express ideas in writing.

LOGOMANIA
Excessive talkativeness; a symptom of certain psychotic states.

LOGOPHASIA
Inability to express ideas in words and speech.

LOGORRHEA
Incoherent rush of words; symptom of mental disorder, or a mere language disorder.

LOGOTHERAPY
A highly directive existential psychotherapy that emphasizes the importance of meaning in the patient's life as gained through spiritual values.

LOIASIS
A form of filariasis found in West Africa, caused by the loa loa worm and transmitted by the bite of the Chrysops fly. The disease is characterized by transient swellings and longer-lasting ones (Calabar swellings) caused by the migration of adult worms in the subcutaneous tissue. It can be treated by taking a specific medicine.

LOIN
The part or parts of the body on either side of the vertebral column between the false ribs and the hipbone.

LONG-ACTING THYROID-STIMULATING HORMONE
An agent with a prolonged effect on the thyroid gland; found in the blood in various thyroid conditions.

LONG BONE
Any of the elongated bones supporting a limb and consisting of an essentially cylindrical shaft that contains marrow and ends in enlarged heads for articulation with other bones.

LONGITUDINALIS LINGUAE
Either of two bands of muscle comprising the intrinsic musculature of the tongue of which one is situated near the dorsal surface and one near the inferior surface of the tongue.

LONG-SIGHTEDNESS
Common name for hypermetropia.

LONG-TERM MEMORY
Memory that involves the storage and recall of information over a long period of time (as days, weeks, or years).

LOOKING-GLASS SELF
The impression of self that an individual obtains from the opinions and responses of other people.

LOOP OF HENLE
The part of the nephron that lies between the proximal and distal convoluted tubules, leaving the cortex of the kidney descending into the medullary tissue, then bending back and reentering the cortex. The loop of H.

LORDOSIS
Abnormal inward curvature of the spine, so that the back is hollowed out and the pelvis is thrust forward. It is a very common fault found in pregnant women and, in fact, is called "pride of pregnancy" when the fetus-filled abdomen protrudes in this way.

LOTION
A liquid preparation that may be applied to large areas of skin.

LOUSE
Any of the small wingless usually flattened insects that are parasitic on warm-blooded animals.

LOUSE-BORNE TYPHUS
Another name for epidemic typhus.

LOVE
A typical sentiment involving fondness for, or attachment to, an object, the idea of which is emotionally

colored whenever it arises in the mind, and capable of evoking any one of the whole gamut of primary emotions, according to the situation in which the object is placed, or represented.

LOW BACK PAIN
Commonly called lumbago: pain in the lumbar and/or sacral region of the back. Although low back pain (with or without pain also radiating down the leg) is an extremely common symptom, there is no general agreement as to its cause. In consequence many doctor's first response to patients with such a complaint is one of despair, and this may be a reasonable response when one considers the list of possible causes: congenital; traumatic; inflammatory; tumors; metabolic; rheumatic; bone disease; pelvic disease.

LOW-DENSITY LIPOPROTEIN
A lipoprotein of blood plasma that is composed of a moderate proportion of protein with little triglyceride and a high proportion of cholesterol and that is associated with increased probability of developing atherosclerosis.

LOWER RESPIRATORY TRACT
The part of the respiratory system including the larynx, trachea, bronchi, and lungs.

LOWE'S SYNDROME
A genetic metabolic disorder that appears to be sex-linked. It results in an excess of amino acids in the urine and acidosis in the blood. The main clinical features are mental retardation, glaucoma, cataracts, rickets, and hypotonia (flaccid muscles).

LOW-PURINE DIET
A diet that avoids high-purine foods, such as liver, sweetbreads, kidneys, sardines, oysters and others.

LOW-SODIUM DIET
A diet restricted to foods naturally low in sodium content and prepared without added salt that is used especially in the management of certain circulatory or kidney disorders.

LSD
Lysergic acid diethylamide; a hallucinogenic drug that induces a state of excitation of the central nervous system and overactivity of the autonomic nervous system, manifested as changes in mood (usually euphoric, sometimes depressive) and perception.

LUCIDITY
Used medically of a sane interval in a mental disorder.

LUDIOMIL
Brand name of a psychoactive drug containing as active compound maprotine prescribed for the treatment of certain depressive conditions.

LUDWIG'S ANGINA
An acute streptococcal or sometimes staphylococcal infection of the deep tissues of the floor of the mouth and adjoining parts of the neck and lower jaw marked by severe rapid swelling that may close the respiratory passage and is accompanied by chills and fever.

LUES
Another name for syphilis.

LUGOL'S SOLUTION
Brand name of an iodine preparation prescribed for the treatment of an overactive thyroid gland.

LUMBAGO
Common name for low back pain.

LUMBAR ARTERY
Any artery of the four or five pairs arising from the back of the aorta, or in the case of the fifth pair from an artery arising from it, opposite

the lumbar vertebrae and supplying the muscles of the loins, the skin of the sides of the abdomen, and the spinal cord.

LUMBAR GANGLION
Any of the small ganglia of the lumbar part of the sympathetic nervous system.

LUMBAR NERVES
The five pairs of spinal nerves arising from the lumbar spinal cord.

LUMBAR PLEXUS
A network of nerves formed by the ventral divisions of some of the lumbar nerves; it is located inside the posterior abdominal wall and supplies the caudal part of the abdominal wall, the front of the thigh, and part of the leg.

LUMBARIZATION
Nonfusion of the first and second segments of the sacrum so that there is one additional articulated vertebra, the sacrum consisting of only four segments.

LUMBAR PUNCTURE
Aspiration of fluid found in the spinal canal through a needle, to diagnose stroke, infection, tumor or other conditions, or to determine the extent of injury after head, neck, or back trauma.

LUMBAR VEIN
Any vein of the four pairs collecting blood from the muscles and integument of the loins, the walls of the abdomen, and adjacent parts and emptying into the dorsal part of the inferior vena cava.

LUMBOSACRAL
Pertaining to the lumbar and sacral region, or to the lumbar vertebrae and sacrum.

LUMBOSACRAL JOINT
The joint between the fifth lumbar vertebra and the sacrum.

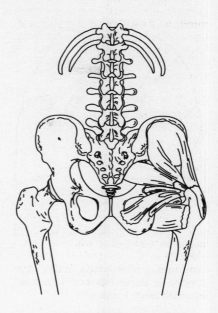

Posterior view of the lower part of the spine with the five lumbar vertebrae, the pelvis and the upper parts of the thigh bones

LUMBOSACRAL PLEXUS
A network of nerves formed by the ventral divisions of the lumbar, sacral, and coccygeal nerves; it supplies the lower limbs, perineum, and coccygeal area.

LUMBRICALIS
One of the worm-like muscles of the hand or foot.

LUMEN
A duct or canal in a tubular organ, as an artery.

LUMEN, VASCULAR
The passageway inside a blood vessel.

LUMINESCENCE
The property of giving off light without a corresponding degree of heat.

LUMPECTOMY
Surgical removal of a tumor without removal of much surrounding

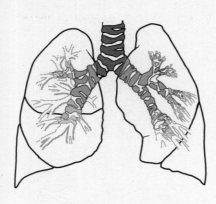

Anterior view of the lungs with the trachea and main bronchi. The right lung consists of three lobes, the left one of two.

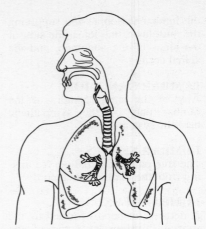

Upper and lower respiratory system with mouth and nose, larynx, trachea, bronchi and lungs.

tissue or nearby lymph nodes; performed in some cases of breast tumor and other tumors.

LUMPY JAW
Another name for actinomycosis.

LUNAR CAUSTIC
Silver nitrate, a compound used in medicine, especially as a cauterizing agent.

LUNATE BONE
One of the carpal (wrist) bones; a crescent-shaped bone that is the middle bone in the proximal row of the carpus between the scaphoid bone and the triquetral bone and that has a deep concavity on the distal surface articulating with the capitate bone.

LUNATE SULCUS
A sulcus of the cerebrum on the lateral part of the occipital lobe that marks the front boundary of the visual area.

LUNG
Either of two largely air-filled organs in the chest, or thoracic cavity, concerned with respiration (breathing), the absorption of oxygen from and release of carbon dioxide into

atmospheric air. The right lung has three lobes, and the left has two lobes.

The lung surfaces are separated from the chest wall by two layers of membrane called the pleura. The small amount of fluid between them allows free movement of the lungs and enables the forced expansion of the chest and diaphragm to fill them with air. Air is drawn into the trachea (windpipe) via the mouth or nose; the trachea divides into the bronchi (airways) which divide repeatedly until the terminal air sacs, or alveoli, are reached.

In the alveoli, air is brought into close contact with deoxygenated blood (i.e., blood from which the oxygen has been extracted in the cells and tissues) in the smallest blood vessels (capillaries) in the lungs. The blood circulation through these comes from the right ventricle of the heart via the pulmonary artery, and returns to the heart's left atrium via the pulmonary veins.

Ventilation of the lungs is the first step in the supply of oxygen to the tissues and the last step in the excretion of carbon dioxide. The oxygen stores of the body are very small, and lung ventilation must supply the body's needs from minute to minute if life is to be continued.

As an organ of excretion, the lung is of great importance; it eliminates more than 50 times as much acid as the kidneys. Although the major role of the lungs is respiratory, they have other diverse and complex activities.

For example, the lungs produce surfactant, an agent that lines the alveoli and prevents them from collapsing; a lack of surfactant is thought to be one of the factors in respiratory distress syndrome in premature babies. Apart from this the lungs participate in the production of several vasoactive substances (i.e., substances that affect the diameter of blood vessels and so the rate of blood flow).

Lung tissue also contains a high concentration of prostaglandins, which it synthesizes; these complex chemicals that act on many parts of the body, such as causing the uterus to contract, etc.

Mast cells are plentiful and the lungs are the richest source of histamine in the body; they are, therefore, greatly affected by allergic reactions. Most of the serotonin (a substance intimately involved in blood clotting and the working of the brain) in the blood is contained within platelets, and the lungs are an important source of megakaryocytes, the large cells that manufacture platelets. In addition, over 90 percent of this vasoactive substance can be removed by the lung in one circulation.

LUNG ABSCESS
Local inflammation with necrosis (death) of lung tissue and surrounding pneumonitis (inflammation of the lungs that does not progress to pneumonia). Lung abscesses are usually due to the breathing in of infected material from the upper airway by an unconscious person or someone who has passed out after drinking alcohol, as well as those who are suffering from a disease of the central nervous system or are under general anesthesia or excessive sedation.

LUNG, BLACK
Pneumoconiosis of coal workers.

LUNG CANCER
One of the most common types of cancer. Predisposing factors include cigarette smoking and exposure to asbestos, vinyl chloride, coal products, and other industrial and chemical products.
Symptoms include:
- cough;
- difficulty in breathing;
- blood-tinged sputum;
- repeated infections.
Treatment depends on the type, site, and extent of the cancer and may include surgery, chemotherapy, and radiation.

LUNG CONGESTION
LUNG, FARMERS
A morbid condition due to inhalation of mouldy hay dust.

LUNG INFARCTION
Death of one or more sections of lung tissue because it has been de-

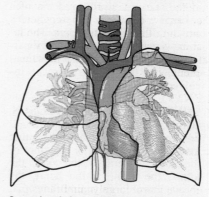

Lungs in relation to the heart and the arterial and venous system in the thoracic cavity. A scan was made of the lung tissue after inhalation of a radioisotope.

prived of an adequate blood supply.

LUNG PERFUSION SCAN
A scanning procedure involving intravenous injection of radioactive albumin (a protein) and examination of lung structure and function, to diagnose pulmonary embolism (a clot or other debris that has travelled to the lung and has blocked an artery).

LUNG VENTILATION SCAN
A procedure in which the person breathes in radioactive gas and the lungs are scanned for areas that do not receive air, or for other abnormalities.

LUPUS
Any of several diseases (as lupus vulgaris or systemic lupus erythematosus) characterized by skin lesions.

LUPUS BAND TEST
A test to determine the presence of immunoglobulins and complement deposits at the junction of the dermal and epidermal skin layers of patients with systemic lupus erythematosus.

LUPUS ERYTHEMATOSUS
A chronic superficial inflammation of the skin marked by red macules covered with scanty adherent scales which fall off, leaving scars. The lesions typically form a butterfly pattern over the bridge of the nose and cheek, but other areas may be involved.

LUPUS ERYTHEMATOSUS, DISSEMINATED
Form of lupus erythematosus that may affect any organ or structure of the body, especially the skin, the joints, the kidneys, the heart, the serous membranes (membranes that moisture, such as those of the joints and those lining the abdomen), and the lymph nodes.

LUPUS ERYTHEMATOSUS PROFUNDUS
A form of lupus erythematosus in which deep browny indurations or subcutaneous nodules occur under normal or less often involved skin; the overlying skin may be erythematous, atrophic, and ulcerated and on healing may leave a depressed scar.

LUPUS ERYTHEMATOSUS, SYSTEMIC
A chronic generalized connective tissue disorder, ranging from mild to fulminating, marked by the following signs and symptoms:
– skin eruptions;
– arthralgia, pain in joints;
– arthritis, inflammation of joints;
– leukopenia, decrease in leukocytes in the peripheral blood;
– anemia;
– vomiting;
– malaise;
– nausia;
– stomach ache;
– visceral lesions;
– neurological manifestations;
– lymphadenopathy;
– fever;
- other constitutional symptoms.
Typically there are many abnormal immunological phenomena.

LUPUS EXUBERANS
A form of lupus vulgaris in which the lesions break down to produce deep, indolent ulcers.

LUPUS HYPERTROPHICUS
A variant of lupus vulgaris in which the lesions consist of a warty vegetative growth, often crushed or slightly exudative, occurring on most areas near body orifices.

LUPUS NEPHRITIS
Glomerulonephritis associated with systemic lupus erythematosus that is typically characterized by proteinuria and hematuria and that often leads to kidney failure.

LUPUS PERNIA
Soft, violaceous skin lesions on the cheeks, forehead, nose, ears, and digits, frequently associated with bone cysts, which may be the first manifestation of sarcoidosis or occur in the chronic stage of the disease.

LUPUS VULGARIS
The most common and severe form of tuberculosis of the skin, most often affecting the face, marked by the formation of reddish brown patches of nodules in a specific part of the skin (corium), which progressively spread peripherally with central atrophy, causing ulceration and scarring and destruction of cartilage in involved sites.

LUPUS SYNDROME
Closely resembling systemic lupus erythematosus, precipitated by prolonged use of certain drugs, most commonly hydralazine, isoniazid, various anticonvulsants, and procainamide.

LURSELLE
Brand name of a drug containing as active compound probucol prescribed for the prevention of atherosclerosis as lipid-lowering drug.

LUSTRAL
Brand name of a psychoactive drug containing as active compound sertraline prescribed for the treatment of certain depressive disorders.

LUTEAL
Pertaining to or having the properties of the corpus luteum or its active principle.

LUTEAL PHASE
The second half of the menstrual cycle during which the corpus luteum secretes the hormone progesterone, which, in turn, causes the endometrium (uterine lining) to become rich in blood vessels and de-

veloped for implantation of a fertilized egg.

If fertilization does not occur, progesterone secretion decreases and about 14 days after ovulation, the endometrium is shed in menstruation.

LUTEIN
A lipochrome from the corpus luteum, fat cells, and egg yolk.

LUTEINIZATION
The process by which a postovulatory ovarian follicle transforms into a corpus luteum through vascularization, follicular cell hypertrophy, and lipid accumulation, the latter giving the yellow color indicated by the term.

LUTEINIZING HORMONE (LH)
A hormone produced by the anterior part of the pituitary gland that stimulates the secretion of sex hormones by the testes and ovaries and is involved in the production of mature sperm and ova. The synthesis shows a cyclic pattern.

LUTEOTROPIC
Stimulating formation of the corpus luteum.

LUXATION
Misalignment, displacement, or dislocation of an organ or joint. (See illustration on next page).

LYASE
A class of enzymes that remove groups from their substrates (other than by hydrolysis), leaving double bonds, or that conversely add groups to double bonds.

LYCANTHROPY
Delusion in which the patient believes himself a wolf. Undoubtedly stimulated by the once widespread superstition that lycanthropy is a supernatural condition in which men actually assume the physical form

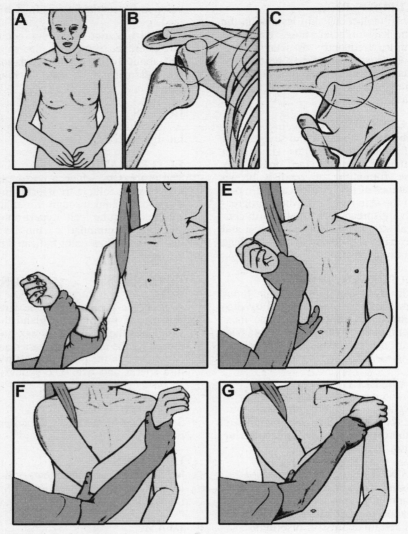

Luxation of the shoulder joint.
A. external view;
B. dislocation of the humerus;
C. in abduction the dislocation is very pronounced:
D, E, F and G: reposition or reduction by the Kocher method: lateral rotation with traction, adduction, and internal rotation.

of other animals, the delusion has been most likely to occur among people who believe in reincarnation and the transmigration of souls.

LYME ARTHRITIS
An acute inflammatory disease, thought to be caused by a tick-borne virus, that affects one or more joints (especially the knees and other large joints), causing heat, swelling and skin redness, often accompanied by chills, fever, and malaise.

Heart abnormalities and neuro-

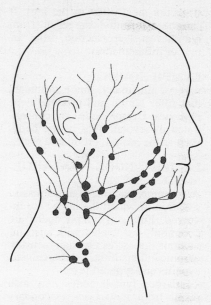

Location of lymph nodes and lymph vessels in the region of the head and neck.

logical complications sometimes occur. Treatment is by pain relievers (for instance, aspirin) and corticosteroids.

LYMPH
A transparent, usually slightly yellow, often opalescent liquid found within the lymphatic vessels, and collected from tissues in all parts of the body and returned to the blood via the lymphatic system. Its cellular components consist chiefly of lymphocytes.

Lymph bathes the tissues of the body, circulates through lymph vessels, and contains chyle and leukocytes (mostly lymphocytes), but otherwise is similar to blood plasma.

LYMPH(ATIC) SYSTEM
Bodily system consisting of lymph nodes and vessels. Fluid located in the tissue spaces is carried into the blood circulation by means of a second system of vessels.

This is a major part of the lymphatic system. Its capillaries admit this interstitial fluid and convey it through increasingly larger vessels to the thoracic lymph vessel, dorsally located in the thorax, from which it is eventually discharged into the left internal jugular or subclavian vein in the root of the neck.

LYMPHADENECTOMY
Surgical removal or one of more lymph glands.

LYMPHADENITIS
Inflammation of the lymph nodes; it usually occurs as a result of systemic neoplastic disease, bacterial infection, or inflammatory condition.

LYMPHADENOGRAPHY
Radiography of lymph nodes after injection of a contrast medium in a lymphatic vessel.

LYMPHADENOPATHY
Another name for Hodgkin's disease.

LYMPHADENOID
Resembling the tissue of lymph nodes.

LYMPHADENOPATHY
Enlargement of the lymph nodes.

LYMPHADENOSIS
Hypertrophy or proliferation of lymphoid tissue.

LYMPHADENOTOMY
Incision of a lymph node.

LYMPHANGIECTASIS
Dilatation of the lymphatic vessels.

LYMPHANGIOGRAPHY
Radiography of lymphatic vessels after introduction of a contrast medium.

LYMPHANGIOLOGY
The scientific study of the lym-

phatic system.

LYMPHANGIOMA
A tumor composed of newly formed lymph vessels; *cavernous lymphangioma*: dilatation of the lymphatic vessels resulting in cavities filled with lymph.

LYMPHANGIOSARCOMA
A malignant tumor of lymphatic vessels, usually arising in a limb that is the site of chronic lymphedema.

LYMPHANGITIS
Inflammation of a lymphatic vessel or vessels that usually results from a streptococcal infection, causing red streaks extending from the infected area, accompanied by fever, headache, and muscle pain. Treatment is by antibiotics.

LYMPHATIC CAPILLARY
Any of the smallest lymphatic vessels that are blind at one end and collect lymph in organs and tissues.

LYMPHATIC DUCT
Any of the lymphatic vessels that are part of the system collecting lymph from the lymphatic capillaries and pouring it into the subclavian veins by way of the right lymphatic duct and the thoracic duct.

LYMPHATIC LEUKEMIA
Malignant disease of the blood-forming tissues, that is marked by abnormal enlargement and productivity of the lymph nodes and other lymphocyte-producing tissues.

LYMPHATOLYSIS
Destruction of some part of the lymphatic system.

LYMPHEDEMA
Chronic swelling of a part due to accumulation of interstitial fluid (edema) secondary to obstruction of lymphatic vessels of lymph nodes.

It occurs most often in the legs. It can be congenital or result from lymph vessel obstruction, from tumor or inflammation.

LYMPH NODES
Any of the many small structures that filter lymph and produce lymphocytes. Lymph nodes are concentrated in several areas of the body, such as the armpit, groin, and neck.

LYMPH NODE ENLARGEMENT
A common reaction to any stressful situation in which the nodes are involved. Enlarged lymph nodes are commonly associated with such infectious disease as German measles, chronic tonsillitis, tuberculosis, syphilis and typhoid fever.

Enlarged lymph nodes may also result from metastases (secondary growth) of malignant tumors.

LYMPH NODULE
Small, localized collection of lymphoid tissue, usually located in the loose connective tissue beneath wet epithelial (covering or lining) membranes, as in the digestive tract, respiratory system, and urinary bladder.

Lymph nodules form in regions of frequent exposure to microorganisms or foreign materials, and contribute to the defense against them.

LYMPHOBLAST
The immature, nucleolated precursor of the mature lymphocyte. The nucleus contains moderately fine chromatin (readily stainable nuclear material) and has a well-defined nuclear membrane. There are one or two nucleoli, and the cytoplasm is yellowish and relatively abundant.

LYMPHOBLASTIC LEUKEMIA
Leukemia characterized by an abnormal increase in the number of lymphoblasts.

LYMPHOBLASTOMA
Any of several diseases of lymph nodes marked by the formation of tumorous masses composed of mature or immature lymphocytes.

LYMPHOBLASTOSIS
An excess of lymphoblasts in the blood.

LYMPHOCYTE
Type of leukocyte (white blood cell), in humans making 20-25 percent of the total leukocytes. Lymphocytes are recycled through the lymph and blood circulatory system repeatedly; their life-spans appear to average one month, but some live as long as nine months. Lymphocytes play a not fully understood role in antibody production and transport and are important to the defense of the body. Lymphocytes occur in two forms: B-cells, the chief agent of the humoral immune system, that recognize the specific antigens and produce antibodies against them; and T-cells, the agents of the cell mediated immune system, that secrete immunological active compounds and assist B-cells in their function. Although the two types of lymphocytes look the same under an ordinary light microscope, they can be distinguished when seen through an electron microscope.

LYMPHOCYTEMIA
Excess of lymphocytes in the blood.

LYMPHOCYTE TRANSFORMATION
A transformation caused in lymphocytes by a mitosis-including agent or by a second exposure to an antigen and characterized by an increase in size and in the amount of cytoplasm, by visibility of nucleoli in the nucleus, and after about 3 days by a marked resemblance to blast cells.

LYMPHOCYTIC CHORIO-

MENINGITIS
An acute viral infection caused by a RNA virus. usually appearing as an influenza-like illness or septic meningitis, which may be associated with rash, arthritis, orchitis or parotitis (e.g., mumps).

LYMPHOCYTIC LEUKEMIA
A leukemia marked by proliferation of lymphoid tissue, abnormal increase of leukocytes in the circulating blood, and enlargement of lymph nodes.

LYMPHOCYTOPENIA
A lower-than-normal number of lymphocytes in the blood circulation, due to malignancy, nutritional deficiency, blood disorder, or certain other diseases.

LYMPHOCYTOMA
A tumor in which lymphocytes are the dominant elements.

LYMPHOCYTOSIS
An excess of normal lymphocytes in the blood or an effusion.

LYMPHOGRANULOMA VENEREUM
An infectious disease, caused by the bacterium Chlamydia trachomatis and transmitted by sexual contact.

It is a relatively common disease, occurring throughout most of the world, especially in tropical and subtropical areas. Incidence of the infection in different sexes is about the same and all races are affected. The disease is characterized by:
- genital lesions;
- swelling of lymph nodes in the groin area;
- headache;
- fever;
- malaise.

LYMPHOGRAPHY
Roentgenography of the lymphatic vessels and lymph nodes after injection of radiopaque material.

LYMPHOID
Resembling or pertaining to lymph or to tissue of the lymphatic system.

LYMPHOID TISSUE
The cells, tissue, and organs that compose the immune system. Among these elements are the bone marrow, thymus, spleen, and lymph nodes.

Lymphoid tissue has several different structural organizations related to its particular function in the immune response. The most highly organized lymphoid tissues are the thymus and lymph nodes, which are well-defined encapsulated organs with easily identifiable architectures.

LYMPHOKINE
Any of various substances (as interferon) of low molecular weight that are immunoglobulins, secreted by T-cells in response to stimulation by antigens, and having a role in cell-mediated immunity

LYMPHOMA
A malignant growth of lymph tissue; one of four types of cancer. Lymphomas differ widely in the types of cells affected and the prognosis; general characteristics include:
- enlarged lymph nodes;
- weakness;
- fever;
- weight loss;
- malaise;
- enlargement of spleen and liver.
Treatment is usually by chemotherapy and radiotherapy.

LYMPHOMA, BURKITT'S
A form of undifferentiated malignant lymphoma, manifested as large osteolytic lesions in the jaw or as an abdominal mass.

LYMPHOMA, FOLLICULAR
Nodular well-differentiated lymphocytic malignant lymphoma, microscopically characterized by multiple, proliferative, follicle-like nodules which disturb the normal architecture of the lymph nodes.

LYMPHOMATOSIS
The formation of multiple lymphomas in the body.

LYMPHOMATOUS
Pertaining to, or the nature of, lymphoma.

LYMPHOPOIESIS
The production of lymphocytes, occurring mainly in the bone marrow, lymph nodes, spleen, and thymus.

LYMPHOSARCOMA
Malignant tumor of the lymphatic tissue.

LYMPHURIA
The presence of lymph in the urine.

LYONIZATION
The process by which or the condition in which all X chromosomes of the cells in excess of one are inactivated on a random basis.

LYOPHILIC
Having an affinity for, or stable in, solution.

LYOPHILIZATION
The creation of a stable preparation of a biological substance by rapid freezing and dehydration of the frozen product under high vacuum.

LYSE
To cause or produce disintegration of a compound, substance, or cell.

LYSIN
An antibody capable of causing dissolution of cells, including, hemolysin, bacteriolysin.

LYSINE
A naturally occurring amino acid, essential for optimal growth in human infants and for the maintenance of nitrogen equilibrium in

adults. Human populations dependent on grains as a sole dietary protein source suffer from lysine deficiency.

LYSINE INTOLERANCE
A disorder in which a lack of or defect in certain enzymes produces an inability to utilize the amino acid lysine, resulting in symptoms of weakness, vomiting and coma. Treatment is by limiting lysine content in the diet.

LYSINEMIA
An inborn error of metabolism in which a defect in or lack of enzymes leads to an inability to metabolize the amino acid lysine; it is characterized by muscle weakness and mental retardation.

LYSIS
(1) Destruction or decomposition, as of a cell or other substance, under influence of a specific agent;
(2) mobilization of an organ by division of restraining adhesions.

LYSOSOME
One of the minute bodies occurring in many types of cells, containing various hydrolytic enzymes and normally involved in the process of localized intracellular digestion.

LYSOZYME
A crystalline basic enzyme present in saliva, tears, egg white, and certain other substances, which functions as an antibacterial agent. Lysozyme catalyzes the breakdown of certain carbohydrates found in capsules of certain bacteria (for instance, cocci) secrete around themselves. It thus has a bacteriolytic (bacteria-killing) action that functions, in the case of lacrimal fluid, to protect the cornea of the eye from infection.

LYSOZYMURIA
Urinary excretion of elevated levels of lysozyme.

LYSSA
Rabies.

LYSSOPHOBIA
Morbid fear of rabies.

LYXOFLAVIN
A yellow crystalline compound isolated from heart muscle and stereoisomeric with riboflavin but derived from lyxose.

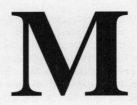

MACERATION
Process of softening a tissue by soaking it in a fluid.

MACLEOD'S SYNDROME
Abnormally increased translucence of one lung usually accompanied by reduction in ventilation and in perfusion with blood.

MACROBIOTICS
Nutritional system based on the production and digestion of so-called "natural" food, especially grains.

MACROBLAST
An erythroblast (red blood cell) destined to produce macrocytes.

MACROCEPHALY
The condition of having an abnormally large head.

MACROCYTE
Extra large-sized red blood cell found in certain forms of anemia, such as pernicious anemia.

MACROGENITOSOMIA
A syndrome characterized by premature physical development and premature appearance of secondary sex characteristics. It is caused by tumors of the pineal gland of the brain.

MACROGLOBULINEMIA
A disorder characterized by increased blood serum viscosity and the presence of macroglobulins in the blood serum.

MACROGLOBULINS
Proteins in the blood that are up to ten times heavier than the usual globulins. They are usually measured as an entity, but can be broken down into separate parts; the largest portion (usually two-thirds) is known as "alpha-2." Macroglobulins comprise about five percent of all globulins.

MACROGLOSSIA
An abnormally large tongue.

MACROLIDES
A class of antibiotics (antibacterial) drugs. They include erythromycin, lincomycin, and vancomycin.

MACROMELIA
Abnormal enlargement of any member of the body.

MACRONUTRIENT
A chemical element or substance (as protein, carbohydrate, or fat) required in relatively large quantities in nutrition.

MACROPHAGE
Large scavenging cell (the name literally means "big eater") concerned with attacking and ingesting germs; large numbers are found in the blood in areas where there is great activity against germ invasion. It is not a true white blood cell, but is produced in the reticulo-endothelial system.

MACROPSIA
An impairment of vision in which objects appear larger than they really are, due to disease of the retina, the light-sensitive coating of the back of the eye.

MACROSCOPIC
Able to be seen with the naked eye.

MACULA
An anatomical structure having the form of a spot differentiated from surrounding tissues.

MACULA ACUSTICA
Either of two small areas of sensory hair cells in the ear that are covered with gelatinous material on which are located crystals or concretions of calcium carbonate and that are associated with the perception of equilibrium.

MACULA CAERULEA
Bluish-gray spot on the skin caused by the body louse

MACULA CORNEAE
Opacities seen in the cornea of the eye.

MACULA DENSA
A group of modified epithelial cells in the distal convoluted tubule of the kidney that lie adjacent to the afferent arteriole just before it enters the glomerulus and control renin release by relaying information about the sodium concentration in the fluid passing through the convoluted tubule to the renin-producing juxtaglomerular cells of the afferent arteriole.

MACULA LUTEA
A small yellowish area lying slightly related to the center of the retina that constitutes the region of maximum visual acuity and is made up almost wholly of retinal cones.

MACULAE
Flat, discolored spots on the skin of varied size and shape. They can be caused by sunburn, pregnancy, old hemorrhages, certain diseases of internal organs, syphilis, and burns.

MACULAR DEGENERATION
A loss of central vision in both eyes produced by pathological changes in the macula lutea and characterized by spots of pigmentation or other abnormalities.

MACULOPAPULAR
Description of a skin rash consisting of both macules (flat spots) and papules (raised spots).

MAGNESIUM
An essential mineral that is important in the formation of bones, the regulation of functions and activities of the nervous system, the metabolism of calcium and potassium and the utilization of all other nutrients.

The body of a healthy man contains about 24 g of magnesium. About two-thirds of this is present as bone mineral and most of the remainder is in the intracellular fluid where it is the most important cation after potassium. The ion plays an important role in many enzymatic reactions.

Magnesium depletion is often present in patients with prolonged diarrhea whatever the cause. The chief features are:
- depression;
- weakness;
- increased irritability.

MAGNETIC RESONANCE IMAGING (MRI)
Also called nuclear magnetic resonance (NMR); new diagnostic method based on the application of specific spectroscopic methods. The new technique allows for obtaining cross-sectional pictures through the human body without exposing the patient to ionizing radiation.

MAGNETOCARDIOGRAPH
An instrument for recording the changes in the magnetic field around the heart that is used to supplement information given by an electrocardiograph.

MAINTENANCE LEVEL
A stage in the development of an organism when growth has virtually stopped and energy is used to keep the condition relatively constant.

MAJOR DEPRESSIVE EPISODE
Mood disorder characterized by

either depressed mood (or possibly, in children or adolescents, an irritable mood) or loss of interest or pleasure in all, or almost all, activities, and associated symptoms, for a period of at least two weeks. The symptoms represent a change from previous functioning and are relatively persistent, that is, they occur for most of the day, nearly every day, during at least a two-week period.

The associated symptoms include:
– appetite disturbance;
– change in weight;
– sleep disturbance;
– psychomotor agitation or retardation;
– decreased energy;
– feelings of worthlessness;
– feelings of inappropriate guilt;
– difficult thinking;
– problems in concentrating;
– recurrent thoughts of death;
– suicidal ideation or attempts.

The average age at onset is in the late 20s, but a major depressive episode may begin at any age, including infancy.

MAJOR HISTOCOMPATIBILITY COMPLEX
A group of genes that function especially in determining the histocompatibility antigens found on cell surfaces and that in man comprise the alleles occurring at four loci on the short arm of the chromosome 6.

MAJOR SURGERY
Surgery involving a risk to the life of the patient; an operation upon an organ within the cranium, chest, abdomen, or pelvic cavity.

MAKE-BELIEVE
The pretense in children's play that fantasy is real, and associated with varying degrees of recognizing the unreality of the situation.

MALABSORPTION SYNDROME
Syndrome resulting from impaired absorption of nutrients from the small intestines. Many different diseases may be responsible:
– chronic pancreatitis;
– cystic fibrosis;
– biliary obstruction;
– alactasia;
– diverticula;
– acute intestinal infections.

MALACIA
Abnormal softening of tissue.

MALADAPTATION
The failure of an organism to develop one or more biological characteristics necessary to ensure success in interaction with the environment.

MALADJUSTMENT
The condition of an individual who is unable to adjust himself adequately to his physical, occupational or social environment, usually with repercussions in his emotional life and behavior.

MALADY
Any disease or ailment of the human body.

MALAISE
Feeling of general discomfort or of being out of sorts. The term is also used to designate an indefinite feeling of debility or lack of health often indicative of or accompanying the onset of an illness.

MALALIGNMENT
Incorrect or imperfect alignment, as of teeth.

MALARIA
Tropical parasitic disease causing malaise and intermittent fever, violent shivering, and sweating, either on alternate days or every third day; bouts often reoccur over many years. One form, cerebral malaria, develops rapidly with encephalitis, coma and shock.

Malaria is due to infection with

the Plasmodium protozoa carried by mosquitos of the genus Anopheles from the blood of infected persons.

The cyclic fever is due to the parasite's life cycle in the blood and liver; diagnosis is by examination of blood. Derivatives of quinine especially chloroquine and primaquine, are used both in prevention and treatment but other drugs may also be used. Mosquito control, primarily by destroying their breeding places (swamps and pools), provides the best method of combatting the disease. Those who are exposed to the infection can protect themselves by taking regular small doses of an antimalarial drug.

MALARIAL CACHEXIA
A generalized state of debility that is marked by:
- anemia;
- jaundice;
- splenomegaly;
- emaciation.
The condition results from long-continued chronic malarial infection.

MALARIA PARASITE
A protozoan of the sporozoan genus Plasmodium that is transmitted to man or to certain other mammals by the bite of a mosquito in which its sexual reproduction takes place, that multiplies asexually in the vertebrate host by schizogony in the red blood cells or in certain tissue cells, and that causes destruction of the red blood cells and the febrile disease malaria or produces gametocytes by sporogony which if taken up by a suitable mosquito initiate a new sexual cycle.

MALE CLIMACTERIC
Change of life in men resulting from an hormonal imbalance that may produce a decrease in body hair and a higher-pitched voice.

MALE HORMONES
Chemical substances secreted by the testicles, ovaries and adrenal glands in humans. Some male hormones used by humans are derived synthetically. Male hormones include testosterone cypionate and estradiol cypionate, testosterone enanthate and estradiol valerate.

MALE-PATTERN BALDNESS
A typical hereditary baldness in the male characterized by loss of hair on the crown and temples.

MALEVOLENCE
Disposition or wish on the part of an individual to harm or distress another.

MALFORMATION
Abnormal structure, especially of a body part.

MALFUNCTION
Functioning imperfectly or badly; failure to operate in the normal and usual manner.

MALIGNANCY
Quality of being malignant. Often refers to a cancerous condition.

MALIGNANT
Severe, evil, or threatening to life; the opposite of being benign. The term is applied to any virulent condition that tends to go from bad to worse.

MALIGNANT CATARRH
A catarrhal fever caused by a virus.

MALIGNANT HYPERTENSION
Severe high blood pressure that may run a rapid course and cause damage to the blood vessel walls in the kidneys, eyes and other organs. Its cardinal feature is central nervous system impairment, for example, coma, seizure, etc.

MALIGNANT HYPERTHERMIA
An inherited condition charac-

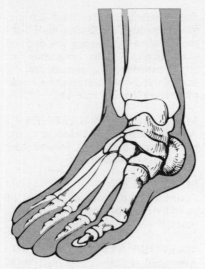

The lower end of the tibia forms the medial malleolus; the lower end of the fibula is the lateral malleolus.

terized by a rapid, extreme, and often fatal rise in body temperature following the administration of general anesthesia.

MALIGNANT PUSTULE
Other term for anthrax; localized anthrax of the skin taking the form of a pimple surrounded by a zone of edema and hyperemia and tending to become necrotic and ulcerated.

MALIGNANT TUMOR
One that invades and destroys surrounding tissues, may produce secondary deposits (metastases) elsewhere in the body, and is likely to recur after removal; a cancerous tumor.

MALINGERING
Intentional production of false or grossly exaggerated physical or psychological symptoms, motivated by external incentives such as avoiding military conscription or duty, obtaining financial compensation, evading criminal prosecution, obtaining drugs, or securing better living conditions.

MALLEOLUS
A rounded process, such as the protuberance on either side of the ankle joint, at the lower end of the fibula, or of the tibia.

MALLEUS
Also called the hammer; one of the three small bones in the middle ear which conduct sound from the eardrum to the organ of hearing (cochlea) in the inner ear.

MALNUTRITION
Inadequate nutrition, especially in children, that may involve all parts of the diet (marasmus), or may be predominantly a lack of protein (kwashiorkor) or vitamins (pellagra, beriberi, scurvy).

   In adults, starvation is less rapid in onset, as the demands of growth are absent, but similar metabolic changes occur.

MALOBSERVATION
Failure to observe, and record adequately and accurately, an event or series of events, because of divided attention.

MALOCCLUSION
Any variation in the normal bite of the teeth, one set upon another. The normal being with the upper front teeth over the bottom teeth.

MALPIGHIAN CORPUSCLE
A small, round body in the cortex substance of the kidney.

MALPIGHIAN LAYER
A layer of cells lying deep within the epidermis, which provides replacements for the outer cells of the epidermis.

MALPOSITION
Out of normal position; refers especially to the position of the baby in the uterus when it assumes a position unsuitable for easy delivery, or to a bad position of a tooth.

MALPRACTICE

Improper, neglectful or illegal performance of a duty by one in a public or professional position, such as a doctor, lawyer or public servant, especially when resulting in injury or loss.

MALPRESENTATION

Any position of the baby during childbirth that impedes delivery.

MALT

The product made from any cereal grain by steeping it in water allowing it to germinate and then drying it.

This activates dormant enzymes such as diastase, which converts the kernel starch to maltose (malt sugar). Malt is used as a source of enzymes and flavoring.

MALTA FEVER

Another name for brucellosis.

MALTASE

An enzyme that acts on maltose, a natural sugar in sprouting plants.

MALTHUSIANISM

The doctrines of Malthus especially with respect to the difference between the rates of increase of a population and its food supply and to the long term effects of this difference on the population.

MALTOSE

Malt sugar; a disaccharide sugar produced by the action of diastase on starch and yielding glucose with the enzyme maltase.

MALT SOUP EXTRACT

Bulk-forming laxative preparation. It acts by absorbing water, stimulating the bowel to form a soft, bulky stool.

MALUNION

Incomplete or faulty union, as of the fragments of a fractured bone.

MAMILLA

Breast nipple or a nipple-like prominence.

MAMILLARY

Strictly pertaining to a breast nipple, but now commonly used to indicate anything to the female breast.

MAMMARY GLAND

Breast; the glands that secrete milk. Each gland consists of branching ducts leading from milk-secreting cells and opening to the exterior through the nipple.

MAMMARY RIDGE

Either of a pair of longitudinal ectodermal thickenings in the mammalian embryo that extend from the base of the anterior to the posterior limb buds and that are the source of the mammary glands.

MAMMECTOMY

Another name for mastectomy or surgical removal of the breast.

MAMMILLARY BODY

Either of two small eminences on the underside of the brain behind the tuber cinereum forming the terminals of the anterior pillars of the fornix in the brain.

MAMMOGRAPHY

X-ray technique to examine breast tissue for tumors or other abnormalities, and to differentiate between benign and malignant tumors.

MAMMOPLASTY

Plastic surgery of the breast.

MANDIBLE

Lower jaw bone.

MANDIBULAR ANGLE

An angle for,med by the junction at the gonion of the posterior border of the ramus and the inferior border of the body of the mandible.

MANDIBULAR ARCH
The first branchial arch of the vertebrate embryo from which in man are developed the lower lip, the mandible, the masticatory muscles, and the anterior part of the tongue.

MANDIBULAR FORAMEN
The opening on the medial surface of the ramus of the mandible that leads into the mandibular canal and transmits blood vessels and nerves supplying the lower teeth.

MANDIBULAR NERVE
The one of the three major branches or divisions of the trigeminal nerve that supplies sensory fibers to the lower jaw, the floor of the mouth, the anterior two-thirds of the tongue, and the lower teeth and motor fibers to the muscles of mastication.

MANDIBULOFACIAL DYSOSTOSIS
Dysostosis of the face and lower jaw inherited as a dominant trait and characterized by bilateral malformations, deformities of the outer and middle ear, and a usually smaller lower jaw.

MANEUVER
A movement, procedure, or method performed to achieve a desired result and especially to restore a normal physiological state or to promote normal function.

MANGANESE
Mineral essential for nursing mothers (lactation), and for various other body functions. Natural sources are whole grains, nuts, green leaf vegetables, prunes, onions and tea. It is an essential trace element for both humans and animals, and occurs in the cells of all living organisms.

It has been shown to be associated with the formation of connective tissue and bone, with growth, carbohydrate and lipid metabolism, the embryonic development of the inner ear, reproductive function and probably brain function.

Manganese deficiency is extremely unlikely to occur in humans because there is a sufficient supply of the metal in the diet.

MANIA
Tremendous enthusiasm or overexcitement, any excessive desire or passion; a mental disorder, characterized by:
- emotional excitement;
- flight of ideas;
- hallucinations;
- delusions;
- disturbance of orientations;
- extreme muscular restlessness;
- increased talking.

MANIC DEFENSE
Form of defensive behavior exhibited by persons who defend themselves against anxiety, guilt and depression. Use of manic defense is not confined to persons liable to develop mania or manic-depressive psychosis.

MANIC-DEPRESSIVE PSYCHOSIS
Psychosis characterized by alternating periods of deep depression and mania. Periods of sanity may intervene. Presently this type of psychosis is usually called a bipolar disorder. The essential feature is one or more manic episodes, usually accompanied by one or more major depressive episodes.

In a bipolar disorder the initial episode that occasioned hospitalization is usually manic. Both the manic and major depressive episodes are more frequent than the major depressive episodes in a major depression. Frequently a manic or major depressive episode is immediately followed by a short episode of the other kind. In many cases there are two or more complete cycles (a manic and a major depressive episode that succeed each other without a period of remission) within a year. Such cases have been called "rapid cycling."

In rare cases over long periods of time, there is an alternation of the two kinds of episodes without any intervening period of normal mood. It is estimated that from 0.4% to 1.2% of the adult population have had bipolar disorder.

MANIC EPISODE
A distinct period during which the predominant mood is either elevated, expansive, or irritable, and there are associated symptoms.

MANIFEST DREAM CONTENT
The parts of a dream that are remembered and reportable, as contrasted with latent dream thoughts.

MANIFEST SCHIZOPHRENIA
A schizophrenic reaction that is observable. A fully developed schizophrenic disorder.

MANIKIN TEST
A performance test that consists of placing together parts of the figure of a wooden man, the pieces being handed to a person without any information of what he or she is making.

MANIPULATION
A treatment method consisting of passive movements using psychologic or accessory motions, which may be applied with a thrust. Manipulation of peripheral joints is applied in the treatment of certain sports injuries and joint conditions. A thrust is a sudden movement performed with a high-velocity short-amplitude motion such that the person cannot prevent the motion.

The motion is performed at the end of the pathologic limit of the joint and is intended to alter positional relationships, to snap adhesions, or to stimulate joint receptors. Pathologic limit means the end of the available range of motion when there is restriction.

MANNERISM
Habitual trick of expression or manner, more or less peculiar to an individual, and so characteristic as often to identify him.

MANNOSIDOSIS
An inherited metabolic disease characterized by deficiency of an enzyme catalyzing the metabolism of mannose with resulting accumulation of mannose in the blood and marked especially by facial and skeletal deformities and by mental retardation.

MANTOUX TEST
A skin test for tuberculosis in which a minute amount of tuberculin (a substance extracted from the tubercle bacillus) is injected into the skin.

After 48 hours a positive test will show swelling surrounded by a pink zone at the injection site. This means that the person has either already been immunized against tuberculosis or has been exposed to the disease; in the latter case, it does not necessarily mean the person has active tuberculosis.

MANUBRIUM
Handle-shaped structure, particularly the manubrium sterni, the upper portion of the breastbone.

MAO
Abbreviation of monoamine oxidase.

MAO-INHIBITORS
Drugs that prevent the activity of the enzyme monoamine oxidase (MAO) in brain tissue, thus affecting mood. MAO inhibitors include antidepressants, the use of which is largely restricted because of severe side effects. These side effects may be interactions with other drugs (such as ephedrine) or foods containing tyramine (such as cheese) and may produce a sudden increase in blood pressure.

MAPLE SYRUP URINE DISEASE

A hereditary metabolic disease in which an excess of amino acids in the urine (amino-aciduria) is associated with mental health. In infants it is associated with muscle rigidity, vomiting, seizures and often death. The disease gets its name from the fact that the overloaded urine smells like maple syrup.

MAP UNIT

A unit that represents a recombination frequency of one percent between genes and that is used as a measure of distance between genes in the construction of genetic maps.

MARASMUS

General wasting of the body, caused by malnutrition; the childhood equivalent of starvation. Marasmus is a condition of chronic undernourishment occurring especially in children and usually caused by a diet deficient in calories and proteins but sometimes by disease or parasitic infection.

MARBLE BONES

Another name for osteopetrosis.

MARBURG DISEASE

Also called green monkey disease; a tropical disease, sometimes also caught by laboratory workers, caused by a virus. It is extremely infectious, has an incubation period of four to nine days and is often fatal.
  Symptoms include:
- nausea;
- severe headache;
- fever;
- diarrhea;
- vomiting;
- rash;
- internal bleeding.

MARCH

The progression of epileptic activity through the motor centers of the cerebral cortex in the brain that is manifested in localized convulsions in first one area and then an adjacent part of the body.

MARCH FRACTURE

Spontaneous fracture of the second metatarsal bone in the foot, which usually occurs suddenly while the person is walking (hence the name). Resting the foot while keeping it immobile will satisfactorily heal the fracture.

MARFAN SYNDROME

An inherited disorder of bones and connective tissue transmitted as an autosomal dominant trait, resulting in abnormalities of the eyes (shortsightedness, detached retina), skeleton (abnormally large, spindle growth) and heart (dilation of the aorta and aortic incompetence). The condition cannot be cured, but the severity of the various disorders can be alleviated.

MARIJUANA

Also called cannabis, pot, grass, Indian hemp; a widely used drug taken in the form of cigarettes. See also Cannabis.

MARROW

Soft substance filling the cavities of the long bones, which manufactures the red blood cells, platelets and granular white blood cells.

MARSH TEST

A sensitive test for arsenic in which a solution to be tested is treated with hydrogen so that if arsenic is present gaseous arsine is formed and then decomposed to a black deposit of arsenic.

MARTINOTTI CELL

A multipolar fusiform nerve cell in the deepest layer of the cerebral cortex with axons ascending into the layer of pyramidal cells.

MASCULINE PROTEST

A tendency attributed especially in the human female in the psychology

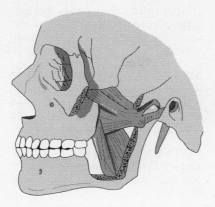

Masseter muscle.

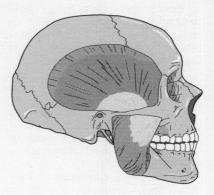

Temporal muscle (originating from the temporal bone and inserting on the mandible) plays an important role in mastication.

of Alfred Adler to escape from the female role by assuming a masculine role and by dominating others. The term is generally used to designate any tendency to compensate for feelings of inferiority or inadequacy by exaggerated overt aggressive behavior.

MASCULINITY
Patterns of behavior, attitudes, etc., presumed to be psychological secondary sex characteristics of the male.

MASCULINIZATION
A change of personality from predominantly feminine to predominantly masculine characteristics, as a result mainly of environmental and social influences.

MASKED EPILEPSY
A type of epilepsy where the convulsions are replaced by integrated, but automatic and unremembered actions, and the period of unconsciousness is brief.

MASOCHISM
Mental state in which the individual gains erotic pleasure from experiencing pain. In psychoanalysis "masochism" describes the unconscious desire to bring humiliation upon oneself, and may again have an erotic basis.

MASSAGE
Manipulation of tissues (as by rubbing, stroking, kneading, or tapping) with the hand or an instrument for remedial or hygienic purposes.

MASTECTOMY
Removal of a breast, including the skin and nipple; lymph nodes from the armpit and some chest wall muscles may also be removed.

Mastectomy, often with radiation therapy, is used to treat breast cancer.

MASSETER
A large muscle that raises the lower jaw and assists in mastication. The muscle arises from the zygomatic arch and the zygomatic process of the temporal bone, and is inserted into the mandibular ramus and angle of the jaw.

MASTITIS
Inflammation of the breast.

MASTOCYTOSIS
Excessive proliferation of mast cells in organs and tissues.

MASTOID
Literally, "breast-shaped", generally used to describe the air spaces lined

by mucous membranes lying behind the middle ear and connected with it; they are situated in the bony protuberances behind the ear (the mastoid process).

MASTOIDITIS
Inflammation of the mastoid air cells behind the ear. The condition may follow middle ear infection; if its drainage is blocked by inflammation and pus; this makes eradication difficult.

Antibiotics have reduced its incidence and surgery to clear or remove the air spaces is now infrequent.

MASTOID PROCESS
The process of the temporal bone behind the ear that is well developed and of somewhat conical form in adults but inconspicuous in children.

MASTURBATION
Production of sexual orgasm by self-manipulation of the genital organs. The term is also applied to designate the erotic stimulation of the genital organs commonly resulting in orgasm and achieved by manual or other bodily contact exclusive of sexual intercourse, by instrumental manipulation, occasionally by sexual fantasies, or by various combinations of these agencies.

MASTURBATION EQUIVALENT
Activity considered to be an equivalent or substitute for masturbation.

MASTURBATION FANTASY
The imaginative activity accompanying masturbation.

MATERIALIZATION
The alleged forming of material objects, or parts of the human body, by superhuman beings.

MATERIA MEDICA
Substances used to treat illness -

primarily drugs, but also herbal medicaments, etc. Also another, older name for pharmacology, the study of drugs.

MATERNAL INHERITANCE
A matriclinous inheritance; inheritance of characters transmitted through the cytoplasma of the egg.

MATERNAL INSTINCT MYTH
The myth that women are predisposed towards childcare, while men are not.

MATERNAL RUBELLA
Rubella in a pregnant woman that may cause developmental anomalies in the fetus when occurring during the first trimester.

MATERNITY
Hospital facilities designed for the care of women before and during childbirth and for the care of newborn babies.

MATING GRADIENT
Practice of women tending to marry above their social class and men marrying below their social class.

MATING TYPE
A strain or clone or other isolate made up of organisms (as certain fungi or protozoans) incapable of sexual reproduction with one another but capable of such reproduction with members of other strains of the same organism.

MATRIX
The intercellular substance in which tissue cells (as of connective tissue) are embedded.

The term is also used to designate the thickened epithelium at the base of a fingernail or toenail from which new nail substance develops.

In dentistry, the term is used for a strip or band place so as to serve as a retaining outer wall of a tooth in filling a cavity.

MATTER
Material, as feces or urine, discharged or for discharge from the living body.

MATTRESS SUTURE
A surgical stitch in which the suture is passed back and forth through both edges of a wound so that the needle is reinserted each time on the side of the egress and passes through to the side of ingress.

MATURATION
The process of becoming mature; the emergence of personal and behavioral characteristics through growth processes. The term is also used to designate the final stages of differentiation of cells, tissues, or organs. Maturation is also the achievement of intellectual and emotional mechanisms.

MATURATION-DEGENERAT ION HYPOTHESIS
The principle that an organism's functions and abilities develop to a certain optimal stage and then decline.

MAXILLA
The upper jaw bone.

MAXILLARY ARTERY
An artery supplying the deep structures of the face, as the nasal cavities, palate, tonsils, and pharynx. The maxillary artery sends a branch to the meninges of the brain

MAXILLARY NERVE
The one of the three major branches of the trigeminal nerve that supplies sensory fibers to the skin areas of the middle part of the face, the upper jaw and its teeth, and the mucous membranes of the palate, nasal cavities, and nasopharynx.

MAXILLARY PROCESS
A triangular embryonic process that grows out from the dorsal end of the mandibular arch on each side and forms the lateral part of the upper lip, the cheek, and the upper jaw except the premaxilla.

MAXILLARY SINUS
An air cavity in the body of the maxilla that communicates with the middle meatus of the nose.

MAXILLARY SINUSITIS
Another name for an inflammatory process in the sinus of the maxilla.

MAXILLARY VEIN
Short venous trunk of the face that is formed by the union of veins from the pterygoid plexus and that joins with the superficial temporal vein to form a vein which contributes to the formation of the external jugular vein.

MAXILLO-ALVEOLAR INDEX
The ratio multiplied by 100 of the distance between the most lateral points on the external border of opposite sides of the alveolar arch to its length.

MAXIMAL SENSATION
That intensity of sensation that is not further increased by increasing the intensity of the stimulus.

MAXIMUM BREATHING CAPACITY
Liters per second of air expelled during forced exhalation; a test of air flow obstruction.

MAXIMUM PERMISSIBLE CONCENTRATION
The maximum concentration of radioactive material in body tissue that is regarded as acceptable and producing significant deleterious effects on the human organism.

MAZZINI'S TEST
A blood test for syphilis.

MBD SYNDROME
Abbreviation for minimal brain dysfunction syndrome.

MEAN CORPUSCULAR HEMOGLOBIN
A measure of the average hemoglobin content in each red blood cell.

MEAN CORPUSCULAR VOLUME
A measure of the average size of red blood cells.

MEASLES
Also called rubeola or morbilli. A high communicable disease caused by a virus and spread by droplet infection (i.e., from tiny droplets of moisture in air that is breathed, sneeze and coughed out) and characterized by sore throat and cold-like symptoms and by a typical rash on the skin.

Possible complications include pneumonia and inflammation of the brain. Measles can be prevented by immunization with the measles vaccine, which is usually given as part of the measles-mumps-rubella (MMR) vaccine.

MEATUS
Any passage or channel or orifice; for example, the external acoustic meatus; the ear canal.

MECHANICAL APTITUDE
Inborn capacity for learning to deal with machine and machinery.

MECHANICAL HEART
A mechanism designed to maintain the flow of blood to the tissues of the body especially during a surgical operation on the heart.

MECHANISM
Physical, chemical, mental, etc. system with limited characteristics. In psychoanalytical theory, it means semi-automatic reaction patterns issuing from repressed emotional complexes, and directed towards ends determined unconsciously.

MECHANISTIC THEORY
The doctrine that all aspects of the universe, including organisms and their psychological processes, can be explained in terms of mechanical laws.

MECHANORECEPTOR
A neural end organ, as a tactile receptor, that responds to a mechanical stimulus (as a change in pressure).

MECHEL-GRUBER SYNDROME
A syndrome inherited as an autosomal recessive trait and typically characterized by:
- occipital encephalocele;
- microcephaly;
- cleft palate;
- polydactyly;
- polycystic kidneys.

MECKEL'S CARTILAGE
The cartilaginous bar of the embryonic mandibular arch of which the distal end ossifies to form the malleus being replaced by fibrous membrane comprising the sphenomandibular ligament and the connective tissue covering most of the remaining part ossifying to form much of the mandible.

MECKEL'S DIVERTICULUM
A congenital hollow sac several inches long, sometimes found attached to the small intestine.

MECONIUM
The sticky, greenish mass, consisting of mucous tissue cells, bile, lanugo hairs and vernix caseosa that collects in the intestines and forms the first fecal discharge of the newborn three or four days after birth.

MECONIUM ASPIRATION SYNDROME
An inflammation of the peritoneum (membrane lining the abdominal cavity) due to the unborn baby breathing in meconium that has entered the amniotic sac in which it lies.

MEDIA
Middle coat of a vein, artery or lymph vessel; the transparent parts of the eye; substances used for culturing germs.

MEDIAL COLLATERAL LIGAMENT
Ligament that connects the medial epicondyle of the femur with the medial condyle and medial surface of the tibia and that helps to stabilize the knee by preventing lateral dislocation.

MEDIAL GENICULATE BODY
A sensory relay nucleus which is part of the auditory system. It is part of the thalamus where the auditory tract synapse joins with auditory fibers which project to the auditory region of the cerebral cortex.

MEDIASTINITIS
Inflammation of the mediastinum.

MEDIASTINOSCOPY
Examination of the mediastinum through an incision above the sternum.

MEDIASTINUM
Space between the lungs, or more accurately between the sacs of pleural membrane containing the lungs.

MEDIASTINUM TESTIS
A mass of connective tissue at the back of the testis that is continuous externally with the tunica albuginea and internally with the interlobular septa and encloses the rete testis.

MEDICAL PSYCHOLOGY
Theories of personality and behavior not necessarily derived from academic psychology that provide a basis for psychotherapy in psychiatry and general medicine.

MEDICATION
Any substance prescribed to treat illness.

MEDICINE
The art and science of healing. Within the last 150 years or so medicine has become dominated by scientific principles, but prior to this, healing was mainly a matter of tradition and magic. Many of these pre-scientific attitudes have persisted to the present day. The term medicine is also used to designate a medication or drug that maintains, improves, or restores health.

MEDICARE
A program of the Social Security Administration which provides medical care for the aged.

MEDITERRANEAN ANEMIA
Another name for thalassemia.

MEDITERRANEAN FEVER
Another name for brucellosis.

MEDULLA
Bone marrow or anything resembling marrow in structure or in relationship to other parts, such as a fatty substance occupying certain cavities; the central part of an organ as distinguished from the cortex, or exterior.

MEDULLA OBLONGATA
Part of the brain stem; the lowest part of the brain. It is also defined as the upward continuation of the spinal cord into the skull.

MEDULLARY CYSTIC DISEASE
A diffuse degeneration of the kidney, either genetic or congenital in origin, usually seen in children or young adults and characterized by the insidious onset of uremia.

MEGACOLON
Also known as Hirschsprung's disease; large, distended colon.

MEGA-ESOPHAGUS
Another name for achalasia.

MEGALOMANIA
An exaggerated overestimation of one's own value, importance and abilities.

MEIBOMIAN CYST
Cyst (painless round lump) caused by blockage of a Meibomian gland. These glands, similar to the grease glands of the skin, are on the inner surface of the eyelids with openings emerging on the free margins of the lids.

MEIOSIS
The division of sex cells, whereby the normal number of chromosomes in a cell is halved, to be combined with another half-set from the other partner during fertilization.

MEISSNER'S CORPUSCLE
Any of the small elliptical tactile end organs in hairless skin containing numerous transversely placed tactile cells and fine flattened terminations.

MELANCHOLIA
Mental disorder characterized by:
extreme depression;
– fear;
– brooding;
– painful delusions;
– disinclination to undertake any mental or physical activity.
In classical times, melancholia was one of the four "humors," and a melancholic personality was one in which there was an excess of black bile, leading to sadness, depression and moodiness.

MELANEMESIS
Black vomit, coffee-ground vomit.

MELANIN
Dark brown pigment that lies in various skin layers and is responsible for skin, hair and eye color.

MELANISM
An excessive development of the dark pigment, melanin, in an animal, as in the panther (a black variety of leopard) and in humans in such conditions as Cushing's disease.

MELANOBLASTOMA
A malignant tumor derived from melanoblasts.

MELANOCYTE
The special cell in the lower layers of the skin, the iris of the eye and the roots of the hair, which produces granules of melanin.

MELANOCYTE-STIMULAT– ING HORMONE
Either of two hormones of the pituitary gland that darken the skin by stimulating melanin dispersion in pigment-containing cells.

MELANOMA
Any tumor characterized by the presence of melanin pigment. Strictly speaking, this is a harmless tumor, such as a pigmented mole, but because some pigmented moles become cancerous the term is now used as an alternative for "melanotic sarcoma."

MELATONIN
Hormone of the pineal gland that produces lightening of the skin by causing contraction of melanophores in pigment-containing cells and that plays a role in sexual development and maturation by inhibiting gonadal development and the estrous cycle.

MELANURIA
Presence of melanin in the urine.

MELENA
Passage of dark, black stools, due to hemorrhage inside the intestinal tract (e.g., from a bleeding peptic ulcer); the blood having been converted by digestive processes.

MELOMANIA
An inordinate liking for music or

melody; excessive or abnormal attraction to music.

MEMBERSHIP CHARACTER
Psychological term denoting the effect on the individuality of an item of experience, sensory or ideational, when it becomes a constituent in a whole.

MEMBRANE
Layer that forms part of the surface of a cell and which encloses organelles within the cell of all animals and plants.

MEMBRANOUS URETHRA
The part of the male urethra that is situated between the layers of the urogenital diaphragm and that connects the parts of the urethra passing through the prostate gland and the penis.

MEMORY
The sum of mental processes that result in the modification of an individual's behavior in the light of previous experience.

Testing of the efficiency of memory may be by recall (e.g., remembering a string of unrelated syllables); recognition (as in a multiple-choice test, where the candidate recognizes the correct answer among alternatives); and relearning, in which comparison is made between the time taken by an individual to commit certain data to memory after a delay.

MEMORY APPARATUS
An apparatus, employed in the study of memorizing to present in regular succession, and at the desired intervals, the material to be memorized.

MEMORY, ASSOCIATIVE
The recalling of a past experience by remembering a fact or incident associated with it that will evoke the experience.

MEMORY CELL
A lymphocyte (a type of white blood cell) that has encountered a specific antigen and is therefore committed to respond in an enhanced fashion on any subsequent encounter with the same antigen; part of the body's defense (immune) system.

MEMORY, KINESTHETIC
Memory that is in terms of ideal presentation of movement sensations.

MEMORY, LONG-TERM
The ability to respond to a stimulus, remember an association, and so on, a long period after the material was first presented.

MEMORY, ORGANIC
A change in living tissue that persists and modifies subsequent activity of that tissue, and which results from the activity of the functioning of the tissue itself.

MEMORY, SCREEN
Fragmentary childhood memories which are similar in structure to manifest dream content in that they have been subjected to the operations of condensation and displacement, and usually serve as a cover for other repressed memories.

MEMORY, SHORT-TERM
The correct recall or appropriate performance
immediately or shortly after the presentation of the material.

MEMORY SPAN
The greatest amount (as the longest series of letters or digits) that can be perfectly reproduced by a subject after a single presentation by the experimenter,

MEMORY TRACE
The changes in the brain that supposedly occur when something is learned.

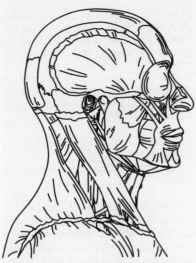

Median section of the head. The dura mater is the outer membrane of the brain and spinal cord. The falx cerebri, between the two hemispheres, is am extension of the cranial dura mater.

MEMORY, UNCONSCIOUS
Repressed ideas and emotions that influence behavior through their derivatives entering consciousness.

MENARCHE
The beginning of the menstrual function; the first menstrual period of an individual.

MENIÈRE'S SYNDROME
A disorder characterized by recurrent prostrating dizziness (vertigo), hearing loss and tinnitus (noises in the ear) associated with excessive fluid in the membranous labyrinth of the inner ear which controls balance. The precise cause of this order is unknown.

MENINGEAL
Pertaining to the meninges or coverings of the brain and spinal cord.

MENINGEAL ARTERY
Any of several arteries supplying the meninges of the brain and neighboring structures.

MENINGEAL VEIN
Any of several veins draining the meninges of the brain and neighboring structures.

MENINGIOMA
Tumor usually situated in the coverings of the brain, but occasionally found in other parts of the central nervous system. It grows by expansion but may be invasive and therefore malignant.

MENINGES
The three membranes covering the brain and spinal cord.
The outer membrane is called the dura mater, the middle one the arachnoid and the innermost the pia mater.

MENINGISMUS
Illness characterized by fever, headache and neck stiffness but without the signs of true meningitis.

MENINGITIS
Inflammation of the meninges (coverings of the brain and spinal cord), most commonly due to bacterial infection, but sometimes caused by viral or fungal infection.
Symptoms include:
- headache;
- stiff neck;
- fever;
- nausea;
- vomiting.
Treatment depends on the cause.

MENINGOCOCCUS
Also called Neisseria meningitides; bacterium that causes meningococcal meningitis.

MENINGO-ENCEPHALITIS
Inflammation of the brain and its coverings.

MENINGO-ENCEPHALOCELE
Protrusion of the brain and its coverings through a bony defect in the skull.

MENINGO-ENCEPHALOMEN INGITIS
Inflammation of the coverings of the brain and the spinal cord.

MENINGOMYELITIS
Inflammation of the spinal cord coverings.

MENINGOMYELOCELE
Also called spina bifida; protrusion of a part of the spinal cord and its membranes through a bony effect in the spinal column.

MENISCUS
One of two crescent-shaped fibro-cartilage discs in the knee joint, which overcome the disparity in the fit of two bone ends. A torn meniscus is the most common knee disorder.

MENOPAUSE
Commonly called "change of life," phase in virtually every woman's life when the activity of her ovaries declines (the climacteric) and then menstrual periods cease altogether (menopause).

MENORRHAGIA
Excessive loss of blood during menstruation. It can only be estimated in relation to the previous history of the woman's menstrual flow and whether the blood loss is excessive enough to produce anemia.

It is sometimes caused by fibroids or a tumor of the uterus or ovary, and all these must be investigated by the doctor; other times, there is no obvious cause. If the excessive blood loss is causing anemia, iron supplements must be taken. If the loss is troublesome, the woman may be prescribed progestogen (a synthetic female hormone) or one of the anti-prostaglandin drugs.

MENORRHEA
Properly, the normal flow of the menstrual periods, but commonly applied to describe an excessive menstrual flow. Strictly speaking, excessive blood loss should be called hypermenorrhea or menorrhagia.

MENSES
Commonly called a "period." The monthly discharge of blood from the uterus.

MENSTRUAL CYCLE
The whole cycle of physiologic changes from the beginning of one menstrual period to the beginning of the next.

MENSTRUAL EXTRACTION
A procedure for shortening the menstrual period or for early termination of pregnancy by withdrawing the uterine lining and a fertilized egg if present by means of suction.

MENSTRUATION
The cyclic, physiologic discharge through the vagina of blood and mucosal tissues from the nonpregnant uterus; it is under hormonal control and normally recurs usually at approximately four-week intervals, except during pregnancy and lactation throughout the reproductive period (puberty through menopause).

MEN SYNDROMES
Abbreviation for multiple endocrine neoplasia syndromes.

MENTAL CHEMISTRY
The doctrine that mental elements are fused by association into complex processes that no longer resemble the original elements.

MENTAL
Of or relating to the mind; of or relating to the total emotional and intellectual response of an individual to his environment.

MENTAL AGE
Measure used in psychological test-

ing that expresses an individual's mental attainment in terms of the number of years it takes an average child to reach the same level.

MENTAL ARTERY
A branch of the inferior alveolar artery on each side that emerges from the mental foramen and supplies blood to the chin.

MENTAL CAPACITY
Sufficient memory and understanding to comprehend in a general way the situation in which pone finds himself and the nature, purpose, and consequence of any act or transaction into which one proposes to enter.

The term is also used to designate the degree of understanding and memory the law requires to uphold validity of or to charge one with responsibility for a particular act or transaction.

MENTAL CONTENT
The total constituents of an individual's experience at any moment.

MENTAL DEFICIENCY
Failure of intellectual development that results in social incompetence and is considered to be the result of a defective central nervous system and to be incurable.

MENTAL DETERIORATION
Progressive degeneration of mental abilities and functions, as seen, for instance, in dementia.

MENTAL DISORDER
Condition characterized by abnormal function of the higher centers of the brain responsible for thought, perception, mood and behavior, in which organic disease has been eliminated as a possible cause.

The borderline between disease and the range of normal variability is indistinct and may be determined by cultural factors.

MENTAL EXAMINATION
The applying of mental tests, either in order to determine an individual's mental level or status, or to diagnose mental disorder.

MENTAL FUNCTION
A particular type of ability such as intelligence.

MENTAL HEALING
The curing of disorders by suggestion or faith.

MENTAL HEALTH
A state of relatively good adjustment, a feeling of well-being and the ability to make the most of one's potentialities and capacities.

MENTAL HOSPITAL
An institution, either state or privately owned, in which rehabilitative care is administered to mentally disturbed persons through various forms of therapy, such as psychotherapy, occupational therapy and chemotherapy.

MENTAL HYGIENE
Investigation of the laws of mental health, and the taking, or advocacy, of measure of its preservation.

MENTAL ILLNESS
A mental or bodily condition marked primarily by sufficient disorganization of personality, mind, and emotion to seriously impair the normal psychological functioning of the individual. It may lead to hospitalization.

MENTAL INCAPACITY
An inability through mental illness or mental deficiency of any sort to carry on the everyday affairs of life or to care for one's person or property with reasonable discretion.

MENTAL MATURITY
The attainment of an adult level of mental development.

MENTAL ORGANIZATION
The organized totality of mental operations in an individual; this term is sometimes used to describe the underlying physiological organization of mental operations.

MENTAL PROCESS
All processes of mental life, conscious and subconscious alike, though most frequently referring only to the former.

MENTAL RETARDATION
Significantly subaverage general intellectual functioning existing concurrently with deficits in adaptive behavior, first showing itself as a child develops.

MENTAL TEST
A standardized procedure for investigating mental capacities and characteristics, which may be either qualitative or quantitative.

MENTHOL
An alcoholic extract from mint oils used as an inhalation and topical antipruritic agent.

MERALGIA PARESTHETICA
An abnormal condition characterized by pain and paresthesia in the outer surface of the thigh.

MERBENTYL
Brand name of a drug containing as active compound diclomine prescribed for the treatment of symptoms of the irritable bowel syndrome.

MERCURY
Metallic element that can be toxic when taken into the body in sufficient amounts. Mercury can enter the body by inhalation if it is in the air; by contact with the skin; by injection, as when it is used as a diuretic; and mostly by ingestion, as when eating fish containing even a trace of the metal.

When small amounts of mercury are taken into the body over long periods of time (i.e., years), no symptoms may appear until they build up to a toxic level.

MERCURY POISONING
The cause of acute gastrointestinal tract and kidney disease if mercury salts are ingested. A chronic form, often from vapor inhalation, causes brain changes with tremor, ataxia (abnormal gait), irritability and social withdrawal.

Organic mercury from fish (e.g., tuna or swordfish) living in contaminated water, or from cereals treated with antifungal agents may cause ataxia, swallowing difficulty, abnormalities of vision and coma. Nephrotic syndrome of the kidney may also be seen.

MERERGASIA
A syndrome consisting of a partial disorganization of personality.

MEROGONY
Development of an embryo by a process that is genetically equivalent to male parthenogenesis and that involves segmentation and differentiation of an egg or egg fragment deprived of its own nucleus but having a functional male nucleus introduced.

MERYCISM
Another term for adult rumination, in which food returns from the stomach to the mouth to be chewed again.

MESCALINE
Hallucinogen derived from the peyote cactus. Peyote is unpleasant, bitter and acrid; it causes a slight burning sensation and itching of mucous membranes.

A few minutes after taking mescaline, the following symptoms may appear:
- nausea;
- dizziness;
- sweating;

- palpitations;
- headache;
- heat or chilliness;
- cramps in chest, neck or abdomen.

MESENTERIC ARTERY
Either of two arteries arising from the aorta and passing between the two layers of the mesentery to the intestine.

MESENTERIC GANGLION
Either of two ganglionic masses of the sympathetic nervous system associated with the corresponding mesenteric plexus.

MESENTERIC NODE
Any of the lymphatic glands of the mesentery.

MESENTERIC PLEXUS
Either of two plexuses of the sympathetic nervous system mostly in the mesentery in close proximity to and distributed to the same structures as the mesenteric arteries.

MESENTERY
The membranous fold in which the intestines is slung from the back wall of the abdomen so that it lies relatively free and mobile in the peritoneal cavity. It consists of a double layer of peritoneum, and within it lie the blood vessels and lymph nodes and vessels of the gut.

MESOCOLON
Fold of the mesentery connecting the colon (large intestine) with the back wall of the abdomen.

MESODERM
Layer of cells in the embryo from which connective tissue, blood, muscle and bone arise.

MESOMORPHY
One of the three basic principal builds that, according to one theory, relate to the three temperaments. According to the classification, the physique is marked by a promi-

nence of muscle, bone and connective tissue.

MESSENGER RNA
A type of ribonucleic acid which transfers genetic information from the cell nucleus to the cytoplasm surrounding it.

METABOLIC ACIDOSIS
A primary fall in the level of bicarbonate in the extracellular fluid; Ph and carbon dioxide combining power are reduced.

METABOLIC ALKALOSIS
A primary increase in the content of bicarbonate in the blood; Ph and carbon dioxide combining power are elevated.

METABOLISM
The sum total of all chemical reactions that occur in a living organism. It can be subdivided into anabolism which describes reactions that build op more complex substances from smaller ones, and catabolism which describes reactions that break down complex substances into simpler ones.

Metabolism provides energy required to keep the body functioning at rest - to maintain breathing, heart beat, and body temperature and to replace worn tissues. It also provides energy needed during exertion. Metabolism provides this energy from breakdown of digested foods.

METACARPUS
Five metacarpal bones that form the palm of the hand.

METAGNOMY
A belief that knowledge can be obtained by superhuman methods from spiritual beings.

METAMORPHOPSIA
The distortion of visually perceived objects when the retina of the eye has been displaced.

METHAMPHETAMINE
A drug of the amphetamine group, sometimes used in the treatment of depression and, in children, in the treatment of hyperactive behavior.

METAPHASE
That stage of cell division during which the chromosomes line up on the spindle equatorial plate.

METAPHORIC LANGUAGE
A form of thinking that resembles the primary process. The metaphor is a device that expresses a vital emotion and experience that originally occurs in the pregenital stage.

METAPHRENIA
Mental stage in which a person directs all his or her energy to personal gain or aggrandizement and completely neglects or ignores his or her family.

METAPHYSICS
The branch of philosophy that is concerned with the ultimate nature of existence.

METAPHYSIS
Growing end of a bone situated between the epiphysis (top of the bone) and the diaphysis (the shaft) of a long bone.

METAPLASIA
Transformation of one tissue into another.

METASTASIS
Transfer of disease from a primary focus to a distant one by conveying the agents or cells causing it through blood vessels or lymph channels. This is the mode by which many cancers spread.

METATARSAL
Relating to any of the five bones constituting the metatarsal region of the foot between the ankle and the beginning of the toes.

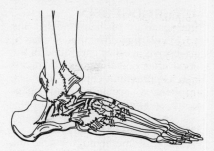

Lateral view of the foot: tarsus (left), metatarsus (middle) and toes (right).

METATARSUS
Region of the foot between the ankle and beginning of the toes. The main structures are the five metatarsal bones.

METEORISM
Gaseous distention of the abdomen.

METHADON
Synthetic narcotic that is slightly more potent than morphine on a weight basis. It is used extensively to prevent withdrawal symptoms in narcotic addicts.

The average maintenance dose (80 to 120 mg) produces no toxic effects in dependent persons. However, this same dose may cause severe respiratory depression or death in non-tolerant adults. Infants and children may suffer from severe respiratory depression after 10 to 15 mg of the drug.

METHANE
An inflammable, explosive gas, from decomposition of organic matter.

METHANOL
A clear, colorless, flammable liquid, used as solvent.

METHAMPHETAMINE
Also called methylamphetamine; generic name of a drug that is a derivative of and similar to amphetamine.

METHEMOGLOBIN
Altered form of hemoglobin (the red blood pigment), that is chocolate-brown in color and found in the blood after poisoning by chemicals such as potassium chlorate, nitrates, nitrobenzol, acetanilid and phenacetin, and in certain diseases.

METHEMOGLOBINEMIA
Presence of methemoglobin in the blood.

METHEMOGLOBINURIA
Presence of methemoglobin in the urine.

METROPATHIA HAEMORRHAGIA
Menstrual periods, usually occurring soon after menarche, that come infrequently but are heavy and last two or three weeks. They usually signify that a girl is not ovulating, and the bleeding can cause iron-deficiency.

METROPERITONITIS
Inflammation of the uterus and peritoneum (the membrane lining of the abdomen); peritonitis resulting from inflammation of the uterus; or inflammation of the peritoneal covering of the uterus.

METRORRHAGIA
Bleeding from the uterus that is not connected with menstruation.

METRORRHEA
Any discharge from the uterus.

MICROBE
Living organism of minute size, a bacterium for instance, but especially one capable of causing disease.

MICROBIOLOGY
Formerly called bacteriology, the study of microorganisms, including bacteria, viruses, fungi and algae. Microbiology embraces the traditional spheres of anatomy, physiology, genetics, taxonomy and ecology, together with various branches of medicine, veterinary sciences and plant pathology, since many microorganisms are pathogenic by nature.

MICROCEPHALY
A condition characterized by the smallness of the head with associated subnormal mental development, produced by an incomplete development of the brain due to a premature closing of the skull.

MICRODETERMINATION
Determination, as of chemical composition, by analysis of minute quantities of material.

MICRODISSECTION
Dissection under a microscope; dissection of cells and tissues by means of fine needles that are precisely manipulated by levers.

MICROGLIA
Neuroglia consisting of small cells with few processes that are scattered throughout the central nervous system. They have a phagocytic function as part of the reticuloendothelial system.

MICROMETASTASIS
The spread of cancer cells from a primary site and the formation of microscopic tumors at secondary sites.

MICRON
Unit of measurement represented by the symbol mu and equal to one-thousandth part of a millimeter.

MICROORGANISM
Another name for microbe; any animal or vegetable organism so small that it is only visible through a microscope.

MICROPSIA
Disorder of visual perception due to disease of the retina of the eye in

which objects are perceived much smaller than they really are.

MICROSCOPE
An instrument for producing enlarged images of small objects. In the compound microscope a magnified, inverted image of an object resting on the "stage" is produced by the objective lens system. This image is viewed through the eyepiece (or ocular) lens system which acts as a simple microscope, giving a greatly magnified virtual image. In most biological microscopy the object is viewed by transmitted light, illumination being controlled by mirror, diaphragm and substance condenser lenses. The near-transparent objects are often stained to make them visible.

MICROSURGERY
Minute dissection or manipulation, as by a micromanipulator or laser beam, of living structures (as cells) for surgical or experimental purposes.

MICROTOME
Instrument used to cut tissue into extremely thin sections for microscopic examination.

MICTURITION
Act of passing urine; another term for urination.

MIDBRAIN
The middle division of the three primary divisions of the developing brain or the corresponding part of the adult brain that includes a ventral part containing the cerebral peduncles and a dorsal tectum containing the corpora quadrigemina and that surrounds the aqueduct of Sylvius, connecting the third and fourth ventricles.

MIDDLE CONSTRICTOR
A fan-shaped muscle of the pharynx that arises from the hyoid bone and from the stylohyoid ligament, inserts into the median line at the back of the pharynx. The muscle acts to constrict part of the pharynx in swallowing.

MIDDLE EAR
The intermediate portion of the ear consisting typically of a small airfilled membrane-lined chamber in the temporal bone continuous with the nasopharynx through the eustachian tube, separated from the external ear by fenestra. The middle ear contains a chain of three ossicles that extends from the tympanic membrane to the oval window.

MIDDLE EAR INFECTION
A common form of ear infection, also called otitis media, that affects the part of the hearing mechanism between the eardrum and the inner ear.

MIDDLE MEATUS
Curved anteroposterior passage in each nasal cavity that is situated below the middle nasal concha and extending along the entire superior border of the inferior nasal concha.

MIDDLE MENINGEAL ARTERY
A branch of the first portion of the maxillary artery that is the largest artery supplying the dura mater, entering the cranium through the foramen spinosum, and dividing into anterior and posterior branches in a groove in the greater wing of the sphenoid bone.

MID-LIFE CRISIS
A period of emotional turmoil in middle age caused by the realization that one is no longer young and characterized by a strong desire for change.

MIGNON DELUSION
The delusional fantasy of a child that his parents are not his real parents and that his true parents are distinguished people.

MIGRAINE
A paroxysmal disorder characterized by recurrent attacks of headache, with or without associated
visual and gastrointestinal disturbances. The cause is unknown, but
evidence suggests a functional disturbance of circulation of blood
vessels within the skull. Headache
may be preceded by a short period
of depression, irritability, restlessness or anorexia, and in some persons by scotomas, visual field defects or hemiparesis. Untreated attacks may last for hours or days.
Nausea, vomiting and photophobia
are common. Specific medicines
may alleviate attacks.

MIKULICZ RESECTION
An operation for removal of part of
the intestine and especially the colon in stages that involves bringing
the diseased portion out of the
body, closing the wound around the
two parts of the loop which have
been sutured together, and cutting
off the deceased part leaving a double opening which is later joined by
crushing the common wall and
closed from exterior.

MILD MENTAL RETARDA-
TION
Mental retardation with an IQ of
50-55 to approximately 70; roughly
equivalent to what used to be referred to as the educational category
"educable." This group constitutes
the largest segment of those with
the disorder - about 85 percent.
People with this level of mental
retardation typically develop social
and communication skills during
the preschool years (ages 0-5), have
minimal impairment in sensorimotor areas, and often are not distinguishable from normal children until a later age.
By their late teens they can acquire academic skills up to approximately sixth-grade level; during
their adult years, they usually
achieve social and vocational skills
adequate for minimum self-support,
but may need guidance and assistance when under unusual social or
economic stress.

MILIARIA
Commonly called prickly heat;
itchy skin rash due to blockage of
the sweat glands.

MILIARY SCLEROSIS
Small hardened areas (sclerosis)
that occur in the spinal cords of
some people with pernicious anemia, accompanied by degeneration
of the spinal cord.

MILIARY TUBERCULOSIS
Acute tuberculosis in which minute
tubercles are formed in one or more
organs of the body by tubercle bacilli usually spread by way of the
blood.

MILIEU INTERIEUR
The bodily fluids regarded as an internal environment in which the
cells of the body are nourished and
maintained in a state of equilibrium.

MILIUM
Small, pearly, non-inflammatory
elevation, situated on the face.
These milia often become hard and
last for years.

MILK
A white liquid containing water,
protein, fat, sugar, vitamins and inorganic salts, which is secreted by
the mammary glands of female
mammals. The secretion of milk
(lactation) is initiated immediately
after birth by the hormone prolactin.
The milk produced by different
mammals all have the same basic
constituents but the proportion of
each ingredient differs from species
to species and within species.

MILK CRUST
Crusty mass seen on the scalp of
very young babies. It is a form of
seborrhea.

MILK FEVER
A fever caused by infection, appearing in women with the onset of lactation following childbirth.

MILK LEG
An inflammation of the veins of the leg that causes pain and swelling, often occurring in women after childbirth.

MILK OF MAGNESIA
Emulsion of magnesium hydroxide, used for its properties as an antacid in ulcers and heartburn, and as a laxative.

MILK SICKNESS
A disease brought about by the consumption of dairy products or of the meat of cattle that have grazed on certain poisonous plants.

MILK TOOTH
Common name for a deciduous tooth; one of the first, temporary teeth in children.

MIL-PAR
Brand name of a drug containing as active compounds magnesium hydroxide and liquid paraffin prescribed for the relief of constipation.

MIMESIS
Imitation with respect to both form and action.

MIMICRY
In biology, the close resemblance of one organism to another which, because the latter is unpalpable and conspicuous, is avoided by certain of the former's predators. The mimic will thus gain a degree of protection on the strength of a predator's avoidance of the mimicked.

MINAMATA DISEASE
A toxic neuropathy caused by the ingestion of methylmercury compounds, as in contaminated seafood and characterized by impairment of cerebral functions, constriction of the visual field, and progressive weakness of muscles.

MIND
The organized totality of physical structures and processes, conscious, unconscious and subconscious, of the brain.

MIND-ALTERING DUGS
Any drugs that decrease alertness, perception, concentration, contact with reality or muscular coordination.

MIND BLINDNESS
Inability to grasp the meaning of objects seen. The term is also used in the sense of cortical blindness.

MIND-BODY-PROBLEM
The philosophical and psychological issue concerning the relation of the mind (or mental processes) to the body (the physical or physiological processes).

MIND READING
The grasping by one individual of what is passing through the mind of another by involuntary signs given by the other.

MIND-SET
A mental inclination, tendency, or habit.

MINERAL
Inorganic elements vital to human health. The required or essential minerals that are absolutely necessary for the body to function are calcium, chlorine, cobalt, copper, fluorine, iodine, iron, magnesium, manganese, phosphorus, potassium, sodium, sulphur, and zinc.

MINERALOCORTICOID
A corticoid, as aldosterone, that affects chiefly the electrolyte and fluid balance in the body.

MINER'S ELBOW
Inflammation of the bursa over the elbow joint. Also known as student's elbow.

MINER'S NYSTAGMUS
Condition seen in coal miners in which the eyes are in a state of uncontrollable constant movement.

MINER'S SPIT
Black spit of the coal miners, which contains particles of coal dust.

MINIMAL BRAIN DYSFUNCTION (MBD-SYNDROME)
A concept that attempts to explain the cause of learning disturbances for which there is no sign of damage to or disease in the brain and nerve pathways. The concept is applied to children with mild to severe learning and/or behavioral disabilities, manifested by impairment in perception, conceptualization, language and control of attention, impulse of motor function.

MINI-PILL
A contraceptive pill that is intended to minimize side effects, containing a very low dose of a progestogen and especially norethindrone but no estrogen.

MINOR SURGERY
Surgery involving little risk to the life of the patient; an operation on the superficial structures of the body or a manipulative procedure that does not involve a serious risk.

MIOTIC
A drug that constricts (narrows) the pupil. Opiate drugs such as morphine have a miotic effect, and someone who is taking one of these drugs has pinpoint pupils. The pupil is sometimes deliberately narrowed by other miotic drugs in the treatment of glaucoma.

MIRAGE
An optical effect that is sometimes seen at sea, in the desert, or over a hot pavement, that may have the appearance of a pool of water or a mirror in which distant objects are seen inverted.

Mirage is caused by the bending or reflection of rays of light by a layer of heated air of varying density.

MIRROR DRAWING
Drawing performed while viewing the design and one's hand in a mirror, used in psychological experiments or to test eye-hand coordination.

MIRROR SPEECH
Speech in which the syllables are spoken backwards.

MIRROR WRITING
Writing produced in the laterally reverse direction, which appears as normal as seen in a mirror. Frequently seen in children as a result of mixed laterality (i.e., they do not have a preference for one side of the body or another).

MISCARRIAGE
Spontaneous abortion. By the roughest of estimates 1 out of every 4 women knows she has had at least one miscarriage. In most cases the cause is unknown.

MISCEGENATION
Marriage or cohabitation between individuals of different races.

MISOGYNY
Hatred of women; phenomenon that one hates women.

MISSED ABORTION
An intrauterine death of a fetus that is not followed by its immediate expulsion.

MISSED LABOR
A retention of a fetus in the uterus beyond the normal period of pregnancy.

MISSIONARY POSITION
A coital position in which the female lies on her back with the male on top and with his face opposite hers.

MITE
Any of numerous small to very minute arachnids of the order Acarina that have a body without a constriction between the cephalothorax and abdomen, mandibles generally chelate or adapted for piercing with usually four pairs of small legs. The Acarina include parasites of insects and vertebrates, some of which are important disease vectors.

MITE-BORN TYPHUS
Another name for scrub typhus.

MITHRIDATISM
The production of immunity against a poison by taking the poison in gradually increased doses.

MITOCHONDRIA
Small rod-like bodies inside cells which contain the enzymes for the generation of energy for the cellular metabolism.

MITOSIS
The process by which a cell divides into two and the normal way in which tissues grow.

MITRAL INSUFFICIENCY
An incomplete closing of the mitral valve between the upper and lower chambers of the left side of the heart (i.e., the left atrium and left ventricle), which permits a backflow of blood in the wrong direction. It is sometimes the result of scar tissue forming after a rheumatic fever infection.

MITRAL STENOSIS
Narrowing of the mitral valve of the heart, causing obstruction of the flow of blood through the left atrioventricular opening -that is, between the upper chamber (atrium)

and lower chamber (ventricle).

MITRAL VALVE
Valve situated between the left atrium and left ventricle of the heart, which, when open, resembles a bishop's miter.

MITRAL VALVULOTOMY
An operation to widen the opening of the mitral valve by means of surgery.

MITTELSCHMERZ
Another name for intermenstrual pain; abdominal pain and other symptoms occurring more or less regularly midway between menstrual periods.

MIXED SCHIZOPHRENIA
A form of schizophrenia characterized by symptoms usually manifested in two or more of the four categories of schizophrenia -hebephrenic, simple, catatonic and paranoid - so that a classification in one of the above categories cannot be made.

MIXTURE
An aqueous liquid medicine; a preparation in which insoluble substances are suspended in watery fluids by the addition of a viscid material, as gum, sugar, or glycerol.

MNEME
Basic memory in the individual or the race; the persistent or recurrent effect of past experience of the individual or of the race.

MNEMON
Theoretical fundamental unit of memory.

MNEMONICS
A technique of improving the memory.

MOBILIZATION
Act of reestablishing mobility in a fixed or stiffened part, a joint, for

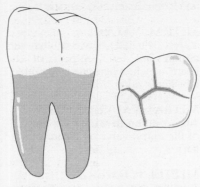

Lateral view (left) and superior view (right) of a molar.

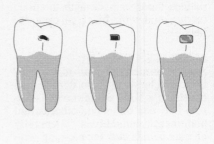

Fillings of molars in case of dental decay.

example. It is also a term used to describe freeing of an organ to make it accessible during surgery; and also the liberation of a substance stored in the body, such as mobilization of the glycogen stored in the liver.

MODERATE MENTAL RETARDATION
Mental retardation characterized by an IQ of 35-40 to 50-55; roughly equivalent to what used to be referred to as the educational level of "trainable." This group constitutes 10% of the entire population of people with mental retardation.

MOGIARTHRIA
A speech defect, due to a disease of or damage to the nervous system, which causes a failure in the coordination of the vocal muscles.

MOGIGRAPHIA
Another name for writer's cramp.

MOHS' TECHNIQUE
A chemosurgical technique for the removal of skin malignancies in which excision is made to a depth of which the tissue is microscopically free of cancer.

MOLAR
Grinding tooth. One of the large double back teeth, of which there

are three on each side of both jaws.

MOIST GANGRENE
Gangrene that develops in the presence of combined arterial and venous obstruction. The condition is accompanied by an infection and is characterized by a watery discharge usually of foul odor.

MOLE
Circumscribed pigmented macule, papule or nodule composed of clusters of melanocytes or nevus cells.

MOLECULAR BIOLOGY
The study of the structure and function of the molecules that make up living organisms. This includes the study of proteins, enzymes, carbohydrates, fats and nucleic acids.

MOLECULAR GENETICS
A branch of genetics dealing with the structure and activity of genetic material at the molecular level.

MOLECULAR LAYER
The outer layer of the cortex of the cortex of the cerebellum and cerebrum consisting of a mass of unmyelinated fibers rich in synapses.

MOLECULE
Entity of atoms linked by chemical bonds and acting as a unity; the smallest particle of a chemical com-

pound that retains the composition and chemical properties of the compound. The composition of a molecule is represented by its molecular formula.

MOLLITES OSSIUM
Another name for osteomalacia.

MOLLUSCUM BODY
Any of the rounded cytoplasmic bodies found in the central opening of the nodules characteristic of molluscum contagiosum.

MOLLUSCUM CONTAGIOSUM
Chronic skin disease, probably of viral origin and highly contagious, characterized by small, pearly, round, flat-topped tumors sometimes with a central depression, containing a cheese-like substance arising from one of the layers of the skin. It is treated by freezing the nodules with liquid nitrogen.

MOLLUSCUM SEBACEUM
Skin tumor occurring mostly on the face and limbs. It grows rapidly for several weeks and then, if left alone, withers and disappears in two or three months.

MOLONEY TEST
Test for determining hypersensitivity to diphtheria toxoid by intradermal injection of a small amount in dilute solution.

MOLYBDENUM
A trace element whose function is not yet established.

MOMISM
An excessive popular adoration and oversentimentalizing of mothers that is held to be oedipal in nature.

MONARTHRITIS
Inflammation of one joint

MONGOLIAN SPOTS
Dark blue, irregular macular spots resembling a bruise, usually found over the lower end of the spine (i.e., the sacrum) of dark-complexioned infants. These spots usually recede spontaneously within the first four years.

MONGOLISM
Another name for Down's syndrome. It is no longer employed.

MONGOLOID
One of the three racial divisions of mankind. Mongoloids generally have straight black hair, little facial hair, yellow to brown skins and the distinctive epicanthic fold; a fold of skin over the eyes that gives them a slanting appearance.

The Amerinds, Eskimos, Polynesians and Patagonians are mongoloid people.

MONILIA VAGINITIS
Infection of the vagina caused by a fungus Monilia or Candida albicans belonging to the yeast family.

MONILIASIS
Also called candidiasis; fungus (Candida albicans) infection, which may affect the skin, mucous membranes, nails, bronchi, lungs, vagina (when it is called Monilia vaginitis) or intestinal tract.

MONILIFORM
Resembling the shape of a string of beads.

MONOAMINE OXIDASE (MAO)
An enzyme that promotes the oxidation of adrenaline, tyramine and other substances (all involved in the transmission of nerve impulses), thus making them inactive. It is suppressed by a group of drugs - called monoamine oxidase inhibitors - that are effective in the treatment of depression, which seems to be associated with a deficiency of these impulse-transmitting substances.

MONOAMINE OXIDASE IN-HIBITOR

Any of various antidepressant drugs which increase the concentration of monoamines in the brain by inhibiting the action of monoamine oxidase.

MONOCROTIC PULSE

A pulse in which dicrotism (double beat) is entirely absent.

MONOCYTE

A large white blood cell.

MONOCYTOPENIA

Abnormal decrease in monocytes in the blood.

MONOGAMY

The state or custom of being married to one person at a time or of having only one mate at a time.

MONOIDEISM

A condition in which the mind is fixed on a single idea, and the individual constantly reverts to the same topic.

MONOMANIA

Mental disorder characterized by a fixed idea.

MONONUCLEOSIS

Short name for infectious mononucleosis, a common virus infection of adolescence causing a variety of symptoms including:
– sore throat;
– headache;
– fever;
– malaise;
– enlargement of lymph nodes and spleen.

Skin rashes, hepatitis with jaundice, pericarditis and involvement of the nervous system may also be prominent. Atypical lymphocytes in the blood and specific agglutination reactions are diagnostic. Severe cases may require steroid therapy and convalescence may be lengthy. It can be transmitted in saliva and has thus been nicknamed the "kissing disease."

MONOPARESIS

Paralysis of a single limb.

MONOPLEGIA

Paralysis of one limb or one group of muscles.

MONOSOMY

A condition in which one chromosome of a pair is missing, resulting in a single member of that pair instead of the normal diploid member.

MONOTONY

Lack of inflection in speaking; continuance of a single, uninteresting operation, situation or occupation.

MONO-UNSATURATED FAT

A fat so constituted chemically that it is capable of absorbing additional hydrogen but not so much hydrogen as poly-unsaturated fat. These fats in the diet have little effect on the amount of cholesterol in the blood.

MONOZYGOTIC TWINS

Twins resulting from the division into two embryos of a single zygote (fertilized egg), following fertilization of a single ovum by a single sperm cell.

MONS PUBIS

Also called mons veneris; rounded eminence of fatty tissue situated beneath the skin in front of the symphysis pubis (the region just above the external genital organs). It becomes covered with hair at puberty.

MONTEGGIA FRACTURE

Fracture of the ulna (the bone on the little finger side of the forearm) and dislocation of the head of the radius (that on the thumb-side of the forearm) at the elbow joint.

MONTGOMERY GLAND

An apocrine gland in the areola of the mammary gland.

MOOD
Emotional condition or attitude, enduring for some time and characterized by particular emotions in a condition of subexcitation, so as to be readily evoked, for instance, an irritable mood.

MOOD DISORDER
Psychic disorder determined by the pattern of mood episodes. Mood disorders are divided into bipolar disorders (manic-depressive disorders) and depressive disorders. The essential feature of bipolar disorders is the presence of one or more manic or hypomanic episodes. The essential feature of depressive disorders is one or more episodes of depression without a history of either manic or hypomanic episodes.

MOOD EPISODE
A mood syndrome that is not due to a known organic factor and is not part of a nonmood psychotic disorder (e.g., schizophrenia).

MOOD SYNDROME
A group of mood and associated symptoms that occur together for a minimal duration of time. For example, the major depressive syndrome is defined as depressed mood or loss of interest, of at least two weeks' duration, accompanied by several associated symptoms, such as weight loss and difficulty concentrating.

Mood syndromes can occur as part of a mood disorder, as part of a nonmood psychotic disorder (e.g., schizoaffective disorder), or as part of an organic mental disorder (e.g., organic mood disorder)

MOOP
A combination of four drugs including mechlorethamine, vincristine, procarbazine, and prednisine that is used in the treatment of some forms of cancer.

MORAL IDIOT
An individual whose ability to sympathize with others is absent while his ability to experience other kinds of emotions is essentially unimpaired.

MORAL FACULTY
The capacity to distinguish between right and wrong.

MORAL IMBECILE
An imbecile whose ability to sympathize with others is inadequately developed while his ability to experience other kinds of emotions is essentially unimpaired.

MORBID
Pertaining to disease or diseased parts

MORBIDITY
Quality of disease or being diseased; the conditions including disease; or the ratio of such individuals to the total population of a community.

MORBIDITY RATE
The ratio of the number of cases of a disease to the number of well people in a given population during a specified period of time, such as a year.

The term "morbidity" involves two separate concepts:

(1) Incidence, the number of new cases of a disease developing in a given population during a specific period of time, such as a year.

(2) Prevalence, the number of cases of a given disease existing in a given population at a specified moment of time.

MORBILLI
Another name for measles.

MORBILLIFORM
Resembling measles. Usually refers to a rash resembling that of measles.

MORGAGNI'S SYNDROME
Congenital heart deformity characterized by an open foramen, stenosis (narrowing) of the pulmonary artery and hypertrophy (abnormally increased size) of the right ventricle of the heart.

MORGUE
A place where the bodies of dead people, particularly accident victims, are kept until identification or disposal.

MORNING SICKNESS
Nausea of pregnant women. Affecting fewer than 50 percent, it mainly occurs during the first three months but may continue throughout the pregnancy, and, despite its name, it can occur any time of the day.

MORON
A level of feeblemindedness that is defined as the range of IQ from 50 to 70, or a mental age between 7 and 9 years. This category includes people who are believed to be capable of supporting themselves by performing simple tasks under supervision.

MORO REFLEX
Startle reflex in infants characterized by a total bodily reaction to a sudden stimulus, for example, a loud noise causes the arms and legs to be flung out, the fingers to fan out, the back to be arched or stretched, extension of the legs, and the head to be drawn back.

MORO TEST
A diagnostic skin test used to detect infection or past infection by the tubercle bacillus.

MORPHEME
Minimal unit of meaning in language.

MORPHINE
Opium derivative used as a narcotic painkiller and also commonly in drug addiction. It decreases respiration and the cough reflex, induces sleep and may cause vomiting and constipation. Medically it is valuable in heart failure; its properties are particularly valuable in terminal malignant disease. Addiction and withdrawal syndromes are common.

MORPHINIZATION
The act or process of treating with morphine. The term is also used to designate the condition of being under the influence of morphine.

MORPHINOMANIA
Morbid desire or craving for morphine.

MORPHOGENESIS
Development of the form and structure of an organ.

MORPHOLOGICAL AGE
Index used to determine height and weight changes compared to data taken from "normal"people.

MORPHOLOGICAL INDEX
The ratio of the volume of the human trunk to the sum of the lengths of one arm and one leg multiplied by a factor 100.

MORPHOLOGY
Branch of biology, dealing with the form and structure of organisms.

MORQUITO'S SYNDROME
A type of mucopolysaccharidose that is transmitted genetically in an autosomal recessive fashion and characterized by normal intelligence, cloudy corneas of the eyes and severe bony changes leading to marked curvature of the spine.

MORTALITY
Death rate; the quality or state of being mortal.

MORTON'S TOE
Metatarsalgia that is caused by compression of a branch of the

plantar nerve between the heads of the metatarsal bones and tends to occur when the second toe is longer than the big toe.

MORTUARY
A place in which dead bodies are kept and prepared for burial or cremation.

MORULA
In embryology, the mass of cells resulting from the division of a fertilized cell during the early cleavage state.

MOSAICISM
A genetic condition in which a person's genes are different in different cells of his or her body. A mosaic individual can pass on normal genes or abnormal genes to offspring.

MOSAIC TEST
A projective instrument used in the assessment of global personality traits in children aged two years and over. The test requires the choice of various ambiguous forms and organization of those forms into something the child wishes to make, using as many pieces as he or she likes.

MOSENTHAL TEST
Test to discover the specific gravity of urine. Normally the specific gravity should be high when the urine is concentrated (i.e., contains more solid material), most frequently on awakening, and lower after a large amount of fluid is ingested.

MOTHER FIGURE
A mature individual with whom a younger, immature person identifies and who comes to exercise such parental functions as advice and encouragement.

MOTHER HYPNOSIS
The concept that submission to hypnotic states can be traced to blind

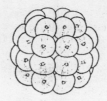

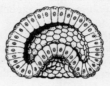
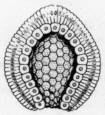

Early stages of the development of an embryo. From top to bottom; early stages in the development of an embryo:
- 32-cell stage:
- morula;
- blastula;
- gastrula

obedience to one's parent; in this case, transference of maternal fixation.

MOTHER YAW
The initial superficial lesion of yaws appearing at the site of infection after an incubation period of several weeks.

MOTILIN
Hormone formed in the duodenum and jejunum (first and second parts of the small intestine). It plays a part in controlling the movements of the stomach and intestines.

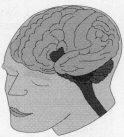

The motor cortex of the brain is located in the frontal lobe.

MOTILITY
Spontaneous movements; ability to perform voluntary movements.

MOTION
Continuous change of position; evacuation of the bowels; the feces, the matter evacuated from the bowels.

MOTION ILLUSION
Appearance of motion in a motionless object; sometimes due to relative movement, and sometimes to the nature of an after-sensation, following a continuous movement of the individual.

MOTION SICKNESS
Also called travel sickness; a disorder caused by repetitive angular and linear acceleration and deceleration and characterized primarily by nausea and vomiting. Sea-, air-, car-, and wing-sickness are specific forms. Prevention is easier than treatment. Excessive stimulation by motion of the controlling apparatus in the inner ear is the primary cause. There is great variation in individual susceptibility.

MOTIVATIONAL HIERARCHY
A hierarchy of human motives that determine behavior. The physical needs are postulated to be the most basic and needs for security and safety are at the next level. Love, affection and a sense of belonging form the next category, followed by needs for esteem, mastery, competence and prestige.
The highest level of need is that for self-actualization which does not appear until the lower-level needs have been satisfied.

MOTIVE
An affective-conative factor that operates in determining direction of an individual's behavior towards an end or goal, consciously apprehended, or unconscious.

MOTONEURON
A neuron that passes from the central nervous system or a ganglion toward or to a muscle and conducts an impulse that causes movement; also called motor neuron.

MOTOR
Pertaining to or that which causes movement, such as a motor cell, center or nerve.

MOTOR APHASIA
Difficulty in articulation, producing retarded, scanty speech, usually associated with defects in writing and understanding and other processes not directly concerned with the production of speech. It is due to disease of or damage to the left cerebral hemisphere.

MOTOR AREA
That part of the brain's surface that controls the movement of muscles, primarily in the frontal lobe of the cerebrum.

MOTOR CENTER
A nervous center that controls or modifies, as by inhibiting or reinforcing, a motor impulse.

MOTOR CORTEX
The cortex of a motor area; the motor areas as a functional whole.

MOTOR DEVELOPMENT
Development of motor skills in the infant and child.

MOTOR END PLATE
The terminal arborization of a motor axon on a muscle fiber.

MOTOR EQUIVALENCE
The principle that a goal can be reached by many different actions requiring different muscular movements.

MOTOR FUNCTION
Any activity resulting from the excitation of muscles and glands by nerve fibers extending from the brain or spinal cord.

MOTOR NEURON
A nerve cell, directly or indirectly exciting or inhibiting the activity of a muscle, and directly in connection with it.

MOTOR NEURON DISEASE
A condition of the nervous system that causes rapid and progressive physical deterioration. Onset is usually in middle age, with weakness and wasting of the arms and weakness of the legs. There may be incontinence, but there is no sensory loss and mental faculties are not affected. The cause for this is not known, and it is, as yet, incurable.

MOTOR POINT
A small area on a muscle at which a minimal amount of electrical stimulation will cause the muscle to contract.

MOTOR ROOT
A nerve root containing only motor fibers; the ventral root of a spinal nerve.

MOTOR SENSATION
Sensations derived from receptor organs in muscles, tendons and joints, sometimes inclusive of sensations from the receptors of the static sense.

MOTOR SET
Tendency on the part of a person to react in a particular way when an anticipated stimulus is presented.

MOTOR SYNDROME
Weak and flabby muscles with loss of power and sometimes exaggerated tendon reflexes due to disease or damage to the cerebral cortex (outer part of the brain).

MOTOR UNIT
The motor neuron, its axon and all branches as well as the muscle fibers that it implies.

MOULDING
Deformation of the baby's head by the
pressure of the birth passage. The head soon takes on a normal appearance after birth.

MOUNTAIN SICKNESS
Altitude sickness experienced especially above 10,000 feet (about 3000 meters) and caused by insufficient oxygen in the air.

MOURNING
The psychological process that are set in train by the loss of a loved-one and that commonly lead to the emotional relinquishing of the person, animal, etc. It follows bereavement, is accompanied by grief, and may or may not be followed by attachment to a new object and is typically accompanied by a degree of identification.

MOUTH
The opening through which humans and animals take food; the cavity containing the parts used in chewing and tasting food.

MOUTH CANCER
Also called oral cancer; malignant tumor of the mouth region. Cancer of the mouth accounts for about 4 percent of all cancers that occur annually in industrialized countries. Usually it can be detected in early stages by routine examination of the

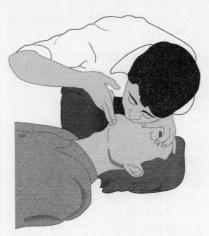

Mouth-to-mouth resuscitation. Attendant forms a tight seal around the patient's mouth with his own mouth and blows forcefully.

mouth. Mouth cancer can occur in men and women of any age, but is most frequently found in men after the age of 40 years.

Cancer of the tongue accounts for about 20 percent of all mouth cancers, and cancer of the salivary glands, 10 percent. About 25 percent are throat cancers that affect that part of the alimentary canal between the mouth and the esophagus.

Regardless of site, mouth cancer, like all cancers, is an uncontrollable, irregular growth of cells.

MOUTH-TO-MOUTH-RESUS– CITATION
Commonly called the "kiss of life," respiration consisting of air being blown directly into the mouth and lungs of an unconscious person by another at short, regular intervals.

MOVEMENT
The act of changing position, of passing from one place to another; said of the entire body or of one or more parts of it.

MOXIBUSTION
Oriental form of treatment, often used as an adjunct to acupuncture, in which moxa, a form of mugwort, is burned on the skin to form a blister. The place where this is done is not necessarily over or even near the affected organ, but its location will be at a point from which the organ is said to be influenced (i.e, an acupuncture point). Sometimes the moxa is burned close to but not directly on the skin.

MS
Abbreviation of multiple sclerosis.

MUCIN
Principal constituent of mucus. It is insoluble in water but soluble in dilute alkali.

MUCOCELE
A cavity of the body that is abnormally dilated because of an accumulation of mucus; this can occur whenever there is mucous membrane.

MUCOCUTANEOUS LYMPH NODE SYNDROME
A syndrome usually occurring in infants and children younger than five years of age, consisting of:
– a characteristic rash that becomes bright red on the hands and feet;
– fever;
– enlargement of lymph glands of the neck;
– polyarteritis (inflammation of arteries) of variable severity.
There is no specific treatment, but 98-99 percent of the patients survive.

MUCOID
Any of a group of substances resembling the mucins, occurring in connective tissue and in cysts.

MUCOLYTIC
Having the property of lessening or destroying stickiness of mucus.

The name is also applied to designate a drug that liquifies mucus secretions in the airways.

MUCOMEMBRANOUS COLIC
Another name for irritable bowel syndrome.

MUCOPOLYSACCHARIDE
Any of a class of polysaccharides that are widely distributed in the body, that bind to water to form thick gelatinous material serving to cement cells together and to lubricate joints and bursae, that are derived from a hexosamine, a uronic acid, and often sulfuric acid.

MUCOPOLYSACCHARIDOSE
Genetic conditions characterized by increased excretion of mucopolysaccharide in the urine and variable symptoms and signs elsewhere in the body, including a typical type of facial appearance, skeletal disorders, mental deficiency, opacity of the cornea of the eye and enlargement of the liver and spleen.

MUCOPROTEIN
Any of the various proteins containing mucopolysaccharide, found in the body's fluid and in connective tissue.

MUCOSA
A mucous membrane.

MUCOUS MEMBRANE
A membrane that lines all the cavities of the body that open externally, such as the mouth, nose or intestines, and which secrete mucus.

MUCOVISCIDOSIS
Another name for cystic fibrosis.

MUCUS
Sticky, aqueous solution of glycoproteins secreted by cells of the mucous membranes of the respiratory and gastrointestinal tract, as well as the salivary and other digestive system glands. It provides a non-living protective layer that is constantly being renewed, allowing removal of any particles absorbed on to it and lubrication of food and feces.

MULTIFACTORIAL INHERITANCE
Inheritance of a trait governed by many genes or multiple factors. Each gene may act independently with cumulative total effect.

MULTIGRAVIDA
Pregnant woman who has been pregnant on a previous occasion.

MULTI-INFARCT DEMENTIA
Type of dementia characterized by demonstrable evidence of impairment in short- and long-term memory. Impairment of short-term memory (inability to learn new information) may be indicated by inability to remember three objects after five minutes. Long-term memory impairment (inability to remember information that was known in the past) may be indicated by inability to remember past personal information (e.g., what happened yesterday, birthplace, occupation) or facts of common knowledge (e.g., past Presidents, well-known dates).

MULTIPARA
Woman, not necessarily a pregnant woman, who has previously given birth to one or more children.

MULTIPLE ALLELE
Any of more than two allele factors located at one chromosomal locus.

MULTIPLE FACTOR
One of a group of nonallelic genes that are inferred to control a hereditary trait which varies in a quantitative manner.

MULTIPLE PERSONALITY DISORDER
The existence within the person of two or more distinct personalities or personality states; personality being defined as a relatively enduring pattern of perceiving, relating to, and thinking about the environment and one's self that is exhibited in a wide

range of important social and personal contexts.

In classical cases, there are at least two fully developed personalities; in other cases, there may be only one distinct personality and one or more personality states. The personalities or personality states each have unique memories, behavior patterns, and social relationships; in other cases, there may be varying degrees of sharing of memories and commonalities in behavior or social relationships.

Several studies indicate that in nearly all cases, the disorder has been preceded by abuse (often sexual) or another form of severe emotional trauma in childhood. Recent reports suggest that this disorder is not nearly so rare as it has commonly been thought to be. In several studies of psychiatric patients, the disorder has been diagnosed about five times more frequently in females than in males.

MULTIPLE SCLEROSIS
A disease of the brain and spinal cord that attacks the myelin sheath covering nerve fibers.

Most of young people diagnosed with MS are between the ages of 20 and 40, and two-thirds of them are women. They have been struck at the prime of life by an unexpected disorder.

The majority of persons with MS can expect to live their normal lifespan. Recent studies have indicated that at least half of those with MS can still engage in a majority of the activities they performed before developing the disease for as long as 15 to 20 years after its onset.

About 50 percent of MS sufferers have a relapsing course, and some - who have mild or infrequent symptoms - may never know they have MS. In the remainder, the degree of severity varies: some persons with chronic MS have a slowly progressive course, while a small percentage develop a more rapid, severely incapacitating form.

This invariability and unpredictability stems from the vary nature of the disorder.

MULTIVITAMIN
Preparation containing several vitamins and all known to be essential to health.

MUMPS
Also called epidemic parotitis; an acute, contagious, generalized viral disease, usually causing painful enlargement of the salivary glands, most commonly the parotids.

After a 14-24 day incubation period, onset occurs with chilly sensations, headache, loss of appetite, malaise and a low to moderate fever that may last 12 to 24 hours before salivary gland involvement is noted. Pain on chewing or swallowing, especially on swallowing acidic liquids such as vinegar or lemon juice, is the earliest symptom of mumps. Both parotid glands are involved in most cases, and the glands are acutely tender during a 24-72 hours fever period.

Prognosis is excellent in uncomplicated cases, although rarely a relapse occurs after about two weeks. Particularly in adults, this disease may affect organs other than the salivary glands. The gonads are involved in about 20 percent of the cases.

Mumps can be prevented by immunization with the mumps vaccine, which is usually given as part of the measles-mumps-rubella (MMR) vaccine.

MUNCHAUSEN'S SYNDROME
Repeated fabrication of illness, usually acute, dramatic and convincing, by a person who wanders from hospital to hospital for treatment. In these persons with a mental illness of psychotic proportions successful treatment is rare.

The name of this syndrome is taken from the name of Baron Munchausen, the hero of a book of fantastic adventures written by R.E. Raspe in 1785.

MUNCHAUSEN'S SYNDROME BY PROXY

Rare syndrome whereby parents fabricate symptoms and signs in their children, leading to innumerable hospital admissions and harmful investigations. The fraudulent medical history and false physical signs generally originate from the mother; some
mothers add their own blood to the child's vomit, urine or feces, or smear blood on to the child's face or genitals.

The children suffer long hospital stays, with painful and damaging investigations and harmful treatments.

MURAL

Of or pertaining to the wall of any cavity of the body.

MURAL PREGNANCY

Pregnancy occurring just inside the Fallopian tube as it enters the uterus.

MURINE TYPHUS

Also called flea typhus, an acute disease similar to, but milder than, epidemic typhus. The cause is an organism called rickettsia mooseri, which is transmitted to humans by rat fleas (Xenopsylla cheopis).

Following an incubation period of 6 to 18 days, a shaky chill develops, associated with headache and fever. The fever lasts about 12 days and terminates gradually. The rash and other manifestations are similar to those of epidemic typhus but are much less severe.

MURMUR

Also called bruit, an extra heart sound, sounding like fluid passing an obstruction, heard between the normal heartbeats. Most murmurs are an indication of a heart disorder (usually of one of the valves), but it is not uncommon to have a murmur in a completely healthy heart.

MUSCLE

The tissue whose contraction produces body movement. Skeletal or striated muscle is the type normally associated with the movement of the body. Its action can either be initiated voluntarily, through the central nervous system or it can respond to reflex mechanisms. Under the microscope this muscle type is seen to be striped or striated. Skeletal muscle functions by being attached via tendons to two parts of

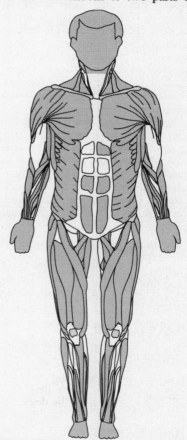

Anterior view of the major skeletal muscles.

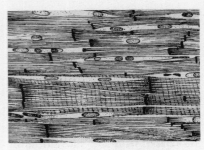

Microscopic view of striated muscle fibers.

the skeleton which move relative to each other.

Smooth type involuntary muscle is under the control of the autonomic nervous system and we are rarely aware of its action. Smooth muscle fibers are constructed in sheets of cells, each with a single nucleus. They are situated in hollow structures such as the gut, bronchi, uterus and blood vessels. Smooth muscle uses the properties of "tone" (continual slight tension) to regulate the diameter of tubes such as blood vessels.

Cardiac muscle, found only in the heart, has the property of never resting throughout life. It combines features of both skeletal and smooth muscle, for it is striped but yet involuntary. The fibers are not discrete but branching and interlinked, thus enabling it to act quickly and in unison when stimulated.

MUSCLE-BOUND
Having some of the muscles tense and enlarged and of impaired elasticity sometimes as a result of excessive exercise.

MUSCLE FIBER
Any of the elongated cells characteristic of muscle.

MUSCLE RELAXANTS
Medicines to lessen painful contractions and spasms of muscles.

MUSCLE SENSE
The part of kinesthesia mediated by end organs located in muscles.

MUSCLE SPASM
Persistent involuntary hypertonicity of one or more muscles usually of central origin and commonly associated with pain and excessive irritability.

MUSCLE SPINDLE
A sensory end organ in a muscle that is sensitive to stretch in the muscle, consisting of small striated muscle fibers richly supplied with nerve fibers, enclosed in a connective tissue sheath.

MUSCULAR COAT
An outer layer of smooth muscle surrounding a hollow or tubular organ (as the bladder, esophagus, large intestine, small intestine, stomach, ureter, and vagina) that often consists of an inner layer of circular fibers serving to narrow the lumen of the organ and an outer layer of longitudinal fibers serving to shorten its length.

MUSCULAR DYSTROPHY
A group of inherited diseases in which muscle fibers are abnormal and undergo atrophy (become wasted). Most develop in early life or adolescence. Duchenne's dystrophy (also called pseudohypertrophic muscular dystrophy) occurs in males although the genes for it are carried by females. It starts in early life and some swelling (pseudohypertrophy) of calf and other muscles may be seen. A similar disease can affect females.

Other types, described by muscles mainly affected, include limb-girdle and facio-scapulo-humeral dystrophies. There are many diverse variants, largely due to structural or biochemical abnormalities in muscle fibers.

Muscular dystrophies usually cause weakness and wasting of muscles, particularly of those close to and in the trunk; a waddling gait and exaggerated curvature of the lower spine are also typical. The muscles of respiration may be affected, with resulting pneumonia and respiratory failure; heart muscle, too, can also be affected.

MUTATION
A sudden and relative permanent change in a gene or chromosome set, which is the raw material for evolutionary change. Chemical or physical agents that cause mutations are known as mutagens. Mutations can occur in any type of cell at any stage in the life of an organism but only changes present in the gametes are passed on to the offspring.

A mutation may be dominant or recessive, viable or lethal. The majority are changes in individual genes (gene mutations) but in some cases changes in the structure or number of chromosomes may be seen. The formation of structural chromosome changes is used to test drugs for mutagenic activity.

Mutation normally occurs very rarely, but certain mutagens - X-rays, gamma rays, neutrons and mustard gas - greatly accelerate mutation.

MUTATION RATE
The frequency of detectable mutations in chromosomes.

MUTE
Not emitting or having sounds of any kind; a person without the power of speech.

MUTISM
The voluntary or involuntary lack of speech due to emotional conflicts.

MUTISM, ELECTIVE
Persistent refusal to talk in one or more major social situations, including school, despite ability to comprehend spoken language and to speak. The refusal to talk is not a symptom of social phobia, major depression, or a psychotic disorder such as schizophrenia.

MYALGIA
Pain in the muscles.

MYASTHENIA GRAVIS
A disease of the junctions between the peripheral nervous system and the muscles, probably due to abnormal immunity, and characterized by extreme fatiguability of muscles. It commonly affects eye muscles, leading to drooping lids and double vision, but it may involve limb muscles. Weakness of the muscles of respiration, swallowing and coughing may lead to respiratory failure and aspiration of bacterial pneumonia. Speech is nasal, regurgitation into the nose may occur and the face is weak, lending its characteristic snarl to the mouth.

The disorder is associated with diseases of the thymus gland and thyroid. Treatment is with cholinesterase inhibitors; steroids and thymus removal may control the causative immune mechanisms.

MYASTHENIC REACTION
That in which the normal contractions of a muscle, stimulated by direct electrical current becomes less intense and of shorter duration.

MYOCARDIAL INFARCTION
The damaging and death of an area of heart muscle (myocardium) resulting from an interruption in the blood supply reaching that area.

MYOCARDITIS
Inflammation of the heart muscle (myocardium). It may be due to a variety of disease, certain chemicals or drugs, injury for instance, electric shock or excessive X-ray treatment, or may be of unknown origin.

MYOCARDIUM
The muscular wall of the heart. The thickest of the three layers of the heart wall; it lies between the inner

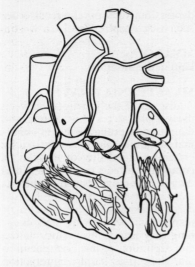

The myocard (muscle layer) of the left ventricle is much thicker than that of the right ventricle.

layer (endocardium) and the outer layer (epicardium).

MYCOLOGY
The study of fungi and the disease they cause.

MYCOPLASMA
Minute organisms in size between bacteria and viruses. Structurally, they consist of an outer three-layered pliable membrane surrounding proteinaceous cytoplasm that contains both RNA and DNA. Mycoplasmas cause diseases in humans, animals and plants.

MYCOSIS
The presence of parasitic fungi in or on the body.

MYCOSIS FUNGOIDES
An uncommon tumor of the reticulo-endothelial system, primarily affecting the skin and occasionally internal organs.

MYCOTOXINS
The toxic product of microscopic fungi (or moulds) which can occur in foodstuffs under certain conditions of humidity and temperature.

MYDRIASIS
Extreme or abnormal dilation of the pupil of an eye.

MYDRIATICS
Eye drops that cause the pupils to dilate to a marked degree. Anticholinergic drugs, such as atropine, have this effect and may cause photophobia as a consequence. Mydriatic drugs may occasionally provoke the onset of glaucoma.

MYELIN
Specialized layering of the membranes of glial cells (in the brain) and Schwann cells (of the peripheral nervous system). The white fat-like substance is wrapped around nerve fibers, producing an electrical insulating sheath.

MYELITIS
Inflammation of the spinal cord or of the bone marrow.

MYELO-ENCEPHALITIS
Inflammation of the spinal cord and the brain.

MYELOGRAPHY
X-ray examination of the spinal cord after the introduction by lumbar puncture of substances that are opaque to X-rays.

MYELOMALACIA
Softening of the spinal cord as a result of injury, pressure, inflammation or disease of the arteries.

MYOCLONIC EPILEPSY
Form of epilepsy in children usually between the ages of five and fifteen years, while in adults it commences between the ages of 25 and 40 years. The characteristic is sudden muscle contractions which may vary in intensity from simple twitching to a contraction that causes a violent movement of the limbs.

MYOCLONUS
Alternating contraction and relaxation of a muscle which usually does not cause movement.

MYOGLOBIN
Molecule found in muscle cells, and which serves as a local store for oxygen. Its affinity for oxygen encourages the transfer of oxygen to it from the blood.

MYOGLOBINURIA
Also called idiopathic paroxysmal myoglobinuria; the presence in the urine of myoglobin, which colors the urine red.

MYOMA
Also called leiomyoma and rhabdomyoma; tumor composed of muscle tissue.

MYOMECTOMY
Surgical removal of a myoma. The term commonly refers to the removal of a fibroid tumor from the wall of the uterus.

MYOMETRITIS
Inflammation of the uterus.

MYOMETRIUM
Muscular wall of the uterus.

MYONEURAL JUNCTION
Termination of a nerve in a muscle.

MYOPATHY
Literally, any disease of the muscle, but now primarily used for a group of rare diseases in which the function of voluntary muscles becomes inadequate due to some disorder of the motor unit (nerve cell, nerve fiber and receptor in the muscle itself). These diseases include:
- muscular dystrophy;
- motor neuron disease;
- myasthenia gravis;
- myotonia.

MYOTONIA ATROPHICA
A disease that runs in families and begins between the ages of 30 and 50. It is characterized by a wasting of muscle unlike that of any other disease, first affecting those of the face and neck, and then extending to the trunk and limbs.

MYOTONIA CONGENITA
Rare hereditary illness of unknown cause, commencing in early childhood, characterized by a striking slowness in the relaxation of the muscles after voluntary effort. Cold, heat, fatigue and hunger makes the condition worse.

MYOTONIC MYOPATHIES
A group of conditions characterized by abnormally slow relaxation of voluntary muscles after contraction.

MYRINGOTOMY
Surgical operation to cut the eardrum to release pus when, due to acute inflammation of the middle ear, there is a risk of the eardrum perforating.

MYSTICISM
Belief in the attainment, through contemplation, of truths inaccessible to the normal understanding.

MYTHOMANIA
Tendency toward the narration of imaginary adventures; elaboration of suggestions given, frequently exhibited in hypnosis.

MYXEDEMA
A disease characterized by swelling and coarsening of the skin and blunting of senses and intellect, because of diminished functioning of the thyroid gland. Treatment involves the taking of maintenance doses of thyroid hormone, usually for the rest of the person's life.

MYXOMA
Tumor arising from connective tissue, containing large quantities of mucus-like juice.

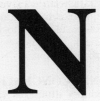

NABOTHIAN CYST
A mucous gland of the uterine cervix especially when occluded and dilated.

NAD (Nicotinamide Adenine Dinucleotide)
A coenzyme of numerous dehydrogenases that occurs in most cells and plays an important role in all phases of intermediary metabolism as an oxidizing agent or when in the reduced form as a reducing agent for various metabolites.

NADP (Nicotinamide Adenine Dinucleotide Phosphate)
A coenzyme of numerous dehydrogenases, as that acting on glucose-6-phosphate, that occurs especially in red blood cells and plays a role in intermediary metabolism similar to NAD but acting often on different metabolites.

NAEGELE'S OBLIQUITY
Inclination of the fetal head, laterally in a flat pelvis.

NAEGELE'S PELVIS
An obliquely contracted pelvis, caused by disease in infancy.

NAEGELE'S RULE
To estimate the day labor will begin, count back three months from the day the last menstrual period began and add seven days.

NAEVUS
Growth composed of blood vessels arising in the skin. Commonly called a birthmark or a mole.

NAEVUS PIGMENTOSUS
Dark-colored spot or mole so frequently seen on the skin.

NAEVUS VASCULOSUS
Bright red, or slightly raised, tiny nodule that may be present from birth or appear within the following two weeks.

NAIL
A horny cell structure of the epidermis of the skin forming flat patches upon the back surface of the terminal phalanges. A nail consists of a body, the proximal portion hidden by the nail fold, both of which rest on the nail bed or matrix.

The crescent-shaped white area near the root is the lunula. The epidermis extending from the margin of the nail fold over the root is called epinychium; that underlying the free border of the distal portion is called hyponychium.

A nail growth in length and thickness through activity of cells in the stratum germinativum of the skin in the region of the root. Average rate of growth in fingernails is about 1 mm per week.

It is slower in toenails and slower in summer than in winter. It varies with age and is affected by disease and certain hormone deficiencies.

NAIL BED
The end of a finger or toe covered by the nail.

NAIL-BITING
Habitual biting at the fingernails usually being symptomatic of emotional tensions and frustrations.

NAIL FOLD
Groove in the cutaneous tissue surrounding the margins and proximal edges of the nail.

NAIL ROOT
Proximal portion of the nail covered by a nail fold.

NAIL WALL
Epidermis covering the edges of the nail.

NAIL-PATELLA SYNDROME
A familial disorder of mesenchymal tissue characterized by abnormalities of bone, joints, fingernails and kidneys.

Management of progressive failure of the kidneys is the same as in other renal diseases. Successful transplants have been done without evidence of recurrence of the disease in the kidney graft.

NANISM
Abnormally small size or stature.

NANOCEPHALISM
Condition of having an abnormally small head.

NANOCORMIA
Abnormally dwarfed chest (thorax) or body.

NANOMELUS
Fetus with congenital abnormality characterized by undersized extremities.

NAPE
The back part of the neck.

NAPKIN RASH
Reddening of the skin in babies caused by constant irritation by wet napkins.

Frequently it is due to a germ which splits up (into various substances) the urea contained in urine; ammonia is one of these and it is this which attacks the skin.

NAPRAPATHY
A system of treatment of disease based on the belief that illness is caused by disordered connective tissue or ligamental tissues, and using massage, manipulation and adjustment of joints and muscles as therapy. The treatment system is closely related to chiropraxy.

NARCISSISM
Erotic gratification derived from love of one's own body, qualities and attributes.

NARCISSISTIC PERSONALITY DISORDER
A pervasive pattern of grandiosity (in fantasy or behavior), hypersensitivity to the evaluation of others, and lack of empathy that begins by early childhood and is present in a variety of contents.

People with this disorder have a grandiose sense of self-importance. They tend to exaggerate their accomplishments and talents, and expect to be noticed as "special" even without appropriate achievement. They often feel that because of their "specialness," their problems are unique, and can be understood only by other special people. Frequently this sense of self-importance alternates with feelings of special unworthiness. For example, a student who ordinarily expects an A and receives a grade of A minus may, at that moment, express the view that he or she is thus revealed to all as a failure. Conversely, having gotten an A, the student may feel fraudulent, and unable to take genuine pleasure in a real achievement.

This disorder appears to be more common recently than in the past, but this may be due only to more professional interest in it.

NARCOANESTHESIA
Anesthesia produced by a narcotic, as scopolamine and morphine.

NARCOANALYSIS
Psychoanalysis whilst the patient is under the influence of drugs and narcotics. It is a form of psychotherapy that is performed under sedation for the recovery of repressed memories together with the emotion accompanying the experience and that is designed to facilitate as acceptable integration of the experience in the patient's personality.

NARCODIAGNOSIS
The use of sedative or hypnotic drugs for diagnostic purposes, as in psychiatry.

NARCOHYPNIA
Numbness following sleep.

NARCOHYPNOSIS
Stupor or deep sleep produced by hypnosis.

NARCOLEPSY
A disease marked by uncontrollable sleepiness. It is a chronic disease which usually begins during puberty and occurs predominantly in males. It is characterized by two elements:
(1) the occurrence, usually several times a day, of attacks of irresistible sleep, lasting on the average 5 to 10 minutes;
(2) the fact that under the influence of certain emotions, the muscles of the body relax acutely, so that the person falls   down and is unable to move for a while. His consciousness remains completely clear throughout and he soon recovers completely.

The emotional loss of tone is a pathological augmentation of a reaction which to a lesser degree is present in many persons.

Narcolepsy, like epilepsy, is a syndrome. As regards to its cause, it is certain that it may develop as a sequence of certain infections of the brain. No sign of such a cause, however, can be found in the majority of cases. Familial elements have repeatedly been reported. Certain drugs have a beneficial effect on the course of the syndrome.

NARCOMA
Coma or stupor from the use of a narcotic.

NARCOMANIA
Abnormal craving for alcohol or narcotics; insanity due to the use of alcohol or narcotics.

NARCOSUGGESTION
The psychoanalytic use of suggestion in subjects who have received sedative or hypnotic drugs.

NARCOSYNTHESIS
Narcoanalysis which has as its goal an integration of the patient's personality.

NARCOTHERAPY
Psychotherapy carried out with the aid of sedating or hypnotic drugs.

NARCOTIC
A drug derived from opium or produced synthetically, that relieves pain, induces euphoria and other mood changes, decreases respiration and peristalsis, constricts the pupils, and produces sleep. The law requires licensed physicians to dispense by prescription.

Stemming from the Greek word for numbness or stupor and once applied only to drugs derived from the opium poppy, the word narcotic no longer has a precise medical meaning. Doctors today use the term narcotic analgesics to refer to opium-derived and synthetic drugs that have pain-relieving properties and other effects similar to those of morphine.

NARCOTIC ANALGESICS
Medicines used to relieve pain. Some of them are also used just before or during an operation to help the anesthetic work better. Codeine and hydrocodone are also used to help some people control their dependence on heroin or other narcotics. Narcotic analgesics may also be used for other purposes as determined by your doctor.

Narcotic analgesics act in the central nervous system to relieve pain. Some of their side effects are also caused by the actions in the central nervous system.

NARCOTISM
An addiction to the use of narcotics.

Addiction may be said to exist when discontinuance causes abstinence symptoms relieved speedily by a dose of the drug. It is this addiction to the original purpose in taking the drug that so readily aggravates the need.

NARIS
The nostril. The anterior naris is the external nostril. The posterior naris is the opening between the nasal cavity and the nasopharynx.

NARRATIVE METHOD
Method of obtaining data in psychological experiments by allowing an observer to give in his own way an account of events.

NASAL
Of or pertaining to the nose.

NASAL BONES
Two small bones forming the arch of the nose.

NASAL CARTILAGES
Cartilages forming the principal portion or framework of the external nose.

NASAL CAVITY
Space in the nostril. The nasal cavity is divided by a septum into a left and a right half. The mucous membrane of the frontal section of the cavity is covered by ciliated and mucus-producing cells. On the side walls are formed three conchae, which narrow the nasal cavity. The mucous membrane of the nasal cavity has a very rich blood supply; under the middle and upper conchae the outlets of other cavities (sinuses) serve to warm inhaled air, while under the lowest concha is located the outlet of the lacrimal canal through which tear fluid from the eye is conducted into the nasal cavity to be evaporated, on inhalation of dry air, in order to elevate the humidity.

Through these structures, the inhaled air is brought to the right levels of temperature and moisture, and is also cleaned of dust and bacteria.

NASAL CONCHA
Any of three thin bony plates on the lateral wall of the nasal fossa on each side with or without their covering of mucous membrane.

NASAL FEEDING
Feeding through a tube in the nasal passage. This is resorted to when it is the only route available to the stomach or when the person refuses to eat. Quite often in the latter case, nasal feeding is necessary to make him realize it is much easier to eat.

NASAL FOSSA
One of the two halves of the nasal cavity.

NASAL CAVAGE
Other term for nasal feeding.

NASAL INDEX
The greatest width of the nasal aperture in relation to a line from the lower curving to the outer side of the orbicularis oris muscle.

NASAL REFLEX
Sneezing resulting from irritation of the mucosa of the nose.

NASAL SINUSES
The air cavities, lined by mucous membrane, which communicate with the nose. The two maxillary sinuses are situated within the cheek bones, the two frontal sinuses within the bone on each side of the root of the nose, and the ethmoid sinuses communicate with the back of the nasal air passages.

NASEPTIN
Brand name of a drug containing as active compound the skin antiseptic chlorhexidine and the aminoglycoside antibiotic neomycin pre-

scribed for the treatment of superficial skin infections.

NASION
The point where the nasofrontal suture is cut across by the median plane.

NASITIS
Inflammation of the mucosa of the nose.

NASOLABIAL
Pertaining to the nose and lips.

NASOLACRIMAL
Pertaining to the nose and lacrimal (tear-producing) apparatus.

NASOPHARYNX
That part of the throat above the soft palate and behind the nose.

NASOTRACHEAL TUBE
A rubber tube or catheter, inserted into the trachea (windpipe) by way of the nose or mouth.

NATAL
Of or pertaining to birth.

NATALITY
The birth ratio; ratio of births to population of a given community.

NATES
Either of the two fleshy protuberances forming the lower and back part of the human trunk.

NATINATALITY
Rate of stillbirths in proportion to birth rate.

NATIVISM
A theory that maintains that practically all functions of an organism, including the mental ones, are inherited.

NATREMIA
The presence of sodium in the blood.

NATRIUM
Sodium; this is found abundantly in plants, animal fluids and minerals, as part of common salt (NaCl).

NATURAL CHILDBIRTH
Refers to training sessions leading to delivery of the child without maternal medication.

NATURAL FAMILY PLANNING
Methods of planning or preventing pregnancy based on observation of naturally occurring signs and symptoms of the fertile and infertile phases of the menstrual cycle.
    Techniques include:
- the basal body temperature method;
- the cervical mucus (Billings') method;
- the symptothermal method;
- the calendar or rhythm method (Ogino-Knaus).

NATURE-NURTURE PROBLEM
One of several controversial issues in psychiatry and psychology related to the relative importance of heredity (called nature) versus environment (called nurture) in the development of normal and abnormal behavior.

NATUROPATHY
A method of treating illness or disease without drugs or surgery, using proper food, heat, exercise and massage to aid natural healing.

NAUSEA
The unpleasant feeling that one is about to vomit.
    It may represent the person's awareness of stimuli to the particular brain center.
    Nausea is associated with altered physiological activity, including the gastric hypomobility and increased parasympathetic tone that precede and accompany vomiting.

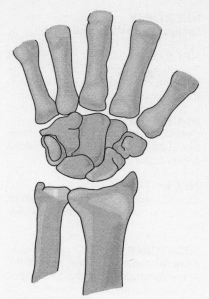

Navicular bone. This small bone of the carpus is the one on the right in the lower row.

NAUSEA GRAVIDARUM
Morning sickness of pregnancy.

NAVEL
The depression or scar in the center of the abdomen, where the umbilical cord was attached to the fetus.

NAVICULAR
Boat-shaped. Also refers to the scaphoid bone, a boat-shaped bone in the hand or foot.

NEAR-SIGHTEDNESS
Myopia, a defect in vision caused by elongation of the eyeball or an error in refraction so that the image comes to a focus in front of the retina; it can be corrected by concave lenses.

NEARTHROSIS
Production of a false joint due to the non-union of a broken bone.

NEBULA
A small cloudy spot on the cornea of the eye.

NEBULIZER
An instrument or apparatus used for spraying a fine mist. In medicine, the term is used to designate a method of administering a drug to the airways and lungs in aerosol form through a face mask. The apparatus includes an electric or hand-operated pump than sends a stream of air or oxygen through a length of tubing into a small canister containing the drug in liquid form.

This inflow of gas causes the drug to be dispersed into a fine mist which is then carried through another tube into the face mask. Inhalation of this drug mist is much easier than inhaling a pressurized aerosol.

NECK
Part of the body between head and shoulders; the constricted portion of an organ, or that resembling a neck.

NECK MANIPULATION
Manipulation of the cervical spine. Cervical hyperextension and/or excessive contralateral rotation poses a threat to the vertebral arteries. The

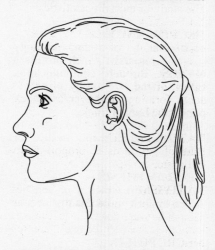

The neck forms the connection between the head and the trunk. It contains the cervical part of the spine, throat, larynx, esophagus and many blood vessels, lymph vessels and nerves.

sites where the arteries are particularly liable to injury are where they pass upwards through foramina of the cervical vertebrae (where stretching and shearing are a special danger); where they pass between the atlas and the axis (where the covering muscles can compress them during rotational movements); and where they cross the arch of the atlas and penetrate the atlanto-occipital ligament (where they can be compressed over the bony arch).

NECRECTOMY
Surgical removal of necrosed tissue.

NECROBIOSIS
Physiological death of a cell or cell group. This is in contrast to necrosis, which is death of cells to a disease process, and to a somatic death, which is death of the entire organism.

NECROCYTOSIS
Death of cells or decomposition of cells.

NECROLOGY
The study of mortality statistics.

NECROMANCY
That branch of parapsychology (psychic research) which professes to work through communication with the dead.

NECROMANIA
Abnormal interest in dead bodies or in death; mania with desire for death.

NECROMIMESIS
A delusion in which a person believes himself to be dead or acts as though he were dead.

NECROPHILIA
Morbid attraction, allegedly sexual, to dead bodies.

NECROPHOBIA
Fear of dead bodies.

NECROPSY
Autopsy or postmortem.

NECROSIS
Pathological death of a cell or organ, which is still in contact with living tissues.

NECROSPERMIA
Condition in which the semen (male ejaculation) contains only dead sperm cells.

NECROTOMY
Dissection of a cadaver; excision of a sequestrum or other necrotic tissue.

NEDOCROMIL
Generic name of an anti-asthmatic, anti-inflammatory drug prescribed for the maintenance treatment of mild to moderate asthma. The drug is not used to treat an active asthma attack. It inhibits inflammatory cells associated with asthma; inhibits reflex reactions to irritants and to exercise and cold.

NEEDLE BIOPSY
A sample of body tissue or fluid obtained via aspiration with a syringe and needle.

NEED-SATISFYING OBJECT
Object which is loved solely for its capacity to satisfy instinctual needs without cognisance being taken of its needs or personality.

NEGATIVISM
An attitude or behavior disorder marked by contrariness.

NELATON LINE
Line from the anterior superior spine of the ilium bone to the tuberosity of the ischium bone of the pelvis.

NEMATODE
Any of a large group (phylum Nematoda) of unsegmented worms, tapered at both ends, including round-

worms, pinworms, and hookworms.

NEMATOSIS
Infestation with threadworms.

NEARTHROSIS
A false joint.

NEGATIVISM
A normal stage of personality development during which a toddler expresses a growing capacity for independence and self-assertiveness by routinely refusing to comply with instructions and requests.

NEOCATHARSIS
A therapeutic method, sometimes used by psychoanalysts, that consists in making conscious childhood sensations.

NEOLALIA
Speech containing many words coined by the speaker, for instance, neologisms. In extreme form a mental disorder.

NEOLOGISM
A mental condition in which the patient coins new words which are meaningless, or words to which he gives special significance without being aware of their normal significance.

NEONATAL
Pertaining to the newborn.

NEONATAL MENINGITIS
Inflammation of the membranous coverings of the brain and/ or spinal cord due to bacterial invasion of the cerebrospinal fluid in the first four weeks of life.

NEONATAL SEPSIS
Invasive bacterial infection that occurs in the first four weeks of life. Bacterial infections are the primary cause in 10 to 20 percent of neonatal deaths and are seen five times more often in low-birth-weight infants than in full-term babies.

NEONATE
A newborn infant.

NEOPATHY
A new complication of a new condition of a disease.

NEOPHILISM
Morbid love or novelty of new persons and scenes.

NEOPHOBIA
Pathological fear of everything that is new.

NEOPLASM
A new and abnormal formation of tissue, as a tumor or growth. It serves no useful function, but grows at the expense of the healthy organism.

A benign neoplasm is a growth not spreading by metastases or infiltration of tissue. A malignant neoplasm is a growth that infiltrates tissue, metastasizes, and often recurs after attempts at surgical removal.

NEOPLASTY
Surgical formation or restoration of parts.

NEOPSYCHOANALYSIS
School of psychoanalysis that repudiates the importance of biology, the instincts, and the role of insight in promoting therapeutic change.

NEOSTOMY
Surgical formation of an artificial opening into an organ or between two organs.

NEPHELOPIA
Dim or cloudy vision from lessened transparency of the media of the eye.

NEPHRECTOMY
Surgical removal of a kidney.

NEPHREMIA
Congested state of the kidney.

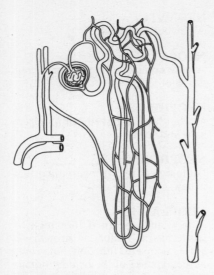

Microscopic structure of a nephron with glomerulus and tubes.

NEPHRITIS
Inflammation affecting the kidneys. The term glomerulonephritis covers a variety of diseases, often involving disordered immunity, in which renal glomeruli are damaged by immune complex deposition (for instance, Bright's disease); by direct autoimmune attack (Goodpasture's syndrome) or sometimes as a part of systemic disease (for instance, lupus, endocarditis, diabetes, or hypertension).

Acute or chronic kidney failure or nephrotic syndrome may result. The treatment is immunosuppressive or with corticosteroids.

NEPHROLITHIASIS
Presence of stones in the kidney.

NEPHROLITHOTOMY
Surgical removal of a stone in the kidney.

NEPHRON
Filtering mechanism of the kidney.

NEPHROPEXY
Surgical fixation of a dropped kidney.

NEPHROSIS
Degeneration of the kidney without signs of inflammation. It is characterized by gross edema (dropsy) and the passage of albumin in the urine.

NEPHROSTOMY
Surgical formation of a fistula (small channel) leading to the kidney pelvis.

NEPHROTIC SYNDROME
A predictable complex that follows a severe and prolonged increase in glomerular permeability for protein in the kidney. The major features are edema, lipids in the urine, increased content of lipids in the blood, all of variable relative severity.

NEPHROTOXIC MEDICATIONS
Medicines that under some circumstances can be toxic to the kidneys.

NEPHROTOXIN
A specific toxin which destroys cells in the kidney.

NEPHRYDROSIS
Distention and dilatation of the pelvis of the kidney resulting from obstruction.

NEPTUNE GIRDLE
Compress of linen covered by flannel that encircles the trunk from the lower end of the breastbone to the pubes. It is used in applying wet packs, especially cold.

NERVE
Collection of bundles of nerve fibers which convey either motor impulses from the brain to the muscles of the body or sensory impulses from one or other part of the body back to the brain.

NERVE-BLOCK ANESTHESIA
That produced by injecting an anesthetic into or near the nerves serving the part to be operated upon.

NERVE CENTER
A group of nerve cells closely connected with one another and acting together in the performance of some function.

NERVE ENDING
The termination of a nerve fiber (axon or dendrite) in a peripheral structure; may be sensory or motor.

NERVE FIBER
One of the primary thread-like fibers or processes known as axons or dendrites of a neuron or nerve cell.

NERVE GAS
A gas, used in chemical warfare, that damages or impairs the central nervous system, resulting in extreme weakness or paralysis.

NERVE IMPULSE
Transmission of a wave of activity (action potential) along a nerve fiber that activates or inhibits a nerve, gland, or muscle fiber.

NERVE ROOT
The beginning of nerve fibers which emerge from the central nervous system and join to form a nerve trunk.

NERVOUS
Pertaining to a nerve, nerves, or nervousness.

NERVOUS BREAKDOWN
Popular term used to describe various kinds of mental illness, often associated with fatigue or emotional stress, which drastically impairs a person's normal efficiency and disturbs his social behavior.

NERVOUS EXHAUSTION
State of fatigue and discomfort due to emotional causes; also called neurasthenia.

NERVOUSNESS
Excessive excitability of the nerv-

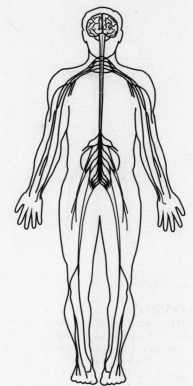

Major peripheral nerves of the upper and lower extremities.

ous system characterized by shaken mental poise and stability, muscle tremor or weakness and an uncomfortable awareness of self.

NERVOUS SYSTEM
The extensive network of cells specialized to conduct information in the form of impulses that control, regulate, and coordinate all functions of the body. The entire nervous system functions as a single unit, receiving and processing information. From sensory receptors, it receives many hundreds of thousands of signals, processes these and sends back tens of thousands of signals to various parts of the body, such as the muscles and glands.

The main functions of the nervous system fall into three groups:
(1) It efficiently integrates the per-

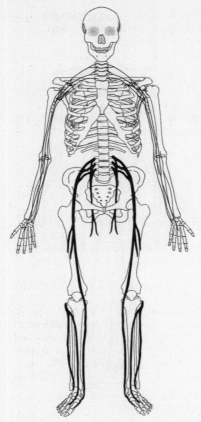

The central (brain and spinal cord) and peripheral part of the nervous system.

formance of diverse organs, each directed to its own function, in a much faster way than would be possible through transportation of substances via the bloodstream. As a result, organ function is integrated to serve a higher order, that of the entire organism.
(2.)The individual can react efficiently and rapidly to changes in the external environment. The ability to adapt to environmental changes contributes to the preservation of the species.
(3) Specific parts of the human nervous system must be regarded as the places where, in a manner yet unknown, the connection is made between mind and body, and where functions as abstract thinking, the emotions and consciousness are located.

NEST
A mass of cells extending from a common center, seen in cancer growth.

NETTLE RASH
Skin rash with intense itching resembling a condition produced by stinging with nettles.

NEURAGMIA
The tearing or rupturing of a nerve trunk.

NEURAL
Pertaining to a nerve or to the nervous system.

NEURAL CONDUCTION
The transmission along a nerve fiber of a wave of excitation in the form of an action potential.

NEURALGIA
Severe pain along the course of a nerve. The pain is sharp, stabbing and comes in paroxysms, lasting usually for a short time; tenderness is often present at the points of exit of a nerve and the paroxysms can be produced by contact with specific areas called trigger zones.

NEURAL PATTERN
The functional arrangement and interconnection of cells active as a result of stimulation from without or within.

NEURAL RIVALRY
Competition between reflex activity and cortical control, for the dominance of some final common path leading to the excitation of a muscle or group of muscles.

NEURAL TUBE
A hollow tubular formation of nerve tissue in the embryo made of joined ectodermal folds on each

side of the neural plate and developing at one end into the brain.

NEURASTHENIA
A state of excessive fatiguability, or lack of vigor, both bodily and mental, often accompanied by hypochondria and sometimes by phobias.

NEURATROPHIA
Atrophy of the nervous system or deficient nutrition of the nervous system.

NEURAXIS
Slender nerve fiber that emerges from a nerve cell, properly called an axis cylinder. That part of the nervous system represented by the brain and spinal cord.

NEURECTOMY
Surgical removal of part of a nerve.

NEURECTOPIA
Abnormal position or displacement of a nerve.

NEURILEMMA
The delicate membranous sheath of a nerve.

NEURINOMA
Tumor arising from the sheath covering a nerve. Also called neurofibroma and neurilemmoma.

NEURITE
The axis cylinder process of a neuron or nerve cell.

NEURITIS
Peripheral neuropathy; any disorder of the peripheral nervous system that interferes with sensation, the nerve control of muscle, or both.

NEUROANASTOMOSIS
Surgical attachment of one end of a severed nerve to the other end.

NEUROARTHROPATHY
Disease of a joint combined with disease of the central nervous system (spinal cord and/or brain).

NEUROBLASTOMA
A malignant hemorrhagic tumor of nerve ganglia.

NEUROCARDIA
Pertaining to the nerves supplying the heart or nervous system and the heart.

NEUROCELE
Ventricles and cavities in the cerebrospinal axis.

NEUROCHORIORETINITIS
Inflammation of the choroid and retina combined with optic neuritis (inflammation of the optic nerve).

NEUROCIRCULATORY ASTHENIA
Sometimes called soldier's heart, effort syndrome or functional heart disease. A complex of nervous and circulatory symptoms, often involving a sense of fatigue, dizziness, shortness of breath, rapid heartbeat and nervousness.

NEUROCRANIUM
The part of the skull enclosing the brain.

NEURODERMATITIS
Skin disease of nervous origin, usually accompanied by severe irritation which causes scratching which in turn provokes a thickening and roughening of the skin called lichenification.

NEURODERMATOSIS
Any skin disease of neural origin, an example being neurofibromatosis.

NEURODERMATROPHIA
Atrophy of the skin due to a disease or disorder of the nervous system.

NEURO-EPITHELIOMA
A relatively rare tumor of neuro-

epithelium in a nerve of special sense.

NEUROFIBRILS
Minute threads or fibrils in the nerve fibers, and also in the cell bodies, regarded as a system for the transportation of molecules from the cell body to the axonal terminals and vice versa.

NEUROFIBROMA
Tumor arising from nerves and nerve tissue, essentially fibrous in nature.

NEUROFIBROMATOSIS
A hereditary (autosomal dominant) disorder that produces pigmented spots and tumors of the skin, tumors of peripheral, optic and acoustic nerves and subcutaneous bony deformities. The various deep tumors are treated by appropriate surgical removal or radiation. The underlying cellular disorder is unknown and no general treatment is available.

NEUROFIBROSITIS
Inflammation of nerve fibers and sensory nerve fibers in muscular tissue.

NEUROGENOUS
Arising from some part of the nervous system.

NEUROGLIA
General term for the fibrous and cellular supporting tissues of the central nervous tissue.

NEUROGLIOMA
Tumor composed of neuroglial tissue.

NEUROGLIOSIS
Development of numerous neurogliomas.

NEUROGRAM
The enduring effect left behind as a result of activity in the nervous system, as, for example, the activity involved in any series of sensory experiences, which forms the basis of memory.

NEUROHUMOR
A chemical substance liberated at a nerve-ending that excites or activates an adjacent structure (neuron or muscle fiber). An example is acetylcholine. These substances are essential for transmission (hence the name neurotransmitter) of impulses across synapses or myoneural junctions.

NEUROHUMORAL
Relating to the interaction of nervous processes and chemical substances, particularly the transmission of neural activity across synaptic membranes with the aid of neurotransmitters.

NEUROHYPOPHYSIS
Back part (posterior lobe) of the pituitary gland.

NEUROKERATIN
The variety of keratin found in myelinated nerve fibers.

NEUROLEPTIC DRUG
Medicine that produces symptoms resembling those of diseases of the nervous system. In general the term is used for those drugs that are prescribed for the treatment of psychotic illnesses and disorders.

NEUROLEPTIC MALIGNANT SYNDROME
Syndrome characterized by ceaseless, involuntary, jerky movements of the tongue, facial muscles and hands.

NEUROLOGY
Branch of medicine concerned with diseases of the brain, spinal cord and peripheral nervous system.

NEUROLYSIS
Exhaustion of a nerve by over-

stimulation; nerve tension; the loosening of adhesions binding a nerve; disintegration of a nerve tissue.

NEUROMA
Tumor arising from a nerve.

NEUROMALACIA
Softening of the nerves.

NEUROMECHANISM
The neural structure controlling organic and systemic function.

NEUROMERE
One of a series of segmental elevations on the ventrolateral surface of the rhombencephalon.

NEUROMIMESIS
Hysterical or neurotic activation of organic disease.

NEUROMOTOR APPARATUS
Interconnected fibrils in lower organisms, probably functioning in the manner in which the nervous system functions in higher organisms.

NEUROMUSCULAR
Relating to both nerves and muscles.

NEUROMUSCULAR BLOCKING AGENTS
A group of drugs prescribed to relax skeletal muscles. They are all given by injection.

NEUROMUSCULAR JUNCTION
The surface of contact, at the end plates, between the fibers of a motoneuron and the muscle fiber that it innervates.

NEUROMYELITIS
Inflammation of nerves and the spinal cord.

NEUROMYOSITIS
Inflammation of nerves complicated by inflammation of muscles which

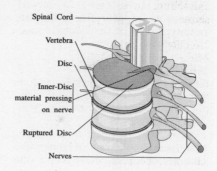

The spinal nerves or neurons in relation to the vertebral column and spinal cord.

come into contact with affected nerves.

NEURON
Nerve cell; the basic unit of the nervous system (including the brain and spinal cord).

Each has a long axon, specialized for transmitting electrical impulses and releasing chemical transmitters that act on muscle or effector cells or other neurons.

Branched processes called dendrites integrate the input to neurons.

NEURONITIS
Inflammation or degenerative changes of nerve cells.

NEURONOPHAGE
A phagocyte that destroys tissue in the nervous system.

NEUROPATHOLOGY
Study of the intrinsic causes of disorders of the nervous system by pathological anatomical methods.

NEUROPHONIA
A tic or spasm of muscles of speech resulting in an involuntary cry or sound.

NEUROPHYSIOLOGY
Study of the physiology of the nervous system.

NEUROPIL
A network of neurofibrils that are nonmyelinated at the synaptic junction between neurons.

NEUROPLASTY
Surgical repair of a nerve, such as nerve grafting.

NEUROPRAXIS
Cessation in function of a peripheral nerve without degenerative changes occurring. Recovery is the usual outcome.

NEUROPSYCHIATRY
Branch of medicine that deals with both nervous and mental disorders.

NEUROPSYCHOPATHY
Neurologic disease combined with a mental disorder.

NEURORADIOLOGY
X-ray studies of the central nervous system, including brain and spinal cord.

NEURORELAPSE
Nervous symptoms in syphilis subsequent to an injection of specific medicines.

NEURORETINITIS
Inflamed condition of the optic nerve and retina.

NEURORRHAPHY
Suturing of ends of a severed nerve.

NEUROSARCOMA
A malignant growth originating from mesodermal cells containing neuromatous components.

NEUROSECRETION
The elaboration and discharge of a chemical substance from a nerve cell.

NEUROSIS
A disorder in which psychological and associated physiological responses to ordinary stress presents in exaggerated form. Neuroses can be regarded as differing from normal conduct mainly quantitatively, in contrast to psychoses, which are marked qualitative departures from normal behavior.

In neuroses contact with reality is undisturbed and neurotic patients retain insight into the morbid character of their impulses and actions, even where these entail bizarre conduct, as in obsessional states or severe phobic anxiety.

If severe neurotic symptoms appear for not discernible reason, further exploration by the general physician or specialist is needed, and the diagnosis should be reviewed if adverse circumstances linked with the neurotic behavior cannot be found, since organic disease and endogenous psychosis may initially present with neurotic features.

NEUROSURGERY
Surgery of the brain, spinal cord and peripheral nervous system.

NEUROSUTURE
Sewing together of the ends of a divided nerve.

NEUROSYPHILIS
Syphilis involving the central nervous system.

NEUROTIC
Relating to or pertaining to the nerve or nervous system. The term is applied to mental disorders.

NEUROTIC CHARACTER
An individual who is attempting in various ways to compensate for some organ inferiority, or, more, generally, to attain superiority, or complete masculinity.

NEUROTIC SYMPTOMS
Some symptoms such as anxiety, apprehension, depressive moods, excessive fatigue, etc., that are common to most if not all neuroses.

NEUROTMESIS
Nerve injury with complete loss of function of the nerve even though there is little apparent damage anatomically.

NEUROTOMY
Division or dissection of a nerve.

NEUROTONY
Nerve stretching, usually to ease pain.

NEUROTOXIC MEDICATIONS
Medicines that cause toxicity to the nerve tissues in the body.

NEUROTOXIN
Toxin (poison) peculiarly destructive to nervous tissue.

NEUROTRANSMITTER
A chemical released from a nerve ending after receiving an electrical impulse. A neurotransmitter may carry a message from the nerve to another nerve so that the electrical impulse passes on, or to a muscle to stimulate contraction, or to a gland to stimulate secretion of a particular hormone. Acetylcholine and noradrenalin are examples of neurotransmitters. Many drugs either mimic or block the action of neurotransmitters.

NEUROTROPHY
Relating to the influence of nerves upon the nutrition and maintenance of the normal condition in tissues.

NEUROTROPIC
Turning towards or having an affinity for nervous tissue.

NEUROVACCINE
A standardized vaccine of specific strength; usually secured by cultivation in a rabbit's brain.

NEUROVARICOSUS
Multiple swellings along the pathway of a nerve.

NEUROVIRUS
Virus that has been modified by its growing in nervous tissue; used in preparing a vaccine.

NEUTRALIZATION
The process by which antibody or antibody in complement neutralizes the infectivity of microorganisms, particularly viruses.

NEUTROPHIL(E)
A leukocyte that stains easily with neutral dyes.

NEUTROPHILIA
Increase in the number of neutrophil leukocytes in the blood.

NEWBORN
An infant recently born.

NIACIN
A crystalline acid that is a member of the vitamin B complex occurring usually in the form of a complex of niacinamide in various animal and plant parts (as blood, liver, yeast, bran, legumes). Niacin is effective in preventing and treating human pellagra and black-tongue disease of dogs.

NIACINAMIDE
A bitter crystalline basic amide that is a member of the vitamin B complex and is interconvertible with niacin in the living organism, that occurs naturally usually as a constituent of coenzymes, and that is sued similar to niacin.

NICHE
A depression or recess on a smooth surface; especially an erosion in the wall of a hollow organ, detected by X-rays.

NICKING
Localized constriction of a retinal vein by the pressure from an artery crossing it; seen especially in arterial hypertension.

NICOLAS-FAVRE DISEASE
Venereal disease marked by involvement of inguinal lymph glands with an exuding lesion.

NICOTINE
A poisonous alkaloid found in all parts of the tobacco plant, but especially in the leaves. When pure, it is a colorless oily fluid with little odor, but a sharp, burning taste. On exposure to air in crude materials, it becomes deep brown with the characteristic tobacco-like smell. Nicotine is one of the most toxic of all poisons.

NICOTINE CHEWING GUM
Also called nicorette. The gum may help in treating smoking addiction. It satisfies physical craving for nicotine in addicted persons and avoids peaks in blood nicotine level resulting from smoking.

NICOTINE DEPENDENCE
Dependence commonly associated with the inhalation of cigarette smoke. Pipe- and cigar-smoking, the use of snuff, and the chewing of tobacco are less likely to lead to nicotine dependence. The more rapid onset of nicotine effects with cigarette-smoking leads to a more intensive habit pattern that is more difficult to give up because of the frequency of reinforcement and the greater physical dependence on nicotine.

People with this disorder are often distressed because of their inability to stop nicotine use, particularly when they have serious physical symptoms that are aggravated by nicotine. Some people who have nicotine dependence may have difficulty remaining in social or occupational situations in which smoking is prohibited.

The difficulty in giving up nicotine use definitely, particularly cigarettes, may be due to the unpleasant nature of the withdrawal syndrome, the deeply entrained nature of the habit, the repeated effects of nicotine, which rapidly follow the inhalation of cigarette smoke (75,000 puffs per year for a pack-a-day smoker), and the likelihood that a desire to use nicotine is elicited by environmental cues, such as the ubiquitous presence of other smokers and the widespread availability of cigarettes. When efforts to give up smoking are made, nicotine withdrawal may develop.

The most common complications are bronchitis, emphysema, coronary artery disease, peripheral vascular disease, and a variety of cancers.

NICOTINE SKIN PATCH
Skin patch with a small amount of nicotine developed as an aid to stop smoking, used in conjunction with a comprehensive behavioral smoking cessation program. The patch delivers a steady but gradually reduced supply of nicotine to the body for the relief of smoking withdrawal symptoms. It reduces the craving for cigarettes.

NICOTINE WITHDRAWAL SYNDROME
Characteristic withdrawal syndrome due to the abrupt cessation of or reduction in the use of nicotine-containing substances (e.g., cigarettes, cigars, and pipes, chewing tobacco, or nicotine gum) that has been at least moderate in duration and amount. The syndrome includes:
- craving for nicotine;
- irritability;
- frustration;
- anger;
- anxiety;
- difficulty concentrating;
- restlessness;
- decreased heart rate;
- increased appetite or weight gain.

The symptoms begin within 24 hours of cessation of or reduction in nicotine use and usually decrease in intensity over a period of a few days to several weeks. Some former nicotine users report that craving for the substance continues for longer periods.

NICOTINIC ACID
Vitamin and generic name of a vasodilator drug. Nicotinic acid may also be prescribed for the prevention of atherosclerosis by lowering blood lipid content.

NICOTINISM
Poisoning from excessive use of tobacco or nicotine.

NICTITATING MEMBRANE
A thin membrane found in many animals at the inner angle or beneath the lower lid of the eye and capable of extending across the eyeball.

NIEMANN-PICK DISEASE
A familial disorder of lipid metabolism in which sphingomyelin accumulates in the reticuloendothelial cells. This disorder may be accompanied by neurological symptoms. Treatment at present is supportive; there is no specific therapy.

NIGHT BLINDNESS
A condition of the eyes in which one can see well by daylight but poorly or not at all by night or dim light.

NIGHTMARE
Dream, marked by acute anxiety. According to psychoanalytical theory, it represents a breaking down of the censorship and the failure of the dream to perform its function of protecting sleep.

NIGHTMARE DISORDER
Dream anxiety disorder; repeated awakenings from sleep with detailed recall of frightening dreams. These dreams are typically vivid and quite extended and usually include threats to survival, security, or self-esteem. Often there is a recurrence of the same or similar themes. The dream experience or the sleep disturbance resulting from the awakenings causes significant distress.

Upon awakening from the frightening dream, the person becomes oriented and alert. Usually, a detailed account of the dream experience can be given, both immediately upon awakening and in the morning. Many people who suffer nightmares have difficulty returning to sleep after awakening from a nightmare.

Over half the cases starts before the age of 10, and in about two-thirds of cases, onset is before age 20. A major stressful life event seems to precede the onset of the disorder in about 60% of cases.

The frequency of episodes is variable both within and among individuals. In many cases three or more nightmares per week are reported. Children frequently outgrow the disorder. If it begins in adulthood, however, the disorder often persists for decades.

The disorder is reported to be particularly common in people with frequent physical and mental health problems.

NIGHT-SCREAMING
State of deep anxiety due to a disturbing dream, from which the person does not awake and for which he later has complete loss of memory. The condition occurs very commonly in children who have enlarged adenoids and nasal obstruction and disappears immediately after the adenoids have been removed.

NIGHT SPASM
Painful contracture of the calf muscles just after getting into bed at night. If not caused by general bodily diseases, many night spasms or night cramps of the legs can be cured by a nightly dose of quinine. It is not known why it should work but it just does.

NIGHT SWEAT
Excessive sweating during the night, sufficient to soak night-clothes, associated with either a toxic state, such as tuberculosis, or a violent anxiety state.

NIGHT TERROR
A form of nightmare, especially in children, causing them to wake up in terror. A night terror is generally a sudden feeling of extreme fear that awakens a sleeping child. Episodes are marked by screaming, inconsolable fear, and panic, but the child generally does not rem,ember such episodes in the morning.

NIGHT VISION
The ability of the eye to see in dim light. Poor bright vision may be due to an inherent defect of the retina of the eye, due to vitamin deficiencies, or to excessive exposure of the eye to sunlight.

NIHILISM
Disbelief in the power of a medicine in modifying a disorder or disease.

NIKOLSKY'S SIGN
Condition of the external layer of the skin in which it is rubbed off by slight friction or injury.

NINHYDRIN REACTION
A reaction of ninhydrin with amino acids or related amino compounds used for the colorimetric determination of amino acids, peptides, or protein by measuring the intensity of the blue to violet to red color formed or for the quantitative determination of amino acids by measuring the amount of carbon dioxide produced.

NIPHABLEPSIA
Blindness caused by light glare or snow.

NIPPLE
Pigmented, conical elevation on the breast, to which converge the 14 to 16 milk ducts from the lobes of the breast.

NIT
Popular name for the egg or larva in the louse.

NITRATE
Any salt of nitric acid; a medicine made from a chemical with a nitrogen base. Nitrates include erythritol tetranitrate, isosorbide dinitrate, nitroglycerin, pentaerythritol tetranitrate.

Nitrates are used for angina pectoris. Depending on the dosage form, they are used either to relieve pain of angina attacks (fast-acting dosage forms) or to prevent angina attacks from occurring (slow-acting dosage forms).

Oral nitrates come in the form of regular tablets, chewable tablets, or extended-release capsules or tablets. When taken orally and swallowed, nitrates are used to prevent angina attacks. They do not act fast enough to relieve the pain of an angina attack.

Nitrates relax blood vessels and increase the supply of blood and oxygen to the heart while reducing its work load.

NITRIC ACID
A corrosive liquid, with powerful oxidizing properties, used in the manufacture of medicine, dyes, explosives and metal products.

NITRITES
A group of chemical compounds, many of which cause dilation of the small blood vessels and lower blood pressure. Examples are amyl nitrite, sodium nitrite, nitroprusside and nitroglycerine.

NITROGEN
A colorless, odorless, tasteless gaseous element occurring free in the atmosphere, forming 4/5 of its volume. It is one of the important ele-

ments in all proteins; nitrogen is essential to plant and animal life for tissue building.

NITROGEN BALANCE
The difference between the amount of nitrogen ingested and that excreted each day. If intake is greater, a positive balance exists; if less, there is a negative balance.

NITROGEN CYCLE
The cycle of chemical changes exchanging nitrogen between the air and the soil. Nitrogen fixation, industrial or by microorganisms, yields combined nitrogen as ammonia and nitrates, which can be absorbed from the soil by plants, which use them to make protein.

NITROGEN EQUILIBRIUM
Condition during which nitrogen excreted in the urine, feces and sweat equals amounts taken in by the body in food.

NITROGEN FIXATION
The metabolic assimilation of atmospheric nitrogen by soil microorganisms and especially rhizobia and its release for plant use by nitrification in the soil on the death of the microorganisms.

NITROGEN LAG
Extent of time required after a given protein is ingested before an amount of nitrogen equal to that in the protein has been excreted.

NITROGEN NARCOSIS
Condition of euphoria, impaired judgement, decreased coordination and motor ability seen in persons exposed to high air pressure such as divers and submariners.

NITROGLYCERINE
Generic name of an anti-anginal agent. The drug is prescribed for prevention and treatment of chest pains associated with angina pectoris.

NITROSUREA
Any of a group of lipid-soluble drugs that function as alkalyting agents, have the ability to enter the central nervous system, and are effective in the treatment of some brain tumors and meningeal leukemias.

NITROUS OXIDE
A combination of nitrogen and oxygen that sometimes produces an exhilarating effect upon being inhaled, used as an anesthetic during dental surgery.

NITRURIA
Presence of nitrates in the urine.

NOCARDIOSIS
An acute or chronic, often disseminated, granulomatous infection caused by the aerobic Gram-negative microorganism Nocardia asteroides.

NOCICEPTIVE
Pertaining to stimuli of a painful nature.

NOCTURIA
Nocturnal enuresis, nycturia and bed-wetting are all synonymous terms.

NOCTURNAL EMISSION
An involuntary discharge of semen during sleep often accompanied by an erotic dream.

NOCTURNAL ENURESIS
Bed-wetting.

NODAL POINT
Either of two points located on the axis of a lens or optical system that any incident ray directed through one will produce a parallel emergent ray directed through the other.

NODDING SPASM
One characterized by nodding of the head; shaking movement of the head. It is seen in several com-

plaints and commonly seen in babies when it is known as spasmus mutans. In this instance it is quite normal, harmless and passes off within the first year. In older children head movements may be due to St. Vitus' dance or to habit spasms of nervous origin.

NODE
Knob or protuberance; a point of construction; a small rounded organ; a lymph gland.

NODES OF RANVIER
Region in a nerve where there is a local constriction of the nerve sheath.

NODULAR
Composed of or characterized by the presence of nodules.

NODULE
Dermatologic condition characterized by a palpable, solid lesion, 5 to 10 mm in diameter, that may or may not be elevated. Examples are keratinous cysts, small lipomas, fibromas, some types of lymphomas, erythema nodosum and a variety of malignant growths.

NOETIC
Of or pertaining to the mind or intellect.

NOISE POLLUTION
Environmental pollution consisting of annoying or harmful noise.

NOMA
A gangrenous ulceration of the mouth and cheeks, occurring mainly in undernourished children.

NOMADISM
Impulse to wander about aimlessly; restlessness.

NOMOGENESIS
A theory of evolution that regards evolutionary change as due to inherent orderly processes fundamental to organic nature and independent of environmental influences.

NON COMPOS MENTIS
Not of sound mind; mentally incompetent to handle one's affairs.

NON-DISJUNCTION
Failure of two chromosomes to separate subsequent to metaphase in meiosis or mitosis so that one daughter cell has both and the other neither of the chromosomes.

NONESSENTIAL AMINO ACID
Any of various amino acids which are required for normal health and growth, whose carbon chains can be synthesized within the body or which can be derived in the body from essential amino acids, and which include alanine, asparagine, aspartic acid, cystine, glutamic acid, glutamine, glycine, proline, serine, and tyrosine.

NON-HODGKIN'S LYMPHOMA
A heterogenous group of diseases, consisting of neoplastic proliferation of lymphoid cells that usually disseminate throughout the body. Non-Hodgkin's lymphoma occurs more frequently than Hodgkin's disease. It occurs in all age groups, the incidence increasing with age. Its cause is unknown, although, as with the leukemias, there is substantial experimental evidence for a viral etiology. Enlarged lymph nodes are rubbery and later become matted. Local disease is apparent in some patients, but the majority have multiple areas of involvement. The prognosis and treatment depend on the type of lymphoma involved.

NON-LAXATIVE DIET
Low residue diet, for instance with boiled milk and toasted crackers. No strained oatmeal, vegetable juice or fruit juice. Dates and concentrated sweets are restricted.

NON-PERMISSIVENESS
In child rearing, preventing the occurrence of undesired behavior by non-punitive means.

NON-PROTEIN NITROGEN
The nitrogen in the blood not appearing as protein; about half is normally present as urea. Blood levels can be managed to determine kidney function.

NONSENSE
In genetics, a genetic information consisting of one or more codons that do not code for any amino acids and usually cause termination of the molecular chain in protein synthesis.

NONSENSE SYLLABLES
Artificial combinations of letters, not forming words, employed as material in learning experiments, so as to exclude associations possibly already formed.

NON-SPECIFIC URETHRITIS
Infection in the urethra not caused by gonorrhea. Discharge due to non-gonorrheal or non-specific urethritis is often identical to gonorrhea symptoms and is often misdiagnosed in both sexes.

NON-STEROIDAL ANTI-INFLAMMATORY DRUGS (NSAIDs)
A family of drugs with pharmacologic characteristics similar to those of cortisone and cortisone-like drugs. They are used for many purposes to help the body deal with inflammation no matter what the cause. Steroidal drugs may be taken orally or by injection (systemic) or applied locally for the skin, eyes, ears, bronchial tubes (topical) and others.

NON-VERBAL TESTS
Intelligence or other mental tests, which do not employ verbal material, or, sometimes, which can be given without en

NORADRENALINE
The neurotransmitter released sympathetic nerve endings exce those supplying the sweat glands and vasodilatory blood vessels in the skeletal muscle.

NOREPINEPHRINE
A catecholamine that is the chemical means of transmission across synapses in postganglionic neurons of the sympathetic nervous system and in some parts of the central nervous system.
It is a vasopressor hormone of the adrenal medulla, and is a precursor of epinephrine in its major biosynthetic pathway.

NORGESTON
Brand name of an hormonal preparation containing as active compound levonorgestrel prescribed as oral contraceptive.

NORLEUCINE
Amino acid manufactured by the body.

NORMAL GIGANTISM
Gigantism in which all body functions are normal.

NORMAL SALINE SOLUTION
A solution prepared by adding approximately one level teaspoonful of common table salt to a pint of water. Much purer and more accurate solutions are employed in surgery. Also called isotonic solution, normal salt solution, physiological salt solution.

NORMERGIC
Having the degree of sensitivity toward an allergen typical of age group and community.

NORMOBLAST
A nucleated red blood corpuscle, similar in size to an ordinary erythrocyte.

NORMOCALCEMIA
The presence of a normal concentration of calcium in the blood.

NORMOCHROMASIA
Average staining capacity in a cell or tissue.

NORMOCHROMIC ANEMIA
An anemia marked by reduced numbers of normal red blood cells in the circulating blood.

NORMOGRAM
Blood possessing normal color and hemoglobin content.

NORMOCYTE
An average-sized red blood corpuscle.

NORMOCYTOSIS
A normal state of the corpuscular elements of the blood.

NORMOTENSIVE
Normal blood pressure; a person with normal blood pressure.

NORMOVOLEMIA
Normal state of the blood volume.

NOSE
The midline organ of the face, concerned with the perception of smell and the preparation of the air stream for respiration.

It is a cartilage extension of the facial bones with two external openings or nostrils. These pass into the nasal cavities, which are separated by a septum and contain turbinates which increase the mucous membrane surface and direct the air flow.

The chemoreceptors for smell lie mainly in the roof of the nasal cavities, but fine nerve fibers throughout the nose contribute to tactile sensation and smell.

The three bony folds of each nasal cavity are covered by a mucous membrane, in which the olfactory sensory receptors are localized.

NOSEBLEED
Hemorrhage from the nose.

NOSOCOMIAL INFECTION
An infection acquired by a patient while in the hospital.

NOSOGENESIS
Classification of a nervous disorder in accordance with the conditions or character of its onset.

NOSOLOGY
A systemic classification or description of diseases.

NOSOMANIA
The delusion of being diseased.

NOSOMYCOSIS
Delusion of being ill.

NOSOPHOBIA
Neurotic fear of being ill.

NOSOTHERAPY
Treatment of one disease by voluntarily introducing another microorganism into the body.

NOSTALGIA
Longing to return to one's native land; may lead to severe condition with psychological and physical symptoms.

NOSTRIL
One of the external apertures of the nose.

NOSTRIL REFLEX
Reduction of opening of the naris on the affected side in lung diseases in proportion to the lessened alveolar air capacity on the affected side.

NOSTRUM
A quack medicine; a cure-all.

NOTALGIA
Painful condition of the back.

NOTCH
A rather deep indentation or narrow

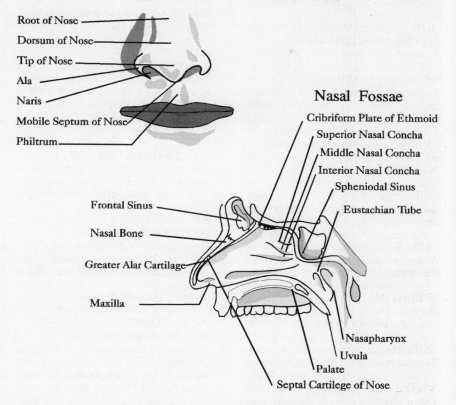

External Nose

Root of Nose
Dorsum of Nose
Tip of Nose
Ala
Naris
Mobile Septum of Nose
Philtrum

Nasal Fossae

Cribriform Plate of Ethmoid
Superior Nasal Concha
Middle Nasal Concha
Interior Nasal Concha
Spheniodal Sinus
Eustachian Tube

Frontal Sinus
Nasal Bone
Greater Alar Cartilage
Maxilla

Nasapharynx
Uvula
Palate
Septal Cartilege of Nose

gap in the edge of an anatomical structure.

NOTIFICATION
The act or an instance of notifying; especially the act or reporting the occurrence of a communicable disease or an individual affected with such a disease.

NOTOCHORD
A rod of cells lying dorsal to the intestine and extending from front to back and forming the axial skeleton in the embryo.

NOURISHMENT
Act of nourishing or of being nourished.

NUBILITY
State of sexual development at which it is possible for sexual intercourse to take place.

NUCHAL LINE
Any of several ridges on the outside of the skull. The superior nuchal line is one on each side of the skull that extends laterally in a curve from the external occipital protuberance to the mastoid process of the temporal bone.

The inferior nuchal line is a line on each side of the skull that extends laterally from the middle of the external occipital crest below and roughly parallel to the superior nuchal line.

NUCLEAR MEDICINE
A branch of medicine that uses radio-isotopes in diagnostic and treatment procedures.

NUCLEAR SCANNING
A diagnostic procedure in which a radioactive substance is administered orally or by injection. A scanning device is then used to detect radioactivity over particular body areas. The size, shape, location and function of body parts can then be recorded via a computer printout.

NUCLEIC ACIDS
The vital chemical constituents of living things; a class of complex threadlike molecules comprising two main types: the deoxyribonucleic acid (DNA) and the ribonucleic acids (RNA). DNA is found almost exclusively in the nucleus of the living cell, where it forms the chief material of the chromosomes. It is the DNA molecule's ability to duplicate itself (replicate) that makes the cell reproduction possible; and it is DNA, by directing protein synthesis, that controls heredity in all organisms other than certain viruses which contain only RNA. RNA performs several important tasks connected with protein synthesis, and is found throughout the cell.

NUCLEOTIDE
Organic chemical of central importance in the life chemistry of all plants and animals. Some nucleotides provide the basic molecular units for the synthesis of various more complex molecules, notably the nucleic acids DNA and RNA; others provide a means of storing and releasing the energy needed to drive biochemical processes.

The nucleotide is a three-part structure, comprising a phosphate group linked to a 5-carbon sugar group (pentose) linked in turn to a nitrogenous side group (base). The four commonest bases are the purines adenine and guanine, and the pyrimidines cytosine and thymine. These serve as the four key "letters" of the genetic code in the DNA molecule.

NUCLEOLUS
A spherical body of the nucleus that becomes enlarged during protein synthesis, being associated with a specific part of a chromosome. It contains the DNA templates for ribosomal RNA.

NUCLEOLUS ORGANIZER
The specific part of a chromosome with which a nucleolus is associated especially during its reorganization after nuclear division.

NUCLEOPROTEIN
A compound that consists of a protein (as a histone) conjugated with a nucleic acid (as a DNA) and that is the principal constituent of the hereditary material in chromosomes.

NUCLEOSIDE
A compound (as guanosine or adenosine) that consists of a purine and pyrimidine base combined with deoxyribose or ribose and is found especially in DNA or RNA.

NUCLEOTIDE
Any of several compounds that consist of a ribose or deoxyribose sugar joined to a purine or pyrimidine base and to a phosphate group and that are the basic structural units of RNA and DNA.

NUCLEUS
(1) A central point about which matter is gathered, as in a calculus.
(2) The vital body in the protoplasm of the cell.
(3) A group of nerve cells or mass of gray matter in the central nervous system.

NULLIPARA
Woman who has never borne a child.

NUMB
Defective sensibility.

NUMBNESS
Local anesthesia (insensibility to touch). Numbness is a loss of sensation in a part of the body, most often caused by pressure on or swelling of the nerve that supplies the area. Nerve damage that produces numbness can be temporary or permanent. Numbness can also be caused by cutting a nerve or by damage to the brain or spinal cord. Persistent or recurrent numbness should be investigated by a doctor.

NUMMULAR
Coin-shaped, or resembling rolls of coins.

NURSE
A person trained to assist a physician or dentist, as in an operating room.

NURSE-ANESTHETIST
A registered nurse who has completed two years of additional training in anesthesia and is qualified to serve as an anesthetist under the supervision of a physician.

NURSE-PRACTITIONER
A registered nurse who has completed advanced training and is qualified to assume some of the duties and responsibilities formerly taken on by a physician.

NURSING
The care of the sick, injured of handicapped. Diagnosis and treatment are the province of the doctor but day-by-day care of the patient is the province of the nurse.

NURSING HOME
A privately operated establishment where maintenance and personal or nursing care are provided for persons (as the aged or the chronically ill) who are unable to care for themselves properly.

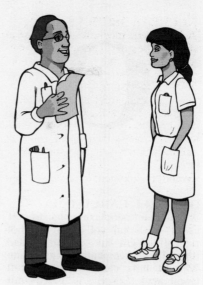

Nurses take care of the sick, injured or handicapped. They play the most important role in the care of hospital patients.

NURTURANCE
Affectionate care and attention.

NUTRITION
The sum of processes involved in taking in nutrients and assimilating and utilizing them.

NUTRITIONAL SUPPLEMENTS
Substances used to treat and prevent deficiencies when the body is unable to absorb them by eating a well-balanced, nutritional diet.

NYMPHOLEPSY
A frenzy of erotic emotion.

NYMPHOMANIA
Excessive sexual desire by a female.

NYSTAGMUS
Rhythmic oscillation of the eyes in a horizontal, vertical or rotatory direction. Nystagmus will blur a person's vision, and he may he able to turn his head into a position to avoid this blur, but the ideal treatment is to remove the cause.

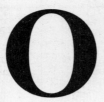

O
Symbol for oxygen.

OAT CELL CARCINOMA
A malignant neoplasm consisting of small epithelial cells that do not typically form masses but spread through the lymphatics; more than 25% of lung cancers are oat cell carcinomas. Surgery is usually not possible; chemotherapy and radiation often ineffective.

OBELION
A point on the sagittal suture that lies between two small openings through the superior dorsal aspect of the parietal bones and is used in craniometric determinations.

OBESITY
Overweight; an increase in the amount of fat in the subcutaneous tissues of the body.

OBEX
A thin triangular lamina of gray matter in the roof of the fourth ventricle of the brain.

OBJECT
Something material that may be perceived by the senses. The term is used to designate something mental or physical toward which thought, feeling, or action is directed.

OBJECTIVE VERTIGO
Vertigo characterized by a sensation that the external world is revolving.

OBJECTIVE LIBIDO
Libido directed toward someone or something other than the self.

OBLIGATE AEROBE
An organism that cannot grow in the absence of oxygen.

OBLIGATE ANAEROBE
An organism that cannot grow in the presence of oxygen.

OBLIQUE
Any of several oblique muscles.

OBLIQUE POPLITEAL LIGAMENT
A strong broad flat ligament that passes obliquely across and strengthens the posterior part of the knee and is derived especially from the tendon of the semimembranous muscle.

OBLIQUUS ABDOMINIS
Either of two flat abdominal muscles on each side that form the middle and outer layers of the lateral walls of the abdomen, that have aponeuroses extending medially to ensheathe the rectus muscle and fusing in the midventral line in the linea alba, and that act to compress the abdominal contents and assist in expelling the content of various visceral organs, as in urination, defecation, parturition, and expiration.

OBLIQUUS EXTERNUS ABDOMINIS
Flat abdominal muscle that forms the outer layer of the lateral abdominal wall; also called external oblique or obliquus externus.

OBLIQUUS INFERIOR
A short eyeball muscle that arises from the orbital surface of the maxilla, moving the eye upward and laterally.

OBLIQUUS INTERNUS ABDOMINIS
Flat oblique abdominal muscle situated under the external oblique muscle in the lateral and ventral

part of the abdominal wall; also called internal oblique or obliquus internus.

OBLIQUUS SUPERIOR
A long thin eyeball muscle that arises just above the margin of the optic foramen, inserted on the upper part of the eyeball and moving the eye downward and laterally.

OBSERVATION
(1) The noting of a fact or occurrence, as in nature, often involving the measurement of some magnitude with suitable instruments;
(2) close watch or examination, as to monitor or diagnose a condition.

OBSESSION
Persistent idea, thought, impulse, or image that is experienced, at least initially, as intrusive and senseless - for example, a parent having repeated impulses to kill a loved child, or a religious person having recurrent blasphemous thoughts.

The person attempts to ignore or suppress such thoughts or impulses or to neutralize them with some other thought or action.

The person recognizes that the obsessions are the product of his or her own mind, and are not imposed from without.

The most common obsessions are repetitive thoughts of violence (e.g., killing one's child), contamination (e.g., becoming infected by shaking hands), and doubt (e.g., repeatedly wondering whether one has performed some act, such as having hurt someone in a traffic accident).

OBSESSIONAL NEUROSIS
Neurosis in which compulsive acts or ideas dominate the person's life.

OBSESSIONAL TYPE
A type, regarded by psychoanalysts as governed by anxiety, arising from a guilty consciousness.

OBSESSIVE-COMPULSIVE NEUROSIS
A neurotic disorder characterized by the presence of recurrent obsessions or compulsions sufficiently severe to cause marked distress, be time-consuming, or significantly interfere with the person's normal routine, occupational functioning, or usual social activities or relationships with others.

Depression and anxiety are common. Frequently there is phobic avoidance of situations that involve the content of the obsessions, such as dirt or contamination. For example, a person with obsessions about dirt may avoid public restrooms; a person with obsessions about contamination may avoid shaking hands with strangers.

The course of the disorder is usually chronic, with waxing and waning of symptoms. Although the disorder was previously thought to be relatively rare in the general population, recent community studies indicate that mild forms of the disorder may be relatively common.

OBSESSIVE COMPULSIVE PERSONALITY DISORDER
A pervasive pattern of perfectionism and inflexibility, beginning by early adulthood and present in a variety of contexts. These people constantly strive to perfection, but this adherence to their own overly strict and often unattainable standards frequently interferes with actual completion of tasks and projects. No matter how good an accomplishment, it often does not seem "good enough." Preoccupation with rules, efficiency, trivial details, procedures, or form interferes with the ability to take a broad view of things. For example, such a person, having misplaced a list of things to be done, will spend an inordinate amount of time looking for the list rather than spend a few moments re-creating the list from memory and proceed with accomplishing the

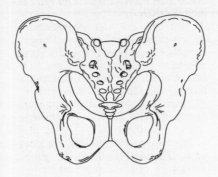

Posterior view of the pelvis. The obturator muscle runs from the margin of the obturator foramen (the big hole in the pelvis), pubis, and ischium to the greater trochanter of the femur.

tasks. Time is poorly allocated, the most important tasks being left to the last moment.

OBSTETRIC FORCEPS
A forceps for grasping the fetal head or other part to facilitate delivery in difficult labor.

OBSTETRICS
The care of women during pregnancy, delivery and then puerperium; a branch of medicine and surgery usually linked with gynecology.

Prenatal care and the avoidance or control of risk factors for both mother and baby - anemia, toxemia, high blood pressure, diabetes, venereal diseases, frequent miscarriages, etc. - have greatly contributed to the reduction of maternal and fetal deaths. The monitoring and control of labor and birth, with early recognition of complications; induction of labor and the prevention of postpartum hemorrhage with oxytocin; safe forceps delivery and cesarean section and improved anesthesia are important factors in obstetric safety.

OBSTIPATION
Extreme constipation, usually caused by an obstruction.

OBSTRUCTIVE BILIARY CIRRHOSIS
Cirrhosis caused by obstruction of the extrahepatic bile ducts by stone, tumor, scar or congenital atresia.

OBSTRUCTIVE JAUNDICE
Form of jaundice due to mechanical obstruction to the bile ducts by gallstones, a growth or by narrowing of the ducts.

OBTURATOR
Either of two muscles arising from the obturator membrane and adjacent bony surfaces. The obturator externus is a flat triangular muscle that arises from the medial side of the obturator foramen made up of the rami of the pubis and ischium and from the medial part of the obturator membrane, inserting by a tendon into the trochanteric fossa of the femur. The muscle acts to rotate the thigh laterally.

The obturator internus arises from the margin of the obturator membrane and from the obturator foramen, inserting into the greater trochanter of the femur, acting to rotate the thigh laterally when it is extended and to abduct it in the flexed position.

OBTURATOR CANAL
The small patent opening of the obturator foramen through which nerves and blood vessels and which is formed by the obturator groove covered over by part of the obturator membrane.

OBTURATOR FORAMEN
An opening that is the largest foramen in the human body, situated between the ischium and pubis of the hipbone, and closed by the obturator membrane except for the obturator canal.

OBTURATOR NERVE
A branch of the lumbar plexus that arises from the second, third, and fourth lumbar nerves and that sup-

plies the hip and knee joints, the adductor muscles of the thigh, and the skin.

OCCASIONALISM
A theory which seeks to explain the apparent causal connection between mental and bodily processes by assuming divine intervention to produce bodily movement on the occasion of the mental idea of movement.

OCCIPITAL
Relating to the occiput (the back part of the skull).

OCCIPITAL BONE
A compound bone that forms the posterior part of the skull and surrounds the foramen magnum, bearing the condyles for articulation with the atlas. The occipital bone is composed of four united elements; the structure is much curved and roughly trapezoid in outline, ending in front of the foramen magnum in the basilar process, and bearing on its external surface behind the foramen magnum the two curved transverse superior and inferior nuchal lines as well as the median external occipital crest and external occipital protuberance.

OCCIPITAL CONDYLE
An articular surface on the occipital bone on each side of the foramen magnum by which the skull articulates with the atlas.

OCCIPITAL CREST
Either of the two ridges on the occipital bone connecting the occipital protuberance and foramen magnum.

OCCIPITAL FONTANEL
A triangular unossified area in the skull of a fetus or infant at the meeting of the sutures between the parietal and occipital bones.

OCCIPITAL LOBE
The dorsal portions of the cerebral hemispheres which contain the centers for vision.

OCCIPUT
The back part of the skull or the head.

OCCLUSION
Closing or shutting up; the absorption, by a metal, of gas in large quantities, as of hydrogen by platinum; the full meeting or contact in a position of rest.

OCCLUSIONAL DISHARMONY
A condition in which incorrect positioning of one or more teeth causing an abnormal increase in or change of direction of the force applied to one or more teeth when the upper and lower teeth are occluded.

OCCLUSIONAL PLANE
An imaginary plane formed by the occlusal surfaces of the teeth when the jaw is closed.

OCCLUSIVE PESSARY
Rubber contraceptive appliance used either to cover the neck of the uterus or to block the upper end of the vagina.

OCCULT BLOOD
Blood which is not apparent to the naked eye but detectable by laboratory tests. "Occult" means present but invisible. Thus occult blood procedures test for blood that can be seen only through microscopic or chemical examination. Virtually all body fluids, excretions and secretions can be tested for occult blood; most often the test is performed on feces and urine.

It has been proposed that if everyone's feces were properly tested for occult blood twice a year, almost all bowel cancer could be eliminated.

OCCUPATIONAL ABILITY
The measurement of an individual's aptitude for a certain vocation or

work by means of a standard test; several different occupational ability tests are usual administered at one time and the results are reported as a profile or pattern.

OCCUPATIONAL ASTHMA
Diffuse, intermittent, reversible airways obstruction caused by inhalation of irritant or allergenic particles or vapors from industrial processes.

OCCUPATIONAL DISEASE
Disease produced by the person's occupation. Frequently a notifiable disease.

OCCUPATIONAL LUNG DISEASE
Lung disorder directly related to the inhalation of dust, fumes, vapors and gases from the occupational environment.

The effects of an inhaled agent depend on a number of factors:
- its physical properties;
- its chemical properties and
- the susceptibility of the exposed person.

OCCUPATIONAL NEUROSIS
Neurosis due to the person's employment and occurring in such people as manual workers, typists, musicians, and in some craftsmen.

OCCUPATIONAL THERAPY
The ancillary specialty to medicine concerned with practical measures to circumvent or overcome disability due to disease. It includes the design or modification of everyday items such as cutlery, dressing aids, baths and lavatory aids and wheelchairs.

Assessment and education in domestic skills and industrial retraining are also important. Diversional activities are arranged for long-stay patients.

OCHLOPHOBIA
Fear of crowds.

OCTREOTIDE
Generic name of a synthetic pituitary hormone prescribed to relieve symptoms of cancer of the pancreas.

OCULAR
Pertaining to the eye, or to the eyepiece of an optical instrument.

OCULAR DOMINANCE
The difference, analogous to right-handedness and left-handedness, between the two eyes with respect to use, preference and efficiency.

OCULOMOTOR
Pertaining to the movement of the eye or to the oculomotor nerve.

OCULOMOTOR NERVE
Either nerve of the third pair of cranial nerves that are motor nerves with some associated autonomic fibers, arising from the midbrain, and supplying muscles of the eye except the superior oblique and the lateral rectus with motor fibers and the ciliary body and iris with autonomic fibers by way of the ciliary ganglion.

ODONTOCLAST
One of the large multinucleate cells that are active during the absorption of the roots of the milk teeth

ODONTOGENESIS
The formation and development of teeth.

ODONTOID PROCESS
A toothlike process that projects from the anterior end of the centrum of the axis in the spinal column, serving as a pivot on which the atlas rotates. The odontoid process is morphologically the centrum of the atlas though detached from that vertebra and more or less perfectly united with the next one behind.

ODONTOLOGY
The branch of anatomical science

that relates to the teeth, their health, growth, structure and disease.

ODONTOMA
A tumor arising from a tooth or dental tissue.

ODONTONECROSIS
Massive decay of a tooth.

ODONTORRHAGIA
Bleeding from the socket of a tooth after its extraction.

OEDEMA
See Edema.

OEDIPUS COMPLEX
Sexual obsession by a son for his mother accompanied by resentment and aggression towards the father. Also called mother complex. Named after the mythological Greek hero who killed his father and married his mother.

OESOPHAGUS
See Esophagus.

OESTROGEN
See Estrogen.

OINTMENT
Any soft, unctuous substance, usually medicated, applied to the skin for medicinal and cosmetic purposes.

OLECRANON
Upper end of the ulna (the inner bone of the forearm) at the elbow joint. On the inner side of this runs the ulnar nerve which, when struck, causes the sensation of pins–and–needles."

OLECRANON FOSSA
The fossa at the distal end of the humerus into which the olecranon fits when the arm is in full extension.

OLEIC ACID
An unsaturated fatty acid, found in animal and vegetable fats.

OLFACTORY
Pertaining to the sense of smell.

OLFACTORY BULB
One of the two oval masses of gray matter located on the bottom of the skull above the nasal cavity extending outward toward the eyes. These bulbs mediate smell and are an extension of the cerebrum.

OLFACTORY LOBE
A lobe of the brain that rests on the lower surface of the temporal lobe and projects forward from the anterior lower part of each cerebral hemisphere, being continuous anteriorly with the olfactory nerve, consisting of an olfactory bulb, an olfactory tract, and an olfactory trigone.

OLFACTORY NERVE
The first cranial nerve which connects the olfactory region in the cerebrum with the olfactory cells.

OLFACTORY SYSTEM
Sensory receptors, neural pathways and brain areas involved in smell. High in the roof of each nasal cavity there is a patch of yellow-brown epithelium in which the olfactory receptors lie.

They are very numerous and consist of a nerve cell with fine processes on its superficial surface and a thin slow conducting axon running from its deep surface up through the cribriform plate of the ethmoid bone.Immediately above the cribriform plate the fibers penetrate the dura and enter the olfactory bulb of the brain. The nose is the peripheral organ of smell, but only a small part is directly olfactory in nature while the remainder is for respiratory purposes.

OLIGOCYTEMIA
Deficiency in the total number of red blood cells present in the body.

OLIGODENDROCYTE
A neuroglial cell resembling an astrocyte but smaller with few and slender processes having few branches.

OLIGODENDROGLIA
Neuroglia made up of oligodendrocytes that is held to function in myelin formation in the central nervous system.

OLIGODENDROGLIOMA
A tumor of the nervous system composed of oligodendroglia.

OLIGOHYDRAMNIOS
Deficiency of amniotic fluid sometimes resulting in embryonic defect through adherence between embryo and amnion.

OLIGOMENORRHEA
Abnormally infrequent or scanty menstrual flow.

OLIGOSPERMIA
Deficiency in the number of spermatozoa (male egg cells) in the semen.

OLIGURIA
Passage of too little urine in relation to the fluid intake. It may be a symptom of kidney disorder.

OLIVE OIL
A pale yellow to yellowish–green nondrying oil obtained from the pulp of olives usually by expression and used chiefly as a salad oil and in cooking, and as a emollient.

OMENTUM
Folds of peritoneal membrane which extend between the stomach and the other abdominal organs.

OMYHOID
A muscle that arises from the upper border of the scapula, inserting in the body of the hyoid bone, and acting to draw the hyoid bone in a caudal direction.

OMNIBUS TEST
A type of group test of intelligence in which items of different kinds are mixed together in place of being arranged separately as in the battery tests and there is one time for the whole test.

OMPHALOCELE
Protrusion of abdominal contents through an opening at the umbilicus occurring as a congenital defect.

OMPHALOMESENTERIC DUCT
The duct by which the yolk sac or umbilical vesicle remains connecting with the alimentary tract of the vertebrate embryo.

ONCHOCERCIASIS
A disease resulting from infection by Onchocerca volvulus and characterized by fibrous noduli in the skin and subcutaneous tissue. Ocular findings are common, blindness may result. The disease, spread by the bite of black flies, occurs in Mexico, Venezuela, Colombia and Central Africa.

ONCOGENE
Gene that is responsible for the origin of cancerous growth.

ONCOLOGY
Study of the factors governing tumor growth.

ONYCHECTOMY
Surgical removal of a nail.

ONYCHIA
Inflammation of the matrix (the tissue under the nail) of the nail, or of the nail substance.

ONYCHOPHAGIA
Nail biting which is thought to be a form of neurotic behavior and a means of releasing inner tension.

OOCYTE
The female egg cell before the

maturation process is complete.

OOGONIA
The first phase in the development of mature female reproductive cells.

OOPHOROPEXY
Surgical fixation of a dropped ovary.

OPACITY
The quality or state of a body that makes it impervious to the rays of light. The term is also used to designate the relative capacity of matter to obstruct by absorption or reflection the transmission of radiant energy, as X-radiation.

OPEN-ANGLE GLAUCOMA
A progressive form of glaucoma in which the drainage channel for the aqueous humor composed of the attachment at the edge of the iris and the junction of the sclera and cornea remaining open in which serious reduction in vision occurs only in the advanced stages of the disease due to tissue changes along the drainage channel.

OPEN FRACTURE
One in which a wound occurs in the skin over the site of the fracture. This may cause an infection.

OPEN-HEART SURGERY
Surgery performed on the opened heart. This phrase is also often used to refer to all heart surgery -whether or not the heart itself is opened.

OPEN REDUCTION
Realignment of fractured bone after incision into the fracture site.

OPERABLE
Refers to a condition in which surgery offers a reasonable hope of improvement.

For instance, in cases of cancer that has not spread and is so localized that it can be removed completely.

OPERANT BEHAVIOR
Behavior which is identified in terms of its effect on the environment.

OPERANT CONDITIONING
Conditioning in which the desired behavior or increasingly closer approximations to it are followed by a rewarding or reinforcing stimulus.

OPERATION
Any surgical procedure. A major textbook or handbook of surgery lists about 3000 operative techniques and procedures.

OPERATOR
In medicine and biology term used in two senses:
(1) One who performs surgical operations.
(2) A chromosomal region that triggers formation of messenger RNA by one or more nearby structural genes and is itself subject to inhibition by a genetic repressor.

OPERCULUM
Any of several parts of the cerebrum bordering the fissure of Sylvius.

OPERON
The closely linked combination of an operator and the structural genes it regulates.

OPHIDIOPHOBIA
Morbid fear of snakes.

OPHTHALMIA
Inflammation of the eye. This may be conjunctivitis, as in neonatal ophthalmia or uveitis as in sympathetic ophthalmia. In this, an inflammatory reaction in both eyes follows injury to one.

OPHTHALMIA NEONATORUM
Acute inflammation of the eyes of a newborn from infection during passage through the birth canal.

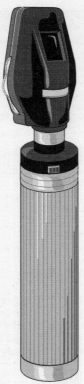

Ophthalmoscope for investigation of the internal parts of the eyeball.

OPHTHALMITIS
Inflammation of the eye.

OPHTHALMOLOGY
The branch of medicine and surgery concerned with diseases of vision and the eye. In infants, congenital blindness and strabismus, and in adults, glaucoma, uveitis, cataract, retinal detachment and vascular diseases are common, as are ocular manifestations of systemic disease such as hypertension and diabetes,

OPHTHALMOPLEGIA
Paralysis of the eye muscles.

OPHTHALMOSCOPE
Instrument for examining the retina and structures of the inner eye. A powerful light and lens system, combined with the cornea and lens of the eye allows the retina and eye blood vessels to be seen at high magnification. It is a valuable aid in diagnosis in ophthalmology, neurology and internal medicine.

OPHTHALMOSCOPY
Direct, visual examination of the interior structures of the eye with a special optic instrument, for diagnostic or other purposes.

OPIATE
Drug that contains opium, is derived from opium, or is produced synthetically and has opium-like characteristics. Opiates are pain-killing medicines derived from opium that have a high index of addiction.

OPIOID
Possessing some properties characteristic of opioid narcotics and not derived from opium.

OPIOID PEPTIDE
Any of a group of endogenous neural polypeptides, as an endorphin or enkephalin, that bind especially to opiate receptors and mimic some of the pharmacological properties of opiates.

OPIOID INTOXICATION
Maladaptive behavioral changes and specific neurologic signs due to the recent use of an opioid. The initial maladaptive behavioral changes from intravenous opioids occur within 2 to 5 minutes after use and often include euphoria that may last 10 to 30 minutes. This is followed by a longer period (two to six hours, depending upon the type of opioid, the dose, and the previous history of drug-taking) of lethargy, somnolence, and apathy or dysphoria.

Other maladaptive behavioral effects during the period of intoxication include impaired judgment and impaired social and occupational functioning.

OPIOID WITHDRAWAL SYNDROME

A characteristic withdrawal syndrome due to recent cessation of or reduction in use of an opioid. The syndrome includes:
- lacrimation;
- rhinorrhea;
- pupillary dilation;
- piloerection;
- sweating;
- diarrhea;
- yawning;
- mild hypertension;
- tachycardia;
- fever;
- insomnia.

OPISTHOTONOS

Violent muscular spasm, which so arches the back that the patient is literally resting on the back of his skull and his heels. It sometimes occurs in cerebrospinal fever, epilepsy, rabies, tetanus (lockjaw) and strychnine poisoning.

OPISTHION

The median point of the posterior border of the foramen magnum.

OPIUM

Narcotic extract from the immature fruits of the opium poppy Papaver somniferum, which is native to Greece and Asia minor. The milky juice is refined to a powder which has a sharp, bitter taste. Drugs obtained from opium include the narcotic analgesics, heroin, morphine and codeine. Synthetic analogues of these include methadone and pethidine.

OPPONENS

Any of several muscles of the hand or foot that tend to draw one of the lateral digits across the palm or sole toward the others.

OPPORTUNISTIC INFECTION

A disease of infection caused by a microorganism that does not ordinarily cause disease but which, un-

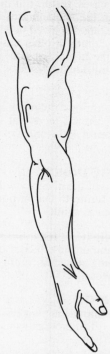

The opposition of the thumb plays an important role in the function of the hand.

der certain conditions (e.g., impaired immune process) becomes pathologic.

OPPOSITIONAL DEFIANT DISORDER

A pattern of negativistic, hostile, and defiant behavior without the more serious violations of the basic rights of others that are seen in a conduct disorder.

Children with this disorder are argumentative with adults, frequently lose their temper, swear, and are often angry, resentful, and easily annoyed by others. They frequently actively defy adult requests or rules and deliberately annoy other people. They tend to blame others for their own mistakes and difficulties.

Manifestations of the disorder are almost invariably present in the home, but may not be present at school or with other adults or peers.

In some cases, features of the disorder, from the beginning of the disturbance, are displayed in areas outside the home; in other cases, they start in the home, but later develop in areas outside the home.

OPSIN
Any of various colorless proteins that are formed in retinal cells by the action of light on a visual pigment.

OPSONIC INDEX
The ratio of the phagocytic index of a tested serum to that of normal serum taken as a unit.

OPSONIFICATION
The action or the effect of opsonins in making bacteria more readily phagocytosed.

OPSONINES
Blood components that enable cells to fight off microorganisms that invade the body.

OPTIC
Pertaining to the eye or vision.

OPTICAL AXIS
A straight line perpendicular to the front of the cornea of the eye and extending through the center of the pupil.

OPTICAL ILLUSION
An illusion of vision; usually refers to an illusion affecting spatial relations, especially of the group designated geometrical illusions.

OPTIC ATROPHY
Atrophy (wasting) of the optic nerve resulting in visual loss proportional to the degree of nerve atrophy. Nothing can be done to restore vision once the optic nerve has atrophied. Therapy, rarely of value, must be directed at the underlying factors causing damage to the nerve.

OPTIC CHIASM
The area in the medial plane at the base of the brain where the nerve fibers of both retinae meet and separate again; those fibers from the nasal side of each retina cross over to the other side of the cortex after this separation.

OPTIC CUP
The optic vesicle after invagination to form a two-layered cup from which the retina and pigmented layer of the eye will develop.

OPTIC DISC
Retinal area where the optic nerve fibers gather before leaving the retina. This area is extremely insensitive to light and is called the blind spot.

OPTIC FORAMEN
The passage through the orbit of the eye in the lesser wing of the sphenoid bone that is traversed by the optic nerve and ophthalmic artery.

OPTIC NERVE
Second cranial nerve which supplies the retina and carries visual stimuli from the eye to the brain.

The optic nerve is either of the pair of sensory nerves that comprise the second pair of cranial nerves, arising from the ventral part of the diencephalon, to form an optic chiasm before passing to the eye and spreading over the anterior surface of the retina. The function of the nerve is to conduct visual stimuli to the brain.

OPTIC NEURITIS
Another name for papillitis.

OPTIC PAPILLA
A slight elevation that is nearly coextensive with the optic disk and is produced by the thick bundles of the fibers of the optic nerve in entering the eyeball.

OPTIC RADIATION
Any of several neural radiations concerned with the visual function; especially one made up of fibers from the pulvinar and the lateral geniculate body to the cuneus and other parts of the occipital lobe.

OPTICS
The branch of physical science that deals with vision, and the properties and phenomena of light, its origin and effects, and its role as a medium of sight.

OPTICAL CONTENT DRAWINGS
A projective technique used with children in which the child is asked to draw whatever he wishes or to complete elaborate already provided stimulus patterns, sometimes being asked to relate a story concerning the drawing.

OPTOMETRY
The measurement and examination of the visual powers. The practice or art of testing the eyes by means of suitable instruments or appliances for defects of vision in order to correct them with eyeglasses or lenses.

ORAL
Pertaining to the mouth. The term is also used in the sense of done, taken or administered by mouth, as an oral medicine.

ORAL CHARACTERISTICS
Traits of a person which reveals a fixation at the oral stage characterized by dependence and passivity.

ORAL CAVITY
Space in the mouth.

ORAL DEPENDENCE
In psychoanalysis the desire to return to the security of the infantile oral stage of development which consisted of the protection of the mother in combination with the intense gratification provided by the mother's breasts and milk.

ORAL LEUKOPLAKIA
A potentially precancerous lesion appearing as an adherent white patch or plaque on the oral mucosa that cannot be characterized clinically or histologically as any other specific disease.

ORAL SADISM
Aggressive, primordial urges toward omnipotent mastery and gratification expressed in fantasy through the oral apparatus.

ORAL SEX
The involvement of the mouth in sex. The oral stimulation of the vulva and vagina (cunnilingus), and the oral stimulation of the penis (fellatio), are the main features of oral sex.

ORAL STAGE
The first psychosexual stage occurring in the first year of life during which the infant's sexual pleasure is derived from the stimulation of the mouth. The infant's first sexual excitations are related in sucking in the feeding process, which becomes the prototype of later sexual satisfaction and the mother, the object involved in the feeding process becomes the prototype of all later love object relations.

ORAL SURGERY
A branch of dentistry that deals with the diagnosis and treatment of oral conditions requiring surgical intervention. The term is also used to designate a branch of surgery that deals with conditions of the jaws and mouth structures requiring surgery.

ORAL TRIAD
Conjoined wishes to be sucked by, sleep with, and be devoured by the breast.

ORAMORPH
Brand name of a narcotic analgesic drug containing active compound morphine sulphate prescribed for severe pain syndromes.

ORBIT
The bony cavity in which the eye is situated. The orbit is perforated for the passage of nerves and blood vessels. The orbit occupies the lateral front of the skull immediately beneath the frontal bone on each side and encloses and protects the eye and its appendages.

ORBITAL FISSURE
Either of two openings transmitting nerves and blood vessels to or from the orbit. The superior orbital fissure is situated superiorly between the greater wing and the lesser wing of the sphenoid bone. The inferior orbital fissure is located between the greater wing of the sphenoid bone and the maxilla.

ORBITAL INDEX
The ratio of the greatest height of the orbital cavity to its greatest width multiplied by 100 where the width is measured from the dacryon to the farthest point on the opposite border and the height is measured along a line perpendicular to the width.

ORBITAL PROCESS
A process of the palatine bone that forms part of the floor of the orbit.

ORCHIDECTOMY
Surgical incision into a testicle.

ORCHIOPLASTY
Plastic surgery of a testicle.

ORCHITIS
Inflammation of a testicle.

ORGAN
A part or member of living organisms, as the heart, having a specific function.

ORGAN BANK
A place where human organs or tissues are stored for future surgical use as transplants.

ORGANELLE
A specialized cellular part, as a mitochondrion, lysosome, or ribosome, that is analogous to an organ.

ORGANIC ANXIETY SYNDROME
Prominent, recurrent, panic attacks or generalized anxiety caused by a specific organic factor. The syndrome is usually caused by endocrine disorders or the use of psychoactive substances.

ORGANIC BRAIN SYNDROME
Any mental disorder, as senile dementia, resulting from or associated with organic changes in brain tissue.

ORGANIC DELUSIONAL SYNDROME
Prominent delusions that are due to a specific organic factor. The nature of the delusions is variable and depends, to some extent, on the etiology. Persecutory delusions are the most common type. Amphetamine use may cause a highly organized paranoid delusional state indistinguishable from the active phase of schizophrenia. Some people with cerebral lesions develop the delusion that a limb of their body is missing.

In organic delusional syndrome, hallucinations may be present, but are usually not prominent.

ORGANIC DISEASE
A disease in which there is a structural alteration in the organ involved, as opposed to functional disease.

ORGANIC HALLUCINOSIS
Presence of prominent persistent or recurrent hallucinations that are due to a specific organic factor. Halluci-

nations may occur in any modality, but certain organic factors tend to produce hallucinations of a particular type. For example, hallucinogens most commonly cause visual hallucinations, whereas alcohol tends to induce auditory hallucinations.

ORGANIC HEART DISEASE
Heart disease caused by some structural abnormality in the heart or circulatory system.

ORGANICISM
The doctrine that symptoms and disease are caused by diseased organs only.

ORGANIC MEMORY
Alteration of living tissue, resulting from any activity in it, involving its functioning in any way, persisting as a condition modifying subsequent activity.

ORGANIC MOOD SYNDROME
A prominent and persistent depressed, elevated, or expansive mood, resembling either a manic episode or a major depressive episode, that is due to a specific organic factor.

The syndrome is usually caused by toxic or metabolic factors. Certain substances, notably reserpine, methyldopa, and some of the hallucinogens, are apt to cause a depressive syndrome. Endocrine disorders are another important etiological factor, and may produce either depressive or manic syndromes.

ORGANIC PERSONALITY SYNDROME
Persistent personality disturbance, either lifelong or representing a change or accentuation of a previously characteristic trait, that is due to a specific organic factor.
The following symptoms are common:
- affective instability;
- recurrent outbursts of aggression;
- marked impaired social judgment;
- marked apathy;
- suspiciousness;
- paranoid ideation.
The syndrome is usually due to structural damage to the brain. Common causes are neoplasms, head trauma, and cerebrovascular disease.

ORGANIC SCOLIOSIS
Spinal curvature due to:
- a disease process such as rickets or inflammation;
- paralysis of the spinal muscles;
- deformities of the chest;
- disease of the hips or the legs.

ORGANIZATION
In medicine, the formation of fibrous tissue from a clot or exudate by invasion of connective tissue cells and capillaries from adjoining tissues accompanied by phagocytosis of superfluous material and multiplication of connective tissue cells.

ORGANIZER
A region of a developing embryo or a substance produced by such a region that is capable of inducing a specific type of development in undifferentiated tissue.

ORGAN OF CORTI
A complex epithelial structure in he cochlea that is the chief part of the ear by which sound is directly perceived and that rests on the internal surface of the basilar membrane and contains two spiral rows of minute rods of Corti which arch over a spiral tunnel of Corti, supporting on the inner side a single row of columnar hair cells and on the outer side several rows having their bases surrounded by nerve cell arborizations.

ORGANOGENESIS
The origin and development of bodily organs.

ORGASM
Sexual climax, usually involving strong involuntary contractions of the genital musculature, perceived as pleasurable.

ORGASMIC DISORDERS, FEMALE
Persistent or recurrent delay in, or absence of, orgasm in a female following a normal sexual excitement phase during sexual activity that the doctor judges to be adequate in focus, intensity, and duration. Some females are able to experience orgasm during noncoital clitoral stimulation, but are unable to experience it during coitus in the absence of manual clitoral stimulation. In most of these females, this represents a normal variation of the female sexual response and does not justify the diagnosis of inhibited female orgasm. However, in some of these females, this does represent a psychological inhibition that justifies the diagnosis.

ORGASMIC DISORDERS, MALE
Persistent or recurrent delay in, or absence of, orgasm in a male following a normal sexual excitement phase during sexual activity that the doctor, taking into account the person's age, judges to be adequate in focus, intensity, and duration. This failure to achieve orgasm is usually restricted to an inability to reach orgasm in the vagina, with orgasm possible with other types of stimulation, such as masturbation.

ORIENTATION
Awareness of one's spatial, temporal, practical or circumstantial situation, with reference particularly to mental orientation in various connections.

ORNITHOSIS
A viral disease occurring in or originating in birds that do not belong to the family containing the parrots; the disease may cause a severe long infection in man.

OROPHARYNGEAL
Relating to the mouth and pharynx.

ORPHAN DRUG
A drug that is effective for a rare condition, but may not be marketed by a drug manufacturer because of the small profit potential compared with the high costs of development and production.

ORTHODONTICS
That branch of dentistry concerned with correction of irregularities in the teeth and malocclusion, and associated abnormalities of the face.

ORTHOGENESIS
Evolutionary change that appears to be directed over a long period of time. Orthogenesis is no longer regarded as an evolutionary mechanism but as the result of consistent selection for the same character in an animal.

ORTHOGNATHISM
Condition in which the jaws, especially the upper jaw, have little or no forward projection.

ORTHOPEDICS
Specialty within surgery, dealing with bone and soft-tissue disease, damage and deformity.

ORTHOPNEA
Inability to breathe except in an upright position, as in congestive heart failure.

ORTHOPRAXY
The correction of physical deformities by means of mechanical appliances.

ORTHOPSYCHIATRY
A cross disciplinary science combining child psychiatry, developmental psychology, pediatrics and family care, devoted to the dis-

covery, prevention and treatment of mental disorders in childhood and adolescence.

ORTHOTICS
System of training techniques which are designed to facilitate cooperative functioning of the two eyes especially in cases of muscular imbalance.

ORTHOSTATIC
Pertaining to or caused by standing upright.

ORTHOTICS
A branch of mechanical and medical science that deals with the support and bracing of weak or ineffective joints or muscles.

ORTHOTONUS
Form of muscular cramp which compels the patient to lie rigid and stretched out.

OS
Bone, mouth, opening or entrance.

OSCILLOGRAM
The tracing or record made by an oscilloscope or oscillograph.

OSCILLOSCOPE
The electronic optical device that pictures changes in electric current of a cathode ray tube.

OSGOOD-SCHLATTER'S DISEASE
Osteochondritis of the tuberosity of the tibia that occurs especially among adolescent males.

OSMIDROSIS
Condition in which the sweat has an abnormally offensive odor.

OSMOLALITY
A measure of the osmotic pressure of a liquid. In medicine osmotic pressure indicates the amount of dissolved material (minerals, hormones, etc.) in a body fluid, most commonly blood or urine.

OSMORECEPTOR
A sensory end organ that is stimulated by changes in osmotic pressure.

OSMOSIS
The process by which fluid passes across a permeable membrane from a solution of lesser, to a solution of greater concentration.

OSMOTIC SHOCK
A rapid change in the osmotic pressure, as by transfer to a medium of different concentration, affecting a living system.

OSSA
Bones; plural of os = bone.

OSSEIN
The soft gluelike protein substance of bone left after the removal of the mineral matter.

OSSICLE
Small bone, especially one of the three small bones in the ear.

OSSIFICATION
Being converted into bone; the process of bone formation usually beginning at particular centers in each prospective bone and involving the activities of special osteoblasts that segregate and deposit inorganic bone substance about themselves.

OSTECTOMY
Surgical removal of a piece or the whole of a bone.

OSTEITIS
Inflammation of a bone.

OSTEITIS DEFORMANS
A slowly progressive bone disorder characterized by an initial osteolytic phase usually followed by an osteoblastic phase, with resulting abnormal histologic patterns and

gross deformity. The cause is unknown.

OSTEITIS FIBROSA
Occurrence in bones of cysts and tumor-like masses caused by a disturbance in calcium and phosphorus metabolism. Also known as Von Recklinghausen's disease.

OSTEOARTHRITIS
Arthritis characterized by degenerative loss of articular cartilage, subchondral bone sclerosis and cartilage and bone proliferation at the joint margins with subsequent osteophyte formation. The cause is unknown but genetic, metabolic, endocrine, biomechanical and other factors have been suggested.

Strictly, this condition is not an inflammation of the bone or joints but a degeneration of tissues characterized by thickening of the joint region with bony outgrowths which lead to roughening and joint deformity, limiting movement and causing pain.

In complete contradiction to most popularly held beliefs, osteoarthritis is not caused by acid, infection, poisons, drugs, food, constipation, cold or damp, but is "old age" of the joints.

OSTEOBLAST
A bone-forming cell.

OSTEOBLASTOMA
A benign tumor of bone.

OSTEOCHONDRITIS
Although the term infers inflammation of both bone and cartilage, the changes most frequently found are degeneration and regeneration of bone (particularly at the growing ends of long bones), and for this reason many doctors prefer to use the term osteochondrosis.

OSTEOCHONDRITIS DEFORMANS JUVENILIS
Disease of the upper end of the thigh bone affecting children between five and ten years of age.

OSTEOCHONDRITIS DISSECANS
Joint affection characterized by partial detachment of fragments of cartilage and underlying bone from the joint surface and frequently resulting in so-called "loose bodies" within the joint. The knee joint is most commonly affected.

OSTEOCHONDROMA
Tumor composed of bone and cartilage.

OSTEOCHONDROPATHY
A disease involving both bone and cartilage.

OSTEOCLASIA
Surgical fracture of a long bone, without opening the tissues, to correct a deformity. The term is also applied to destruction of bony tissue and to the resorption of bone.

OSTEOCLAST
Any of the large multinucleated cells in developing bone that are associated with the dissolution of unwanted bone, as in the formation of canals or the healing of fractures.

OSTEOCLASTOMA
Giant-cell tumor arising in bone, regarded as harmless, but may recur after removal.

OSTEODYSTROPHIA
Defective bone formation. It includes such bone defects as are seen in rickets, dwarfism and the like.

OSTEOGENESIS
Development of bony tissue.

OSTEOGENESIS IMPERFECTA
Hereditary condition characterized by abnormal fragility of the bones, resulting in "spontaneous" fractures associated with striking blueness of

the whites of the eyes and sometimes with deafness.

OSTEOGENETIC SARCOMA
Malignant tumor arising from the deep layers of periosteum (the membrane covering a bone).

OSTEOID
Resembling bone. Also the young matrix (layer) of true bone in which calcium salts are deposited to form proper bone.

OSTEOLOGY
The study of the structure, function and disease of bone.

OSTEOMA
Tumor arising in bony tissue.

OSTEOMALACIA
Disease due to vitamin D deficiency in adult life, characterized by softening of the bones, a low concentration of calcium and phosphorus in the blood, together with an increased secretion of calcium and phosphorus in the urine. The bones become curved and deformed and there is liability to "spontaneous" fractures.

OSTEOMYELITIS
Bacterial infection of bone, usually caused by staphylococcus, streptococcus and salmonella carried to the bone by the blood, or gaining access through open fractures. It commonly affects children, causing fever and local pain. If untreated or partially treated, it may become chronic with bone destruction and a discharging sinus. Antibiotics and surgical drainage are frequently necessary.

OSTEOPATHY
System of treatment based on the theory that disease arises from the mechanical and structural disorder of the body skeleton. Prevention and treatment are practiced by manipulation, often of the spine.

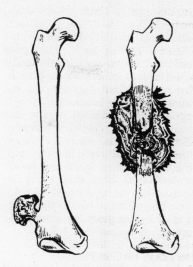

Benign (left) and malignant (right) osteoma of the femur.

OSTEOPERIOSTITIS
Inflammation of both the bone and periosteum (the surrounding membrane).

OSTEOPETROSIS
Congenital disease characterized by increased density of the bones, "spontaneous" fractures, enlargement of the spleen and anemia. Symptoms usually begin in childhood, with fractures following injury, and general backwardness.

OSTEOPHYTE
Small local outgrowth of bone from the periosteum commonly seen in osteoarthritis.

OSTEOPLASTY
Repair operations on bone; replacement of lost bone tissue or reconstruction of defective bony parts.

OSTEOPOROSIS
Softening of the bones. It is the almost universal disease of older people. Osteoporosis affects the entire skeleton. The back, legs and feet are affected. The disease may be noted first in the mouth, for, as jaw bones

weaken due to lack of minerals, teeth loosen and the condition called periodontal disease brings eventual loss of teeth. The spine tends to collapse because the small bones are too weak to support it. The ribs may fall forward onto the rim of the pelvic bones, thus crowding all the abdominal organs and creating much digestive distress. Osteoporosis is more common among women than among men. The average man loses five to six percent of his bone mass every ten years after the age of 35. At 65, bone loss slows to two to three percent every ten years. In women the rate of loss is doubled.

OSTEOSARCOMA
A sarcoma derived from bone or containing bone tissue; also called osteogenic sarcoma.

OSTEOSYNTHESIS
The operation of uniting the ends of a fractured bone by mechanical means, as a wire or metal plate.

OSTEOTOMY
Surgical division or removal of a part of a bone.

OTC
Abbreviation for over-the-counter. Over-the-counter drugs can be bought in a drug store, a chemists's shop or elsewhere without a prescription.

OTECTOMY
Removal of the auditory ossicles (three little bones in the middle ear).

OTHEMATOMA
Blood-filling swelling on the outer ear.

OTHEMORRHEA
Blood containing discharge from the ear.

OTIC GANGLION
A small parasympathetic ganglion that is associated with the mandibular nerve, located just below the foramen ovale of the sphenoid bone, receiving preganglionic fibers from the glossopharyngeal nerve by way of the lesser petrosal nerve, and sending postganglionic fibers to the parotid gland by way of the auriculotemporal nerve.

OTITIS
Inflammation of the ear.

OTITIS EXTERNA
Inflammation of the external ear (that part from the eardrum outwards).

OTITIS INTERNA
Inflammation of the internal ear.

OTITIS MEDIA
Inflammation of the middle ear, marked by pain, fever, dizziness, and abnormalities of hearing.

OTOCONIA
Small crystals of calcium carbonate in the saccule and utricle of the ear that under the influence of linear acceleration cause stimulation of the hair cells by their movement relative to the gelatinous supporting substrate containing the embedded cilia of the hair cells.

OTOLITH
Stone formed within the membranous labyrinth of the ear.

OTOPHARYNGEAL
Pertaining to the ear and pharynx (the back part of the throat).

OTOPHARYNGEAL TUBE
Tube that runs from the back of the nose to the middle ear and equalizes the atmospheric pressure on both sides of the eardrum. Also called Eustachian tube and otosalpinx.

OTOPIESIS
Deafness resulting from abnormal pressure on the labyrinth.

OTORRHAGIA
Discharge of blood from the ear hole.

OTORRHEA
Discharge from the ear hole.

OTOSCLEROSIS
Condition in which there is progressive deafness due to abnormal bone formation in the hearing apparatus interfering with the conduction of sound.

OTOSCOPE
An instrument for examining the internal parts of the ear.

OTOSCOPY
Examination or auscultation of the ear with an otoscope.

OUTER EAR
The outer portion of the ear that collects and directs sound waves toward the tympanic membrane by way of a canal which extends inward through the temporal bone.

OUTLET
An opening or a place through which something is let out, as the pelvic outlet.

OUTPATIENT CARE
The provision of mental health treatment on an outpatient basis that does not include any overnight stay in an inpatient facility.

OUTPUT
The amount of energy or matter discharged usually within a specified time by a bodily system or organ.

OVAL WINDOW
An oval opening between the middle ear and the vestibule having the base of the stapes or columella attached to its membrane.

OVARIAN
Pertaining to or resembling the ovary.

OVARIAN CANCER
Malignant growth of the female sex gland. Of the cancers of the female genital organs, 18-20 percent are ovarian cancers; the peak incidence occurs in women in their 50s. Since an ovarian cancer usually remains occult until it enlarges or extends enough to produce symptoms, early detection is difficult, and the disease has become extensive within or beyond the pelvis in a large number of patients before diagnosis. This, if routine pelvic examination reveals an ovary enlarged more than 2 inches (5 cm) in diameter, careful follow-up is required.

Any enlargement of the ovary in a postmenopausal woman should signify a malignancy that requires prompt surgical excision. The disease is known as the "silent killer" because the symptoms rarely show until the disease has reached an advanced stage.

OVARY
Any of a pair of female gonads, located in the lower abdomen. The ovaries are very delicate and important organs. They store the potential eggs throughout a woman's life and develop each month into a mature egg or ovum. The ovaries also produce hormones such as estrogen and progesterone, which develop and maintain a woman's secondary sexual characteristics. These hormones prepare the uterus for pregnancy and regulate the menstrual cycle. The ovaries are very active organs undergoing constant internal changes. All these functions interre-

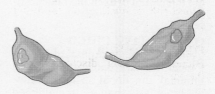

Morphology of the ovaries.

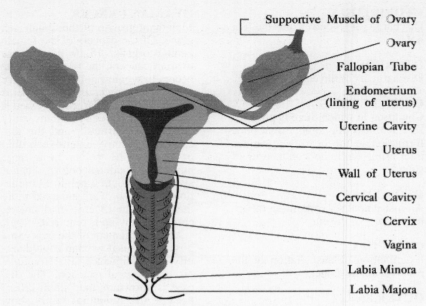

The internal female genital organs.

late like biochemical clockwork, and a delicate balance is necessary for a woman's body to work correctly. If this mechanism is disturbed or fails to work correctly one months, ovulation might not occur and a cyst could develop.

On cross-section the ovary is seen to be composed of an outer cortex and an inner medulla although these two areas are not sharply demarcated. The cortex forms the bulk of the ovary and consists of a dense cellular stroma in which are situated numerous germ cells arranged in cellular formations known as follicles. The medullary stroma is loose and more vascular and within it may be found a number of hilus cells which may be homologous to the interstitial cells in the male testicles.

OVERACTIVE CHILD
Child with a syndrome of pathological activity mostly due to a minimal functional disturbance of the brain. Overactivity in childhood can have a variety of causes. For example, any child who is anxious

rather than depressed due to troubles, either at home or at school, is often restless. The degree of the restlessness usually depends on individual circumstances; for instance, hyperkinesis may be particularly marked in the classroom or in the hospital waiting room, but much less evident when the child is on holiday. A detailed history may indicate possible causes for anxiety and the attitudes and remarks of the mother when discussing the child can be revealing.

OVERCOMPENSATION
Using more effort than is necessary to make up for weakness or deficiency.

OVERDETERMINATION
The assumption that mental processes are caused by more than one factor.

OVER-LEARNING
Learning in which repetition practice has proceeded beyond the point necessary for the retention or recall required.

OVERT RESPONSE
Any response that can be observed by another person.

OVIDUCT
Fallopian duct or tube.

OVUM (plural: ova)
Female egg which is contained on the organs known as the ovaries. Reproduction is accomplished by the successful fertilization of the ovum with a sperm and the subsequent development of the fertilized ovum into a baby.

Ova (and sperm) are unlike other cells in the human body because each have only 23 chromosomes. When they join they can produce an offspring with the correct number, 46 chromosomes.

OXALATE
Oxalic acid. Eating many foods that naturally contain the chemical oxalate (sorrel, spinach, cabbage, tomatoes, rhubarb and even chocolate) usually has no adverse effect; in some people, however, it can cause hyperoxaluria (an abnormally excessive amount of oxalate in the urine). If it then combines with calcium, oxalate can on occasion cause kidney stones.

OXIDE
A compound of oxygen with an element or radical.

OXYGEN
A gas which is the most important component of the air we breathe. It is vital to energy-producing chemical reactions in the living cells of the body. Breathed into the lungs, it enters the blood stream and is carried by the blood to the body tissues.

OXYGEN TENT
Enclosed space, often made of plastic, in which a patient may be nursed in an atmosphere enriched with oxygen. It is mainly used for

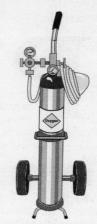

Oxygen in tanks is used in emergency situations in a hospital.

small children with acute respiratory diseases, or in adults when the use of a face mask is impractical.

OXYHEMOGLOBIN
Combination of oxygen and hemoglobin in the red blood cells. This combination gives arterial blood its bright red color, compared with the darker red of venous blood in which the hemoglobin is deficient in oxygen.

OXYURIS
Threadworm.

OZENA
Chronic disease of the nose, accompanied by a bad smelling discharge.

OZONE
Tri-atomic allotrope of oxygen; blue gas with a pungent odor. It is a very powerful oxidizing agent, and yields ozonides with olefins.

The upper atmosphere contains a layer of ozone, formed when ultraviolet radiation acts on oxygen; this layer protects the earth from the sun's ultraviolet rays. Ozone is made by subjecting oxygen to a high-voltage electric discharge. It is used for killing germs, bleaching, removing unpleasant odors from food and sterilizing water.

PABULUM
Any food or nutrient.

PACEMAKER
A small mass of specialized cells in the right atrium of the heart which gives rise to the electrical impulses that initiate contractions of the heart muscle. Also called sinoatrial node or S-A node of Keith-Flack. Under abnormal circumstances, other heart tissues may assume the pacemaker role by initiating electrical impulses that stimulate contraction.

PACEMAKER, ARTIFICIAL
An electrical device which can substitute for a defective natural pacemaker and control the beating of the heart by a series of rhythmic electrical discharges. If the electrodes which deliver the discharges to the heart are placed on the outside of the chest, it is called an "external pacemaker." If they are placed within the chest wall, it is called an "internal pacemaker."

PACEMAKER, DEMAND
An implanted heart pacemaker in which the generator stimulus is inhibited by a signal derived from the heart's electrical activation, thus minimizing the risk of pacemaker-induced fibrillation of the heart muscle.

PACEMAKER, FIXED-RATE
An implanted heart pacemaker in which the generator stimulates the heart at a predetermined rate, regardless of the heart rhythm.

PACHYBLEPHARON
Thickening of the eyelids.

PACHYCEPHALY
Abnormal thickness of the bones of the skull.

PACHYCHEILIA
Thickening of the lips.

PACHYDERMA
Abnormal thickening of the skin.

PACHYGLOSSIS
Abnormal thickness of the tongue.

PACHYMENINGITIS
Inflammation of the dura mater, the outermost of the three membranes (the meninges) covering the brain.

PACHYONYCHIA
Abnormal thickening of the nails.

PACHYSOMIA
Abnormal thickening of parts of the body.

PACHYVAGINITIS
Chronic inflammation of the vagina with thickening of the vaginal walls.

PACINIAN CORPUSCLES
Small, bulblike sensory end organs attached to the end of nerve fibers in subcutaneous and submucous tissue, especially in the palms, soles, joints, and genitals.

PACK
To treat the body or any part of it by wrapping it (for instance, with blankets or sheets).

PACKED CELLS
A preparation of blood cells separated from the liquid plasma, used in the treatment of some cases of severe anemia to restore adequate levels of red blood cells overloading the circulatory system with too much fluid.

PACKING
The filling of a wound or cavity with gauze, sponges, pads, or other material; also, the material used for this purpose.

PAD
A cushion-like mass of soft material.

PAGE'S DISEASE
Form of neurosis that develops in a casualty which is consciously or subconsciously determined to obtain compensation.

PAGET'S DISEASE
A disease of unknown cause, seldom occurring under the age of forty, in which one or more bones gradually become thick and soft and occasionally fractures spontaneously.

PAIN
The detection by the nervous system of harmful stimuli. The function of pain is to warn the individual of imminent danger; even the most minor tissue damage will cause pain, so that the avoiding action can be taken at a very early stage. The receptors of pain are unencapsulated nerve endings, distributed variably about the body: the back of the knee has about 230 per square centimeter, the tip of the nose about 40.

Deep pain, from the internal organs, may be felt as surface pain or in a different part of the body. This phenomenon, referred pain, is probably due to the closeness of the nerve tracts entering the spinal cord.

PAINKILLER
Something, as a drug, that relieves pain.

PAIN SENSE
A special sense found in all parts of the body, free nerve endings being the supposed receptors. Points can be localized in the skin especially sensitive to pain stimuli, that are usually called pain spots.

PAIN SPOT
A small area of the skin especially sensitive to pain.

PAIN THRESHOLD
The point at which a stimulus activates pain receptors to produce a feeling of pain. Individuals differ in pain threshold, some experiencing pain sooner than others with a higher pain threshold.

PAINTED SICKNESS
A tropical skin disease characterized by thickened patches of skin and color changes caused by a germ (a spirochete).

PAINTER'S COLIC
Lead poisoning in painters that produces abdominal pain.

PALATE
Structure dividing the mouth from the nose and bounded by the upper gums and teeth; it is made of bone and covered by mucous membrane. At the back is a soft mobile connective-tissue structure which can close off the naso-pharynx during swallowing and speech.

PALATE, CLEFT
Congenital fissure in the medial line of the palate.

PALATE, HARD
The front portion of the palate, separating the oral and nasal cavities, consisting of the bony framework and covering membranes.

PALATE, SOFT
The fleshy part of the palate, extending from the posterior edge of the hard palate; the uvula projects from its free inferior border.

PALATINE BONE
Either of a pair of roughly L-shaped bones of the skull that form the pos-

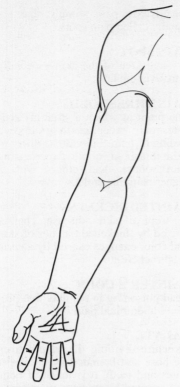

Arm with the palmar surface of the hand.

terior part of the hard palate, part of the floor of the orbit, and part of the nasal cavity.

PALATITIS
An inflamed condition of the palate.

PALATOGLOSSAL
Pertaining to the palate and tongue.

PALATOPLASTY
Plastic surgery of the palate, usually to repair a cleft palate.

PALATOPLEGIA
Paralysis of the palate.

PALATOSCHIZIS
Cleft palate.

PALEOCEREBELLUM
A phylogenitically old part of the cerebellum concerned with maintenance of normal postural relationships and made up chiefly of the anterior lobe of the vermis and of the pyramid.

PALEOCORTEX
The olfactory cortex of the cerebrum.

PALEOPALLIUM
Phylogenetically old part of the cerebral cortex that develops along the lateral aspect of the hemispheres giving rise to the olfactory lobes.

PALILALIA
A condition in which a phrase or word is repeated with increasing rapidity.

PALIDROMA
A recurrence or relapse.

PALIGENESIS
The stages in the development of the individual, so far as they present an epitome in the stages in the evolution of the species or race.

PALIGRAPHIA
Pathologic repetition of letters or words in writing.

PALLIATIVE
Something that soothes; something that relieves pain but does not cure.

PALLIUM
The cortex (superficial layer of cells) of the brain hemispheres.

PALLOR
Paleness, as of the skin.

PALM
The part of the inner surface of the hand from the wrist to the base of the fingers.

PALMATURE
An abnormal condition in which the fingers are webbed.

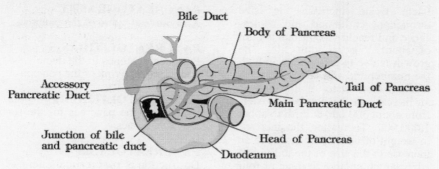

Morphology and topography of the pancreas.

PALMISTRY
Study of the palm of the hand for diagnostic or therapeutic purposes.

PALMUS
Clonic spasm of leg muscles, producing jumping motion.

PALPABLE
Perceptible by touch.

PALPATE
To examine by the sense of touch.

PALPATION
Examination by touch or feeling, as with the hand, to assist in diagnosing an illness.

PALPEBRA
Eyelid; *palpebra inferior*: the lower eyelid; *palpebra superior*: the upper eyelid.

PALPEBRATION
Winking, especially if uncontrolled and persistent.

PALPITATION
A sensation of fluttering of the heart or abnormal rate or rhythm of the heart as experienced by the person.

PALSY
Paralysis, especially a progressive form of paralysis culminating late in life, characterized by tremors of the limbs, muscular weakness and rigidity, and a peculiar gait and attitude.

PANACEA
A remedy for all diseases.

PANAGGLUTININ
An agglutinin which agglutinates the red blood cells of all human blood groups.

PANANGITIS
Inflammation involving all the coats of a vessel.

PANCARDITIS
Diffuse inflammation of all layers of the heart wall.

PANCREAS
Organ consisting partly of exocrine gland tissue, secreting into the duodenum, and partly of endocrine gland tissue (the islets of Langerhans), whose principal hormones include insulin and glucagon.

The pancreas lies on the back wall of the upper abdomen, much of it within the duodenal loop. Powerful digestive enzymes (pepsin, trypsin, lipase, amylase) are secreted into the gut; this secretion is in part controlled by intestinal hormones (secretin) and in part by nerve reflexes. Insulin and glucagon have important roles in glucose and fat metabolism; other pancreatic hormones affect gastrointestinal tract secretion and activity.

Islets tissue increases in size throughout childhood and adolescence and reaches a constant weight of about 1 g in adult life. The growth is due to an increase in both the number and size of the islets. In the first three years of life there is an increase in the number of islets from about 300,000 at birth to about 1,000,000. Thereafter, the increase in weight of islet tissue is due to an increase in the size of the individual islets which enlarge to three or four times their size at birth.

PANCREATALGIA
Pain in the pancreas or region of the pancreas.

PANCREATECTOMY
Surgical removal of the pancreas or part of it.

PANCREATIC CHOLERA
Constant diarrhea due to a disorder of the pancreas. The major clinical features are prolonged massive watery diarrhea and symptoms of hypokalemia and dehydration. The condition should be treated by a specialist in a hospital.

PANCREATIC DUCT
Pancreas-juice-carrying duct leading from the pancreas and joining with the common bile duct to empty its secretions into the duodenal part of the small intestine.

PANCREATIC JUICE
An alkaline fluid containing a mixture of digestive enzymes, discharged by the pancreas into the duodenum.

PANCREATIN
A preparation made from the pancreas of cattle or dogs, used as a digestive. The preparation contains a number of enzymes from the pancreas.

PANCREATITIS
Inflammation of the pancreas.

PANCREATOGRAPHY
X-ray investigation of the pancreas.

PANCREATOLITHIASIS
Presence of stones in the ductal system of parenchyma of the pancreas.

PANCREATOLITHOMY
Incision of the pancreas for the removal of stones.

PANCREATOLYSIS
Destruction of pancreatic tissue.

PANCREATOZYMIN
A hormone of the mucosa of the duodenum that stimulates the external secretory activity of the pancreas, especially its production of amylase.

PANCYSTITIS
Cystitis involving the thickness of the wall of the urinary bladder.

PANCYTOPENIA
Abnormal depression of all he cellular elements of the blood (red blood cells, platelets, white blood cells), usually associated with aplastic anemia or bone marrow.

PANDEMIC
A widespread epidemic disease.

PANDICULATION
Yawning and stretching actions, as when first awakening.

PANENCEPHALITIS
Inflammation of brain tissue, probably of viral origin, which produces inclusion bodies in the nerve cells of both the gray and white matter.

PANESTHESIA
The sum of the sensations experienced.

PANHYPOPITUITARISM
Generalized secretory deficiency of the anterior lobe of the pituitary gland; a disorder characterized by such deficiency.

PANHYSTERECTOMY
Total removal of the uterus.

PANHYSTEROSALPINGECT OMY
Excision of the body of the uterus, cervix, and Fallopian tubes.

PANIC
Extreme and unreasoning fear and anxiety.

PANIC ATTACK
Discrete periods of intense fear or discomfort. The panic attacks usually last minutes or, more rarely, hours. The attacks, at least initially, are unexpected; they do not occur immediately before or on exposure to a situation that almost always causes anxiety.

PANIC DISORDER
A term which is usually synonymous with panic attack but which may take such specific and unrelated forms as, for instance, homosexual panic. Panic disorder is a separate diagnostic entity within the group of anxiety states.

PANIC STATES
A sustained condition of overwhelming morbid anxiety affecting either an individual or group to which the panic has been transmitted.

PANIMMUNITY
Immunity to several bacterial and viral infections.

PANNICULITIS
Inflammation of the panniculus fat tissue, especially of the abdomen.

PANNICULUS ADIPOSUS
The fat under the skin; a layer of fat underlying the corium of the skin.

PANNUS
(1) Superficial vascularization of the cornea with infiltration of granulation tissue;

(2) an inflammatory exudate overlying the synovial cells on the inside of a joint.

PANOSTEITIS
Inflammation of every part of a bone.

PANOTITIS
Inflammation of all the parts or structures of the ear.

PANPHOBIA
Fear of everything; vague and persistent dread of an unknown evil.

PANPSYCHISM
Belief that only psychological or mentalistic reality exists.

PANSEXUALISM
The view that human behavior and motivation can be fully explained in terms of the sex drive or motive.

PANTHOTENIC ACID
Also called vitamin B_5, a member of the vitamin B complex. Preparations of the vitamin are used for the prevention and treatment of deficiency states.

PANTOTROPIC
Having affinity for tissues derived from all three germ layers.

PAPAIN
An enzyme found in papaya which acts on protein. Available in tablets and as a powder to tenderize meat.

PAPANICOLAOU SMEAR
Microscopic examination of cells taken from different parts of the body, often the cervix of the uterus and vagina, to detect abnormalities such as cancer, infection and effects of irradiation, and to determine cellular hormonal activity.

The test was named after Dr. G. Papanicolaou who worked for many years to perfect and quantify the test.

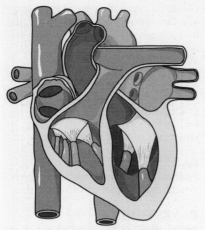

The papillary muscles inside the ventricles of the heart play an important role in the function of the valves.

PAP TEST
Abbreviation for Papanicolaou smear.

PAPILLA
A small nipple-shaped projection or elevation.

PAPILLA, DENTAL
The small mass of condensed mesenchyme capped by each of the enamel organs.

PAPILLA, DUODENAL
Either of the small elevations on the mucosa of the duodenum, the major papilla at the entrance of the conjoined pancreatic and common bile ducts, the minor at the entrance of the accessory pancreatic duct.

PAPILLA, FILIFORM
Nipple-shaped threadlike elevation covering most of the tongue.

PAPILLA, FOLIATE
One of the parallel mucosal folds on the tongue margin at the junction of its body and root.

PAPILLA, FUNGIFORM
One of the knoblike projections of the tongue scattered among the filiform papillae.

PAPILLARY MUSCLES
Small, cone-shaped muscles projecting from the walls of the lower heart chambers (the ventricles) to which are attached fibrous cords (chordae tendineae) stretching up to the flaps of the valves between upper and lower chambers.

When the ventricles fill with blood and contract, the papillary muscles also contract and tighten the cords, allowing the valves to be pressed shut, but preventing them from being pushed back and open into the upper chambers (the atria) by the surging blood.

PAPILLEDEMA
Edema (swelling) of the optic disk.

PAPILLITIS
Inflammation of the optic disk of the retina.

PAPILLOMA
A benign tumor derived from epithelium.

PAPOVAVIRUS
A group of relatively small, ether-resistent DNA viruses, many of which are oncogenic or potentially oncogenic.

PAPULATION
The formation of papules.

PAPULE
A small, firm raised skin lesion, as in chickenpox.

PAPULOSIS
The presence of multiple papules.

PARA–
Word element: beside, beyond, apart from, against.

PARA-AMINOBENZOIC ACID
Part of folic acid, one of the members of the vitamin B complex; a

drug used as a sunscreen in many lotions and creams.

PARABIOSIS
The union of two individuals, as conjoined twins, or of experimental animals by surgical operation.

PARABLEPSIA
False or perverted vision.

PARACENESTHESIA
Any disturbance of the general sense of well-being.

PARACENTESIS
Surgical puncture of a cavity for the aspiration of fluid, most often the abdomen, through a hollow needle; it is performed for therapeutic or diagnostic purposes.

PARACEPHALUS
A fetus with a defective head and imperfect sense organs.

PARACERVICAL BLOCK
A type of regional anesthesia in which a local anesthetic agent is injected on each side of the cervix to achieve anesthesia during labor and childbirth.

PARACRINE
Denoting the influence of the secretion of one kind of endocrine cell on that of another kind which is not the normal target cell.

PARACUSIS
Any perversion of hearing.

PARACYSTITIS
Inflammation of tissues around the urinary bladder.

PARADIDYMIS
A small, vestigial structure found occasionally in the adult in the spermatic cord.

PARADOXICAL PULSE
A pulse that is weaker during inspiration, a condition sometimes observed in compression of the heart.

PARADOXIA SEXUALIS
Manifestation of sexual impulses or behavior not characteristic of the chronological age of the individual.

PARADOXICAL COLD
The sensation of coldness when a relatively warm object stimulates a cold receptor or spot on the skin.

PARAFFIN
A purified hydrocarbon wax used for embedding histological specimens.

PARAFFINOMA
A chronic granuloma produced by prolonged exposure to paraffin.

PARAGEUSIA
Perversion of the sense of taste, or a taste hallucination.

PARAGLOSSIA
Inflammation of the oral tissues under the tongue.

PARAGRAMMATISM
Disorder of speech, with confusion in the use and order of words and grammatical forms.

PARAGRANULOMA
The most benign form of Hodgkin's disease, largely confined to the lymph nodes.

PARAGRAPHIA
Slight impairment of ability to express thoughts in writing, as a result of a pathological condition of some areas of the cerebral cortex of the brain.

PARAHORMONE
A substance, not a true hormone, which has a hormone-like action in controlling the functioning of some distant organ.

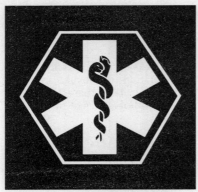
Symbol for paramedic assistance.

PARAINFLUENZA VIRUS
A virus causing upper respiratory infections, including the common cold, bronchiolitis, croup, and other disorders, most commonly in children.

PARAKERATOSIS
Persistence of the nuclei of keratinocytes as they rise into the horny layer of the skin. It is normal in the epithelium of the true mucous membrane of the mouth and vagina.

PARAKINESIA
Perversion of motor function; irregular action of an individual eye muscle. The term is also used for the assumption or suggestion of supernormal forces, for levitation with mere contact.

PARALALIA
Distortion of speech sounds, as in lisping, usually due to a disorder of the peripheral speech systems.

PARALEXIA
The misreading of words and phrases, as a result of a pathological condition of some areas of the cerebral cortex of the brain.

PARALLEL PLAY
The situation in which a child rather plays next to than with other children and no attempt is made to influence the play of others nearby.

PARALOGIA
Difficulty in the expression of ideas in speech, and consequent illogicality or irrelevance.

Paralogia is a reasoning disorder characterized by inappropriate responses to questioning and based on underlying autistic or dereistic processes, as in schizophrenia.

PARALYSIS
Temporary or permanent loss of muscle power or control. It may consist of inability to move a limb or part of a limb or individual muscles; paralysis of the muscles of breathing, swallowing and voice production being especially serious.

Paralysis may be due to:
- disease of the brain (e.g., stroke, tumor);
- disorders of the spinal cord (poliomyelitis);
- nerve roots (slipped disc);
- peripheral nervous system (neuritis);
- neuromuscular junction (myasthenia gravis);
- muscular tissue (muscular dystrophy).

Disturbance of blood potassium levels can also lead to paralysis.

PARALYSIS AGITANS
Another name for Parkinsonism.

PARALYTIC STROKE
Sudden loss of muscular power from some disease of the brain or spinal cord.

PARAMAX
Brand name of a drug containing as active compounds paracetamol and metoclopramide prescribed for the treatment of severe headaches such as migraine.

PARAMEDIC
A person who supplements the work of professional medical personnel.

PARAMIMIA
A behavioral disorder in which gestures are distorted and do not express feelings.

PARAMNESIA
The sensation or illusion of remembering something that has never been experienced; a basic disorder of memory.
(1) A condition in which the proper meaning of words cannot be remembered.
(2) The illusion of remembering scenes and events when experienced for the first time.

PARANOIA
A psychosis characterized by delusions of persecution (hence the popular term, persecution mania) and grandeur, often accompanied by hallucinations. The delusions may form a self-consistent system that replaces reality.

PARANOID DEFENSES
Feelings that others are hostile to oneself.

PARANOID DEMENTIA
Mental disorganization with systematized delusion formation on the basis of dementia. The disorder is seen at old age as a specific form of dementia.

PARANOID DISORDER
State of heightened self-awareness with a marked tendency to self-reference and projection of the person's own ideas to others. Paranoid states range imperceptibly from a circumscribed delusional system with no loss of affect or associative processes, to the more complete disorganization seen in paranoid schizophrenia.

PARANOID PERSONALITY DISORDER
A pervasive and unwarranted tendency, beginning by early adulthood and present in a variety of contexts, to interpret the actions of people as deliberately demeaning or threatening.

Almost invariably there is a general expectation of being exploited or harmed by others in some way. Frequently a person with this disorder will question, without justification, the loyalty or trustworthiness of friends and associates. Often the person is pathologically jealous, questioning without justification the fidelity of his or her spouse or sexual partner.

Since people with this disorder rarely seek help for their personality problems or require hospitalization, the disorder seldom comes to clinical attention. Because of a tendency of some of them to be moralistic, grandiose, and extrapunitive, people with this disorder may be over-represented among leaders of cults and other fringe groups.

PARANOID SCHIZOPHRENIA
A form of schizophrenia with severe paranoia. Of the people admitted to mental hospitals as schizophrenics about half are characterized as suffering from the paranoid form of this disorder. The victim harbors delusional notions that he is being persecuted or threatened. He may believe his food is being laced with arsenic or that an invisible gas is poisoning the air in his bedroom.

PARAOLFACTORY
A small area of the cerebral cortex situated on the medial side of the frontal lobe below the corpus callosum and considered part of the limbic system.

PARAPHILIA
Sexual disorder characterized by recurrent intense sexual urges and sexually arousing fantasies generally involving either:
- nonhuman objects;
- the suffering or humiliation of oneself or one's partner (not merely simulated);

– or children or other nonconsenting persons.

For some people with a paraphilia, paraphiliac fantasies or stimuli may always be necessary for erotic arousal and are always included in the sexual activity, if not actually acted out alone or with a partner. In other cases the paraphiliac preferences occur only episodically, for example, during periods of stress; at other times the person is able to function sexually without paraphilia fantasies or stimuli.

PARAPLEGIA
Total or partial paralysis of both lower limbs. This condition is caused by injury or disease involving the spinal cord. Below the level of the lesion or damage, there is locomotor paralysis and sensory loss. Bladder and bowel functions can be affected. About half of the people whose paraplegia is the result of an accident, have a complete lesion, meaning that paralysis is symmetrical and complete below the level of injury. For the other half the lesion is incomplete and paralysis uneven so that, for example, one leg may be more severely affected than the other.

PARAPRAXIS
A faulty action due to the interference of some unconscious wish, conflict or train of thought. Slips of the tongue and pen are the classic parapraxes.

PARAPROTEINEMIA
A heterogenous group of diseases characterized by the presence in blood serum or urine of a monoclonal immunoglobulin.

PARAPSORIASIS
A group of slowly developing, persistent, skin diseases, characterized by maculopapular scaly erythrodermas; devoid of subjective symptoms and resistant to treatment.

PARAPSYCHOLOGY (Psychic research)
A field of study concerned with scientific evaluation of two distinct types of phenomena: those collectively termed ESP (extrasensory perception), and those concerned with life after death, reincarnation, etc., particularly including claims to communication with souls of the dead (spiritism or, incorrectly, spiritualism).

Tests of the former have generally been inconclusive, of the latter almost exclusively negative. But in both cases many "believers" hold that such phenomena, being beyond the bounds of science, cannot be subjected to laboratory evaluation.

PARASEXUAL
Relating to or being reproduction that results in recombination of genes from different individuals but does not involve meiosis and formation of a zygote by fertilization as in sexual reproduction.

PARASITE
An organism that is for some part of its life-history physically dependent on another, the host, from which it obtains nutrition and which may form its total environment.

Nearly all the major groups of animals and plants from viruses to vertebrates and bacteria and angiosperms, have some parasitic members. The most important parasites, besides the viruses which are of a wholly parasitic group, occur in the bacteria, protozoa, flatworms and roundworms.

Bloodsucking arthropods, such as mosquitos, tsetse flies and ticks, are also important because they transmit parasitic diseases and serve as vectors or transport-hosts for other parasites.

PARASITEMIA
The presence of parasites in the blood.

PARASITIC DISEASE
Infestation or infection by parasites, usually referring to non-bacterial and non-viral agents. Malaria, leishmaniasis, trypanosomiasis, filariasis, schistosomiasis, toxoplasmosis, amebiasis and tape worm are common examples.

PARASITICIDE
Destructive to parasites; also, an agent that destroys parasites.

PARASITISM
Symbiosis in which one population (or individual) adversely affects another, but cannot live without it.

PARASITOLOGY
The scientific study of parasites and parasitism.

PARASITOPHOBIA
A delusion that one is infested with parasites.

PARASOMNIA
An abnormal event that occurs either during sleep or at the threshold between wakefulness and sleep; the predominant complaint focusses on the disturbance, not on its effect on sleeping or wakefulness. Examples are:
- dream anxiety disorders;
- sleep terror disorders;
- sleepwalking disorders.

PARASUICIDE
An apparent attempt at suicide, as by self-poisoning or self-mutilation, in which death is not the desired outcome.

PARASYMPATHETIC NERVOUS SYSTEM
One of the two divisions of the autonomic nervous system (the other being the sympathetic nervous system), consisting of nerve fibers that leave the brain and sacral portion of the spinal cord, extend to nerve cell clusters (ganglia) at specific sites, from which fibers are distributed to blood vessels, glands, and other internal organs.

Generally parasympathetic nerves show the following actions and functions:
- stimulate peristalsis;
- slow the heart rate;
- induce the secretion of bile, insulin and digestive juices;
- dilate peripheral blood vessels;
- contract the bronchioles, pupils, and esophagus.

The system works in balance with the sympathetic nervous system, often opposing its actions.

PARASYMPATHETIC
Anticholinergic; producing effects resembling those of interruption of the parasympathetic nerve supply of a part; having a destructive effect on the parasympathetic nerve fibers or blocking the transmission of impulses to them.

PARASYMPATHICOMIMETIC
Having an effect (as from a medicine) similar to that caused by stimulation of the parasympathetic nervous system. The term is usually applied to a drug that stimulates the parasympathetic part of the autonomic nervous system. These drugs are used as mitotics and to stimulate bladder contraction in urinary retention.

PARASYSTOLE
A heart irregularity attributed to the interaction of two foci independently initiating heart impulses at different rates.

PARATAXIC MODE
The second stage in perceiving. The child in parataxic mode perceives the world in a prelogical order viewing himself as the center of the universe.

PARATHYMIA
Display of an inappropriate reaction or of the opposite mood from what would be expected from the situ-

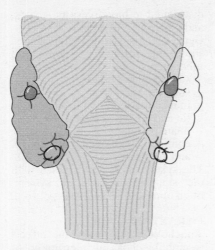

Localization of the parathyroids in close association with the thyroid.

ation. This is an affect disturbance characteristic of schizophrenia.

PARATHYROID GLANDS
A set of four small endocrine glands lying behind the thyroid which regulate calcium metabolism. As a rule, there are four parathyroid glands but there may be more and, very occasionally, fewer than four. They are small, yellow, oval bodies, about 5 mm long and 4 mm wide, situated on the posterior surface of the lobes of the thyroid gland. On each thyroid lobe, there are two parathyroid glands, one being placed superiorly about the middle of the lobe at the level of the lower border of the cricoid cartilage, behind the junction of the pharynx and esophagus. The inferior gland may be situated at the lower edge of the thyroid lobe or may lie in relation to one of the inferior thyroid veins.

Parathyroid hormone releases calcium from bone and alters the interstitial absorption and kidney excretion of calcium and phosphorus.

PARATHYROID HORMONE
A hormone synthesized and released into the bloodstream by the parathyroid gland. It regulates calcium and phosphorus distribution in the body and functions in neuromuscular excitation and blood clotting.

PARATYPHOID
Infection due to Salmonella of all groups except Salmonella typhosa. The infection is accompanied by:
- fever;
- diarrhea;
- rash;
- spleen and lymph node enlargement.

Spread is by cases or carriers and contaminated food; antibiotics may be helpful in treatment.

PARAURETHRAL
Near the urethra.

PARAVAGINITIS
Inflammation of the tissues alongside the vagina.

PARENCHYMA
The essential or functional elements of an organ, as distinguished from its stroma or framework.

PARENTAL ATTITUDES
Attitudes which parents exhibit towards their children, which have a great effect upon the shaping of the child's development from infancy and subsequent personality characteristics.

PARENTERAL
Not through or in the intestine. The term is generally applied to a medicine introduced in a way other than through the digestive tract.

PARENTERAL NUTRITION
The administration of nutrients by a route other than the digestive system, say, for example, by intravenous administration of fluids.

PARESIS
Incomplete paralysis, either due to partial paralysis of a nerve innervating a muscle or to a complete pa-

ralysis of a small nerve in such a way that other nerves may partially take over the nerve supply to a muscle group.

PARESTHESIA
Morbid or perverted sensation; an abnormal sensation, as burning, prickling, formication, etc., usually associated with partial damage to a peripheral nerve.

PARIES
A wall, as of an organ or cavity.

PARIETAL
Pertaining to the pair of bones forming part of the top and sides of the skull; pertaining to parieties or structural walls of hollow organs.

PARIETAL BONE
Either of two skull bones forming the top and sides of the cranium.

PARIETAL LOBE
One of the main divisions of each hemisphere of the cerebral cortex, located beneath the crown of the head and concerned with sensory and associative nerve functions.

PARINAUD'S SYNDROME
Paralysis of the upward movements of the two eyes that is associated especially with a lesion or compression of the superior colliculi of the midbrain.

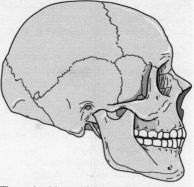

The parietal bone of the skull is located between the frontal bone (right) and the occipital bone (left).

PARITY
The condition of a woman with respect to having borne viable offspring.

PARKINSONISM
A group of neurological disorders marked by hypokinesia, tremor, and muscular rigidity. The major neurological symptoms include tremor of the hands and muscle rigidity that resemble Parkinson's disease. It may be caused by prolonged treatment with an antipsychotic drug.

PARKINSON'S DISEASE
Also known as paralysis agitans, parkinsonian syndrome, shaking palsy or parkinsonism. Parkinson's disease is a chronic, progressive

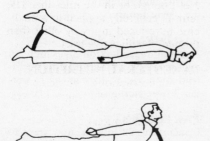
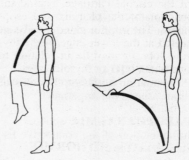

Exercises for a patient with Parkinson's disease to improve mobility.

disorder of the brain characterized by slowness and poverty of purposeful movement, muscular rigidity and tremor.

The disease itself is idiopathic, meaning it is a disease without recognizable cause, as of spontaneous origin.

Symptoms resembling Parkinson's disease -generally known as parkinsonism - may also result from various causes such as:
- certain psychotropic drugs;
- carbon monoxide poisoning;
- manganese poisoning;
- infarcts of the basal ganglia;
- hydrocephalus;
- tumors near the basal ganglia;
- brain trauma;
- aftereffect of encephalitis.

There seems no doubt that the neuronal degeneration responsible for the idiopathic disease is situated in the basal ganglia of the cerebral hemispheres and brain stem. The constant pathological finding concerns loss of melanin pigment and degeneration of nerve cells in the substantia nigra in the midbrain. Nerve cells from the substantia nigra pass to the striatum (part of the basal ganglia) of the cerebral hemispheres which has the highest dopamine content of the brain. This is reduced in Parkinson's disease, the loss paralleling the loss of nerve cells in the substantia nigra.

Dopamine-drugs may alleviate the symptoms of Parkinson's disease.

PARODONTISM
Inflammation of the tissues around a tooth.

PARONYCHIA
Inflammation involving the folds of tissue around the fingernail.

PAROPHTHALMIA
Inflammation of the connective tissue around the eye.

PAROREXIA
Nervous perversion of the appetite, with craving for special articles of food or for articles not suitable for food.

PAROSMIA
Any disorder of the sense of smell; a distortion of the sense of smell, as when affected with a cold.

PAROTID GLAND
Either of the two salivary glands on the sides of the face, one in front of each ear.

PAROTITIS
Inflammation of the parotid gland.

PAROXYSM
A sudden and violent access of passion or emotion. The term is also used in the sense of any sudden intensification of a disease or symptom, especially one occurring with regularity.

PAROXYSMAL SUPRAVENTRICULAR TACHYCARDIA
A condition in which the heart rate suddenly increases to 140-200 beats per minute and a 1:1 atrioventricular conduction is maintained.

PAROXYSMAL TACHYCARDIA
A period of rapid heartbeats which begins and ends suddenly.

PARROT FEVER
An acute feverish illness caused by a virus and transmitted by birds of the parrot family.

PARTHENOGENESIS
Asexual reproduction in which an egg develops without it being fertilized by a spermatozoan, as in certain lower animals.

PARTURIENT
Concerning childbirth; may refer to a woman who is to give birth.

PARTURITION
Act of giving birth.

PART-WHOLE TEST
A type of association experiment or test, where the subject is required to specify the whole of which the name of a part is presented.

PARULIS
An abscess beneath a tooth pocket.

PASSIVE IMMUNITY
Immunity created by injecting into a person serum obtained from a person, sometimes an animal, who has recovered from the disease and who has produced and has circulated in his blood vast quantities of antibodies.

PASSIVE FEELINGS
Delusional feelings of being acted upon by various forces or influences, electrical, hypnotic, etc., characteristic particularly of schizophrenia.

PASSIVE MOVEMENT
Movement of the body parts by a therapist or other agent and not by efforts of the person.

PASSIVE TRANSPORT
The movement of small molecules across a cell membrane by diffusion; it does not require the expenditure of energy.

PASTE
A semisolid preparation, generally for external use, of a fatty base, a viscous or mucilaginous base, or a mixture of starch and petrolatum.

PASTEURELLA
A genus of gram-negative bacteria, including Pasteurella multicida, the etiologic agent of the hemorrhagic septicemias.

PASTEURELLOSIS
Infection with organisms of the genus Pasteurella.

PASTEURIZATION
Heating of milk or other liquids to moderate temperature for a definite time, often 60 degrees for 30 minutes, which kills most pathogenic bacteria and considerably delays other bacterial development.

PASTEUR TREATMENT
A treatment for preventing certain diseases, especially hydrophobia (rabies), by a series of inoculations with a virus of gradually increasing strength.

PAST-POINTING TEST
A test for defective functioning of the vestibular nerve in which the subject is asked to point at an object with his eyes open and then closed first after rotation in a chair to the right and then to the left and which indicates an abnormality if the subject does not past-point in the direction of rotation.

PATCH
A small area differing from the rest of a surface.

PATCH, PEYER'S
Oval elevated patch of closely packed lymph follicles on the mucosa of the small intestines.

PATCH TEST
A skin test for identifying an allergen. A paper or cloth patch containing suspected allergens (for instance, pollen, animal hair) is applied to the skin; the appearance of a red, swollen skin or any rash when the patch is removed - usually one or two days later - usually indicates allergy to that particular substance.

PATELLA
Flat, triangular bone at the front of the knee joint. (See illustration on next page)

PATELLAR REFLEX
Reflex produced by a blow just below the patella (kneecap), with the leg relaxed and bent at the knee,

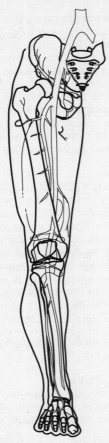

The patella is located in front of the knee joint and embedded in the tendon of the quadriceps muscle.

which is normally an upward kick, caused by the contraction of the quadriceps muscle.

PATELLECTOMY
Excision of the patella.

PATENCY
The condition of being wide open.

PATENT DUCTUS ARTERIO-SUS
A congenital heart defect in which a small duct between the artery leaving the left side of the heart (aorta) and the artery leaving the right side of the heart (pulmonary artery), which normally closes soon after birth, remains open.

PATENT FORAMEN OVALE
One type of congenital heart defect. An oval hole (foramen ovale) between the left and right upper chambers of the heart, which normally closes shortly after birth, remains open.

PATENT MEDICINE
A drug or other therapeutic substance that carries a specific trademark and is available without a prescription.

PATERNITY TEST
Comparison of blood types among mother, child, and a man suspected of being the father of the child in an effort to determine the father of the child.
   If the child blood group could not have resulted from the combination of the man's blood group in combination with that of the woman, then the man is definitely not the father of the child. A DNA-test will show a direct relationship between father and child.

PATHO–
Word element: disease.

PATHERGASIA
Mental malfunction, implying functional or structural damage, marked by abnormal behavior.

PATHERGY
A condition in which the application of a stimulus leaves the organism unduly susceptible to subsequent stimuli of a different kind.

PATHOCLISIS
Specific sensitivity to specific toxins, or a specific affinity of certain toxins for certain systems or organs.

PATHOGENESIS
The production or development of disease.

PATHOGENICITY
The quality of producing or the ability to produce pathologic changes or disease.

PATHOGNOMONIC
Indicative or characteristic of a particular disease.

PATHOGRAPHY
The study of personality in the light of the disorders and ailments from which an individual suffers or has suffered.

PATHOLOGICAL
Of or pertaining to the cause of disease.

PATHOLOGICAL DIAGNOSIS
Diagnosis based on the structural lesion present.

PATHOLOGICAL GAMBLING
Chronic and progressive failure to resist impulses to gamble, and gambling behavior that compromises, disrupts, or damages personal, family, or vocational pursuits. The gambling preoccupation, urge, and activity increase during periods of stress. Problems that arise as a result of the gambling lead to an intensification of the gambling behavior.

PATHOLOGICAL MALINGERING
Another name for Munchausen's syndrome.

PATHOLOGY
Study of the anatomy of disease. Morbid anatomy, the dissection of bodies after death with a view to discovering the cause of disease and the nature of its manifestations is complemented and extended in histology. In addition to autopsy, biopsies and surgical specimens are examined; these provide information that may guide treatment. It has been said that pathology is to medicine what anatomy is to physiology.

PATHOPHYSIOLOGY
The physiology of disordered function.

PATHOPSYCHOLOGY
The psychology of mental disease.

PATHWAY
A course usually followed. In neurology, the nerve structures through which impulses are traveling.

PATIENT
Person who is ill or is undergoing treatment for a disease. A patient usually consults a doctor because he or she feels unwell or because there is a problem for which one requires help. It is fundamental to an effective therapeutic relationship that the doctor establishes rapport with his patient. This basis of a sound relationship is established during the medical interview. Rapport is the end result of a complex psychological mechanism involving both the patient and the doctor.

PATHOMETER
An instrument that records such physical indications of emotional strain as fluctuating blood pressure, and may be employed as a lie detector.

PATHONEUROSIS
A neurotic disorder following a disease or injury and interpreted as withdrawal from the external world and concentration of the disease or injured part, or on the part of the libido.

PAUL-BUNEL TEST
A blood test for heterophil antibodies, used to confirm the diagnosis of infectious mononucleosis.

PAVOR
Terror.

PAVOR DIURNUS
Attacks of fear in children during a daytime nap.

PAVOR NOCTURNUS
A nightmare of children causing them to cry out in fright and awake in panic.

PEAK
The highest value of a measurement or recording, as the top temperature of a patient's fever period or the sharp elevation during an electrocardiographic tracing.

PEARL
A small medicated granule, or a glass globule with a single dose of volatile medicine.

PECTEN
A narrow zone in the anal canal, bounded above by the pectinate (comb-shaped) line.

PECTIC SUBSTANCE
Any of a group of complex colloidal carbohydrate derivatives of plant origin that contain a large proportion of units derived from galactorunic acid and include protopect-

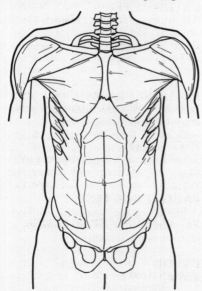

The major and minor pectoral muscles run from the thorax to the upper arm. Contraction of these muscles causes adduction of the arm.

ins, pectins, pectinic acid, and pectic acids.

PECTINOSIS
Stenosis of the anal canal due to an inelastic ring of tissue between the anal groove and anal crypts.

PECTIN
(1) Any of various water-soluble substances that bind adjacent cell walls in plant tissues and yield a gel which is the basis of fruit jellies.
(2) A product containing mostly pectin and used chiefly in making jelly and other foods, in pharmaceutical products, especially for the control of diarrhea.

PECTINASE
An enzyme or complex of enzymes that catalyze the hydrolysis of pectic substances.

PECTINEUS
A flat quadrangular muscle of the upper front and inner aspect of the thigh that arises mostly from the iliopectineal line of the pubis and is inserted along the pectineal line of the femur.

PECTORAL
Pertaining to the chest or the breast.

PECTORALIS
Either of the muscles that connect the ventral walls of the chest with the bones of the upper arm and shoulder of which in man there are two on each side. The pectoralis major muscle is a large muscle arising from the clavicle, the sternum, the cartilages of most or all of the ribs, and the aponeurosis of the external oblique muscle, inserting by a strong flat tendon into the posterior bicipital ridge of the humerus. The pectoralis minor muscle is a muscle that lies beneath the larger one, arising from the third, fourth, and fifth ribs, and inserting by a flat tendon into the coracoid process of the scapula.

PECTUS
The breast, chest or thorax.

PEDAL
Pertaining to the foot or feet.

PEDERASTY
Homosexual anal intercourse, especially between a man and a young boy who is the passive partner.

PEDIATRICS
Branch of medicine concerned with care of children. This starts with newborn, especially premature, babies in whom intensive care is required to protect the baby from and adapt it to the environment outside the uterus.

An important aspect is the recognition and treatment of congenital diseases in which structural or functional defects occur due to inherited diseases (e.g., mongolism) or diseases acquired during development of the embryo or fetus (e.g., spina bifida). Otherwise, infectious diseases, failure to grow or develop normally, mental retardation, diabetes, asthma and epilepsy form the bulk of pediatric practice.

PEDICLE
A narrow stemlike part of an organ.

PEDICULAR
Pertaining to or caused by lice.

PEDICULOSIS
Infestation with lice. Symptoms include intense itching, which often produces skin irritation that becomes secondarily infected.

PEDIGREE
A table, chart, diagram, or list of an individual's ancestors, used in genetics in the analysis of mendelian inheritance.

PEDODONTICS
That branch of dentistry dealing with the teeth and mouth conditions of children.

PEDOPHILIA
A preference for repetitive sexual activity with prepubertal children. The age difference between the adult with this disorder and the child victim may be set at 10 years or more.

Sexual offenses against children constitute a significant proportion of reported criminal sexual acts. The recidivism rate for homosexual pedophilia is second to exhibitionism, and ranges from 15 to 30 percent of those apprehended roughly twice the rate of heterosexual pedophilia.

PEDORTHICS
The design, manufacture, fitting, and modification of shoes and related foot appliances as prescribed for the amelioration of painful or disabling conditions of the foot and leg.

PEDUNCLE
Narrow process serving as a support or a stalk. The term is mostly descriptive of types of tumors hanging free on a stalk and certain features of brain anatomy.

PEER GROUP
Consistent interaction of two or more people who share norms and goals, and have developed some type of role and status divisions governing their interactions.

PEG TEETH
Term applied to the permanent teeth of those suffering with congenital syphilis, from the peg-like aspect of the tops of the teeth.

PELIZAEUS-MERZBACHER DISEASE
A familial degenerative disease of the central nervous system that is characterized by slowly progressive demyelination of white matter resulting in mental deterioration and the occurrence of various motor disorders, as ataxia and nystagmus.

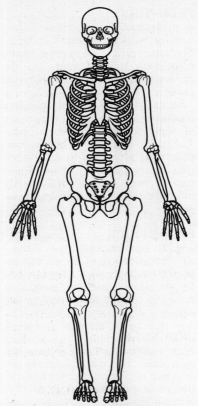

Pelvis or pelvic girdle consists of the two coxal bones. The pelvic girdle provides a strong and stable support for the lower extremities on which the weight of the body is carried

PELLAGRA
Vitamin deficiency disease (due to lack of niacin), often found in maize- or millet-dependent populations. A dermatitis, initially resembling sunburn, but followed by thickening, scaling and pigmentation, is characteristic; internal epithelium is affected (sore tongue, diarrhea). Confusion, delirium, hallucinations and ultimately dementia may ensue. Niacin replacement is essential and food enrichment is an important preventive measure.

PELOTHERAPY
Use of medicated mud in the treatment of disease.

PELVIC
Pertaining to the pelvis.

PELVIC CAVITY
That within the pelvis.

PELVIC GIRDLE
The bony structure, made up of the left and right hipbones, the sacrum and coccyx, to which the bones of the legs are attached.

PELVIC INFLAMMATORY DISEASE (PID)
Term given for any extensive infection of the organs of the pelvic area. Vaginal or uterine infections can spread up into the Fallopian tubes, causing an infection in the tubes, or salpingitis. The infection occasionally spread into the abdomen and to the ovaries.

This can lead to an abscess in the Fallopian tubes or ovaries, or can spreads to the peritoneum, causing peritonitis. This is an extremely serious condition that can lead to death if left untreated.

The disease is often caused by gonorrheal infection. The condition can also be of non-venereal origin due to other bacteria, including streptococcus, staphylococcus or coli bacteria.

PELVIC PLEXUS
A plexus of the autonomic nervous system that is formed by the hypogastric plexus, by branches from the sacral part of the sympathetic chain, and by visceral branches of the second, third, and fourth sacral nerves and that is distributed to the viscera of the pelvic region.

PELVIMETRY
Manual measurement or X-ray studies of the pelvic bones to determine of the space is adequate for giving childbirth.

PELVIOTOMY
Incision or transection of a pelvic bone.

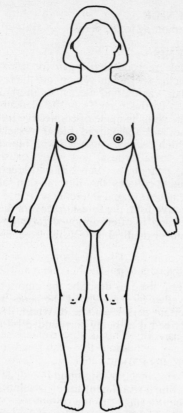

The female pelvis is broader than the male pelvis.

PELVIS
Lowest part of the trunk, bounded by the pelvic bones and in continuity with the abdomen. The principal contents are the bladder and lower gastrointestinal tract (rectum) and reproductive organs, particularly in females the uterus, ovaries, Fallopian tubes and vagina. The pelvic floor is a powerful muscular layer that supports the pelvic and abdominal contents and is important in urinary and fecal continence. The pelvic bones articulate with the legs at the hip joints.

PEMPHIGOID
Any condition characterized by the appearance of bullae, often on reddish macules. Treatment is by corti-

costeroids, but there may be spontaneous remission.

PEMPHIGOID, BENIGN MUCOSAL
A chronic bullous disease of elderly persons, involving primarily the mucous membranes, particularly the conjunctiva and oral mucosa, with scarring.

PEMPHIGUS
Disease of the skin, characterized by thin-walled bullae arising from normal skin or mucous membrane; the bullae frequently rupture, leaving raw patches that often become infected. Treatment is by corticosteroids.

PEMPHIGUS ERYTHEMATOSUS
A relatively benign form of chronic pemphigus that is characterized by the eruption on the face and trunk of lesions resembling those which occur in systemic lupus erythematosus.

PEMPHIGUS FOLIACEUS
A chronic affection characterized by the eruption of flat bullae (blisters) followed by universal redness and scaling of the skin, leaving denuded, raw areas.

PEMPHIGUS NEONATORUM
A condition seen in newborn infants and usually due to a streptococcal germ affecting the skin. Frequently the contamination is from an attendant who is carrying the germ in the throat.

PENECTOMY
Surgical removal of the penis.

PENETRANCE
A term used to refer to the frequency with which the effects of a gene (whether dominant or recessive) known to be present are actually seen in the individuals carrying it.

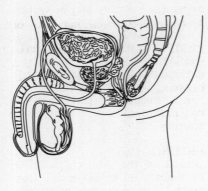

The external male genital organs consist of penis and scrotum.

PENICILLIN
Substance produced by a class of fungi which interferes with cell wall production by bacteria and which was one of the first, and remains among the most useful, antibiotics.

Since the discovery in 1928 and the beginning of its medical use in 1940, numerous derivatives have been manufactured, extending the range of activity, overcoming resistance in some organisms and allowing some to be taken by mouth.

Staphylococcus, streptococcus and the bacteria causing the venereal disease of gonorrhea and syphilis are among the organisms sensitive to natural penicillin, while bacilli negative to Gram's stain, which cause urinary tract infection, septicemia, etc., are destroyed by semisynthetic penicillins.

PENICILLINASE
An enzyme produced by certain bacteria, especially staphylococci strains, that inactivates penicillin, and causes resistance to the antibiotic.

PENICILLINASE- RESIST-ANCE ANTIBIOTIC
An antibiotic that is not rendered inactive by penicillinase; included are such preparations as nafcillin, cloxacillin, oxacillin.

PENILE
Pertaining to the penis.

PENIS
Male reproductive organ for introducing sperm and semen into the female vagina and uterus; its urethra also carries urine from the bladder. The penis is made of connective tissue and specialized blood vessels which become engorged with blood in sexual arousal and which cause the penis to become stiff and erect; this facilitates the intromission of semen in sexual intercourse. A protective fold, the foreskin, covers the tip and is often removed for religious or medical reasons in circumcision.

PENIS AWE
Term used to describe the emotion evoked by the sight of the penis in certain persons, some of whom described it as being surrounded by a halo.

PENIS ENVY
Term coined by Sigmund Freud, denoting a reaction of little girls at the phallic stage to the discovery of sexual differences. The girls feel they have been deprived of the penis (castrated) and wish to have it back.

PENTOSE
A monosaccharide containing five carbon atoms in a molecule.

PENTOSURIA
A benign inborn error of metabolism due to a defect in the activity of the enzyme l-xylulose, resulting in high levels of l-xylulose in the urine.

PEP PILL
Any of various stimulant drugs, as amphetamine, in pill or tablet form.

PEPSIN
The proteolytic enzyme of gastric juice which catalyzes the hydrolysis

of native or denatured proteins to form a mixture of polypeptides.

PEPSINOGEN
An active compound secreted by the chief cells of the stomach glands and converted to pepsin in the presence of gastric acid or of pepsin itself.

PEPTIC
Relating to pepsin or to digestion.

PEPTIC ULCER
A circumscribed ulceration of the mucous membrane of the stomach or duodenum, penetrating through the muscular mucosa and occurring in areas bathed by acid and pepsin.

Peptic ulcers occur only if the stomach secretes acid. Most people secrete acid; some develop ulcers and others do not.

There appears to be a balance between ulcer-promoting factors, such as the secretion of acid or pepsin into the stomach, and factors protecting the stomach's mucosal lining, such as mucus production, membrane barriers to permeability, and replacement of shed or damaged mucosal cells. Many influences can disturb this balance. Stress is implicated as a common precipitating factor.

The usual peptic ulcer has a chronic, recurrent course. Symptoms vary with its location and the person's age; complaints may be atypical in children and minimal in the elderly. Some ulcer patients may not have symptoms, others report them for the first time when a complication develops.

The typical pain is described as burning, gnawing or aching, but the distress may also be described as soreness, an empty feeling or hunger. The typical pain is steady, mild or moderately severe, located in a well-circumscribed area, and relieved by antacids or milk. The treatment is designed to neutralize or decrease gastric acidity.

PEPTIDE
A compound containing two or more amino acids linked through the amino group of one acid and the carboxyl group of the other. The linkage -NH-CO- is termed a peptide bond.

PEPTIDE BOND
The chemical bond between carbon and nitrogen in a peptide linkage.

PEPTIDE LINKAGE
The bivalent CONH that unites the amino acid residues in a peptide.

PEPTIDERGIC
Of or pertaining to nerve cells that secrete peptide hormones.

PEPTONE
Any of a class of dissolvable and soluble substances into which proteins are converted by the action of pepsin or trypsin.

PER ANUM
Through or by way of the anus or anal opening.

PERCEPTION
The process of recognizing or identifying something. The term is usually employed of sense perception, when the thing which we recognize or identify is the object affecting a sense organ.

PERCEPTION TIME
The time which elapses between the presentation of the object, and the indication by the subject, that he has perceived it.

PERCEPTUAL
Of, or relating to, or involving perception, especially in relation to immediate sensory experience.

PERCEPTUAL DEVELOPMENT
Acquisition of perceptual skills in the infant.

PERCEPTUAL FIELD
All those elements of the external environment which an organism perceives or experiences as he experiences them.

PERCEPTUAL LEARNING
Learning to see things or events differently; this kind of learning is usually taken to fall between ideational and motor learning.

PERCEPTUAL SCHEME
The cognitive pattern which serves as a frame of reference against which an organism reacts to the environment and external stimuli.

PERCEPTUALIZATION
Organization of sensory elements into a meaningful whole.

PERCUSSION
Tapping the body as an aid in diagnosing the conditions of parts beneath by the sound obtained.

A physician will often tap the chest to determine the state of the heart and lungs

For instance, whether there may be a fluid accumulation or an enlarged heart.

PERFORMANCE TEST
A type of mental test which the subject is asked to do something, rather than to say something, the use of language being greatly reduced.

PERFUSION
A pouring of fluid into or through or the forcing of a liquid through, organs by way of blood vessels.

PERI–
Word element: around, near.

PERIADENITIS
Inflammation of tissues around a gland.

PERIANAL
Around the anus (back passage).

PERIANGIITIS
Inflammation of the tissue around a blood or lymph vessel.

PERIAPICAL
Pertaining to tissues around the apex of a tooth.

PERIAPICAL ABSCESS
An infection around the root of a tooth.

PERIAPPENDICITIS
Inflammation of the tissues around the vermiform appendix.

PERIARTERITIS
Inflammation of the outer coats of one or more arteries.

PERIARTERITIS NODOSA
A progressive disease of connective tissue characterized by nodules (often large) along arteries that may cause blockage of the artery and resulting in inadequate circulation to the affected area.

Symptoms include:
– visceral pain;
– fever;
– signs of lung, kidney and intestine damage.

Treatment is by corticosteroids.

PERIARTHRITIS
Inflammation of tissues around a joint.

PERIBRONCHIAL
Around a bronchus or bronchi.

PERIBRONCHITIS
A form of bronchitis consisting of inflammation and thickening of the tissues around the bronchi.

PERICARDIAL TAMPONADE
An accumulation of excess fluid between the two layers of the membrane sac surrounding the heart (pericardium). This can happen rapidly or gradually and impairs the normal functioning of the heart.

PERICARDIOCENTESIS
Surgical puncture of the pericardial cavity for the aspiration of fluid.

PERICARDIOLYSIS
The operative freeing of adhesions between the visceral and parietal pericardium.

PERICARDIOTOMY
Surgical opening of the sac surrounding the heart.

PERICARDITIS
Inflammation of the pericardium (the membranous sac surrounding the heart). It may be due to infection, trauma, neoplastic disease, or myocardial infection; or it may result from unknown causes.
Symptoms include:
- fever;
- dry cough;
- difficulty in breathing;
- pain below the breastbone, often radiating upward;
- rapid pulse;
- increasing anxiety and fatigue.

If untreated it can lead to restricted heart action due to effusion. Treatment depends on the cause; it may include antibiotics, analgesics, removal of accumulated fluid, oxygen, and steps to lower fever.

PERICARDIUM
The double-layered membranous sac surrounding the heart. The layer adjacent to the heart (visceral pericardium) is of serous membrane, and the outer layer (parietal pericardium) is of fibrous membrane.

PERICARDIUM, PARIETAL
Outer part of the sac surrounding the heart, anchored to other chest structures such as the breastbone. It is a protective membrane.

PERICARDIUM, VISCERAL
Inner part of the sac surrounding the heart. It forms the outermost layer of the heart wall and is also called the epicardium.

PERICHOLANGITIS
Inflammation of the tissues around the bile ducts.

PERICHOLECYSTITIS
Inflammation of tissues surrounding the gallbladder.

PERICHONDRIUM
The tissues covering the surface of cartilage.

PERICYSTITIS
Inflammation of tissues around the urinary bladder.

PERIMYSIUM
The connective tissue demarcating a fascicle of skeletal muscle fibers.

PERINATAL
Occurring in the period immediately preceding, during of following birth.

PERINATOLOGY
That branch of medicine concerned with the anatomy, physiology, and diagnosis and treatment of disorders of the mother and fetus or newborn child during late pregnancy, childbirth, and the puerperium.

PERINEAL
Relating to the perineum (the area between the anus and genital organs).

PERINEOTOMY
Surgical incision into the perineum.

PERINEUM
The region between the anus (back passage) and the vulva (vaginal opening) or scrotum (the bag containing the testicles).

PERINEURITIS
Inflammation around a nerve.

PERINEURIUM
Connective tissue covering around bundles of nerve fibers; the sheath surrounding each bundle of

fibers in a peripheral nerve.

PERIOD
Colloquial, the menses; an interval of division of time.

PERIODIC
Occurring at intervals.

PERIODIC APNEA OF THE NEWBORN
A condition of newborn infants characterized by an irregular breathing pattern with periods of rapid breathing followed by brief periods of not breathing (apnea); it is normal in most infants, often associated with REM (rapid eye movements) sleep.

Frequent episodes of apnea, not associated with REM sleep or periodic breathing patterns, may be a sign of neural, respiratory, circulatory or other disorder and are thought to be associated with sudden infant death syndrome (SIDS).

PERIODICITY
Recurrence at regular intervals of time.

PERIODONTAL
Surrounding a tooth; pertaining to the periodontium.

PERIODONTAL DISEASE
Inflammation or degeneration of tis-

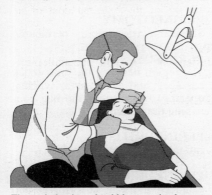

The periodontium should be examined regularly to prevent the occurrence of gum diseases.

sues that surround and support the teeth: gingiva, alveolar bone, periodontal ligament and cementum.

PERIODONTITIS
Inflammation or degeneration, or both, of the dental periosteum, alveolar bone, cementum and adjacent gingiva.

Chronic gingivitis often progresses to periodontitis in which the bone supporting the teeth and the connecting ligament (the periodontal membrane) are both damaged. On superficial examination the gingivae may appear fairly normal, there is destruction of tissue and the attachment of gingiva to tooth is lost leaving a space (pocket) between.

PERIODONTIUM
The tissues investing and supporting the teeth, including the cementum, periodontal ligament, alveolar bone, and gingiva.

PERIODONTOSIS
An uncommon widespread degeneration of the periodontal tissues with loss of alveolar bone so that teeth may be lost at an early age.

PERIORAL DERMATITIS
A red papular eruption of unknown cause occurring around the mouth and on the chin. The condition predominantly occurs in women aged 20 to 60. Tetracycline is the most effective treatment.

PERIOSTAL
Pertaining to the periosteum.

PERIOSTEUM
The fibrous membrane covering the surfaces of all bones, except at joint surfaces.

PERIOSTITIS
Inflammation of the periosteum.

PERIOSTOSIS
Abnormal deposition of periosteal

bone; the condition manifested by development of periosteomas.

PERIPARTUM
Occurring during the last month of gestation or the first few months after delivery, with reference to the mother.

PERIPHERAL
Pertaining to or situated near the periphery (outer edge).

PERIPHERAL NERVE
Those which connect the central nervous system to the rest of the body.

Some are sensory nerves, carrying sensation of pain, heat, cold, touch and the like from the body to the central nervous system. Some are motor nerves which carry impulses from the central nervous system to the muscles causing them to contract.

PERIPHERAL NERVOUS SYSTEM
The sensory and motor nerves outside the brain and spinal cord; it consists of 12 pairs of cranial nerves and 31 pairs of spinal nerves and the branches of these nerves that innervate the organs of the body.

PERIPHERAL NEUROPATHY (NEURITIS)
A syndrome of sensory, motor, reflex and vasomotor symptoms, single or in any combination, produced by disease of a single nerve, two or more nerves in separate areas, or many nerves simultaneously.

The lesions, usually degenerative and rarely accompanied by signs of inflammation, may be in the nerve roots or peripheral nerves.

PERIPHERAL RESISTANCE
The resistance by the arterioles to the flow of blood. An increase in peripheral resistance causes a rise in blood pressure.

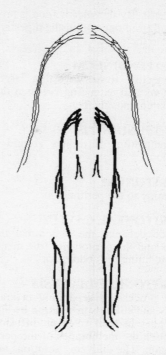

The peripheral nervous system consists of many nerve bundles carrying motor and sensory signals.

PERIPHERY
An outward surface or structure; the portion of a system outside the central region.

PERIPHLEBITIS
Inflammation of tissues around a vein, or of the external coat of a vein.

PERISALPINGITIS
Inflammation around the Fallopian tubes.

PERISTALSIS
A progressive wave of contraction occurring in alimentary tubes within the body which have longitudinal and transverse muscle fibers. There is a narrowing and shortening of a portion of the tube, which then relaxes while a lower portion becomes shortened and narrowed so that the tube's contents are forced

onwards. By this means food is propelled from one end of the digestive tract to the other.

PERITENDINEUM
Connective tissue investing larger tendons and extending between the fibers composing them.

PERITENDINITIS
Inflammation of tissues around a tendon.

PERITONEAL
Relating to the peritoneum.

PERITONEAL CAVITY
Space between the abdominal organs and the peritoneum (the membrane lining the abdomen).

PERITONEAL DIALYSIS
The process of separating crystalloids and colloids in solution by differences in their rates of diffusion through the membranes of the peritoneum. The dialyzing solutions are introduced into and removed from the peritoneal cavity, as either a continuous or an intermittent procedure.

PERITONEAL LAVAGE
Another name for peritoneal dialysis.

PERITONEUM
Serous membrane that covers the entire abdominal wall (parietal peritoneum) and envelops the organs contained in the abdomen (visceral peritoneum).

PERITONITIS
Acute inflammation of the visceral and parietal peritoneum. Although chemical and mechanical stimuli can cause peritoneal irritation, the most common causes are the infecting bacteria Escherichia coli and Streptococcus faecalis. Organisms or irritants escape from the intestinal tract most often following perforation of the appendix or a peptic ulcer. Peritonitis may also complicate any operation in the abdominal cavity, or may result from the spread of pelvic infection into the peritoneal cavity.

Clinical manifestations vary according to the cause and extent of the peritonitis. Onset is marked by severe localized or diffuse abdominal pain. In the early stages, as paralytic ileus develops, moderate abdominal distention is present, usually with nausea and vomiting and, occasionally, diarrhea, Direct abdominal tenderness, and marked muscle spasm are present. Sepsis will be shown by the following symptoms:
- fever;
- tachycardia;
- chills;
- rapid breathing;
- leukocytosis.

Treatment should be in the hands of a specialist in the hospital.

PERNICIOUS
Dangerous or likely to lead to death, as in pernicious anemia.

PERNICIOUS ANEMIA
A type of anemia characterized by defective red blood cell production, in the presence of megaloblasts in the bone marrow, and deterioration of nerve tissue in the spinal cord. It is caused by lack of intrinsic factor essential for the absorption of vitamin B12 or to a deficiency of vitamin B12 in the diet.

Symptoms include:
- pallor;
- anorexia;
- weight loss;
- fever;
- weakness;
- tingling of the extremities.

Treatment includes the administration of vitamin B12, folic acid, and iron.

PERONEAL NERVE
Nerve of the leg consisting of the deep peroneal nerve and the superfi-

cial peroneal nerve and originating from the common peroneal nerve.

The common peroneal nerve is the smaller of the branches into which the sciatic nerve divides, passing obliquely outward and downward from the popliteal space and to the neck of the fibula where it divides into the deep peroneal nerve and the superficial peroneal nerve.

The deep peroneal nerve is a nerve that arises as a branch of the common peroneal nerve where it forks between the fibula and the peroneus longus muscle and innervates or gives off branches innervating the muscles of the anterior part of the leg, the extensor digitorum brevis of the foot, and the skin between the big toe and the second toe.

The superficial peroneal nerve arises as a branch of the common peroneal nerve where it forks between the fibula and the peroneus longus muscle ends, innervates or supplies branches innervating the muscles of the anterior part of the leg and the skin on the lower anterior part of the leg, on the dorsum of the foot, on the lateral and medial sides of the foot, and between the toes.

PERONEUS
Any of three levels of the lower leg that arise especially from the fibula, inserting on one of the metatarsal bones of the foot, and including the peroneus brevis, peroneus longus, and peroneus tertius.

PERONEUS BREVIS
A peroneus muscle that arises from the side of the lower part of the fibula, ending in a tendon and assisting in everting and pronating the foot.

PERONEUS LONGUS
A peroneus muscle that arises from the head and side of the fibula, ending in a long tendon that inserts on the side of the first metatarsal bone

and the cuneiform bone on the medial side, and assisting in eversion and pronation of the foot.

PERONEUS TERTIUS
A branch of the extensor digitorum longus muscle that arises from the lower portion of the fibula, inserting on the dorsal surface of the base of the fifth metatarsal bone, and moving the foot dorsally and assisting in everting it.

PERSONALITY
The unique organization of traits, characteristics and mode of behavior of an individual, setting him apart from other individuals and at the same time determining how others react to him. Personality refers to the mental aspects of an individual in contrast to physique. Personality is thus shown to be the pattern of traits, characterizing an individual person, trait here meaning any psychological characteristic of a person, including dispositions to perceive different situations similarly and to react consistently despite changing stimulus conditions, values, abilities, motives, defenses and aspects of temperament, identity and personal style.

PERSONALITY DISORDER
A psychopathological condition or group of conditions in which an individual's entire life pattern is considered deviant or nonadaptive although he shows neither neurotic symptoms nor psychotic disorganization.

PERSONALITY INVENTORY
Any of several tests that attempt to characterize the personality of an individual by objective scoring of replies to a large number of questions concerning his own behavior and attitudes.

PERSONALITY TEST
Any of several tests that consists of standardized task designed to deter-

mine various aspects of the personality or the emotional status of the individual examined.

PERSPIRATION
Watery fluid secreted by the skin as a means of reducing body temperature. Sweating is common in hot climates, after exercise and in the resolution of fever, where the secretion and subsequent evaporation of sweat allow the skin and thus the body to be cooled.

PERTHES' DISEASE
A fairly common condition occurring in young people in which the growing bony center in the head of the femur (thigh bone) first becomes necrotic and is then absorbed and replaced by new bone. It is probably the result of a disorder of the blood vessels in the part, possibly by an injury, cutting off the blood supply to the growing center, which then dies.

PERTURBATION
A disturbed and unpleasant emotional state, usually connected with some state of mental confusion.

PERTUSSIS
An acute, highly communicable bacterial disease, characterized by a paroxysmal or spasmodic cough that usually ends in a prolonged, high-pitched, crowing inspiration. Pertussis is caused by Borderella pertussis and is endemic throughout the world. In a given locality it becomes epidemic every two or four years. In occurs in all ages, but about half of all cases occur before age two, since infants usually have no protective antibodies. Active immunization is very reliable. Erythromycin therapy commencing during the incubation period and continuing for 10 to 14 days may abort the infection in contact.

PERVERSION
A socially disapproved or prohibited form of conduct, particularly in sexual life. Interpretation varies and the term itself is becoming outmoded.

PES
The terminal organ of the leg, or lower limb; any footlike part.

PESSARY
(1) An instrument placed in the vagina to support the uterus or rectum or as a contraceptive device;
(2) a medicated vaginal suppository.

PESSIMISM
An inclination to emphasize adverse aspects, conditions, and possibilities or to expect the worst possible outcome.

PETECHIA
A minute red spot due to escape of a small amount of blood.

PETIT MAL
Epilepsy seen especially in children, in which there is sudden momentary unconsciousness with only minor myoclonic jerks.

PETROSAL BONE
The petrous portion of the temporal bone in man.

PEXIS
The fixation of matter by a tissue.

PEYER'S PATCHES
Collections of lymphoid tissue in the submucosa of the small intestine which contain lymphocytes, plasma cells, germinal centers and T-cell-dependent areas.

PEYRONIE'S DISEASE
Dysplasia of the cavernous sheath consisting of the investing fascia of the corpora of the penis.

PFANNENSTIEL'S INCISION
A long, horizontal abdominal incision made below the line of the pu-

bic hair and above the mons veneris down to and through the sheath of the rectus abdominis muscles but not the muscles themselves which are separated in the direction of their fibers.

PFEIFFER'S BACILLUS
A minute bacillus of the genus Haemophilus (Haemophilus influenzae) associated with acute respiratory infection and meningitis.

PFEIFFER'S PHENOMENON
Demonstration that cholera vibrio introduced into the peritoneal cavity of an immune guinea pig lose their mobility and are lysed regardless of the presence of cells.

pH
A measure of how much hydrogen gas is in the blood; it reflects the number of hydrogen ions that are present per liter. A pH of 7, which is neutral (neither acid nor alkaline), means there are 100 nano-equivalents of hydrogen ions per liter of blood. The body functions best when the blood pH is 7.40, that is, when it contains about 40 nano-equivalents of hydrogen ions per liter. Therefore, the blood is normally very slightly alkaline (on the base when considered on an acid-base relationship).

The pH is also measured in urine, spinal fluid, lung fluid, semen and many other body secretions.

PHACOCELE
Hernia of the eye lens.

PHACOLYSIS
Dissolution or discission of the eye lens.

PHACOSCLEROSIS
Hardening of the eye lens.

PHACOSCOPE
Instrument for viewing accommodative changes of the eye lens.

PHACOTOXIC
Exerting a deleterious effect upon the crystalline lens.

PHAGE TYPING
Identification of bacteria by testing their susceptibility to bacterial viruses.

PHAGOCYTE
A cell that consumes bacteria and other foreign matter. Fixed phagocytes, including macrophages, do not circulate in the blood but are found in the liver, bone marrow, spleen, and other areas. Free phagocytes, such as leukocytes, circulate in the blood.

PHAGOCYTIC INDEX
A measure of phagocytic activity determined by counting the number of bacteria ingested per phagocyte during a limited period of incubation of a suspension of bacteria and phagocytes in blood serum.

PHAGOCYTOSIS
Destruction of bacteria by phagocytes; the process of ingestion and usually of isolation or destruction of particulate material by cells that is a characteristic function of various leukocytes and reticuloendothelial cells and serves as an important bodily defense mechanism against infection by microorganisms and against occlusion of mucous surfaces or tissues by foreign particles and tissue debris.

PHAGOMANIA
An insatiable craving for food or an obsessive preoccupation with the subject of eating.

PHAGOPHOBIA
Neurotic fear of eating.

PHAKOMA
An occasional small, grayish–white tumor seen microscopically in the retina in tuberous sclerosis.

PHAKOMATOSIS
Any of four hereditary syndromes marked by disseminated hamartomas of the eye, skin, and brain.

PHALANGES
The bones of the fingers and toes.

PHALLIC CHARACTER
An individual with permanent and consistent patterns of functioning which reflect reaction formation to castration fear experienced during the oedipal stage.

PHALLICISM
The worship of the generative principle as symbolized by the phallus.

PHALLIC PHASE
In psychoanalytic theory, the period in psychosexual development between the ages of 2 and 6, when awareness of or self-manipulation of the genitals is a prime source of pleasure.

PHALLIC SADISM
Aggressive urges in the phallic phase of development during which the child interprets the sexual act as a violent, aggressive activity.

PHALLIC WOMAN
The idea of women with phallic attributes, usually either an infantile conception of the mother during the pre-oedipal phase of development, or a neurotic conception of women found in men with an aversion to women.

PHALLITIS
Inflammation of the penis.

PHALLOPLASTY
Surgical repair or reconstruction of the penis done to treat congenital abnormalities or injury.

PHALLUS
The penis.

PHANEROSIS
The process of becoming visible.

PHANTASM
An illusion, a phantom, an element of the imagination or disordered mind. The term is also used to designate an apparition of a living or dead person.

PHANTOM
(1) An image or impression not evoked by actual stimuli;
(2) a model of the body or a specific part thereof.

PHANTOM LIMB SYNDROME
A sense of pain, discomfort, or other sensation at a site where an arm or leg has been amputated.

PHANTOM PAIN
The sensation of having pain in a limb or part of a limb that was amputated.

PHANTOM TUMOR
An artificial swelling produced by gaseous distention of the intestine or contraction of a muscle.

PHARMAC(O)–
Word element: drug, medicine.

PHARMACEUTICAL
Pertaining to pharmacy or drugs.

PHARMACIST
One who is licensed to prepare and sell or dispense drugs and compounds, and to make up prescriptions. A pharmacist is a licensed, trained health professional concerned with the preparation and dispensing of drugs. Pharmacists may advise on the correct use of nonprescription drugs and may answer questions about the use of prescribed medication.

PHARMACODIAGNOSIS
Use of drugs or medicines in diagnosis.

PHARMACODYNAMICS

The study of biochemical and physiological effects of drugs and the mechanisms of their action, including the correlation of actions and effects of drugs with their chemical structure.

The term is also used to describe the effects or actions that a drug produces in the body.

For example, pain relief or bronchoconstriction are pharmacodynamic effects that stem from the chemical make-up of the drug concerned.

PHARMACOGENETICS

The study of the relationship between genetic factors and the nature of responses to drugs.

PHARMACOGNOSY

The branch of pharmacology dealing with natural drugs and their constituents; possible uses of medicinal substances in their natural or unprepared state.

PHARMACOKINETICS

The action of drugs in the body over a period of time, including the processes of absorption, distribution, localization in tissues, transformation, and excretion. The term is usually used to describe how the body deals with a drug, including how it is absorbed into the bloodstream, distributed to different tissues, broken down, and finally excreted from the body.

PHARMACOLOGIST

A scientist concerned with the study of drugs and their actions. Pharmacologists are responsible for research into new drugs. Clinical pharmacologists are usually qualified doctors.

They are primarily concerned with the actions of drugs in the treatment of specific disorders and with monitoring their effects on patients in clinical trials and in medical practice.

PHARMACOLOGY

The study of drugs, their chemistry, mode of action, routes of absorption, excretion and metabolism, drug interactions, toxicity and side-effects.

PHARMACOPEIA

A text containing all available drugs and pharmacological preparations, providing a vital source for accurate prescribing in medicine. It lists the following parameters of drugs:
- their properties and formulation;
- routes and doses of administration;
- mode of action;
- metabolism and excretion;
- known interaction with other drugs;
- contraindications;
- precautions in particular disease;
- toxicity and side effects.

Used as a reference book by doctors and pharmacists, a pharmacopeia describes sources, preparations, doses and tests that can be used to identify individual drugs and to determine their purity. It may also contain information about mechanisms of action, possible adverse effects, comments about the relative effectiveness and safety of a drug in treating a particular disorder, and price comparisons between similar drugs.

PHARMACOPSYCHOSIS

Any of a group of mental diseases due to alcohol, drugs, or poisons.

PHARMACOTHERAPY

Treatment of diseases with medicines.

PHARMACY

The preparation or dispensing of drugs and pharmacological substances used in medicine; also, the place where this is practiced. Most drugs are now formulated by drug companies and the pharmacist needs only measure them out and instruct the patient in their use. In the past, however, the pharmacist mixed numerous basic substances to prepare a variety of medicines, tonics, etc.

The term is not only used to describe the practice of preparing drugs and making up prescriptions, but it is also used to refer to the place where these activities are carried out.

PHARYNGALGIA
Pain in the throat (pharynx).

PHARYNGEAL BURSA
A crypt in the pharyngeal tonsil that represents a communication existing during fetal life between the pharynx and the tip of the notochord.

PHARYNGEAL CAVITY
The cavity of the pharynx that consists of a part continuous anteriorly with the nasal cavity by way of the nasopharynx, a part opening into the oral cavity by way of the isthmus of the fauces, and a part continuous posteriorly with the esophagus and opening into the larynx by way of the epiglottis.

PHARYNGEAL PLEXUS
A plexus formed by branches of the glossopharyngeal, vagus, and sympathetic nerves supplying the muscles and mucous membranes of the pharynx and adjoining parts.

PHARYNGEAL TONSIL
Either of two masses of lymph tissue at the back of the nasopharynx behind the posterior nares.

PHARYNGECTOMY
Surgical excision of the pharynx.

PHARYNGISMUS
Spasm of the muscles of the pharynx.

PHARYNGITIS
Inflammation of the pharynx (back part of the throat).

PHARYNGOLARYNGITIS
Inflammation of the pharynx and larynx (voice apparatus).

PHARYNGOPARALYSIS
Paralysis of the muscles of the throat (pharynx).

PHARYNGOSCOPE
An instrument for inspecting the throat (pharynx).

PHARYNGOSPASM
Spasm of the muscles of the throat (pharynx).

PHARYNX
The back of the throat where the mouth (oropharynx) and nose (nasopharynx) pass back into the esophagus. It contains specialized muscles for swallowing. The food and air channels are kept functionally separate so that swallowing does not interfere with breathing and speech.

PHENOCOPY
An individual with all the hallmarks of a particular genetic disorder but with no hereditary cause apparent in his pedigree.

PHENODEVIANT
An individual whose phenotype differs significantly from that of the typical phenotype in the population.

PHENOL
An extremely poisonous compound, obtained by distillation of coal tar; used as an antimicrobial. Ingestion or absorption of phenol through the skin causes colic, weakness, collapse, and local irritation and corrosion. In low concentration phenol is used in throat lozenges and sprays.

PHENOLPHTHALEIN
A white crystalline compound formed by the interaction of phenol and phthalic anhydride, used medically and to indicate the presence of

alkalis, which turn it red, and of acids, which decolorize. The drug is also used for the relief of constipation.

Possible side effects include:
- potassium loss (thirst, weakness, heartbeat irregularity)
- belching;
- cramps;
- burning on urination.

PHENOL RED
A red crystalline acid-base indicator, also used in medicinal analysis.

PHENOLSULFONPHTHALEIN
A dye used in kidney function tests. Urine levels are measured at regular intervals after injection of 6 mg, to test the excretory capacity of the kidney tubules. Rate of excretion is decreased in kidney and some urinary tract diseases, increased in some liver diseases.

PHENOMENAL SELF
Image of the self that each person perceives in his own way, based on the evidence he senses.

PHENOMENOLOGY
The way in which an individual perceives and interprets events and his relationship to them in contrast both to his objective responses to stimuli and to any inferred unconscious motivation for his behavior. The term is also used to designate a psychology based on the theory that an individual's behavior is determined by his phenomenology.

PHENOMENON
Any sign of objective symptom; any observable occurrence or fact.

PHENOMENOLOGY
The systematic investigation of conscious experience as experience, regarded by some as the true method of approach to psychology.

PHENOTYPE
The appearance of, and charac-

teristics actually present in an organism, as contrasted with its genotype (its genetic make-up). heterozygotes and homozygotes with a dominant gene have the same phenotype but differing genotypes. Organisms may also have an identical genotype but differing phenotype due to environmental influences.

PHENYLALANINE
An amino acid that accumulates in excessive amounts in phenylketonuria, an inherited enzyme deficiency disease that causes mental retardation if not diagnosed and treated soon after birth.

PHENYLKETONURIA
An inborn error of metabolism, characterized by a virtual absence of phenylalanine hydroxylase activity and an elevation of phenylalanine in the blood. This condition frequently results in mental retardation. With untreated phenylketonuria, prognosis, while not life-threatening, is poor for intellectual development. Early and well-maintained treatment makes normal development possible and prevents involvement of the central nervous system.

Treatment consists in limiting the phenylalanine intake of the child so that his essential amino acid requirement is met but not exceeded.

PHENYLPYRUVIC ACID
An intermediate product of phenylalanine metabolism; present in the urine in certain metabolic diseases of the newborn.

PHEOCHROMOCYTOMA
A tumor which arises in the adrenal glands. It produces and releases into the bloodstream large quantities of norepinephrine and epinephrine. These powerful natural stimulants may then create such symptoms as high blood pressure, elevated heart rate, headaches, anxiety and excessive sweating.

PHERESIS
Any procedure in which blood is withdrawn from a donor, a portion (plasma, leukocytes, etc.) is separated and retained, and the remainder is retransfused into the donor.

PHEROMONE
A substance secreted to the outside of the body and perceived (as by smell) by other individuals of the same species, releasing specific behavior in the percipient.

PHILADELPHIA CHROMO-SOME
An abnormal short chromosome 22 that is found in the hematopoietic cells of persons suffering from chronic myelogenous leukemia and lacking the major part of its long arm which has usually undergone translocation to chromosome 9.

PHILTRUM
The vertical groove in the median portion of the upper lip.

PHIMOSIS
Excessive narrowing of the foreskin in front of the penis so that it cannot be withdrawn over the glans (the bulbous tip).

PHI PHENOMENON
Apparent motion resulting from an orderly sequence of stimuli, as lights flashed in rapid succession a short distance apart on a sign, without any actual motion being presented to the eye.

PHLEBITIS
Inflammation of the veins, usually causing thrombosis (thrombophlebitis) and obstruction to blood flow. It is common in the superficial veins of the legs, especially varicose veins, and visceral veins close to inflamed organs or abscesses.

PHLEBOGRAM
A radiogram of a vein with contrast medium.

PHLEBOGRAPHY
Radiography of a vein filled with contrast medium; the graphic recording of the venous pulse.

PHLEBOLITH
A venous calculus or concretion.

PHLEBOPLASTY
Plastic repair of a vein.

PHLEBOSCLEROSIS
Fibrous thickening of the walls of a vein.

PHLEBOSTASIS
Retardation of blood flow in veins; temporary sequestration of a portion of blood from the general circulation by compressing the veins of an extremity.

PHLEBOTHROMBOSIS
An abnormal condition marked by the formation of a clot within a vein without prior inflammation of the wall of the vein; it is associated with prolonged bed rest, surgery, pregnancy, and other conditions in which blood flow coagulates more quickly than normal. The affected area, usually the leg, may become swollen and tender. The danger is that the clot may become dislodged and travel to the lungs.

PHLEBOTOMY
The act or practice of opening a vein for letting blood.

PHLEGM
Viscid mucus excreted in abnormally large quantities from the respiratory tract.

PHLEGMATIC PERSONALITY
Characterized by slowness, apathy and listlessness due to an excess of phlegm.

PHLEGMON
An inflammation characterized by a spreading cellulitis (affecting superficial tissues).

PHOBIA

A neurosis characterized by exaggerated anxiety on confrontation with a specific object or situation, or the anxiety itself. Classic phobias are agoraphobia (an abnormal fear or dread of open or public places) and claustrophobia (an abnormal dread of being confined in closed rooms or small places).

Specialists classify phobias into three major groups:
- agoraphobia;
- social phobias, such as extreme stage fright;
- simple phobias, or fear of a specific object or situation, such as thunderstorms or height.

It is only very recently that doctors have begun to make real strides in helping phobics overcome their fears and live normal lives. Two new paths for treating phobics are being taken: medication and behavioral therapy.

PHOBIC ANXIETY

Anxiety produced by some external object or situation out of all proportion to its real dangerousness.

PHOBIC REACTION

The unconscious neurotic pattern of attempted defense, characterized by a phobia or phobias as the most prominent feature of the neurotic reaction and by the predilection to develop phobic manifestations under appropriate conditions of physical stress.

Displacement from the original internal source of threat and danger has taken place to an external object-source.

PHOTOPHOBIA

Morbid fear of being afraid; excessive fear of acquiring a phobia.

PHOCOMELIA

Congenital absence of the proximal portion of a limb or limbs, the hand or feet being attached to the trunk by a small irregular bone.

PHON

The unit of loudness on a scale beginning at zero for the faintest audible sound and corresponding to the decibel scale of sound intensity with the number of phons of a given sound equal to the decibels of a pure 1000-cycle tone judged by the average listener to be equal in loudness to the given sound.

PHON(O)–

Word element: sound, voice, speech.

PHONASTHENIA

Weakness of the voice; difficult phonation from fatigue.

PHONATION

The utterance of vocal sounds.

PHONEME

The smallest unit of sound in speech; the basic unit of spoken language; a member of the set of the smallest units of speech that serve to distinguish one utterance from another in a language or dialect.

PHONEMICS

A branch of linguistic analysis that consists of the study of phonemes.

PHONETICS

Science of vocal sounds; the study and classification of the sounds made in spoken utterances. The term is also used to designate the system of speech sounds of a language or group of languages.

PHONIATRICS

The treatment of speech defects.

PHONICS

The science of sound; a method of teaching beginners to read and pronounce words by learning the phonetic value of letters, letter groups, and syllables.

PHONIC SPASM

Spasms of the throat muscles

when attempting to speak.

PHONISM
A sensation of hearing produced by the effect of something seen, felt, tasted, smelled, or thought of.

PHONOCARDIOGRAPHY
The graphic representation of heart sounds and murmurs; by extension, the term also includes pulse tracings.

PHONOCATHETER
A device similar to a conventional catheter, with a microphone.

PHONOMETER
A device for measuring intensity of sounds.

PHORIA
Tendency of the visual axis of one eye to deviate when the other eye is covered and fusion is prevented.

PHOSE
Any subjective visual sensation.

PHOSPHATASE
An enzyme in milk which acts on calcium and phosphorus. It is believed pasteurization destroys it.

PHOSPHATE
Any of numerous chemical compounds related to phosphoric acid.

PHOSPHATEMIA
An excess of phosphates in the blood.

PHOSPHATURIA
An excess of phosphates in the urine.

PHOSPHENE
A sensation of light due to a stimulus other than light rays, for instance, a mechanical stimulus.

PHOSPHOCREATINE
An organic compound, found in muscle tissue, which furnishes the energy for contractions.

PHOSPHOLIPID
One of a group of lipoidal compounds, such as lecithin and cephalin, which are phosphoric esters and are found in living cells throughout nature.

PHOSPHORIC ACID
The most important oxygen acid of phosphorus, used to make phosphate salts for fertilizers and detergents.

PHOSPHORISM
Chronic phosphorus poisoning. Ingestion or inhalation to phosphorus produces the following symptoms:
- toothache;
- anorexia;
- weakness;
- anemia.

PHOSPHORURIA
The presence of free phosphorus in the urine.

PHOSPHORUS
An essential mineral; important to the strengthening of bones and teeth, maintaining the acid-alkaline balance in the blood and the functioning of brain cells. Phosphorus and calcium are closely linked and must be absorbed in proper proportions in order to be effective. Rich natural sources are nuts, meats, legumes (especially soybeans), milk products and bone meal. Phosphorus is also available as a supplement, usually in combination with other minerals.

PHOSPHORUS CYCLE
The process by which phosphorus is circulated through the biosphere, or living world, and returned to an inorganic state for recycling.

PHOSPHORYLATION
The metabolic process of introducing a phosphate group into an organic molecule.

PHOSPHORYLATION, OXIDATIVE

The formation of high-energy phosphate bonds by phosphorylation of ADP to ATP; it occurs in the mitochondria of the cell.

PHOT(O)–

Word element: light.

PHOTOACTIVATION

The process of activation of a substance by means of radiant energy and especially light.

PHOTALGIA

Pain, as in the eye, caused by light.

PHOTISM

A visual sensation produced by the effect of something heard, felt, tasted, smelled, or thought of.

PHOTOACTIVE

Reacting chemically to sunlight or ultraviolet radiation.

PHOTOCATALYSIS

Promotion or stimulation of a chemical reaction by light.

PHOTOCHEMISTRY

The branch of chemistry dealing with the chemical properties or effects of light rays or other radiation.

PHOTOCOAGULATION

Condensation of protein material by the controlled use of an intense beam of light (for instance, argon laser) used especially in the treatment of retinal detachment and destruction of abnormal retinal vessels of tumor masses inside the eyeball.

PHOTODERMATITIS

An abnormal state of the skin in which light is an important causative factor.

PHOTOINACTIVATION

The retardation or prevention of a chemical reaction by radiant energy (as light).

PHOTOLYSIS

Chemical decomposition by light.

PHOTOLUMINESCENCE

The quality of being luminescent after exposure to light.

PHOTOMETER

A device for measuring intensity of light.

PHOTOMICROGRAPH

A photograph of an object as seen through an ordinary light microscope.

PHOTON

A particle (quantum) of radiant energy.

PHOTO-OPHTHALMIA

Inflammation of the eye caused by intense light, such as that produced in oxyacetylene welders who forget to wear goggles.

PHOTOPAROXYSMAL

Denoting an abnormal electroencephalographic response to photic stimulation (brief flashes of light), marked by diffuse paroxysmal discharge recorded as spike-wave complexes; the response may be accompanied by minor seizures.

PHOTOPERIOD

The period of time per day that an organism is exposed to daylight.

PHOTOPERIODISM

The physiologic and behavioral reactions brought about in organisms by changes in the duration of daylight and darkness.

PHOTOPHOBIA

Abnormal visual intolerance to light, often associated with albinism, drug-induced pupil dilation, migraine, encephalitis, measles, and other diseases.

PHOTOPHTHALMIA

Ophthalmia due to exposure to intense light, as in snow blindness.

PHOTOPSIA
Appearance as of sparks or flashes, in irritation of the retina.

PHOTOPSIN
The protein moiety of the cones of the retina that combines with retinal chemicals to form photochemical pigments.

PHOTOPTARMOSIS
Sneezing caused by the influence of light.

PHOTOPTOMETER
An instrument for measuring visual acuity by determining the smallest amount of light that will render an object just visible.

PHOTORECEPTIVE
Sensitive to stimulation by light.

PHOTORECEPTOR
A nerve end-organ or receptor sensitive to light.

PHOTORETINITIS
Damage to the retina caused by looking at the sun without adequate protection.

PHOTOSENSITIVE
Exhibiting abnormally heightened sensitivity to sunlight.

PHOTOSENSITIZATION
The development of abnormally heightened reactivity of the skin to sunlight.

PHOTOSENSITIZING MEDICATIONS
Medicines that can cause abnormally heightened skin reactions to the effects of sunlight.

PHOTOSYNTHESIS
A chemical combination caused by the action of light; specifically, the formation of carbohydrates from carbon dioxide and water in the chlorophyll tissue of plant under the influence of light.

PHOTOTAXIS
The movement of cells and microorganisms under the influence of light.

PHOTOTHERAPY
The use of strong light to treat disorders such as acne and hyperbilirubinemia of the newborn.

PHOTOTOXIC
A toxic effect triggered by exposure to light.

PHOTOTROPHIC
Capable of deriving energy from light.

PHOTOTROPISM
The tendency of an organism to turn or move toward or away from light.

PHREN
The diaphragm (the muscular sheet separating the chest and abdominal cavity); the mind.

PHRENALGIA
Depression, melancholia; pain in the diaphragm.

PHRENASTHENIA
Paralysis of the diaphragm; feebleness of mind.

PHRENOLOGY
The theory that the various faculties of the mind occupy distinct and separate areas in the brain cortex, and that the predominance of certain faculties can be predicted from modifications of the parts of the skull overlying the areas where these faculties are located.

PHRENOSPASM
Spasm of the diaphragm.

PHRICTOPATHIC SENSATIONS
Tactual sensations, indefinitely lo-

calized, and of tingling and peculiarly irritating character.

PHTHIRIUS
A genus of lice, including Phthirius pubis (the pubic, or crab, louse), which infests the hair of the pubic region, and sometimes the eyebrows and eyelashes.

PHTHISIS
Wasting of the body; an almost obsolete term for tuberculosis.

PHTHISIS BULBI
Shrinkage of the eyeball.

PHYCOMYCETES
A group of fungi comprising the common water, leaf, and bread moulds.

PHYCOMYCETES
Any of a group of acute fungal diseases caused by members of Phycomycetes.

PHYCOMYCOSIS
Any infection caused by fungi of the order Phycomycetes. These fungi inhabit soil and do not usually produce disease in humans.

PHYLAXIS
The activity of the body in defending itself against infection.

PHYLOGENY
The complete developmental history of a race or group of organisms.

PHYMA
A skin tumor or tubercle.

PHYSICAL
Pertaining to the body, to material things, or to physics.

PHYSICAL ANTHROPOLOGY
Anthropology concerned with the comparative study of human evolution, variation, and classification especially through measurement, examination and observation.

PHYSICAL DIAGNOSIS
Diagnosis made after inspection, palpation, percussion or auscultation.

PHYSICAL ALLERGY
A condition in which allergic symptoms and signs are produced by exposure to cold, sunlight, heat or mild trauma.
   The underlying cause is unknown in most cases.

PHYSICAL DIAGNOSIS
Diagnosis made after inspection, palpitation, percussion or auscultation.

PHYSICAL EDUCATION
Instruction designed to further the health, growth and athletic capacity of the body. It may include gymnastics, sports and Oriental techniques such as yoga.

PHYSICAL EXAMINATION
Examination of the body by auscultation, palpitation, percussion and inspection.

PHYSICAL SIGN
An indication of bodily condition that can be directly perceived, as by auscultation, by an examining physician.

PHYSICAL THERAPY
Another name for physiotherapy; the treatment of disease by physical and mechanical means, as massage, regulated exercise, water, light, heat, and electricity.

PHYSICIAN
One legally qualified to practice medicine.

PHYSIOGNOMY
Study of personality that involves determining a person's personality from the general configuration of the body.

PHYSIOLOGICAL AGE
Rating, on the analogy of mental age, of an individual, on the basis of a scale determined by the condition of important physiological terms, such as the vascular system, reproductive system, etc.

PHYSIOLOGICAL COMPENSATION
Enlargement of an organ in an attempt to compensate for a deficiency caused by the failure of another organ.

PHYSIOLOGICAL JAUNDICE
Mild yellowing that occurs at birth in the baby and passes off in a few days.

PHYSIOLOGICAL LIMIT
Maximum speed of efficiency attainable in a motor act, because of the physiological nature of the neuromuscular mechanisms involved.

PHYSIOLOGICAL PSYCHOLOGY
A branch of psychology that deals with the effects of normal and pathological physiological processes on mental life.

PHYSIOLOGY
The study of function in living organisms. Based on anatomy, physiology seeks to demonstrate the manner in which organs, tissue, and cells perform their tasks, and in which the body is organized and maintained in a state of homeostasis.

PHYSIOPATHOLOGY
A branch of biology or medicine that combines physiology and pathology especially in the study of altered bodily function in disease.

PHYSIOTHERAPY
An aid to the treatment of the sick or injured by means of physical agents. This includes massage, physical or therapeutic exercises, various forms of light, heat, and electricity, ultraviolet light, air and water. Physiotherapy is used extensively in restoring function of wasted, stiff or contracted muscles after injury.

PHYSIQUE
The body organization, development, and structure.

PHYTOPARASITE
Any parasitic vegetable organism or species.

PHYTOTHERAPY
The use of vegetable drugs in medicine.

PHYTOTOXIN
An exotoxin produced by certain species of higher plants; any toxin of plant origin.

PIA MATER
The innermost of the three meninges covering the brain and spinal cord. It is highly vascularized and closely applied to the brain and spinal cord, nourishing the nerve cells.

PICA
Persistent eating of a nonnutritive substance. Infants with this disorder typically eat paint, plaster, string, hair, or cloth. Older children may eat animal droppings, sand, insects, leaves, or pebbles. There is no aversion to food.

PICK'S DISEASE
A form of presenile dementia occurring in middle aged people, characterized by the following symptoms:
- early, slowly progressive changes of character and social deterioration;
- leading to impairment of intellect, memory and language functions;
- apathy;
- euphoria.

Women are more affected than men and there may be a hereditary pattern of transmission, probably determined by an incompletely penetrant autosomal gene.

The brain suffers a generalized atrophy with circumscribed shrinkage of the frontal and temporal lobes but without occurrence of senile plaques and neurofibrillary tangles.

PICKWICKIAN SYNDROME
An abnormal condition in which there is extreme obesity, often with decreased lung function and sleepiness.

PICORNAVIRUS
An extremely small, ether-resistant RNA virus, one of the group comprising the enteroviruses and rhinoviruses.

PICROTOXIN
A poisonous bitter crystalline compound found especially in cocculus that is a compound of picrotoxinin and picrotin and is a stimulant and convulsant drug administered intravenously as an antidote for poisoning by overdoses of barbiturates.

PICTURE COMPLETION TEST
A type of intelligence test in which the subject is required to find the missing parts in a picture. It is regarded to be a performance form of the completion test.

PICTURE INTERPRETATION TEST
A type of intelligence test in which the subject is required to say what a picture is about, the grade of mental level being assessed according to the nature of the response.

PIEDRA
A fungal disease of the hair in which white or black nodules of fungi form on the shafts.

PIERRE ROBIN SYNDROME
A congenital defect of the face characterized by micrognathia, abnormal smallness of the tongue, cleft palate, absence of the gag reflex, and sometimes accompanied by bilateral eye defects, glaucoma, or retinal detachment.

PIESESTHESIA
The sense by which pressure stimuli are felt.

PIESIMETER
Instrument for testing the sensitiveness of the skin to pressure.

PIGEON BREAST
A congenital condition in which there is abnormal forward projection of the breastbone; it is usually harmless and requires no treatment.

PIGMENT
Any coloring matter of the body; a paint-like medicinal preparation to be applied to the skin.

PIGMENTATION
The deposition of coloring matter; the coloration or discoloration of a part by a pigment.

PIGMENTOPHAGE
Any pigment-destroying cell, especially such a cell of the hair.

PILE(S)
Hemorrhoid(s).

PILL
A small globular or oval medicated mass to be swallowed.

PILL, ENTERIC-COATED
One enclosed in a substance that dissolves only when it has reached the intestines.

PILLAR
A body part likened to a pillar or column, as the margin of the external inguinal ring.

PILLAR OF THE FAUCES
Either of two curved folds on each

side, that bound the fauces and enclose the tonsil,

PILLAR OF FORNIX
Either of the anterior and posterior diverging extensions of the fornix of the brain.

PILLION
A temporary artificial leg.

PILOCYSTIC
Hollow or cyst-like, and containing hair.

PILOERECTION
Erection of a hair.

PILOMOTOR
Pertaining to the arrector muscles, the contraction of which produces goose flesh and piloerection.

PILOMOTOR REFLEX
Erection of the hairs of skin in response to emotional stress, skin irritation, or cold.

PILONIDAL FISTULA
An abnormal tract containing hairs extending from an opening of the skin, usually near the cleft at the top of the buttocks.

PILOSE
Hairy; covered with hair.

PILOSEBACEOUS
Pertaining to the hair follicles and the sebaceous glands.

PIMPLE
A small, inflamed, pus-containing swelling on the skin usually due to infection of a pore obstructed with sebaceous secretions.

PIN
In orthopedics, a rodlike metal device used to secure fragments of a bone.

PINCEMENT
Pinching of the flesh in massage.

PINEAL
Pertaining to the pineal body.

PINEAL BODY
Pineal gland, a gland-like structure situated over the brain stem and which appears to be a vestigial remnant of a functioning endocrine gland in other animals. It has no known function in man.

PINEALOBLASTOMA
Tumor of the pineal gland in which the pineal cells are not well differentiated.

PINEALOCYTE
An epithelioid cell of the pineal body.

PINEALOMA
A tumor of the pineal body composed of tumor nests of large epithelial cells.

PINKEYE
Contagious inflammation of the mucous membrane of the eyelids, affecting humans and certain animals.

PINK SPOT
The appearance of pulp through the attenuated hard tissue of the crown of a tooth affected with resorption of dentine.

PINNA
The largely cartilaginous projecting portion of the external ear.

PINOCYTOSIS
The ingestion of soluble materials by cells.

PINTA
A chronic skin disease that is endemic in tropical America, occurring successively as an initial papule, a generalized eruption, and a patchy loss of pigment, and that is caused by a spirochete of the genus Treponema (Treponema careteum), morphologically indistinguishable

from the causative agent of syphilis.

PINWORM INFESTATION
An intestinal infestation by Enterobius vermicularis, characterized by perianal itching.

The pinworm is the most common parasite infecting children in temperate climates. The prevalence of Enterobius in the general childhood population is at least 20 percent; for institutionalized children it is as high as 85 percent.

Since the parasitic relationship is seldom harmful, prevalence is high, and reinfestation is probable, treatment is usually not indicated.

However, most parents are shocked by the concept of infestation and actively seek treatment even when their children have had pinworms many times. Specific drugs will eradicate the infection in most cases.

PIPETTE
A glass or transparent plastic tube used in measuring or transferring small quantities of liquid or gas.

PIRIFORMIS
A muscle that arises from the front of the sacrum, passes out of the pelvis through the greater sciatic foramen, inserting into the upper border of the greater trochanter of the femur. The function of the piriformis is rotating the thigh laterally.

PIRIFORM LOBE
The lateral olfactory gyrus and the hippocampal gyrus taken together.

PIRIGOFF'S AMPUTATION
Amputation of the foot through the articulation of the ankle with retention of part of the calcaneus.

PISIFORM
Resembling a pea in shape and size.

PITCH
(1) A dark, more or less viscous residue from distillation of tar and other substances;
(2) the quality of sound dependent on the frequency of vibration of the waves producing it.

PITCHER'S ELBOW
Pain and disability associated with the tearing of tendons from their attachment on the epicondyle of the humerus often with involvement of tissues within and around the elbow joint.

PITTING
The action or process of forming pits, as in acned skin, a tooth, or a dental restoration.

PITTING EDEMA
Edema of such severity that pressure on the surface by the fingers leaves behind small depressions or pits.

PITUICYTE
One of the pigmented more or less fusiform cells of the stalk and posterior lobe of the pituitary gland that are usually considered to be derived from neuroglial cells.

PITUITARY GLAND
Major endocrine gland just below the brain, under the control of the adjacent hypothalamus and in its turn controlling other endocrine glands.

The posterior pituitary is a direct extension of certain cells in the hypothalamus and secretes vasopressin and oxytocin into the blood stream.

The anterior pituitary develops separately and consists of several cell types which secrete different hormones including:
- growth hormone;
- follicle stimulating hormone (FSH);
- luteinizing hormone (LH);
- thyreotropic hormone;
- adrenocorticotropic hormone (ACTH);
- prolactin.

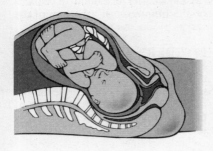

The exchange of materials between fetal and maternal circulation occurs through a structure called the placenta. It is attached to the navel of the fetus by the umbilical cord, and it communicates with the mother through countless small blood vessels that emerge from the uterine wall.

PITUITARY MYXEDEMA
Myxedema caused by deficiency of thyrotropin secreted by the anterior of the pituitary gland.

PITUITARY PORTAL SYSTEM
A portal system supplying blood to the anterior lobe of the pituitary gland through veins connecting the capillaries of the median eminence of the hypothalamus with those of the anterior lobe.

PITYRIASIS
Originally, a group of skin diseases marked by the formation of fine, branny scales, but now used only with a modifier.

PITYRIASIS ALBA
A chronic condition with patchy scaling and hypopigmentation of the skin of the face, occurring most often in children and young adults characterized by circumscribed round or oval patches of depigmentation or less than normal pigmentation.

PITYRIASIS ROSACEA
A self limited, mild, inflammatory skin disease characterized by scaly lesions, possibly due to an unidentified infectious agent. It may occur at any age but is seen most frequently in young adults. In temperate climates, incidence is highest during spring and autumn.

PITYROSPORUM
A genus of yeast-like fungi, including Pityrosporon orbiculare, a species customarily found on normal skin but capable of causing a specific skin disease (Tinea versicolor) in susceptible host.

PIVOT JOINT
An anatomical articulation that consists of a bony pivot in a ring of bone and ligament, as that of the odontoid and atlas, and that permits rotatory movement only.

PIVOT TOOTH
An artificial crown attached to the root of a tooth by a usually metallic pin.

PKU
Abbreviation of phenylketonuria.

PLACEBO
A tablet, syrup or other form of medication which is inactive and is prescribed in lieu of active preparations, e.g., in experimental studies of drug effectiveness. Placebos are frequently used in clinical trials of new drugs. A physician may sometimes administer a placebo because of the emotional or psychological uplift it may give to a patient convinced that his or her condition calls for some form of drug treatment.

PLACENTA
Specialized structure derived from the uterus lining and part of the embryo after implantation; it separates and yet ensures a close and extensive contact between the maternal (uterine) and fetal (umbilical) blood circulation. This allows nutrients and oxygen to pass from the mother to the fetus, and waste products to

pass in the reverse direction.

The placenta thus enables the embryo and fetus to live as a parasite, dependent on the maternal organs. Gonadotropins are produced by the placenta which prepares the maternal body for delivery and the breasts for lactation.

The placenta is delivered after the child at birth (the afterbirth) by separation of the blood vessel layers; placental disorders may cause hemorrhage or fetal immaturity.

PLACENTA ACCRETA
One abnormally adherent to the muscle of the womb (myometrium), with partial or complete absence of the decidua basalis.

PLACENTA CIRCUMVALLATA
One encircled with a dense, raised, ring, the attached membranes being doubled back over the edge of the placenta.

PLACENTAL BARRIER
A semipermeable membrane made up of placental tissue and limiting the character and amount of material exchanged between mother and fetus.

PLACENTAL LACTOGEN
Human placental lactogen (HPL), also known as chorionic somatomammotropin (HCG), is a hormone produced by the placenta (the blood supply around the fetus during pregnancy). It first appears in the blood after about the fifth week of pregnancy and gradually increases in amount until the baby is born, after which it disappears.

Its appearance and gradual increase are an indication of normal pregnancy. Blood is taken from a vein and the serum is tested.

PLACENTAL SCAN
A scanning procedure performed on a pregnant woman after intravenous injection of a radioactive substance to locate the fetus and placenta and detect intrauterine bleeding, which would require immediate treatment.

PLACENTAL TRANSMISSION
The conveyance of medicines or disease products through the placental circulation of the mother into her baby.

PLACENTA PREVIA
One located in the lower uterine segment, so that it partially or entirely covers or adjoins the internal opening of the cervix canal. The placenta is implanted abnormally in the uterus so that it partially or completely covers the outlet from the uterus to the vagina; it is a common cause of bleeding in late pregnancy. If severe hemorrhage occurs immediate Cesarean section is required to save the mother's life. If the placenta is next to, but not blocking, the uterine outlet, vaginal delivery may be attempted.

PLACENTATION
The series of events following implantation of the embryo and leading to development of the placenta.

PLACENTOGRAPHY
Radiological visualization of the placenta after injection of a contrast medium.

PLAGUE
An acute febrile, infectious, highly fatal disease due to Yersinia pestis, beginning with chills and fever, quickly followed by prostration, and frequently attended by delirium, headache, vomiting, and diarrhea. The disease is transmitted to man by flea bites, or communicated from patient to patient.

PLAGUE, BUBONIC
Infectious disease caused by a bacillus (Yersinia pestis) and characterized by:
– inguinal, axillary or cervical adenitis;

– rarely without fever;
– complication: hemorrhages.
The incubation period amounts to 2-6 days. The transmission is by bites of fleas of wild rodents in rural areas; bites of rat fleas, cat fleas and human fleas in urban plague; person-to-person transmission by airborne droplets and fomites in pneumonic plague. The treatment is by antibiotics.

PLAGUE, PNEUMONIC
Lung disease caused by a bacillus (Yersinia pestis) and characterized by:
– sudden onset;
– sputum at first mucous and then rusty or bright red;
– cough developing in 24 hours;
– fever;
– severe chills.
When untreated death occurs within 48 hours. The incubation period amounts to 2-3 days. The transmission is by respiratory droplets and freshly solid articles. The disease occurs in general as a complication of bubonic plague. The treatment is by antibiotics.

PLANE, AXIAL
One parallel with the long axis of a body structure.

PLANIGRAPHY
Roentgenographic technique that makes on a film sharp images of structures in a predetermined plane and blurs images of other structures below and above.

PLANNED PARENTHOOD
The practice of birth control measures, as contraception, designed to regulate the number and spacing of children in a family.

PLANOMANIA
An abnormal desire to wander and to have no social restraints.

PLANTA PEDIS
The sole of the foot.

PLANTALGIA
Pain in the sole of the foot.

PLANTAR
Relating or belonging to the sole of the foot.

PLANTAR FLEXION
Movement of the foot that flexes the foot or toes downward toward the sole.

PLANTAR INTEROSSEUS
Any of three small muscles of the plantar aspect of the foot each of which lies along the plantar side of one of the third, fourth, and fifth toes facing the second toe, arising from the metatarsal bone of the toe along which it lies, inserting into its proximal phalanx, and acting to flex the proximal phalanx and extend the distal phalanges of its toe and to abduct its toe toward the second toe.

PLANTAR REFLEX
Reflex in which drawing a blunt instrument or stroking the outer part of the sole from the heel toward the little toe causes the toes to bunch and curl downward. In those over the age of 1.5-2 years, an upward movement of the big toe after this stimulus is usually a sign of neurological damage, the Babinski sign.

PLANTAR WART
A wart occurring on the sole that, because of pressure, develops a callus ring around its soft center and becomes painful. Treatment includes cryosurgery, electro-desiccation, and application of topical aids.

PLAQUE
A small, flat, rounded, abnormal formation or area, as on the skin.

PLASMA
The fluid portion of the blood, including fibrinogen; distinguished from serum from which fibrinogen has been separated.

PLASMA CELL

A mononuclear cell with abundant, strongly basophilic cytoplasm, prevalent in the extracellular plasma of lymphoid tissue but relatively uncommon in peripheral blood.

PLASMA CELL DYSCRASIAS

A group of clinically and biochemically diverse disorders characterized by the disproportionate proliferation of one clone of cells normally engaged in immunoglobulin synthesis.

The disorders vary from asymptomatic and apparently stable conditions to progressive, overtly neoplastic disorders. The cause is unknown.

No treatment of these disorders is recommended; patients are being observed for change in status at four- to six-months intervals.

PLASMACYTOMA

A neoplasm of plasma cells, occurring in bone marrow usually in association with multiple myeloma, or less commonly occurring in soft tissues, especially those of the upper respiratory tract.

PLASMACYTOSIS

An excess of plasma cells in the blood.

PLASMA MEMBRANE

A semipermeable limiting layer of cell protoplasm consisting of three molecular layers of which the inner and outer are composed of protein while the middle layer is composed of a double layer of fat molecules.

PLASMAPHERESIS

The removal of plasma from withdrawn blood, which has been used to identify and analyze plasma proteins for diagnostic purposes and has been tried experimentally in the treatment of certain diseases.

PLASMA PROTEIN

Any of various proteins in blood plasma, including fibrinogen and prothrombin, important for blood coagulation and gamma globulins, which are important in immune responses.

PLASMA RENIN ACTIVITY

The action of renin, an enzyme secreted by the kidney that influences salt and water balance; measured to detect adrenal disease associated with high blood pressure, and to evaluate various predictive factors concerning treatment.

PLASMA VOLUME

Measurement of total volume of plasma; elevated in liver and spleen diseases and vitamin C deficiency, decreased in dehydration, shock and Addison's disease.

PLASMID

Any extrachromosomal self-replicating genetic element of a cell.

PLASMIN

A proteolytic enzyme with a high specificity for fibrin and the particular ability to dissolve formed fibrin clots.

PLASMINOGEN

The inactive precursor of plasmin, occurring in plasma and converted to plasmin by a specific enzyme.

PLASMODIUM

Genus of protozoa responsible for malaria. The organism is transmitted to the bloodstream of man by the bite of a special type of mosquito.

Four main types are recognized:
– Plasmodium falciparum;
– Plasmodium vivax;
– Plasmodium ovale;
– Plasmodium malariae.

PLASMOLYSIS

Shrinkage and dissolution of the protoplasm in a living cell when excessive water loss occurs by exosmosis.

PLASMOTROPISM
Destruction of red blood cells in the liver, spleen, or bone marrow, as contrasted with their destruction in the circulation.

PLASTER
A paste-like mixture which can be spread over the skin and which is adhesive at body temperature.

PLASTER OF PARIS
Calcined calcium sulfate; on addition of water it forms a porous mass that is used in making casts and bandages to support or immobilize body parts, and in dentistry for taking dental impressions.

PLASTICITY
(1) The ability to retain a shape attained by pressure deformation.
(2) The capacity of organisms with the same genotype to vary in developmental pattern, in phenotype, or in behavior according to varying environmental conditions.

PLASTIC SURGERY
The branch of surgery devoted to reconstruction or repair of deformity, surgical defect or the results of injury.

PLATELET
Thrombocyte, minuscule body, essential to the blood clotting process. They are manufactured in bone marrow at the rate of about 100,000 each day. When bleeding occurs, platelets group or clump together (aggregate), swell up, stick to the injured area, and attempt to act as plugs to stop the bleeding. The normal life span of platelets is about eight days. Only one drop of blood is necessary for examination and may be taken from the fingertip, heel or earlobe or from a tube of blood drawn for other tests.

PLATELET-ACTIVATING FACTOR
A substance that is produced by immunological reaction and that produces clumping of blood platelets.

PLATELET COUNT
The number of platelets in a sample of blood. Platelets, essential in blood clotting, may be reduced in number in some blood diseases and after chemotherapy. Normal values in whole blood amount to 150,000-400,000/microliter.

PLATYCORIA
A dilated condition of the pupil of the eye.

PLATYSMA MUSCLE
Muscle that wrinkles the skin of the neck and chest and depresses the jaw and lower lip. The origin is the clavicle, acromion and fascia over the deltoid muscle, and pectoralis muscle.
The insertion is the lower border of the mandible and the opposite platysma. The muscle is innervated by the cervical branches of the facial nerve.

PLEASURE PRINCIPLE
The biologic principle by which man ordinarily and automatically seeks to avoid pain and discomfort, and strives for gratification and pleasure.

PLAY THERAPY
A form of psychotherapy for children in which play with games and toys is used to gain insight into the child's feelings and thoughts and to help treat conflicts and psychological problems.

PLAY VALUE
The degree to which a toy or object suits the interests and abilities of a child at a particular stage in development.

PLEIOTROPISM
The production of a single gene of multiple phenotypic effects.

PLEOCYTOSIS
The presence of a greater than normal number of cells in the cerebrospinal fluid.

PLEOMORPHISM
The occurrence of various distinct forms by a single organism or within a species.

PLETHORA
An excess of blood or other body fluid.

PLETHYSMOGRAPHY
The recording of changes in the size of an organ, part, or limb as blood circulates through it. However, lung volumes can also be measured with the technique.

PLEURA
A thin membrane that covers the inside of the thorax and also invests the lungs.

PLEURAL CAVITY
Potential space between the membrane enveloping the lungs and that lining the inside of the chest (the pleural membranes).

PLEURALGIA
Pain coming from the pleura.

PLEURAL SPACE
The small space between the visceral and parietal layers of the pleura.

PLEURECTOMY
A surgical excision of part of the pleura.

PLEURISY
Inflammation of the pleura, the two thin connective tissue layers covering the outer lung surface and the inner chest wall.

It causes characteristic chest pain, which may be localized and is made worse by deep breathing and coughing. It may be caused by infection (e.g., pneumonia, tuberculosis) or tumors and inflammatory disease.

PLEURODYNIA
Paroxysmal pain in the intercostal muscles.

PLEURODYNIA, EPIDEMIC
An epidemic disease due to coxsackievirus B, marked by sudden attack of violent pain in the chest, fever, and a tendency to recrudescence on the third day.

PLEUROLITH
A concretion in the pleura.

PLEUROLYSIS
Surgical separation of the pleura from its attachments.

PLEUROPNEUMONIA
An inflammation of the pleura and of the lungs.

PLEXITIS
Inflammation of a nerve plexus.

PLEXOR
A small hammer with a soft rubber head or the like, used in percussion for diagnostic purposes.

PLEXUS
A network or tangle, chiefly of vessels or nerves.

PLICA
A fold or folding, as of skin.

PLICATION
The operation of taking tucks in a structure to shorten it.

PLUG
An obstructing mass.

PLUMBISM
Chronic lead poisoning.

PLUMMER-VINSON SYNDROME
A condition that is marked by difficulty in swallowing, atrophic changes in the mouth, pharynx, and

upper esophagus, and hypochromic anemia and is considered to be due to an iron deficiency.

PLURI–
Word element: many.

PLURIGLANDULAR
Pertaining to several glands or their secretions.

PMA INDEX
A measure of the incidence and severity of gingivitis in a given population based on examination and rating of the degree of involvement of the interdental gingival papilla and the marginal and attached portions of the gingiva in each individual.

PNEUMATIC
Pertaining to air or respiration.

PNEUMATIZATION
The formation of pneumatic cells or cavities in tissue, especially such formation in the temporal bone.

PNEUMATOCELE
A usually benign, thin-walled air-containing cyst of the lung.

PNEUMATOMETRY
Measurement of the air inspired and expired.

PNEUMATOSIS
Air or gas in an abnormal location in the body.

PNEUMATURIA
Gas or air in the urine.

PNEUMOCOCCURIA
Presence of pneumococci in the urine.

PNEUMOCOCCAL VACCINE
An active immunizing agent effective against many strains of Pneumococcus associated with most cases of pneumococcal pneumonia.

PNEUMOCOCCUS
An individual organism of the species Streptococcus pneumoniae.

PNEUMOCONIOSIS
Any lung disease, for instance, anthracosis, silicosis, due to permanent deposition of substantial amounts of particulate matter in the lungs, inhaled during years of exposure, often in extractive industries. Characteristic changes are seen in the lungs.

PNEUMOCYSTITIS
A genus or organism of uncertain status, but considered to be protozoa. Pneumocystitis carinii is the causative agent of interstitial plasma cell pneumonia, one of the opportunistic infections accompanying final stages of AIDS.

PNEUMOCYSTITIS CARINII PNEUMONIA
Lung infection caused by a protozoan (Pneumocystitis carinii) which is endemic in America and Europe. The disease has become well known as a very serious complication of AIDS.

Under normal conditions the protozoan may cause outbreaks of acute or subacute pulmonary disease in infants in hospitals and institutions or opportunistic infections in adults. The incubation period is 1-2 months.

PNEUMOGRAPHY
Medical term with two different meanings:
(1) graphic recording of the respiratory movements;
(2) radiography of a part after injection of a gas.

PNEUMOHEMOTHORAX
Air or gas and blood in the pleural cavity.

PNEUMOHYDROMETRA
Gas and fluid in the uterus.

PNEUMOHYDROTHORAX
Air or gas with effused fluid in the thoracic cavity.

PNEUMOLITHIASIS
The presence of concretions in the lungs.

PNEUMOMYCOSIS
Any fungal disease of the lungs.

PNEUMECTOMY
Excision of lung tissue; it may be total, partial, or of a single lobe.

PNEUMONIA
Inflammation and consolidation of lung tissue. It is usually caused by bacteria (pneumococcus, staphylococcus, Gram's stain negative bacilli), but rarely results from pure virus infection (influenza, measles); other varieties occur if food, secretions or chemicals are aspirated or inhaled.

The inflammatory response causes lung tissue to be filled with exudate and pus, which may center on the bronchi (bronchopneumonia) or be restricted to a single lobe (lobar pneumonia). Cough with yellow or green sputum (sometimes containing blood); fever, malaise and breathlessness are common. Antibiotics and physiotherapy are essential in treatment.

PNEUMONITIS
Inflammation of the lung, caused by a virus or allergic reaction. Treatment includes removal of the offending agent, if possible, and corticosteroids.

PNEUMONOCENTESIS
Surgical puncture of a lung for aspiration.

PNEUMONOCYTE
Collective term for the alveolar epithelial cells (great alveolar cells and squamous alveolar cells) and alveolar phagocytes of the lungs.

PNEUMOTHORAX
Presence of air in the pleural space between the lung and the chest wall. This may result from trauma, rupture of lung bullae in emphysema or in asthma, tuberculosis, pneumoconiosis, cancer, etc., or in tall thin athletic males, it may occur without obvious cause. Drainage of the air through a tube inserted in the chest wall allows the lung reexpansion.

POCK
A pustule raised on the surface of the body in an eruptive disease.

POCKMARK
A mark or scar on the skin made by smallpox or other disease.

PODAGRA
Gouty pain in the great toe.

PODALGIA
Pain in the foot.

PODARTHRITIS
Inflammation of the joints of the feet.

PODIATRY
Chiropody; care of the feet, concerned with the nails, corns and calluses, bunions and toe-deformities. Care of the skin of the feet is especially important in the elderly and in diabetics.

PODODYNIA
Neuralgic pain of the heel and sole; burning pain without redness in the sole of the foot.

PODOPHYLLIN
A resin obtained from podophyllum and used in medicine as a caustic.

PODOPHYLLUM
A small genus of herbs (family Berberidaceae) that have poisonous rootstocks, large palmate leaves, and large fleshy sometimes edible berries.

POIKILOCYTE
An abnormally shaped erythrocyte.

POIKILODERMA
A condition characterized by pigmentary and atrophic changes in the skin, giving it a mottled appearance.

POISON
A substance which, on ingestion, inhalation, absorption, application, injection, or development within the body, in relatively small amounts, may cause structural damage or functional disturbance. Many drugs are poisonous if taken in overdose.

POISONING
The morbid condition produced by a poison.

POLIOMYELITIS
Infantile paralysis; viral disease causing muscle paralysis as a result of direct damage to motor nerve cells in the spinal cord or brain stem. The virus usually enters by the mouth or gastrointestinal tract and causes a mild feverish illness, after which paresis or paralysis begins, often affecting mainly those muscles that have been most used in preceding days.

Treatment is with bed rest and avoidance of complications: contracture, bed sores, venous thrombosis, secondary infection, myocarditis, respiratory failure and swallowing difficulties.

Current polio vaccine is either a live attenuated strain taken by mouth or a dead strain given by injection. Poliomyelitis vaccination has been one of the most successful developments in preventive medicine.

POLIOMYELOPATHY
Any disease of the gray matter of the spinal cord.

POLIOSIS
Depigmentation of the hair; premature grayness of the hair.

POLIO VACCINE
A vaccine intended to confer immunity to poliomyelitis.

POLIOVIRUS
An organism that causes poliomyelitis. On the basis of specificity of neutralizing antibody, poliovirus can be distinguished into three serotypes 1,2 and 3.

POLIOVIRUS VACCINE
Vaccine prepared from poliovirus to provide immunity to poliomyelitis. The live oral form of the vaccine, called the Sabin vaccine, is routinely given to children under the age of 18; inactivated polio vaccine, known as the Salk vaccine, is given subcutaneously, usually to infants and unvaccinated adults.

POLLEN
The male fertilizing element of the flowering plants; often the cause of an allergy.

POLLEX VAGUS
Deviation of the thumb toward the ulnar side.

POLLEX VARUS
Deviation of the thumb toward the radial side.

POLLINOSIS
Hay fever; an allergic reaction to pollen.

POLLUTION
The contamination of one substance by another so that the former is unfit for an intended use; or, more broadly, the addition to any natural environmental resource on which life or the quality of life depends or any substance or form of energy at a rate resulting in abnormal concentrations of what is then termed the "pollutant." Air, water and soil may be resources chiefly affected.

POLY–
Word element: many, large amount.

POLYADENOSIS
Disorder of several glands, particularly endocrine glands.

POLYARTERITIS
Inflammation of several arteries; multiple sites of inflammatory and destructive lesions in the arterial system.

POLYARTERITIS NODOSA
A progressive disease of connective tissue characterized by nodules (often large) along arteries that may cause blockage of the artery and resulting in inadequate circulation to the affected area.
   Symptoms include:
- visceral pain;
- fever;
- malaise;
- signs of lung, kidney and intestinal damage.
Treatment is by corticosteroids.

POLYCYSTIC KIDNEY DISEASE
An abnormal condition in which the kidneys are enlarged and contain many cysts. It occurs in childhood and adult forms and often leads to kidney failure.

POLYCYTHEMIA
An abnormal increase in the number of erythrocytes in the blood, often associated with pulmonary or heart disease, or exposure to high altitudes for a long period, but in many cases of unknown cause.

POLYNEURITIS
General inflammation of the nerve of the peripheral nervous system, extending from the spinal cord and brain to the skin, muscles and other parts of the body.
   It may be caused by a virus infection, diabetes, alcoholism, chemical poisoning, and allergy or malnutrition. Varying degrees of paralysis are associated with the condition.

POLYNEUROPATHY
A noninflammatory degenerative disease of nerves usually caused by toxins.

POLYOPIA
Abnormality of the refractive visual mechanisms which cause several images of an object to form on the retina.

POLYP
Benign tumor of epithelium extending above the surface, usually on a stalk. Polyps may cause nasal obstruction and some (as in the gastrointestinal tract) may have a tendency to become a cancer.

POLYPECTOMY
The surgical excision of a polyp.

POLYTAR
Brand name of a preparation containing as active compound coal tar, prescribed for a variety of non-inflammatory skin disorders such as eczema, psoriasis and dandruff.

PONDERAL INDEX
A measure of relative body mass expressed as the ratio of a cube root of body weight to height multiplied by 100.

PONDERAX
Brand name of a drug containing as active compound fenfluramine prescribed as appetite suppressant for the treatment of obesity.

PONS
A broad mass of chiefly transverse nerve fibers conspicuous on the ventral surface of the brain at the anterior end of the medulla oblongata of the brain stem.

PONTINE FISSURE
A flexure of the embryonic hindbrain that serves to delimit the developing cerebellum and medulla oblongata of the brain stem.

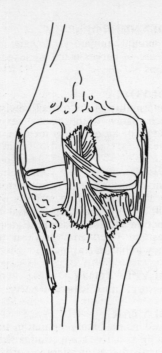

Posterior view of the lower extremity with the popliteal space between thigh and leg.

PONTINE NUCLEUS
Any of various large groups of nerve cells in the basal part of the pons that receive fibers from the cerebral cortex and send fibers to the cerebellum by way of the middle cerebellar peduncle.

POPLITEAL SPACE
A lozenge-shaped space at the back of the knee joint.

PORENCEPHALY
The presence of cavities in the brain.

POSITRON EMISSION TOMOGRAPHY (PET)
Type of scanner that is being used to identify small areas of tissue in organs.

PET is a computerized radiographic technique that allows examination of the metabolic activity of various tissues.

Radioactively tagged substances taken by the patient give off positively charged particles that interact with certain cells, giving off gamma rays, which are detected by special devices and converted through computer analysis into color-coded images.

POSTCENTRAL GYRUS
A gyrus of the parietal lobe located just posterior to the central sulcus, lying parallel to the precentral gyrus of the temporal lobe, and comprising the somesthetic area.

POSTENCEPHALITIS
Symptoms or residual abnormality remaining after recovery from epidemic encephalitis.

POSTERIOR
Directed toward or situated at the back; opposite to anterior.

POSTERIOR HORN
The cornu of the lateral ventricle of each cerebral hemisphere that curves backward into the occipital lobe. The term is also used to designate the dorsal horn of the spinal cord.

POSTERIOR ROOT
A bundle of nerve fibers arising from a spinal ganglion and passing to the central nervous system.

Also called sensory roots because they carry sensory impressions from the body to the central nervous system.

POSTFEBRILE
Occurring after a fever.

POSTHERPETIC NEURALGIA
Neuralgia following an attack of herpes zoster. It persists in the area concerned long after the shingles and blisters have been healed and can be most trying for elderly people to endure.

POSTHYPNOTIC DEPRES-SION

A suggestion given an individual in the hypnotic state to perform an act after coming out of the state, usually on a signal being given.

POSTINFECTIOUS PSYCHO-SIS

A mental disorder which follows an acute disease such as influenza, pneumonia, typhoid fever and acute rheumatic fever. Its characteristics include mild confusion and suspicion, irritability and depressive reactions.

POSTMATURITY

The condition of an infant after a prolonged gestation period.

POSTMORTEM

After death, as an examination of the body.

POSTNATAL

Occurring after birth, with reference to the newborn.

POSTNATAL DEPRESSION

Depressive condition after delivery. If the depression lasts longer than 72 hours, is associated with lack of interest in the infant, suicidal or homicidal thoughts, hallucinations or psychotic behavior, it is pathologic and requires professional guidance.

True psychosis is probably the emergence of pre-existing mental illness in response to the physical and psychological stress of pregnancy and delivery.

POSTOPERATIVE

After a surgical operation.

POSTPARTUM

Occurring after childbirth, with reference to the mother.

POSTPARTUM PSYCHOSIS

A psychotic episode precipitated by giving birth.

POST-TRAUMATIC

Following injury.

POST-TRAUMATIC STRESS DISORDER

Development of characteristic symptoms following a psychologically distressing event that is outside the range of usual human experience (i.e., outside the range of such common experiences as simple bereavement, chronic illness, business losses, and marital conflict). The stressor producing this syndrome would be markedly distressing to almost anyone, and is usually experienced with intense fear, terror, and helplessness. The characteristic symptoms involve re-experiencing the traumatic event, avoidance of stimuli associated with the event or numbing of general responsiveness, and increased arousal. The most common traumata involve either a serious threat to one's life or physical integrity; a serious threat or harm to one's children, spouse, or other close relatives and friends; sudden destruction of one's home or community; or seeing another person who has recently been, or is being, seriously injured or killed as the result of an accident or physical violence. In some cases the trauma may be learning about a serious threat or harm to a close friend or relative, e.g., that one's child has been kidnapped, tortured, or killed.

Symptoms usually begin immediately or soon after the trauma. Reexperiencing symptoms may develop after a latency period of months or years following the trauma, though avoidance symptoms have usually been present during this period.

POSTHALLUCINOGENIC PERCEPTION DISORDER

The reexperiencing, following cessation of use of a hallucinogen, of one or more of the same perceptual symptoms that were experienced

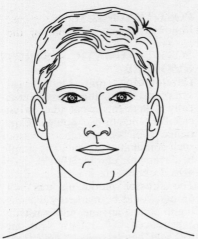

Posture is being determined by the structural integrity of the skeleton and neuromuscular system.

while intoxicated with the hallucinogen. Usually the symptoms last for just a few seconds.

POSTURE
The position or carriage of the body and limbs as a whole. Posture may also be defined as the position or bearing of the body whether characteristic or assumed for a special purpose.

POTASSIUM
A mineral necessary - usually in combination with sodium - for maintaining body fluids and to enable the nervous and muscular systems to function properly. Best natural sources are legumes, whole grains, meats, fish, backstrap molasses, almonds, leafy green vegetables and dried fruits; however, it is the mineral most easily lost by refining and overcooking foods.

POTASSIUM FOODS
Foods high in potassium content, including dried apricots and peaches, lentils, raisins, citrus and whole-grain cereals.

POTENTIATION
Enhancement of one agent by an-

other so that the combined effect is greater than the sum of the effects of each one alone.

POTT'S FRACTURE
External rotation fracture of the tibia and fibula (lower leg bones) at the ankle joint.

POULTICE
A soft, moist, mass about the consistency of cooked cereal, spread between layers of muslin, linen, gauze, or towels and applied hot to the given area in order to create moist local heat or counterirritation.

POWDER
Aggregation of particles obtained by grinding or triturating a solid.

POX
Any eruptive or pustulate disease, especially one caused by a virus, for instance, chickenpox, cowpox.

POXVIRUS
Any of a group of morphologically similar and immunologically related DNA viruses, including the virus of vaccinia (cowpox), smallpox, and those producing pox diseases in lower animals.

PRADER-WILLY SYNDROME
A congenital disorder characterized by;
- short stature;
- mental retardation;
- abnormally small hands;
- abnormally small feet;
- hypogonadism;
- uncontrolled appetite leading to obesity.

PRECANCEROUS
Pertaining to a tumor or growth that is not malignant but probably will become so if left untreated.

PRECENTRAL GYRUS
The gyrus containing the motor area immediately anterior to the central sulcus.

PRECIPITANT
A substance that causes precipitation.

PRECIPITATION
The act or process of precipitating; to cause settling in solid particles or substance in solution.

PRECIPITIN
An antibody that combines with its antigen to form a complex that settles out of solution as a precipitate. This reaction is used to identify an unknown antigen or to establish the presence of antibodies to a known antigen.

PRECLINICAL
Before a disease becomes clinically recognizable.

PRECOCIOUS
Pertaining to earlier-than-expected development of physical or mental abilities; clairvoyance relating to an event or state not yet experienced.

PRECOGNITION
Knowledge of a future event which could not have been rationally inferred.

PRECONDITIONING
Presentation of two stimuli consecutively without reinforcement. The conditioning of the experimental subject to the second stimulus is preconditioning.

PRECONSCIOUS
A psychoanalytical term for mental processes of which the individual is unaware but which he can recall as opposed to unconscious processes which he cannot recall.

PRECONVULSIVE
Relating to or occurring in the period just prior to a convulsion.

PRECUNEUS
A somewhat rectangular gyrus bounding the mesial aspect of the parietal lobe of the cerebrum and lying immediately in front of the cuneus.

PRECURSOR
Something that precedes. In biological processes, a substance from which another, usually more active or mature substance is formed. In clinical medicine, a sign or symptom that heralds another.

PREDIABETES
A state of latent impairment of carbohydrate metabolism in which the criteria for diabetes mellitus are not all satisfied.

PREDICTIVE TEST
A medical test generally applied to asymptomatic individuals to provide information regarding the future occurrence of disease.

PREDISPOSITION
A congenital condition in an individual, favoring development in a certain direction or of certain characteristics; or of a tendency favoring the acceptance of certain beliefs.

PREECLAMPSIA
An abnormal condition of pregnancy characterized by:
- hypertension;
- edema;
- presence of protein in the urine.
Abnormal metabolic functioning, ocular disorders, and other complications frequently occurring in the pregnant woman; fetal malnutrition and lowered birth weight in the child.

Untreated severe preeclampsia can lead to eclampsia and convulsions that threaten the life of both the mother and fetus.

PREEXISTING CONDITION
A condition existing before an insurance policy goes into effect and commonly defined as one which would cause an ordinary prudent

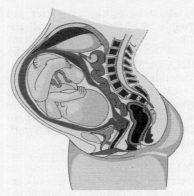

Localization of the fetus in the uterus in the latter part of pregnancy.

person to seek diagnosis, care, or treatment.

PREFRONTAL LOBE
The region of the brain at the front part of each cerebral hemisphere; it is concerned with learning, memory, emotions and behavior.

PREFRONTAL LOBOTOMY
Lobotomy of the white matter in the frontal lobe of the brain.

PREGANGLIONIC
Anterior or proximal to a ganglion; being, affecting, involving, or relating to a usually myelinated efferent nerve fiber arising from a cell body in the central nervous system and terminating in an autonomic ganglion.

PREGENITAL PHASE
Psychoanalytical term for the early, undifferentiated sexuality of the child, before there is attachment to, or predominance of the genital zone.

PREGNANCY
Gestation; the period during which a woman carries a developing fetus in the uterus, from the time of conception to the birth of the child. Pregnancy lasts 266 days from the day of fertilization but is usually calculated as 280 days from the first day of the last menstrual period. Pregnancy involves changes in virtually every system of a woman's body, including:
- an increase in total blood volume;
- an increase in kidney filtration;
- increased urination;
- enlargement of the breasts;
- changes in the color of the nipple area;
- gastrointestinal changes, often manifested as heartburn, nausea, vomiting and constipation;
- increased nutritional need;
- increased bodyweight;
- endocrine changes.

PREHENSION
Visually directed reaching.

PREMARIN
Brand name of a drug containing as active compounds conjugated estrogens. These female sex hormones are prescribed for various hormonal deficiency states.

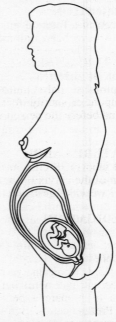

Schema of the relationship between pregnant uterus and abdominal wall

PREMATURE
Happening, arriving, existing or done before the proper time.

PREMATURE APNEA
Periodic breathing associated with short ventilatory pauses and true apnea (longer breathing pauses of ten seconds or more associated with slow heart activity and/or cyanosis) frequently found in premature infants.

PREMATURE BIRTH
Birth of a baby before the 40th week and after the 28th week of pregnancy. Prior to the 28th week it is called an abortion or miscarriage.

PREMATURE INFANT
Any infant born before 37 weeks of gestation. Previously, any infant weighing less than 2.5 kg (5.5 lb) was termed premature; this definition was inappropriate since many newborns weighing less than 2.5 kg are actually mature or postmature but small for gestational age and have a different appearance and different problems than do premature infants.

PREMATURE EJACULATION
Persistent or recurrent ejaculation with minimal sexual stimulation or before, upon, or shortly after penetration and before the person wishes it.

PREMATURE LABOR
Onset of labor with effacement and dilatation of the cervix of the uterus before 37 weeks of gestation.

PREMEDICATION
The giving of a drug to induce a sleepy state prior to administering a general anesthetic. Generally, the term applied to drugs given between one and two hours before an operation to prepare a person for surgery. Premedication usually contains a narcotic analgesic to help relieve pain and anxiety and to reduce the dose of anesthetic needed to produce unconsciousness. An anticholinergic drug is also sometimes included to reduce secretions in the airways.

PREMENSTRUAL TENSION
A condition characterized by nervousness, irritability, emotional instability, depression and which may include headaches, edema and pain in the breasts that occurs during the seven to ten days before menstruation and disappears a few hours after the onset of menstrual flow.

This syndrome seems to be related to fluctuations in estrogen and progesterone and to the fluid-retaining action of estrogen. Most women have a combination of symptoms. Younger women in their late twenties and up tend to have them premenstrually.

Treatment involves fluid retention and some psychoactive drugs. Hormonal manipulation is less helpful than would be expected from the theoretical cause.

PREMOLAR
One of the two teeth between the canine and the first molar, a bicuspid. Also incorrectly applied to a molar tooth of the first dentition. The premolars replace these so-called deciduous molars.

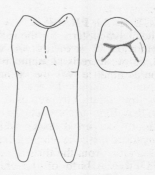

Lateral and superior view of a premolar.

PREMONITION
The thought, usually with anxiety, of a coming event, derived from some experience of suggestion, which may be quite irrelevant, but is regarded as a warning.

PRENATAL
Before birth.

PRENATAL CARE
The care of the pregnant woman during the period of gestation. Ideally, all persons should be examined between six and eight weeks of pregnancy (i.e., when a menstrual period is two or four weeks late) so that duration of pregnancy can be estimated early.

PRENATAL DEVELOPMENT
The process of growth, differentiation, development, and maturation between fertilization and birth.

PRENATAL DIAGNOSIS
Any of various diagnostic procedures to determine if the fetus has a genetic or other abnormality. The procedures involve X-rays and ultrasonography (sonograms), which can reveal structural abnormalities and allow growth to be followed; amniocentesis in which amniotic fluid is withdrawn for analysis and identification of chromosome and metabolic defects, and fetoscopy in which fetal blood can be withdrawn and analyzed.

PREOPERATIVE
Pertaining to the period prior to surgery, when the patient is prepared for surgery by limitations on food and fluids by mouth, by removal of fluids by mouth, by removal of body hair from the area to be incised, by premedication, and/or other procedures.

PREOPTIC AREA
A region of the brain that is situated immediately below the anterior commissure, above the optic chiasm, and anterior to the hypothalamus although it is not clearly demarcated from the hypothalamus and that regulates certain autonomic activities often with the hypothalamus.

PREOPTIC NUCLEUS
Any of several groups of nerve cells located in the preoptic area in the lateral and the medial portions.

PREPERCEPTION
The prepared set or attitude of readiness for an expected perception, or other experience, generally involving an anticipatory idea, which identifies the clearness of the experience itself.

PREPRANDIAL
Before a meal.

PREPSYCHOTIC
Preceding or predisposing to psychosis; possessing recognizable features prognostic of psychosis.

PREPUBERTY
Period of about two years immediately before puberty when growth and changes leading to sexual maturity occur.

PREPUCE
The fold of skin that is a retractable cover over the glans of the penis or the fold around the clitoris.

PRESBY–
Word element: old age.

PRESBYCUSIS
Progressive, double-sided symmetrical perceptive hearing loss occurring with age.

PRESBYOPIA
Farsightedness developing with advancing age as the lens of the eye becomes less elastic.

PRESCHIZOPHRENIC
One whose behavior and personal-

ity traits are prognostic of schizophrenia.

PRESCRIPTION
A written order for medication, therapy or a device given by a properly authorized medical practitioner, especially a written order for a medicine given by a physician to a pharmacist. A prescription is written and signed by a doctor and carries the name and address of the patient for whom the drug is prescribed. The pharmacist keeps a record, often computerized, of all prescriptions dispensed.

PRESCRIPTION MEDICINE
A medicine that can only be dispensed to the public with a prescription.

PRESENILE DEMENTIA
Another name for Alzheimer's dementia.

PRESENILITY
Premature old age; pertaining to a condition resembling senility, but occurring in early or middle life.

PRESENT
Said of the part of a baby that first appears at the mouth of the uterus.

PRESENTATION
The position of the baby in the uterus with reference to the part of the baby directed toward the birth canal. Normally the head appears first (cephalic presentation), but in some cases the buttocks, feet, shoulder, or side may present first.

Abnormal presentations may cause difficulty in childbirth and attempts to turn the baby may be made, or if normal delivery is deemed hazardous a Cesarean section is performed.

PRESERVATIVE
An agent that is added to fluid (as in food or medicine) that prevents the growth of microbial organisms.

PRESSOR
Tending to increase blood pressure, as a pressor substance.

PRESSORECEPTIVE
Sensitive to stimuli due to vasomotor activity.

PRESSURE
Force or stress applied to a surface.

PRESSURE PATTERN
A perceptual experience of relative roughness or smoothness, dependent on simultaneous or successive pressure sensations within a cutaneous area.

PRESSURE POINT
A region of the body in which the distribution of soft and skeletal parts is such that a static position, as a part of a cast, tends to cause circulatory deficiency and necrosis due to local compression of blood vessels.

PRESSURE SORE
Another name for decubitus ulcer.

PRESTHESIA
An abnormal exceptional cutaneous sensation such as tingling, itching and burning occurring in spinal cord lesions, and as a conversion system of psychogenic origin.

PRESYSTOLE
The period of time before systole (contraction beat of the heart).

PRETECTAL
Occurring in or being the transitional zone of the brain stem between the midbrain and the diencephalon that is situated rostral to the superior colliculus and is associated with the analysis and distribution of light impulses.

PREVALENCE
The number of instances of a given disease or other condition in a given population at a designed time;

sometimes used to mean prevalence rate.

When used without qualification the term usually refers to the situation at a specific point in time (point prevalence).

PREVALENCE RATE
The total number of all individuals who have an attribute or disease at a particular time (or during a particular period) divided by the population risk of having the attribute or disease at the point in time or midway through the period.

PREVENTIVE MEDICINE
That branch of medicine concerned primarily with the prevention of disease; it concerns itself with immunization, the eradication of disease carriers (for instance, malaria-carrying mosquitos), screening programs, and other factors.

PREVERTEBRAL
Situated in front of the vertebrae (bones of the spine).

PRIAPISM
Persistent painful erection of the penis due to disease and injuries of the spinal cord, stone in the bladder or injury to the penis.

PRICKLY HEAT
A mild skin condition caused by temporary blockage of the sweat gland openings in the skin. It occurs when a child is overheated.

PRIMAL
Psychoanalytical term for a fragmentary recalled experience or scene from early childhood, the apparent first stage in the production of a neurosis.

PRIMAL SADISM
The part of the death instinct which remains within the person, partially bound with the libido and partially directed at the self.

PRIMAL SCREAM THERAPY
Psychotherapy in which the patient recalls and reenacts a particularly disturbing past experience and expresses normally repressed anger or frustration especially through spontaneous and unrestrained screams, hysteria, or violence.

PRIMARY DEFENSE
The psychotic symptom in emotional illness. The symptom, a psychologically intended defense, is primary, as opposed to the defense of the symptom which constitutes a secondary defense.

PRIMARY DYSMENORRHEA
Cyclic pain associated with menses during ovulatory cycles, but without demonstrable lesions affecting the reproductive cycle.

The pain is thought to be the result from uterine contractions and ischemia.

PRIMARY FOLLICLES
Tightly packed aggregates of lymphocytes, found in the cortex of the lymph node or in the white pulp of the spleen after antigenic stimulation.

PRIMARY HEALTH CARE
Health care provided by a physician, nurse, or other health care professional in the first contact of the patient with health care.

PRIMARY SYPHILIS
The first stage of syphilis that is marked by the development of a chancre and the spread of the causative spirochete in the tissues of the body.

PRIMATES
The highest order of mammals, including man, apes, monkeys, and lemurs.

PRIMIGRAVIDA
A woman pregnant for the first time.

PRIMIPARA
A woman who has been delivered of a child (or children) for the first time.

PRIMIPARITY
The state of being a primipara.

PRIMITIVE
Undeveloped, undifferentiated, rudimentary.

PRIMORDIAL
Pertaining to underdeveloped or primitive state.

PRIMORDIUM
The first recognizable state in the differentiation and development of a particular organ or structure.

PRIVILEGED COMMUNICATION
A communication between parties to a confidential relation, as between physician and patient, such that the recipient cannot be legally compelled to disclose it as a witness.

PROCESS
A course of action; a group of phenomena, as an inflammatory process; a prominence or outgrowth, such as the spinous process of a vertebra or the axis cylinder of a nerve; in chemistry, a method of procedure, reaction or test.

PROCTALGIA
Pain in the rectum.

PROCTATRESIA
A congenital condition in which there is no opening for the anus or rectum.

PROCTASIA
Dilatation of the rectum or anus.

PROFOUND MENTAL RETARDATION
Mental retardation with an IQ below 20 or 25. This group constitutes approximately 1%-2% of people with mental retardation. During the early years, these children display minimal capacity for sensorimotor functioning. A highly structured environment, with constant aid and supervision, and an individualized relationship with a caregiver are required for optimal development. Motor development and self-care and communication skills may improve if training is provided. Currently, many of these people live in the community, in group homes, intermediate care facilities, or with their families. Most attend day programs, and some can perform simple tasks under close supervision in a sheltered workshop.

PROGENESIS
Precocious sexual reproduction in a trematode worm in which metacercariae or sometimes cercariae may lay eggs capable of repeating the life cycle.

PROTECTOMY
Excision of the rectum.

PROCTITIS
Inflammation of the rectum characterized by blood in the stool, frequent urge to defecate but inability to do so, and sometimes diarrhea.

Increasing in incidence, proctitis may result from rectal gonorrhea, non-specific transmitted infection, candidiasis, primary and secondary syphilis, genital warts and a variety of skin conditions.

PROCTOCELE
Protrusion of the rectum, usually into the vagina in cases of uterine prolapse.

PROCTODYNIA
Pain in or about the anus or rectum.

PROCTOLOGIST
A physician who specializes in proctology.

PROCTOLOGY
That branch of medicine concerned with the diagnosis and treatment of disorders of the colon, rectum, and anus.

PROCTOPEXY
Surgical fixation of the rectum.

PROCTOPHOBIA
A morbid dread or apprehension about diseases of the back passage, common in persons suffering with disorders of the rectum and anus. In some neurotic personalities it may become obsessional.

PROCTOPLASTY
Plastic repair of the rectum.

PROCTOPOSIS
Prolapse of the rectum.

PROCTOSCOPE
An instrument (a type of endoscope) used to examine the rectum and the end portion of the colon.

PROCTOSTOMY
Surgical creation of a permanent artificial opening into the rectum.

PRODROME
The earliest sign of a disease or a developing condition; a symptom indicating the onset of a disease.

PROGERIA
Premature aging. Is a rare condition also known as Hutchinson-Gilford progeria syndrome. Signs begin to appear in the individual soon after birth, and the average life expectancy is approximately 12 years.

PROGESTERONE
A hormone derived from the corpus luteum in the ovary, adrenals, or placenta. The hormone is responsible for uterine endometrial changes preparatory for implantation of the blastocyst, for development of the maternal placenta and for development of mammary glands.

PROGESTERONE RECEPTOR TEST
A test of a tumor's response to progesterone, to predict whether the tumor is likely to respond to hormonal therapy.

PROGESTINS
Female sex hormones prescribed for a number of medical conditions.
(1) Treatment for menstrual or uterine disorders caused by progestin imbalance.
(2) Contraceptive, when combined with estrogens in birth control pills.
(3) Treatment for cancer of breast and uterus.
(4) Treatment for toxic sleep apnea.
(5) Treatment for female hormone imbalance.
(6) Treatment for weight loss.
The drug creates a uterine lining similar to that of pregnancy that prevents bleeding. The drug also suppresses a pituitary gland hormone responsible for ovulation. It also stimulates cervical mucus, which stops sperm penetration and prevents pregnancy.
  Possible side effects include:
- appetite or weight changes;
- swollen feet or ankles;
- unusual tiredness or weakness;
- menstrual cycle changes.
Particularly dangerous is the forming of blood clots in leg, brain or lung.

PROGNATHISM
Prognathous condition.

PROGNATHOUS
Having projecting jaws; having the jaws projecting beyond the upper part of the face.

PROGNOSIS
A prediction of the outcome of an activity or process, especially a disease or mental disorder, including an indication of the duration, severity and course.

PROGRESSIVE
Steadily advancing; going from bad to worse.

PROGRESSIVE MUSCULAR ATROPHY
Progressive muscular wasting, due to degeneration in certain cells of the spinal cord, resulting in degeneration of anterior nerve routes and wasting of the muscles supplied by them. Sometimes called chronic anterior poliomyelitis.

PROGRESSIVE SPINAL MUSCULAR ATROPHY
A group of progressive neuromuscular disorders classified as infantile, juvenile and adult. The infantile form is severe and rapidly progressive, beginning before or after birth or in the first few months, characterized by a general weakness and atrophy of the muscles.

The juvenile type, affecting children and adolescents, is only slowly progressive, with a relatively benign course permitting walking as long as twenty years after onset.

The adult type initially affects the hands, but slow progression may lead to complete paralysis of the arms and spastic symptoms of other muscles.

PROJECT
To attribute or assign, something in his own mind or a personal characteristic, to a person, group, or object. The term is also used to designate to connect by sending nerve fibers or processes.

PROJECTION
The objective reference of sensations; reference to an object, as the origin or source of the stimuli, or their localization within or without the body.

PROJECTION AREA
An area of the cerebral cortex having connection through projection fibers with subcortical centers that in turn are linked with peripheral sense or motor organs.

PROJECTION CENTER
The region of the cerebral cortex of the brain, connecting directly with sensory or motor centers in other parts of the brain and spinal cord.

PROJECTION FIBER
A nerve fiber connecting some part of the cerebral cortex with lower sensory or motor centers.

PROJECTION TEST
A type of mental test aiming at the determination of personality traits through the completion of sentences, interpretation of ink-blots and the like.

PROJECTIVE PLAY
Play in which the child is using play materials such as dolls and a doll house, expressed unconscious ideas, attitudes and feelings that the child would otherwise be unable to express and that are useful in coming to an understanding of dynamics and mental disturbances of the child.

PROLACTIN
A pituitary hormone that stimulates milk secretion; measured in new mothers with lactation problems, women with menstrual problems or when brain tumor is suspected.

PROLAMIN
One of a group of simple proteins obtained from gluten of grain, as wheat or oats, and insoluble in pure water, absolute alcohol and neutral solvents.

PROLAPSE
A falling of an organ or part as the uterus, from its normal position.

PROLAPSED UTERUS
Condition in which the uterus slips down and may even protrude into and out through the vagina. Early

symptoms are:
- a feeling of dragging in the lower abdomen;
- backache while standing or during exertion or exercise;
- frequency of urination;
- a feeling of large internal weight between the vulva and anus.

Late symptoms are:
- swelling of the vulva;
- uncomfortable to painful sexual intercourse;
- vaginal pain;
- sometimes discharge.

The cause is often weakness and/or stretching of the pelvic ligaments and muscles due to childbearing.

PROLIFERATION
Growth and production by multiplication.

PROLINE
An amino acid manufactured by the body.

PROMETAPHASE
A stage sometimes distinguished between the prophase and metaphase of mitosis or meiosis and characterized by disappearance of the nuclear membrane and formation of the spindle.

PROMISCUITY
Sexual behavior not restricted to one sexual partner.

PROMONOCYTE
A cell in an intermediate stage of development between a monoblast and a monocyte.

PROMONTORY
A bodily prominence:
(1) the angle of the central side of the sacrum where it joins the vertebra;
(2) a prominence on the inner wall of the tympanum of the ear.

PROMOTER
A substance that in very small amounts is able to increase the activity of a catalyst. The term is also used to designate the region of a genetic operon where transcription is initiated by binding with an appropriate polymerase.

PRONATION
The condition of being prone; the act of placing in a prone position; the turning of the palm of the hand downward.

PRONATOR
A muscle which produces the movement of pronation.

PRONE
Lying face downward; the position of the hand with the palm turned downward.

PRONE PRESSURE METHOD
A method of artificial respiration consisting essentially of alternate pressure and release of pressure on the back of the thorax of the prone patient by means of which water if present is expelled from the lungs and air is allowed to enter.

PRONUCLEUS
The haploid nucleus of a male or female gamete (as an egg or sperm) up to the time of fusion with that of another gamete in fertilization.

PROPHAGE
An intracellular form of a bacteriophage in which it is harmless to the host, and reproduces when the host does.

PROPHASE
The third phase of mitosis in which chromosomes are condensed from the resting form and split into paired chromatids.

PROPHYLACTIC
A drug, procedure, or piece of equipment used to prevent disease. For example, a course of drugs given to a traveller to prevent

malarian infection, is termed malaria prophylaxis.

PROPHYLAXIS
The prevention of disease; measures designed to preserve health and prevent the spread of disease.

PROPRIETARY
Manufactured and distributed under a trade name. The term proprietary is now generally applied to a drug that is sold over the counter, its name being registered to a private manufacturer, i.e., a proprietor.

PROPRIOCEPTOR
A nerve-ending located in a muscle, tendon or joint, whose impulses, together with those of the labyrinth (organ of balance in the ear) supply information by which we are informed of our attitude in space or the position of various parts of the body.

PROPTOSIS
A falling downward; prolapse; exophthalmus (forward projection of the eyeballs).

PROPULSION
The act of propelling or pushing forward; a tendency to fall forwards in walking such as is seen in paralysis agitans (Parkinson's disease).

PROSENCEPHALON
The forebrain; the anterior part of the brain.

PROSOPTOSIS
Personation, spontaneous or induced, of a discarnate personality, from the characteristics of the individual when living, preserved in the memories of the living, and collected by supernormal means.

PROSPECTIVE REFERENCE
Reference of thought in the present, to some future situation, as a partial analysis of purpose.

PROSTAGLANDINS
A variety of naturally occurring aliphatic acids with various biological activities including increased vascular permeability, smooth muscle contraction, bronchial constriction and alteration in the pain threshold.

It has been known for a number of years that seminal fluid contains lipid-soluble substances which stimulate smooth muscle and it has been suggested that the active substance should be called prostaglandin.

While prostaglandins are present in highest concentration in seminal fluid they have been found in numerous other tissues such as kidneys, iris, pancreas, lung, brain and human menstrual fluid.

PROSTALGIA
Pain in the prostate gland.

PROSTATE GLAND
Male reproductive gland which surrounds the urethra at the base of the bladder and which secretes semen. This organ is formed of fibrous muscular and glandular tissue.

It is described as having the shape of a chestnut, and as being an inverted pyramid whose base is applied to the neck of the bladder.

The normal gland usually measures about 1 inch (2.5 cm) from front to back, 1.3 inch (2.5-3 cm) from above downward and nearly 2 inches (5 cm) from side to side. The connective tissue around the gland is condensed to form a fibrous capsule.

There is a groove between the neck of the bladder and the base of the prostate gland which contains a venous plexus.

The prostate gland is traversed from top to bottom by the urethra. The glandular tissue consists of secretory acini. After middle age, acini may contain concretions or secretion and desquamated cells.

PROSTATECTOMY
Surgical removal of the prostate gland. The operation usually results in male sterility but does not preclude sexual intercourse.

PROSTATIC URETHRA
The part of the male urethra from the base of the prostate gland where the urethra begins as the outlet of the bladder to the point where it emerges from the apex of the prostate gland.

PROSTATIC UTRICLE
A small blind pouch that projects from the wall of the prostatic urethra into the prostate gland.

PROSTATITIS
Inflammation of the prostate gland.

PROSTATORRHEA
An abnormal discharge of secretion from the prostate gland especially when more or less continuous.

PROSTATOTOMY
Surgical incision, as for drainage of an abscess, into the prostate gland.

PROSTHETICS
Mechanical or electrical devices inserted into or onto the body to replace or supplement the function of defective or diseased organs. Artificial limbs designed for persons with amputations were among the first prosthetics; but metal or plastic joint replacements or bone fixations for subjects are now also available.

PROSTHESIS
An artificial substitute for a part that has been removed surgically or is missing, for instance, a denture or artificial limb.

PROSTHODONTICS
The branch of dentistry dealing with the making of artificial teeth and other oral structures needed to replace missing or injured parts of the chewing apparatus.

PROTANOPIA
Type of partial color blindness, characterized by confusion of red and green, and insensitivity to the extreme red of the spectrum.

PROTEASE
Any enzyme that exerts a digestive action on proteins.

PROTEIN
Any of a large group of complex compounds, containing carbon, hydrogen, oxygen, nitrogen, and sometimes phosphorus and sulfur. Proteins consist of chains of amino acids, joined by peptide bonds. All the protein in any living organism is undergoing a continual process of breakdown and resynthesis.

Protein synthesis takes place within the cells of an organism guided by RNA.

PROTEINASE
A protein-splitting enzyme.

PROTEINEMIA
An abnormal amount of protein in the blood.

PROTEINURIA
The presence of protein in the urine.

PROTEOCLASTIC
The splitting up of proteins.

PROTEOLYSIS
The conversion of proteins into simpler substances by the action of enzymes.

PROTHROMBIN
A substance in blood plasma and essential for the clotting of blood. In the presence of thromboplastin and calcium, prothrombin is converted to thrombin, which in turn, converts fibrinogen into fibrin which then contract to form a clot.

PROTHROMBIN CONSUMPTION TEST
A test of one of the phases in the

blood clotting process; a measure of the blood's ability to generate a normal amount of thromboplastin.

PROTHROMBIN TIME
Time required for clot formation in blood plasma; a measure of the activity of several coagulation factors.

PROTHROMBIN TIME TEST (QUICK TEST)
Prothrombin (Factor II) is one of the 12 known factors necessary to stop bleeding (normal body coagulants). Like four other clotting factors, it is manufactured in the liver from vitamin K, which is obtained in the diet primarily from green leafy vegetables, fish and liver.

Although the prothrombin time test indicates the level of prothrombin in the blood, it is more a measure of the overall blood coagulation response to the taking of cumarin anticoagulant medicines.

PROTOPATHIC
Responding solely and indiscriminately to gross stimuli, as extreme pain.

PROTOPATHIC EMOTION
The earliest or most primitive affective or emotional experience of a child, a pure or simple unpleasantness.

PROTOPLASM
The substance including and contained within the plasma membrane of animal cells but in plants forming only the cell's contents. It is usually differentiated into the nucleus and the cytoplasm.

The latter is usually a transparent viscous fluid containing a number of specialized structures; it is the medium in which the main chemical reactions of the cell take place. The nucleus contains the cell's genetic material.

PROTOPORPHYRIN
An important natural compound that occurs as an iron complex in hemoglobin and other blood pigments. Elevated levels indicate porphyria (a congenital metabolic disease), lead poisoning, liver disease or certain cancers.

PROTOTAXIC MODE
The earliest stage in perceiving. The infant's prototaxic mode is a state of unconscious and diffused experience.

PROTOZOA
The lowest form of animal life which consists of unicellular organisms, which have neither a nervous system nor a circulatory system. Some are pathological to humans and produce such diseases as amebic dysentery, Leishmaniasis, kala-azar, etc.

PROVIRUS
The genome of an animal virus integrated into the chromosome of the host cell, and thereby replicated in all of the host's daughter cells.

PROXIMAL CONVOLUTED TUBULE
The convoluted portion of the nephron that lies between Bowman's capsule and the loop of Henle, made up of a single layer of cuboid cells with striated borders, and held to be concerned especially with resorption of sugar, sodium and chloride ions, and water from the glomerular filtrate.

PROXIMODISTAL LAW
Development proceeds from the center of the body to the periphery.

PRURIGO
A group of itching, papular eruptions (small, raised spots) of the skin.

PRURITUS
Itching, a sensation that the person instinctively attempts to relieve by scratching.

PRURITUS ANI
Extreme itching around the anus. Although popularly believed to be due to piles it seldom is, the condition is always being associated with anxiety, nervousness and emotional instability.

PRURITUS VULVAE
Intense itching about the vulva. It may also be associated with emotional stress and worry or be precipitated by vaginal discharge, such as leucorrhea.

PSEUDO–
Word element: false.

PSEUDOARTHROSIS
A pathologic condition in which failure of callus formation following pathologic fracture through an area of ossification in a weight-bearing long bone results in formation of a false joint.

PSEUDOCLONUS
Rhythmical contractions of ankle muscles on bending toes inward. This condition occurs in excessive fatigue, hysteria and toxic conditions.

PSEUDOCYESIS
A hysterical manifestation in which a woman shows all the superficial signs and symptoms of pregnancy but is not, in fact, pregnant. Also called false pregnancy.

PSEUDODEMENTIA
Extreme apathy, without intelligence defect. In older people, it is sometimes due to metabolic or toxic conditions.

PSEUDODOMINANCE
Appearance of a recessive phenotype in a heterozygote containing the recessive gene on one chromosome and a deletion or only part of the dominant gene on the corresponding part of the homologous chromosome.

PSEUDOENCEPHALUS
A fetus with a tumor in place of a brain.

PSEUDOESTHESIA
A subjective sensation occurring in the absence of the appropriate stimuli.

PSEUDOEXSTROPHY
A developmental anomaly marked by the characteristic musculoskeletal defects of exstrophy of the bladder but with no major defect of the urinary tract.

PSEUDOFOLLICULITIS
A chronic disorder, most often in the submandibular region of the neck, the characteristic lesions of which are erythematous papules, less commonly pustules, containing buried hairs; in contrast to sycosis barbae, it affects exclusively those who shave.

PSEUDOGLOTTIS
The aperture between the false vocal cords.

PSEUDOGOUT
A joint disease with protean manifestations which may include intermittent attacks of acute arthritis; a degenerative arthropathy that is often severe but can be asymptomatic; and X-ray evidence of calcinosis of the articular cartilage in characteristic sites.

PSEUDOHEMATURIA
The presence in the urine of pigments that impart a pink or red color, but with no detectable hemoglobin or blood cells.

PSEUDOHERMAPHRODITISM
A state in which the gonads are of one sex, but one or more contradictions exist in the morphological criteria of sex.

PSEUDOHERNIA
An inflamed sac or gland simulat-

ing strangulated hernia.

PSEUDOHYPERTROPHIC MUSCULAR DYSTROPHY

The most common form of muscular dystrophies. It is a sex-linked recessive disorder, typically presenting in boys aged three to seven years as proximal muscles weakness causing waddling gait, toe-walking, lordosis, frequent falls and difficulty in standing up and climbing stairs. The pelvic girdle is affected first; then the shoulder girdle.

PSEUDOHYPERTROPHY

Apparent increase in the size of an organ not due to enlargement of essential functional tissue. For instance, apparent enlargement of a muscle due to deposits of fat within it.

PSEUDOLOGIA FANTASTICA

A tendency to tell extravagant and fantastic falsehoods centered about one's self, easily renounced when confronted with facts.

PSEUDOMENSTRUATION

A bleeding from the uterus which is not a true menstrual period.

PSILOCYBIN

Hallucinogenic drug derived from a Mexican fungus (Psilocybe mexicanus) and related to LSD.

PSILOSIS

Falling out of hair.

PSITTACOSIS

An infectious atypical form of pneumonia caused by Chlamydia psittaci and transmitted by certain birds. Human infection usually occurs by inhaling dust from feathers or excreta of infected birds; it may also be transmitted to humans by a bite from an infected bird or, rarely, by cough droplets of infected persons.

The onset may be insidious or abrupt, with fever, chills, general malaise and anorexia. The temperature gradually rises and cough develops, initially dry but at times becoming mucopurulent. During the second week pneumonia and frank consolidation may occur with secondary purulent lung infection.

Convalescence is gradual and may be prolonged, especially in severe cases. Tetracycline is effective.

PSORIASIS

Common skin condition characterized by patches of red, thickened and scaling skin. It often affects the elbows, knees and scalp but may be found anywhere.

Several forms are recognized and the manifestations may vary in each individual with time. The cause is unknown. Various treatment approaches may diminish the symptoms.

PSYCHE

Greek word meaning soul. In the fifth century BC the soul was personified as a beautiful woman, whom the god of love, Eros, fell in love with and tormented. In the present context it means the mind, including conscious and unconscious processes; in psychoanalysis, the total of the ID, EGO, SUPEREGO.

PSYCHEDELIC

Of, relating to, or being drugs (as LSD) capable of producing abnormal psychic effects (as hallucinations) and sometimes psychic states resembling mental illness.

PSYCHIATRY

The branch of medicine concerned with the study and treatment of mental illness. It has two major branches; one is psychotherapy, the application of psychological techniques to the treatment of mental illnesses where a physiological origin is either unknown or does not exist; the other, medical therapy, where attack is made either on the organic source of the disease or, at least, on its physical or behavioral symptoms.

PSYCHIC, PSYCHICAL
Pertaining to the mind; of or relating to the psyche; psychogenic; sensitive to nonphysical or supernatural forces and influences.

PSYCHIC BLINDNESS
Inability to see because of a lesion in the cerebral cortex of the brain or functional disorder, the sensory apparatus of the eye being unimpaired.

PSYCHIC DEAFNESS
Inability to hear because of a lesion in the cerebral cortex of the brain or functional disorder, the auditory apparatus being unimpaired.

PSYCHIC DETERMINISM
Principle of psychoanalytic theory that states all behavior is motivated or directed toward some specific goal.

PSYCHIC DISTANCE
Degree of detachment of an individual from the practical significance or appeal of an object.

PSYCHIC FORCE
Parapsychological term referring to the hypothetical cause of an alleged telekinetic phenomenon.

PSYCHO
A victim of several mental or emotional disorder; especially a psychoneurotic person.

PSYCHOACOUSTICS
A branch of science dealing with hearing, the sensations produced by sounds, and the problems of communication.

PSYCHOACTIVE
Affecting the mind or behavior.

PSYCHOACTIVE AGENT
A chemical substance that affects the mind, a mood altering drug.

PSYCHOANALYSIS
A system of psychology having as its base the theories of Sigmund Freud; also, the psychotherapeutic technique based on that system. The distinct forms of psychoanalysis developed by Jung and Adler are more correctly termed respectively analytical psychology and individual psychology.

Freud's initial interest was in the origins of neuroses. On developing the technique of free association to replace that of hypnosis in this therapy, he observed that certain patients could in some cases associate freely only with difficulty. He decided that this was due to memories of certain experiences being held back from the conscious mind and noted that the most sensitive areas were in connection with sexual experiences. He thus developed the concept of the unconscious (later to be called the ID), and suggested (for a while) that anxiety was the result of repression of the libido.

He also defined "resistance" by the conscious to acceptance of ideas and impulses from the unconscious, and transference, the idea that relationships with other people or objects in the past affect the individual's relationships with other people or objects in the present.

PSYCHOANALYST
One who practices or adheres to the principles of psychoanalysis; a psychotherapist trained at an established psychoanalytic institute.

PSYCHOANALYTICAL PSYCHOTHERAPY
A simplified and shorter method of treatment based on modified principles of psychoanalysis.

PSYCHOBIOGRAPHY
A biography written from a psychodynamic or psychoanalytic point of view.

PSYCHOBIOLOGY
The study of mental life and behavior in relation to other biological processes.

PSYCHOCULTURAL
Of or relating to the interaction of psychological and cultural factors in the individual's personality or in the characteristics of a group.

PSYCHODIAGNOSTICS
The use of the individual's behavior and results on psychological tests for the study of the individual's personality.

PSYCHODRAMA
A projective technique and form of group psychotherapy in which a person is asked to act out meaningful situations in the presence of people who act as auxiliary egos confronting the person on various issues, the therapist and the audience.

PSYCHODYNAMICS
(1) The study of mental and developmental processes from a dynamic point of view, as a branch of psychology and psychiatry.
(2) Explanation or interpretation, as of behavior or mental states, in terms of mental or emotional forces or processes.
(3) Motivational forces acting especially at the unconscious level.

PSYCHOGALVANIC RESPONSE
The apparent diminution of the electrical resistance of the skin, due in reality to the production of an electromotive force in the skin, resulting from mental activity.

PSYCHOGENESIS
The development and origin of mental characteristics; the development from mental as distinguished from physical origins.

PSYCHOGERIATRICS
A branch of psychiatry concerned with behavioral and emotional disorders among the elderly.

PSYCHOGNOSIS
The study of mental phenomena by means of hypnosis.

PSYCHOGRAM
A description of the mental life of an individual. The term is also used to designate the pattern of responses to a projective technique, as the Rorschach test.

PSYCHOKINESIS
Movement of physical objects by the mind without use of physical means.

PSYCHOKINETICS
A branch of parapsychology that deals with psychokinesis.

PSYCHOLEPSY
An attack of hopelessness and mental inertia especially following elation and occurring typically in psychasthenic individuals.

PSYCHOLINGUISTICS
The study of linguistic behavior as conditioning and conditioned by psychological factors.

PSYCHOLOGICAL
(1) Relating to, characteristic of, directed toward, influencing, arising in, or acting through the mind especially in its affective or cognitive functions.
(2) Directed toward the will or toward the mind specifically in the conative function.
(3) Relating to, concerned with, deriving from, or used in psychology.

PSYCHOLOGICAL PRIMARY
Any of the set of colors which are perceived as belonging to objects, which include red, yellow, green, and blue and sometimes black and white, and in terms of which all other colors belonging to objects can be described.

PSYCHOLOGICAL TEST

A general term for a test which either measures or evaluates abilities, general or specific, or personality traits.

It may be part of a general medical examination in cases of involvement of the brain in disorders and diseases of the nervous system. In general not a single test is applied, but a complete psychometric examination is performed.

PSYCHOLOGIST

A specialist in one or more branches of psychology; a practitioner of clinical psychology, counseling, or guidance.

PSYCHOLOGY

Originally the branch of philosophy dealing with the mind, then the science of mind, and now, considered in its more general context, the science of behavior, whether human or animal.

PSYCHOMETRIC FUNCTION

A mathematical formula which expresses the relation between the quantitative variation in a stimulus and the judgments of a subject who is reporting about the stimulus.

PSYCHOMETRICS

A branch of clinical or applied psychology dealing with the use and application of mental measurement. The term is also used to designate the technique of mental measurements; the use of quantitative devices for assessing psychological tendencies and traits.

PSYCHOMIMETIC

Producing effects (as hallucinations or paranoid delusions) that resemble or are identical with psychotic symptoms.

PSYCHOMOTILITY

Bodily movement proceeding from mental processes and indicating psychological tendencies and traits.

PSYCHOMOTOR

Of or relating to motor action directly proceeding from mental activity. The term is also used in the sense of or relating to psychomotor epilepsy.

PSYCHOMOTOR ATTACK

Form of epileptic seizure characterized by short attacks of extreme motor activity, sometimes violent, of which the individual has no consciousness, and which usually originates in the temporal lobe.

PSYCHOMOTOR EPILEPSY

Epilepsy characterized by partial rather than generalized seizures that typically originate in the temporal lobe and are marked by impairment of consciousness, automatism, bizarre changes in behavior, hallucinations (as of odors), and perceptual illusions, as visceral sensations.

PSYCHOMOTOR RETARDATION

Psychiatric term for gross slowing-down of both mental and physical processes occurring in deep depression.

PSYCHONEUROSIS

Group of functional nervous and mental disorders, less serious and less fundamental than psychoses, of which hysteria may be taken as the type.

PSYCHONOMIC

Of, relating to, or constituting the laws of mental life.

PSYCHOPATHIC

Of, relating to, or characterized by psychopathy or psychopathic personality.

PSYCHOPATHIC PERSONALITY

An emotionally and behaviorally disordered state characterized by clear perception of reality except for the individual's social and moral obligations and often by the pursuit of immediate personal gratification in criminal acts, drug addiction, or sexual perversion.

PSYCHOPATHOLOGY
The study of psychological and behavioral dysfunction occurring in mental disorder or in social disorganization; disordered psychological and behavioral functioning, as in mental illness.

PSYCHOPATHY
Mental disorder; psychopathic personality.

PSYCHOPHARMACOLOGY
The study of the effects of drugs on the mind and behavior.

PSYCHOPHONASTHENIA
A hysterical symptom in which the voice becomes tremulous, choked, and irregular in pitch with overall difficulty in vocalization.

PSYCHOPHYSICS
A branch of psychology that studies the effects of physical processes, as intensity of stimulation, on the mental processes and especially sensations of an organism.

PSYCHOQUACK
An unqualified psychologist or psychiatrist.

PSYCHOSEXUAL
Of or relating to the mental, emotional, and behavioral aspects of sexual development. The term is also used in the sense of relating to mental or emotional attitudes concerning sexual activity.

PSYCHOSEXUALITY
The psychic factors of sex and sexual behavior.

PSYCHOSIS
A term formally applied to any mental disorder, but now generally restricted to those disturbances of such magnitude that there is personality disintegration and loss of contact with reality. The disturbances are psychogenic in origin, or without clearly defined physical cause.

The psychoses include:
- organic psychoses;
- schizophrenic disorders;
- paranoid disorders;
- manic depressive psychosis.

PSYCHOSOMATIC DISEASE
Any illness in which some activity, usually anxiety or the inhibition of emotions, causes physiological malfunction. There is debate as to which disorders are psychosomatic, but among the most likely candidates are:
- gastric ulcers;
- heart failure;
- ulcerative colitis;
- certain types of asthma.

PSYCHOSURGERY
Cerebral surgery employed in treating psychic symptoms.

PSYCHOTECHNOLOGY
The application of psychological methods and results to the solution of practical problems especially in industry. The term is also used to designate the application of technology for psychological purposes, as personal growth or behavior change.

PSYCHOTHERAPY
The application of the theories and discoveries of psychology to the treatment of mental illness. Psychotherapy does not usually involve physical techniques, such as the use of drugs or surgery. The term is sometimes used misleadingly to distinguish other forms of therapy from psychoanalysis. Almost all psychotherapeutic interventions are some type of support, confrontation or interpretation. Each of these may be powerful facilitators when used correctly, but may be damaging when untimely or unprofessional.

PSYCHOTOXIC
Of, or relating to, or being an habituating drug, as amphetamine, which is not a true narcotic but the abuse of which may be correlated with deleterious personality and behavioral changes.

PSYLLIUM
Plant of the genus Plantago. Herbal preparations are used in the treatment of constipation. The name is also used to designate a drug used for the relieve of constipation and the prevention of straining for bowel movement. The drug acts by absorbing water, stimulating the bowel to form a soft, bulky stool.

PTOMAINE
Any of an indefinite class of toxic bases, usually considered to be formed by the action of bacterial metabolism or proteins.

PTERYGIUM
A triangular fleshy mass of thickened conjunctiva occurring usually at the inner side of the eyeball, covering part of the cornea, and causing a disturbance of vision.

PTERYGOID FOSSA
A V-shaped depression on the posterior part of each pterygoid process that is formed by the divergence posteriorly of its medial and lateral pterygoid plates and that contains the medial pterygoid muscle and the tensor veli palatini.

PTERYGOID PLATE
Either of two vertical plates making up a pterygoid process of the sphenoid bone.

PUBERTY
The time during the growth of a person at which sexual development occurs, commonly associated with a growth spurt. Female puberty involves several stages - the acquisition of breast buds, of sexual hair, and the onset of menstruation -

which may each begin at different times.
Male puberty involves sexual hair development, voice change, and growth of the testes and the penis.

PUBLIC HEALTH
The practice and organization of preventive medicine within a community. Many threats are beyond individual control. Disease, epidemics, pollution of the air and purity of water can only be effectively regulated by laws and health authorities. Among the strictest controls are those on sewage and waste disposal. Most advanced countries have pure food laws controlling food purity, freshness and additives.

PUDENDAGRA
Pain in the genitals, especially the female genital organs.

PUDENDAL BLOCK
Regional anesthesia produced by injecting a local anesthetic agent into the pudendal nerve plexus either transvaginally or through the buttock.

PUDENDAL NERVE
A nerve that arises from the second, third, and fourth sacral nerves and that supplies the external genital organs, the skin of the perineum, and the anal sphincter muscles.

PUDENDUM
The external genital organs, especially the female.

PULMONARY ARCH
Either the right or the left sixth aortic arch that in the human fetus persists on the right side as the right pulmonary artery and on the left side as the ductus arteriosus and part of the pulmonary trunk.

PULMONARY ARTERY
An arterial trunk or other of its two main branches that carry blood to the lungs. The pulmonary trunk is a

large arterial trunk that arises from the conus arteriosus of the right ventricle, ascending in front of the aorta, and branching into the right and left pulmonary arteries.

The right pulmonary artery is a branch of the pulmonary trunk that passes under the arch of the aorta to the right lung where it divides into branches. The left pulmonary artery is a branch of the pulmonary trunk that passes to the left in front of the descending part of the aorta, giving off the left in front of the descending part of the aorta, giving off the ductus arteriosus in the fetus which regresses to the ligamentum arteriosum in the adult, and passes to the left lung where it divides into branches.

PULMONARY PLEXUS
Either of two nerve plexuses associated with each lung that lie on the dorsal and ventral aspects of the bronchi of each lung and distribute fibers mainly from the vagus nerve to the lungs.

PULMONARY VEINS
The veins which conduct oxygenated blood from the lungs into the left upper chamber of the heart (left atrium).

PULP
The soft interior of an organ.

PULPITIS
Inflammation of the dental pulp (containing vascular, connective and nervous tissue) and the adjacent periodontal tissues, resulting in toothache.

PULSE
The throb in an artery due to an increase in the tension of its walls following a heart beat. The pulse is usually counted on the thumb side of the wrist, but may be taken over any artery that can be felt. The normal pulse is regular, even and occurs some 70 to 80 times a minute.

PULSE PRESSURE
The difference between the blood pressure in the arteries when the heart is in contraction (systole) and when it is in relaxation (diastole).

PULVINAR
A rounded prominence on the back of the thalamus.

PUNCH-DRUNK
Suffering cerebral injury from many minute brain hemorrhages as a result of repeated head blow's received in boxing.

PUPIL
The round, contractile aperture in the middle of the iris of the eye through which the rays of light pass to the retina.

PUPILLARY REFLEX
The variation of the size of the pupil, depending on the intensity of light falling on the retina, and controlled by muscle fibers in the iris.

PUPILLOGRAPHY
The measurement of the reactions of the pupil.

PUPILLOMOTOR
Having a motor influence on or involving alteration of the pupil of the eye.

PURGATIVE
A medicine that evacuates the bowels. The term is generally applied to a drug that helps eliminate feces from the body, either to relieve constipation or to empty the bowel/intestine before surgery.

PURINE
The parent compound of a class of organic bases of major biochemical importance. The purines adenine and guanine are part of DNA.

PURINE FOODS
Foods that are metabolized into uric acid. Foods high in purines include:

anchovies, liver, brains, sweet-breads, sardines, kidney, oysters, gravy and meat extracts.

PURKINJE CELL
Any of numerous nerve cells that occupy the middle layer of the cerebellar cortex and are characterized by a large globose body with massive dendrites directed outward and a single slender axon directed inward.

PURKINJE FIBER
Any of the modified cardiac muscle fibers with few nuclei, granulated central cytoplasm, and sparse peripheral striations that make up Purkinje's network.

PURKINJE NETWORK
A network of intracardiac conducting tissue made up of syncytial Purkinje fibers that lie in the myocardium and constitute the bundle of His and other conducting tracts which spread out from the sinoatrial node.

PURKINJE PHENOMENON
A shift of the region of apparent maximal spectral luminosity from yellow with the light-adapted eye toward violet with the dark-adapted eye that is permanently associated with predominance of cone vision in bright and red vision in dim illumination.

PURULENT
Pertaining to pus.

PURULENT EFFUSION
Liquid composed of pus.

PUS
Off-white or yellow liquid consisting of inflammatory exudate, the debris of white blood cells and bacteria resulting from localized inflammation, especially abscesses. Pus contained in cavities is relatively inaccessible to antibiotics and may require drainage by surgery.

Pus suggests but does not prove the presence of bacterial infection.

PUSTULE
Dermatologic condition characterized by a superficial, elevated lesion containing pus. Pustules may result from infection or seropurulent evolution of vesicles. Possibilities include
- impetigo;
- acne;
- furuncles;
- carbuncles;
- certain deep fungus infections;
- kerion;
- pustular miliaria;
- pustular psoriasis of the palms and soles.

PUTAMEN
An outer reddish layer of gray matter in the lentiform nucleus; part of the basal ganglia of the cerebrum.

PYCNOSIS
Thickening or inspissation; a degenerative change in body cells, whereby the nucleus of the cells is condensed and shrinks to a dense, structureless mass.

PYELITIS
Inflammation of the pelvis of the kidney.

PYELOCYSTITIS
Inflammation of the pelvis, of the kidney and of the urinary bladder.

PYELOGRAPHY
X-ray examination of the kidney and ureter after they have been filled with a substance opaque to X-rays.

PYELONEPHRITIS
Inflammation of both the pelvis and the substance of the kidney.

PYELOPHLEBITIS
A suppurative condition which originates in the appendix or rectal areas and spreads via the portal vein

to the liver, where abscesses are formed.

PYELOTOMY
Surgical incision into the pelvis or the kidney.

PYKNOLEPSY
A condition marked by epileptiform attacks resembling petit mal.

PYRAMID
Either of two large bundles of motor fibers from the cerebral cortex that reach the medulla oblongata and are continuous with the corticospinal tracts of the spinal cord. The term is also used to designate a conical projection making up the central part of the inferior vermis of the cerebellum.

PYRAMIDAL CELL
Any of numerous large multipolar pyramid-shaped cells in the cerebral cortex.

PYRAMIDALIS
A small triangular muscle of the lower front part of the abdomen that is situated in front of and in the same sheath with the rectus muscle and functions to tense the linea alba.

PYRAMIDOTOMY
A surgical procedure in which a corticospinal tract is severed, as for relief or parkinsonism.

PYROMANIA
A mad, recurring impulse to set fire to objects and buildings.

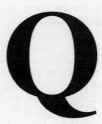

Q FEVER
Infectious disease caused by a rickettsia (Coxiella burnetti) and characterized by:
- sudden chills;
- chest pain;
- headache;
- fever;
- weakness;
- severe sweating;
- sore throat;
- cough;
- pneumonitis signs.

The fatality rate is less than 1 percent.The incubation period is 2-3 weeks. Transmission mechanisms are by contacts with infected animals, dust, contaminated material (e.g., wool, fertilizer, raw milk).

Treatment and control: antibiotics (tetracyclines); secretion precautions, search for source of infection, pasteurization of milk.

QRS COMPLEX
The series of deflections in an electrocardiogram (ECG) that represent electrical activity generated by ventricular depolarization prior to contraction of the ventricle.

Q-T INTERVAL
The interval from the beginning of the QRS complex to the end of the T wave on an electrocardiogram (ECG) that represents the time during which contraction of the ventricles occurs.

QUACK
A pretender to medical skill; an ignorant or dishonest practitioner.

QUADRANT
Any of the four more or less equivalent segments into which an anatomic structure may be divided by vertical and horizontal partitioning through its midpoint.

QUADRATE LOBE
A small lobe of the liver on the underside of the right lobe to the left of the fissure for the gallbladder.

QUADRATUS
Any of several skeletal muscles more or less quadrilateral in outline.

QUADRICEPS
A large muscle in the front of the thigh that controls the extension of the leg. The quadriceps is a large

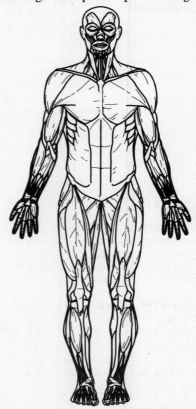

The quadriceps muscle occupies the major part of the anterior portion of the thigh. The common tendon inserts on the tibia.

extensor muscle of the front of the thigh divided above into four parts which include the rectus femoris, vastus lateralis, vastus intermedius, and vastus medialis, and which unite in a single tendon to enclose the patella as a sesamoid bone at the knee and inserting as the patellar ligament into the tuberosity of the tibia.

QUADRIGEMINAL PULSE
A pulse in which there is a pause after every fourth beat.

QUADRIPARA
A woman who has borne her fourth child or is in her fourth confinement.

QUADRIPLEGIA
Paralysis of all four limbs, caused by traumatic injury or disease to the nerve cells of the spinal cord in the neck. The most common cause of injury are diving accidents, falls, traffic accidents, where the head is thrown forward following deceleration of the body, and war injuries.

QUANTITATIVE ANALYSIS
Chemical analysis designed to determine the amounts or proportions of the components of a substance.

QUANTITATIVE CHARACTER
An inherited character that is expressed phenotypically in all degrees of variation between one often indefinite extreme and another.

QUANTITATIVE INHERITANCE
Genic inheritance of a character, as skin color, controlled by a group of genes at different loci with each allelic pair having a specific quantitative effect.

QUARANTINE
Period during which a person or animal must be kept under observation in isolation from the community after having been in contact with a severe infectious disease. The term derives from the period of 40 days that ships from the Levant had to wait before their crews could disembark at Medieval European ports, from fear of their carrying plague.

QUARTAN MALARIA
Type of malaria, caused by the Plasmodium malariae; the paroxysms occurring every 72 hours.

QUASIA
A drug consisting of the heartwood of various tropical trees (family Simaroubaceae) used in medicine as a bitter tonic and as a remedy for roundworms, as an insecticide, and in brewing as a substitute for hops.

QUELLADA
Brand name of a topical antiparasitic preparation containing as active compound lindane prescribed for superficial parasitic skin infections.

QUESTIONNAIRE
A series of questions dealing with some psychological, social, educational, etc. topic or topics, with the object of obtaining data with regard to some problem.

QUICKENING
The first feeling by a pregnant woman of the baby's movements within the womb. It usually occurs about the twentieth week of pregnancy and may feel to the mother like a feather brushing across the abdomen or there may occur convulsive movements as the child moves its limbs.

QUICK PULSE
A pulse that strikes the finger rapidly but leaves it just as rapidly.

QUINCY
Another name for peritonsillar cellulitis.

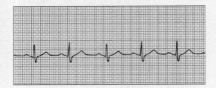 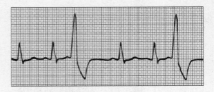

Normal (left) and pathological (right) electrocardiograms with PQRST-waves.

QUININE

Substance derived from cinchona bark from South America and Asia, for long used in treating a variety of ailments. It was pre-eminent in early treatment of malaria until the 1930s when atabrine was introduced; after this more suitable quinine derivatives such as chloroquine was synthesized.

Quinine is also a mild analgesic and may prevent cramps and suppress heart rhythm disorders. Now rarely used, its side effects include vomiting, deafness, vertigo and vision disturbances.

QUININE FEVER

A disease marked by high temperature and skin rashes, occurring in people exposed to quinine during its manufacture.

QUINONE

Any of various usually yellow, orange, or red quinonoid compounds including several that are biologically important as coenzymes, hydrogen acceptors, or vitamins.

QUINSY

An abscess behind the tonsil that pushes the swollen tonsil right across the midline of the throat and makes speaking and swallowing almost impossible until the abscess bursts.

QUINTESSENCE

The highest concentration extract which can be made of any substance.

QUINTUPLET

One of five children or offspring born at one birth.

QUOTIDIAN

Recurring each day; an intermittent fever which recurs each day.

QUOTIENT

The numerical ration multiplied by 100 between a test score and a measurement on which that score might be expected largely to depend; for example, intelligence quotient.

Q-WAVE

The electrocardiographic wave associated with the contraction of the ventricles (lower chambers of the heart).

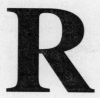

RA
Abbreviation of rheumatoid arthritis.

RABIES
An acute infectious disease of mammals including men, characterized by irritation of the central nervous system.

The etiological agent is a virus present in the saliva of some animal species. These animal species transmit the infection by biting animals or humans. In humans, the incubation period varies from ten days to over a year. It is usually shortest in persons with extensive bites or bites about the head or trunk.

The disease commonly begins with a short period of mental depression, restlessness, malaise and fever. Restlessness increases to uncontrollable excitement, with excessive salivation and painful spasms of the laryngeal and pharyngeal muscles. As a result, the person cannot drink, though his thirst is great (hence hydrophobia).

Rabies rarely occurs in humans if proper local and systemic prophylaxis is carried out immediately after exposure. If rabies develops, treatment is symptomatic. Vigorous supportive treatment is recommended and expert consultation should be sought to assist in clinical management. Although death from rabies was once considered inevitable if symptoms developed, recovery has occurred following aggressive, vigorous, supportive treatment to control respiratory, circulatory and nervous symptoms.

RACHIALGIA
A pain in the spine.

RACHIOPATHY
Any disease or illness of the vertebral column.

RACHIOTOMY
Surgical operation of cutting into or through the vertebral column or spine.

RACHITIC
Pertaining to rickets.

RAD
A unit of absorbed dose of radiation; it represents the absorption of 100 ergs of nuclear (or ionizing) radiation per gram of absorbing material such as body tissue.

RADIAL
A body part, as an artery or nerve, lying near or following the course of the radius.

RADIAL NERVE
A large nerve that arises from the posterior cord of the brachial plexus and passes spirally down the humerus to the front of the lateral epicondyle where it divides into a superficial branch distributed to the skin of the back of the hand and arm and a deep branch to the underlying extensor muscles.

RADIAL KERATOTOMY
A multiple incision of the cornea forming a series of slits in a radial pattern resembling the spokes of a wheel that is performed to correct myopia.

RADIATION
The emission and propagation through space of electromagnetic radiation or subatomic particles. Exposure to X-rays and gamma rays is measured in roentgen units; absorbed dose of any high-energy radiation in rad.

RADIATION ABSORBED DOSE

A unit of radiation exposure that measures the absorbed dose.

RADIATION, IONIZING

Any radiation consisting of directly or indirectly ionizing particles or a mixture of both. Directly ionizing particles are charged particles (electrons, protons, alpha particles, etc.) having sufficient kinetic energy to produce ionization by collision; indirectly ionizing particles are uncharged particles (neutrons, photons, etc.) which can liberate directly ionizing particles or can initiate nuclear transformation.

Ionizing radiation occurs in the atmosphere both naturally (e.g., cosmic rays and disintegration of radioactive elements in the earth) and through the activities of man (e.g., the explosion of nuclear devices and accidental escape of material from nuclear reactors, for instance, the disaster in Chernobyl).

It can cause severe cell damage and lead to cancer, and exposure to it must be strictly controlled.

RADIATION SICKNESS

Malaise, nausea, loss of appetite and vomiting occurring several hours after exposure to ionizing radiation in large doses. This occurs as an industrial or war hazard, or more commonly following radiation therapy for cancer, lymphoma or leukemia. Large doses of radiation may cause bone marrow depression with anemia, agranulocytosis and bleeding, or gastrointestinal disturbance with distention and bloody diarrhea. Skin erythema and ulceration, lung fibrosis, nephritis and premature atherosclerosis may follow radiation and there is a risk of malignancy developing.

RADIATION THERAPY

Use of ionizing radiation, as rays from an outside source or from radium or other radioactive metal implants, in treatment of malignant disease - cancer, lymphoma and leukemia.

The principle is that rapidly dividing tumor cells are more sensitive to the destructive effects of radiation on nucleic acids and are therefore damaged by doses that are relatively harmless to normal tissues.

Certain types of malignancy indeed respond to radiation therapy but radiation sickness may also occur.

RADICOTOMY

Surgical division of nerve roots.

RADICULAR

Pertaining to a radicle or spinal nerve root.

RADICULITIS

Inflammation of nerve roots, usually spinal nerve roots.

RADIOACTIVE

A property of certain substances of spontaneous emitting alpha, beta or gamma rays from the nucleus of the atom. It is a natural phenomenon in such substances as radium or it can be artificially induced by placing a substance inside a thermonuclear pile and bombarding it with high-velocity particles, thus producing radioactive isotopes.

RADIOACTIVE ISOTOPES

Elements which have been rendered radioactive by being placed in an atomic pile. Chemicals known to migrate specifically to certain parts of the body can be used as tracers which can be followed by a Geiger counter for the effect their radioactive rays exert on the part to which they migrate.

RADIOAUTOGRAPHY

A method by which graphic records are obtained by placing a radioactive material in contact with a photographic emulsion and developing the exposed film or plate.

RADIODIAGNOSIS
Diagnosis by means of radiography.

RADIOGRAPH
Any X-ray photograph; to take such photographs.

RADIOGRAPHY
The making of film records (radiographs) of internal structures of the body by exposure of film specially sensitized to X-rays or gamma rays.

RADIO-IMMUNOASSAY
A variety of immunologic techniques in which a radioisotope is used to detect antigens or antibodies in some form of immunoassay.

RADIO-IMMUNOSORBENT ASSAY TEST
A test using serum immunoglobulin E to detect allergic reactions to environmental substances such as animal hair, grasses, cosmetics and dust.

RADIO-ISOTOPE
An isotope that is radioactive; radio-isotopes are used clinically in diagnostic and therapeutic procedures.

RADIO-ISOTOPIC SCANNING
A diagnostic technique involving radioactive labelling of tissues and organs by the injection of radio-isotopes into the bloodstream. The emitted radioactivity is detected by a scanner and a record or scan of the labelled area is made.

RADIOLOGY
The use of radioactivity, gamma rays and X-rays in medicine, particularly in diagnosis but also in treatment.

RADIONECROSIS
The destruction of tissues caused by exposure to radium or X-rays.

RADIONUCLIDE
A type of radioactive substance made up of atoms that disintegrate, emitting electromagnetic radiation.

RADIOPAQUE
Any substance which stops the passage of X-rays.

RADIOSENSITIVITY
Capable of being damaged or destroyed by radiation, as a tumor, cell or tissue.

RADIOSURGERY
Originally the term meant the surgical use of radium but is now also applied to many other forms of irradiation.

RADIOTHERAPY
See: Radiation Therapy.

RADIUM
A highly radioactive metal element discovered in 1898 by Pierre and Marie Curie, who separated it from pitchblende. The chloride and bromide salts of radium are usually used in treatment.

RADIUS
The bone of the thumb inside of the forearm. The radius movably articulates with the ulna at both ends so as to permit partial rotation about that bone, that bears on its inner aspect somewhat distal to the head a prominence for the insertion of the biceps muscle tendon, and that has the lower end broadened for articulation with the proximal bones of the carpus so that rotation of the radius involves also the hand. (See illustration on next page).

RAMIFICATION
Branching of any organ or part.

RAMISECTION
Surgical division of some of the rami (branches) of the sympathetic nervous system.

RAMUS
A branch, usually of a nerve or

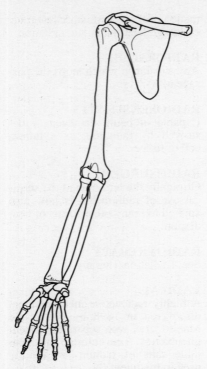

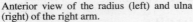

Anterior view of the radius (left) and ulna (right) of the right arm.

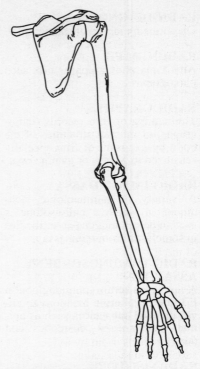

Posterior view of the radius (right) and ulna (left) of the right arm.

blood vessel; a slim process projecting from a large bone, such as the ramus of the lower jaw.

RAMUS COMMUNICANS
Any of a bundle of nerve fibers connecting a sympathetic ganglion with a spinal nerve and being divided into two kinds:
(1) one consisting of myelinated preganglionic fibers, called also white ramus communicans;
(2) one consisting of unmyelinated postganglionic fibers; called also gray ramus communicans.

RANULA
A cystic tumor beneath the tongue, due to blockage of the duct of either the sublingual or submaxillary salivary gland.

RAPE
Sexual intercourse with a woman without her consent.

RAPHE
A seam or ridge, especially one indicating the line of junction of two symmetrical halves.

RAPHE NUCLEUS
Any of several groups of nerve cells situated along or near the median plane of the tegmentum of the mesencephalon.

RAST
Abbreviation of radio-immunosorbent assay test.

RAT-BITE FEVER
Condition that may occur after the bite of an infected rat, even though the wound healed normally. The syndrome is characterized by the following symptoms:
- sudden onset;

- general pains;
- maculopapular or petechial rash.

The condition may be caused by Streptobacillus moniliformis or Spirillum minor. The incubation time is 3-10 days.

Transmission: rat–bite or indirect contact with rats and contaminated food (milk), no person-to-person transmission. The treatment is by antibiotics (tetracyclines).

RATIONALIZATION
An effort to distort reality in order to protect one's self-esteem. It is an attempt to mediate between the ID and reality, the weak EGO ascribed rationally to the irrational demands of the ID.

RAUWOLFIA SERPENTINA
Tropical shrub from which reserpine, a drug used in hypertension and some mental illness, is extracted. The drug affects the heart and nervous system by reducing the supply of noradrenalin.

RAYNAUD'S DISEASE
Intermittent attacks of pallor or congestion of the extremities, with the return of the skin to normal color in between the attacks.

A common disease among young women, it is an excessive reaction to cold in otherwise normal blood vessels, which go into spasm and cut off the blood supply to the fingers or toes.

The symptoms are: sudden onset of intense pallor and/or cyanosis of the tips of the fingers following exposure to cold or, occasionally, emotional upset.

The fingers are usually uncomfortable, with burning pain, tingling or numbness. When this kind of attack, which can recur frequently, ends, the skin turns bright red, and there may be slight swelling, throbbing and pain.

Drugs that dilate the peripheral arteries can be useful. Sometimes surgery to sever the lumbar sympa-thetic nerves is suggested for intractable arterial spasm.

REACTION
The response to stimulation; in chemistry, the interaction of two or more chemical substances; in psychiatry, the mental response to a particular condition or event.

REACTION FORMATION
In psychoanalytical theory a defense mechanism which consists of counteracting the unconscious drive derivative with the opposite conscious attitude such as feeling conscious aversion toward a person toward whom the individual feels unconscious attraction.

REACTION TIME
The interval between the application of a stimulus and the beginning of a response, or, alternatively, the time it takes between seeing a situation and making some muscular movement, such as applying the brakes of a car when sighting an obstruction. In a normal healthy young adult this is approximately one-fifth of a second.

REACTIVE SCHIZOPHRENIA
Schizophrenia characterized by a radical onset, oscillations between excitement and stuporous depressions and by periods of almost normal functioning alternating with states of confusion.

READING DISABILITY
Problem or disturbance in the reading ability or progress of a child. It can be due to a number of factors including developmental neurological disturbances; slow development of vocabulary; difficulty with auditory-visual integration and with perception of auditory stimuli; an inadequate resolution of internal and external conflicts.

READING SPAN
The number of words that can be

perceived and comprehended by the subject in a single fixation period, that is, the period of time when the eye is not moving in the reading process.

REAGENT
Any substance involved in a chemical reaction, or used for the detection or determination of another substance by chemical or microscopical means.

REALISM
A toddler's inability to distinguish dreams.

REALITY ADAPTATION
The process of becoming adapted to the external environment.

REALITY FEELING
The feeling or consciousness of the need for motor adaptation.

REALITY PRINCIPLE
According to Sigmund Freud, the guiding principle of the eye in contradistinction of the ID's pleasure principle; it is the ability to postpone or renounce immediate gratification in order to avoid unpleasant consequence and/or secure a greater reward in the future.

REALITY TESTING
The capacity to distinguish between mental images and external percepts, between fantasy and external reality, to correct subjective impressions by reference to external facts.

REALITY TEST
Type of mental test where the subject is required to draw conclusions from certain data, or to check conclusions already drawn.

REBIRTH FANTASY
A characteristic fantasy, symbolizing one's birth, motivated by an unconscious wish, and expressing itself in dreams and day-dreams of swimming or emerging from water.

REBOUND
Sudden contraction of a muscle after it has relaxed and not been excited by a further stimulus.

REBOUND EFFECT
Return of a condition, often with increased severity, once the prescribed drug is withdrawn.

REBOUND TENDERNESS
A sensation of pain felt when pressure, as to the abdomen, is suddenly removed.

RECALL METHOD
A method of measuring retention, or the rate of forgetting, by the percentage of items recalled after various intervals of time since they were learned.

RECEPTIVE LANGUAGE DEVELOPMENT
The process of acquiring the ability to understand the spoken word.

RECEPTOR
Peripheral nerve endings in the skin and special sense organs. The term is also used to designate a cellular entity, as a beta-receptor or alpha-receptor, that is a postulated intermediary between a chemical agent, as a neurohormone, acting on nervous tissue and the physiological or pharmacological response. Natural body chemicals such as neurotransmitters bind to cell receptors to initiate a response in the cell. Many drugs also have an effect on cells by binding to a receptor. They may promote cell activity or may block it.

RECESSIVE CHARACTERISTICS
A characteristic of one parent found in a minority of the offspring, in contrast to the dominant characteristic of the other parent. It is a part of the rules that govern the characteristics a child will inherit from its ancestors.

RECESSIVE INHERITANCE
Inherited characteristic that fails to show in the child because the corresponding dominant characteristic has suppressed it and taken precedence.

RECIDIVISM
Repeated or habitual relapse into crime or antisocial behavior.

RECIPE
A doctor's prescription.

RECIPIENT
The receiver of a blood transfusion or organ donation.

RECIPROCAL INHIBITION
A term that indicates that elicitation of a particular spinal reflex is accompanied by the inhibition of another, and vice versa.

RECOMBINANT
An animal which has experienced a recombinational event during meiosis, consisting of cross-over and recombination of parts of two chromosomes.

RECOMBINATION
The presence of offspring of gene combinations not found in either parent.

Such new combinations may be formed by the crossing over of chromosomes in meiosis, this being present in either gamete, unite randomly at fertilization.

RECONSTRUCTIVE PSYCHO-THERAPY
A form of psychotherapy which focuses on the reconstruction of childhood and adult experiences which are instrumental in the person's experiences.

RECORD LINKAGE
A method for assembling the information contained in two or more records, e.g., in different sets of medical charts, and in vital records such

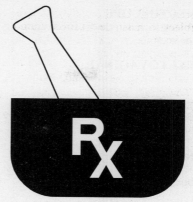

Symbol of a recipe of a drug or medicament.

as birth and death certificates, and a procedure to ensure that the same individual is counted only once.

RECREATIONAL THERAPY
A kind of therapy in which the person is encouraged to participate in some form of play or recreation in order to enjoy it for its own sake.

RECREMENT
Any secretion, such as saliva, that is reabsorbed into the body after it has fulfilled its function.

RECTAL
Pertaining to the rectum.

RECTAL ANESTHESIA
That induced by introducing the anesthetic into the rectum.

RECTALGIA
Pain in the rectum. Also called proctalgia.

RECTAL REFLEX
The mechanism by which the feces are evacuated from the rectum, characterized by contraction of the rectal muscles and relaxation of the internal and external sphincter valves of the anus.

RECTECTOMY
Surgical removal of the rectum.

RECTOSCOPE
A surgical instrument for examining the rectum.

RECTOVAGINAL
Pertaining to rectum and vagina.

RECTOVESICAL
Pertaining to rectum and urinary bladder.

RECTUM
The distal portion of the large intestine.

RECURRENT INFECTION
Repeated bouts of the same type of infection in the same person.

RED BLOOD CELL
Erythrocyte; one of the three kinds of formed elements found in the blood.

Their most important function is to carry oxygen by means of hemoglobin, the red pigment these cells contain.

RED BLOOD CELL INDICES
Parameters of red blood cells. New electronic equipment has made determination of the red blood cell (erythrocyte) indices a valuable aid not only in classifying anemias but in determining the basic cause of the anemia and in helping to decide the specific therapy. The three main indices are:
- mean corpuscular volume (MCV);
- mean corpuscular hemoglobin (MCH);
- mean corpuscular hemoglobin concentration (MCHC).

RED CROSS
International agency for the relief of victims of war and disaster. Its two aims are to alleviate suffering and to maintain a rigid neutrality so that it may cross national borders to reach those otherwise ignitable.

RED INDURATION
Chronic fibrosis of the lung associated with a deposit of red oxide of iron and also seen in marked passive congestion of the lungs.

RED NUCLEUS
A nucleus of gray matter in the tegmentum of the midbrain on each side of the middle line that receives fibers from the cerebellum of the opposite side by way of the superior cerebellar peduncle and gives rise to fibers of the rubrospinal tract of the opposite side. The red nucleus is involved in motor activity.

REDUPLICATION
The doubling of paroxysms in some forms of intermittent fever; the doubling of the first and second sounds of the heart beat.

REEDUCATION
(1) Training in the use of muscles in new functions or of prosthetic devices in old functions in order to replace or restore lost functions.
(2) Training to develop new behaviors, as attitude or habits, to replace others that are considered undesirable.

REFERRED SENSATION
A sensory experience localized at a point quite different from the part effected by the stimulation.

REFLEX
A reflected action or movement; the sum total of any particular automatic response mediated by the nervous system. (See illustration on next page)

REFLEX ARC
The path followed by an impulse from afferent neurons through intermediate neurons to efferent neurons, in the production of a reflex response; the basic unit of function of the nervous system.

REFLEXOGENOUS ZONE
The area of skin and mucous membranes, the stimulation of which gives rise to more or less generalized motor response.

REFLEXOLOGY
A system of laws in the field of learning experiments, in which a simple reflex connection, such as might be due to a neurological reflex arc, is supposed to exist between the stimulus and the response.

REFRACT
To cause deviation; to estimate the extent of visual defect in an eye.

REFRACTION
The process of deviating; the deviation of a ray of light passing through one transparent medium to another of different density, as for instance an object that is half in and half out of water; the process of correcting errors of defective vision by providing spectacles.

REFRACTORY
Resistant to treatment.

REFRACTORY PERIOD
A brief period of time, following the passage of a nerve impulse in a nerve fiber, during which it fails to respond, either absolutely, or relatively.

REFSUM'S SYNDROME
A recessive familial disorder of lipid metabolism characterized by peripheral neuropathy, ataxia, retinitis pigmentosa and bone and skin changes. Prolonged treatment with a diet deficient in phytanic acid is beneficial.

REFUSION
Injection of blood into the circulation after its prior removal from the same person.

REGENERATION
The regrowing of a lost or damaged

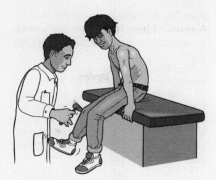

Investigation of the knee jerk reflex.

part of an organism. In plants this includes the production of, for instance, dormant buds and adventitious organs.

All animals possess some power to regenerate, but its extent varies from that in sponges, in which all the cells in a piece of the body can be almost completely separated and will yet come together again to build up new but smaller sponges, to that in higher animals, in which regeneration is limited to the healing of wounds.

REGIME
A systematic course or plan to maintain or improve health. This may include diet, sanitary arrangements, hygiene, exercise and drug medication.

REGIONAL ANESTHESIA
Anesthesia of a region of the body accomplished by a series of encircling injections of an anesthetic.

REGIONAL ILEITIS
Chronic inflammatory disease usually affecting the last part of the ileum, and characterized by the development of granulomatous tissue in the intestinal walls which sometimes leads to obstruction. It is also known as Crohn's disease.

REGRESSION
Return or reversion to an earlier or more primitive stage, type or phase.

It means the tendency on the part of the individual organisms or social groups to revert towards the typical form.

The psychoanalytical usage of the reverting of the libido to a channel of expression, belonging to an earlier phase of development, or the reverting of the individual to interests and forms of behavior characteristic of an earlier or infantile phase, often as a result of fixation.

REGRESSIVE BEHAVIOR
Behavior more appropriate to an earlier level of development.

REGULATOR GENE
A gene that synthesizes a repressor substance which inhibits the action of a specific operator gene, thus preventing the synthesis of messenger RNA by that operon.

REGURGATION
A backflow of blood through a defective heart valve; return from the stomach to the mouth soon after eating without the ordinary expulsive efforts of vomiting.

REHABILITATION
Means of enabling the handicapped to lead lives which are as normal as possible considering their disability. The term can cover social disability (treatment of prisoners) as well as physical or mental difficulty.

REHABILITATION THERAPY
Therapy aimed at restoring or maintaining the greatest possible function and independence.

Rehabilitation therapy is especially useful for persons who have suffered from stroke, an injury, or disease by helping them recover the maximum use of the affected area of the body.

REIMPLANTATION
Replacement of a tissue or organ into its original site or at a new site; in dentistry, replacement of an extracted tooth into its original socket.

REINFECTION
A second infection by the same type of germ.

REINFORCEMENT
A situation that takes place when the conditioned stimulus is presented simultaneously or at an effective level before the unconditioned stimulus.

REINFORCEMENT MECHANISM
Areas of the brain which are positively or negatively reinforcing.

REINFORCEMENT OF AFFECT
The process in which the suppressed ideas and the mechanisms of suppression combine their forces producing mutual cooperation.

REINFORCEMENT WITHDRAWAL
A therapeutic method of withholding reinforcement for responses to reduce the probability of the recurrence of these responses.

REINTEGRATION
Repeated or renewed integration, as of the personality and mental activity after mental illness.

REITER'S SYNDROME
Arthritis associated with nonbacterial urethritis and conjunctivitis, usually seen in adult males following recent sexual exposure. It may also follow an acute attack of unexplained diarrhea.Only a few are disabled by chronic persistent disease.

Treatment is nonspecific, with anti-inflammatory agents such as aspirin or indomethacin.

REJECTION
A type of avoiding behavior on the part of an organism; a negative attitude toward a judgment, suggestion or belief.

RELAPSING FEVER
Infectious condition caused by various species of the genus Borrelia. The condition is characterized by a sudden onset, periods of fever during 2-9 days with general symptoms, relapses (2-10), possible delirium, transitory rash during the initial period. The incubation time is from 5 to 15 days, usually 8 days.

Transmission mechanisms: in epidemic form, by crushing the body of an infected louse on the skin abrasion; in endemic form, by the bite of infected agrasid ticks on vertebrate animals. Treatment by antibiotics (tetracyclines).

RELATIONSHIP PSYCHO-THERAPY
Psychotherapy in which the relationship between the psychotherapist and the client serves as the means and end of psychotherapy.

RELATIONSHIP SYSTEM
System of designation, classification and social significance of kinship or other relationship, sanctioned by tradition.

RELATIVE RISK
The ratio of the risk of disease or death among the exposed to the risk among the unexposed. This usage is synonymous with risk ratio.

RELAXANT
An agent that reduces tension; a loosening.

RELAXATION
A diminution of tension in a part; a diminution in functional activity.

RELAXATION PRINCIPLE
An aspect of psychoanalytical procedure, where the analyst, in order to keep the atmosphere easy, adopts the mood of the client.

RELEARNING
The reacquisition of some skill or some memory material already acquired, but lost as a result of disease, injury or obliviscence.

RELEASE PHENOMENON
The activity in a lower center of the brain when a higher controlling center is not functioning.

RELAPSE THERAPY
A short-term child therapy concerned with specific symptoms resulting from a traumatic event. It consists of the expression of the traumatic situation which caused the symptoms through play, allowing the child to master his repressed emotions.

REM
A unit of biological dose of radiation; the name is derived from the initial letters of the term "roentgen equivalent man (or mammal)". The number of rems of radiation is equal to the number of rads absorbed multiplied by the relative biological effectiveness of the given radiation (for a specified effect).

The rem is also the unit of dose equivalent, which is equal to the product of the number of rads absorbed and the quality factor of the radiation.

REMEDIAL TRAINING
Attempts to train defectives and delinquents, so as to make them, as far as possible, useful and efficient members of the community.

REMEDIATION
Intervention intended primarily as a response to a dysfunctional state or condition once it has been identified.

REMEDY
Something that cures or relieves a disease or bodily disorder.

REMISSION
A period of time during which there is no evidence of a previously existing disease.

REMITTENT FEVER
A paroxysmal fever in which the daily differences in temperature vary by more than one degree.

REM SLEEP
A state of sleep that recurs cyclically several times during a normal period of sleep and that is characterized by increased neural activity of the forebrain and midbrain, by depressed muscle tone, and especially by dreaming, rapid eye movements, and vascular congestion of the sex organs.

RENAL
Pertaining to the kidneys.

RENAL ANGIOGRAPHY
X-ray studies of the blood vessels surrounding or supplying the kidneys, after injection of a contrast medium.

RENAL CIRCULATION
The circulation of the blood through the kidneys. Important in heart diseases because of its function in the elimination of water, certain chemical elements and waste products from the body.

RENAL COLIC
Colic due to the presence of stones in the kidney or ureter, the tube carrying urine from the kidney to the bladder.

RENAL GLUCOSURIA
Excretion of glucose in the urine in the presence of normal or low blood glucose levels.

RENAL HYPERTENSION
High blood pressure caused by damage to or disease of the kidneys or their blood vessels.

RENAL SCAN
A scan of the kidneys for size, shape and exact location, to diagnose a tumor or other abnormalities; done after intravenous injection of a radioactive substance.

RENAL SCLEROSIS
Involvement of the kidney in high blood pressure vascular disorders, causing disturbances in kidney function and a clinical picture identical to that of chronic nephritis. Also called nephrosclerosis.

RENAL TUBULAR ACIDOSIS
Impaired ability to secrete hydrogen ions in the distal part of the nephron or to reabsorb bicarbonate ions proximally, leading to chronic metabolic acidosis which, in the distal form, may be accompanied by potassium depletion and by rickets or osteomalacia.

RENIN
An enzyme produced by the kidney. It regulates the production of the hormone aldosterone, which in turn controls the salt and water balance in the body. It also metabolizes to form other compounds that cause the muscles around arteries to tighten and become smaller in size, thus raising the blood pressure.

REGRESSION
In psychopathology a psychic mechanism by which shameful impulses or experiences are deliberately thrust back from a conscious into a subconscious level and become part of the unconscious.

REPLICATION
The duplication of genetic material (DNA or RNA) in a cell as part of the process of cell division which enables a tissue to grow or a virus to multiply.

REPRODUCTION
The process by which an organism produces offspring, an ability that is a unique characteristic of animals and plants. There are two kinds of reproduction: asexual and sexual.

In asexual reproduction, parts of an organism split off to form new individuals, a process found in some animals but which is more common in plants.

In sexual reproduction, special (haploid) cells containing half the normal number of chromosomes, called gametes, are produced. The joint of the male and female gametes (fertilization) produces a (diploid) cell with the normal number of chromosomes, the zygote, which grows to produce an individual with genes inherited from both parents.

REPUGNANCE
An emotional attitude toward an action or object, with the impulse toward strong opposition or rejection.

RESECTION
The surgical removal of a section of a bone or a piece of an organ or tissue.

RESENTMENT
An emotional attitude characterized by anger against someone, because of real or imagined obstruction of one's interest, or injury to oneself or one's friends.

RESIDENTIAL TREATMENT
Psychotherapeutical treatment offered in an institutional setting which involves a total program for supporting the client's ego strengths, reinforcing his ego weakness.

RESIDUAL TYPE SCHIZOPHRENIA
Type of psychosis characterized by at least one episode of schizophrenia, but the clinical picture that occasioned the evaluation or admission to clinical care is without prominent psychotic symptoms, though signs of the illness persist. Emotional blunting, social withdrawal, eccentric behavior, illogical thinking, and mild loosening of associations are common. If delusions or hallucinations are present, they are not prominent, and are not accompanied by strong affect.

RESIDUAL URINE
The urine remaining in the bladder after urination. This damming back of urine is due to an obstruction pressing on the outlet. In the male it may be due to enlargement of the prostate gland and in the female due to dropping of the bladder into the vagina, as the result of stretching of the vagina at childbirth.

RESISTANCE
In psychoanalysis a continuation of repression which interferes, often actively, with the progress of the analysis. The person resists in various ways, working for or reaching the goal for which he entered analysis.

RESISTANCE SENSATION
A complex of pressure and kinesthetic sensory impressions, when muscles are being contracted against opposing pressure.

RESONANCE
The prolonged, non-musical, composite sound which results from vibration of the normal chest; the attribute of relatively long duration possessed by certain sounds.

RESORPTION
The removal by absorption; in dentistry, the process which causes the disappearance of the roots of the first set of teeth.

RESPIRATION
The exchange of oxygen and carbon dioxide between the atmosphere and the body cells, including inspiration and expiration, diffusion of oxygen from alveoli to the blood and of carbon dioxide from the blood to the alveoli, and the transport of oxygen to and carbon dioxide from the body cells.

RESPIRATOR
An appliance which filters the air

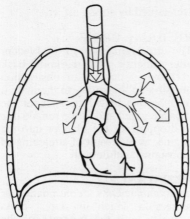

Flow of air during inhalation.

breathed through it, or which provides artificial respiration for paralyzed or unconscious patients.

RESPIRATORY ACIDOSIS
A primary increase in arterial carbon dioxide pressure; Ph is low and carbon dioxide combining power increases if kidney function is intact.

RESPIRATORY ALKALOSIS
A primary decrease in carbon dioxide pressure; blood Ph is increased and carbon dioxide combining power is reduced.

RESPIRATORY DISTRESS SYNDROME
A disorder primarily of prematurity, manifested clinically by respiratory distress and pathologically by pulmonary hyaline membranes and atelectasis of the lungs. The disease is the leading cause of morbidity and mortality in prematurely born infants.

RESPIRATORY PULSE
The modification in the pulse during respiration.

RESPIRATORY SOUNDS
Any sound heard through the stethoscope placed over any portion of the respiratory tract.

RESPIROMETER
An instrument which determines the character of respiration.

RESPONDENT LEARNING
No new responses are learned; rather available responses come under the control of a new stimulus through the conditioning process; also referred to as classical conditioning.

RESPONSE
The reaction of the body to a stimulus.

REST-CURE
A method of treatment not widely used or recognized, which stresses the importance of rest, environmental change, fattening diet, massage and mild exercises.

RESTITUTION
Rotation of the baby's head immediately after its delivery; a return to the normal condition.

RESTLESSNESS
A general state of the organism, reflecting itself in a feeling which is being regarded as one of the elementary dimensions of feeling.

REST PAUSE
A pause introduced during a working period, with the object of eliminating or reducing fatigue, and usually forming a regular part of the organization of the work.

RESUSCITATION
Restoring to life those near death, by artificial respiration and external cardiac massage (cardiopulmonary resuscitation). (See illustration on next page)

RESUSCITATOR
An apparatus for giving artificial respiration.

RETARDATION
The slowing up of movement or de-

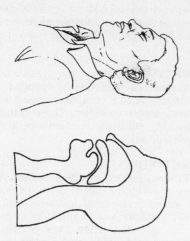

Resuscitation. Establishing an open airway; closed airway.

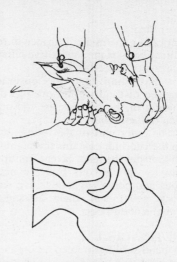

Resuscitation. Establishing an open airway; open airway.

velopment; applied usually to the mental development of a child, where the mentality is defined below normal, and even below an IQ of 70.

RETENTION
The persisting trace left behind as an after-effect by any experience, forming the basis of learning, habit and skill.

RETICULAR
Resembling or pertaining to a network.

RETICULOCYTE
A net-like red blood cell observed during the process of blood regeneration.

RETICULOCYTE
A test to determine the number of reticulocytes in a specimen of whole blood, a measure of bone marrow activity; decreased in hemolytic disease; elevated after hemorrhage, or when recovering from anemia.

RETICULOCYTOSIS
An excess of reticulocytes in the blood.

RETICULO-ENDOTHELIAL SYSTEM (RES)
Generic name for those cells in the body that take up dyes and other foreign material from the blood stream and other body fluids; they are also known as macrophages.

Blood monocytes are functionally part of the system as are macrophages in the lymph nodes, spleen, bone marrow, liver (Kupffer cells) and lung alveoli.

RETINA
The innermost tunic of the eyeball containing the neural elements for reception and transmission of visual stimuli. The retina comprises the innermost of the three coats of the eyeball:
- an outer, fibrous tunic, made up of the sclera behind and the cornea in front;
- an intermediate, pigmented vascular tunic;
- an internal, nervous tunic (retina) continuous with the optic nerve.

The retina as a whole can be divided into three concentric zones:
(1) Extending from the posterior pole to a level well forward of the equator is the truly nervous portion, also called the optic portion of

the retina.

(2) Lining the internal surface of the ciliary body is the insensitive ciliary portion of the retina.

(3) Extending onto the posterior surface of the iris, and even to the margin of the pupil is the iris portion of the retina.

The outer part of the retina, next to the choroid, contains the pigment rhodopsin; the inner layers, continuing to the vitreous body, contain rods and cones (light-sensitive sensory cells) and their associated ganglia and fibers.

RETINACULUM
A band serving to keep an organ in its place.

RETINAL DETACHMENT
A condition of the eye in which the retina has separated from the choroid.

RETINAL DISPARITY
The slight difference in the two retinal images due to the angle from which each eye views an object.

RETINAL RIVALRY
The oscillating perception of first one than the other of two visual stimuli which differ radically in color or form when they are presented simultaneously to congruent areas of both eyes.

RETINENE
Either the orange or the yellow carotenoid pigment of the retina.

RETINITIS PIGMENTOSA
A slowly progressive, bilateral, tapeto-retinal degeneration. No therapy is effective.

RETINITIS PROLIFERANS
Neovascularization of the retina associated with neuropathy due to diabetes.

RETINOBLASTOMA
A congenital malignant tumor that arises from the nuclear layers of the retina. If diagnosed early more than 80 percent of the cases can be cured.

RETINOIDS
A group of drugs that are synthetic vitamin A-like compounds used to treat skin conditions. These drugs include etretinate, isotretinoin and retinoic acid.

RETINOL
Vitamin A. Deficiency of vitamin A (a fat-soluble alcohol) is considered a major problem of nutrition. Usually vitamin A is supplied in minimal amounts in the average diet. Some health faddists who eat excessive amounts of food high in vitamin A may display symptoms of hair loss, fatigue, irritability, cerebral edema and yellowish skin color.

Vitamin A deficiency is a major cause of blindness in young children in parts of the world where the diet is inadequate. Night blindness and "dry eye" are early indications of the deficiency.

RETINOPATHY
Damage to the retina of the eye (the back portion on which the image of what we see is projected). The symptoms are blurriness, then progressive loss of vision. The visual loss may be generalized over the eye or may be worse in some parts than in others.

Damage to the retina is usually caused by damage to the blood vessels of the eye, with narrowing and loss of blood supply, congesting of veins with formation of aneurysms, and rupture of blood vessels, leading to blockage of vision in front of the retina. There are many possible causes for these changes including hypertension, diabetes mellitus and generalized atherosclerosis.

The treatment consists of all measures needed to control the underlying problem.

RETINOSCOPE
The apparatus used for measuring the refraction of the eye.

RETINOSCOPE
The examination of the retina to determine the degree of any faulty refraction of the eye.

RETRACTOR
An instrument used to draw back wound edges or an organ so that the surgeon has a clear operative field.

RETRACTION
Effect of a new experience or piece of learning on retention of a previous experience or piece of learning.

RETROACTIVE ASSOCIATION
A connection established between an item in a series and another item which has preceded it in the series.

RETROBULBAR
Situated behind the eyeball.

RETROBULBAR NEURITIS
Inflammation of the optic nerve behind the eyeball.

RETROFLEXED
Bent backwards.

RETROFLEXION OF THE UTERUS
One which is displaced backwards but has its cervix (neck) in the normal position.

RETROGRADE AMNESIA
Inability to remember events prior to an accident in which the brain was damaged.

RETROGRADE PYELOGRAPHY
A method of pyelography in the urinary system in which the opaque medium is introduced into the ureter via the urinary bladder.

RETROGRESSION
The passing from a higher to a lower type of structure in the development of an animal; in medicine, a going backwards, degeneration, involution, atrophy or the subsidence of a disease or its symptoms.

RETROLENTAL FIBROPLASIA
A bilateral disease characterized by abnormality of the retinal vessels that occur in premature infants in whom the immature retina was exposed to high postnatal incubation oxygen concentrations. Careful monitoring of the oxygen content of the incubator is necessary to minimize the incidence of this complication or prematurity.

RETROSPECTION
The systematic review and observation of an experience after it has already happened, especially as soon after its occurrence as possible.

RETROVERSION
A turning backwards.

RETROVERSION OF THE UTERUS
Backward displacement of the uterus with forward displacement of the cervix (neck).

RETROVIRUSES
Viruses that contain RNA, not DNA, and that produce a DNA analog of their DNA through the production of an enzyme known as "reverse transcriptase". The resulting DNA is incorporated in the genetic structure of the invaded cell in a form referred to as the "provirus".

REVASCULARIZATION
Restoration of sufficient bloodflow to body tissues when supplying arteries are narrowed or blocked by injury or disease. Such surgery can be done on the legs, kidneys, brain, neck or (most commonly) the heart.

REVERSION
A character of trait which appears in one generation, but is not present in the immediately preceding generation.

REVULSION
A sudden and strong emotional reaction or chance of feeling, usually in the direction of extreme displeasure.

REYE'S SYNDROME
Acute encephalopathy and fatty degeneration of the viscera, which tends to follow some acute viral infections. The cause is unknown, but some viruses have been implicated as associated or contributing factors.
The major symptoms are:
– vomiting;
– hepatic dysfunction;
– change in mental status;
– progressing rapidly in severe forms of coma;
– respiratory arrest;
– gastrointestinal bleeding is possible.
The syndrome may occur in children under 18 years of age, clusters of cases or outbreaks linked to influenza B virus, sporadic cases after varicella, enterovirus and myxovirus infections.

RHABDOMYOMA
A tumor composed of striated (striped) muscle fibers.

RHABDOMYOSARCOMA
A malignant tumor composed of striated muscle fibers.

RHABDOVIRUS
Any of a group of RNA-containing rod- or bullet-shaped viruses found in plants and animals and including the causative agents of rabies and vesicular stomatitis.

RHACHISCHISIS
A congenital cleft in the vertebral column (spine).

RHAGADES
Cracks or fissures in skin that has lost its elasticity through infiltration and thickening. Seen in syphilis, intertrigo (moist eczema), keratoderma (hard skin) and other affections.

RHEOBASE
The minimal electrical current required to excite a tissue, as nerve or muscle, given indefinitively long time during which the current is applied.

RHESUS FACTOR
A substance discovered in 1940 to be present in the blood of 85 percent of human beings and so named because it was first found in the blood of Rhesus monkeys. See Rh-factor.

RHEUMATIC CHOREA
Another name for chorea minor.

RHEUMATIC DISEASE
Any of several diseases, as rheumatic fever or fibrositis, characterized by inflammation and pain in muscles or joints.

RHEUMATIC FEVER
An acute inflammatory complication of streptococcal infection, characterized mainly by arthritis, chorea or heart disorders alone or in combination, with residual heart disease as a possible sequel of the inflammatory process of the heart (carditis).
The mixture of manifestations arbitrarily diagnosed as acute rheumatic fever occurs as an inflammatory complication (without pus formation) of streptococcal infection (Group A streptococci) and can affect one or more of five major sites:
– joints (arthritis);
– brain (chorea);
– heart (carditis);
– subcutaneous tissue (nodules);
– skin (erythema marginatum).
The attack rates of rheumatic fever

range from 0.1 percent in untreated people with mild or symptomatic streptococcal infections to 3 percent in those with inflammatory processes of the throat accompanied by fever.

To prevent rheumatic heart disease, rheumatic fever must be prevented. Rheumatic fever occurs most often in children. The first stage is a streptococcal infection of the beta-hemolytic type which may manifest itself as a strep throat, scarlet fever or infection of the middle ear. Sometimes it may be an infection which has no outward manifestations at all, a so-called "silent" strep.

RHEUMATIC HEART DISEASE

The damage to the heart, particularly the heart valves, by one or more attacks of rheumatic fever. The valves are sometimes scarred so they do not open and close normally.

RHEUMATIC NODULE

Nodule, especially near the wrist or elbow, which can be felt through the skin, occurring in limited numbers in the graver cases of rheumatic fever in childhood. It is nearly always an indication that the heart has been involved in a rheumatic process.

RHEUMATISM

A much abused name, popularly applied to any pain affecting muscles, tendons, joints, bones or nerves, which produces discomfort or disability in such widely varied disorders as rheumatoid arthritis, degenerative joint disease, spondylitis, bursitis, fibrositis, myositis, neuritis, lumbago, sciatica and gout.

RHEUMATOID ARTHRITIS

Contrary to popular belief this is really a disease of the whole body which attacks the joints as a complication, so that the person may feel ill, depressed, lose his appetite and become anemic as well as having swollen and painful joints. The origin of the disease is unknown.

RHEUMATOID FACTOR

An anti-immunoglobin antibody directed with rheumatoid arthritis and other rheumatoid diseases.

The majority of those suffering with rheumatoid arthritis have an immunoglobin antibody called rheumatoid factor.

The more rheumatoid factor detected in the blood, the greater the possibility that rheumatoid arthritis exists. Unfortunately, a number of other diseases can also elevate RF levels (liver, lung, and heart conditions, syphilis and some worm infestations).

RH FACTOR

A blood factor present in most, but not all people. An Rh-positive person can develop antibodies to the Rh-factor if exposed to it through blood transfusion or pregnancy. An Rh-positive infant of a woman with Rh antibodies may be born with a serious blood disease.

Administration of an immune human globulin to an Rh-negative mother within 72 hours of giving birth to an Rh-positive infant will prevent the development of antibodies and protect her future pregnancies.

RHINALGIA

Pain in the nose.

RHINENCEPHALON

The olfactory portion of the brain; the anterior inferior part of the forebrain that is chiefly concerned with olfaction and that is considered to include the olfactory bulb together with the forebrain olfactory structures receiving fibers directly from it and often formerly the limbic system which is now known to be concerned with emotional states and affective behavior.

RHINITIS
The most frequent of the acute upper respiratory infections, characterized by edema and vasodilation of the mucous membrane of the nose, nasal discharge and obstruction.

RHINOLALIA
A nasal tone of voice such as is heard when the nose is obstructed in the course of a head cold.

RHINOPHARYNX
The nasopharynx (the area which includes the nose and throat).

RHINOPHYMA
Acne of the nose, associated with a marked degree of connective tissue hypertrophy.

RHINOPOLYP
Polyp of the nose. A benign tumor arising from the lining of the nose and resulting in obstruction to the nasal airway.

These tumors may precipitate attacks of hay fever, and even though they can be removed surgically, there is, unfortunately, a tendency for them to recur.

RHINORRHEA
The discharge of mucus from the nose, a "runny" nose.

RHINOSCLEROMA
A chronic inflammatory disease of the nasopharyngeal mucosa that is characterized by the formation of granulomas and by dense induration of the tissues and nodular deformity.

RHINOSCOPE
An instrument used to examine the inside of the nose.

RHINOTRACHEITIS
Inflammation of the nasal cavities and trachea; particularly a disease of the upper respiratory system, usually caused by a virus.

RHIZOTOMY
The surgical section of the posterior roots of the spinal nerves, performed as treatment for pain and spastic paralysis.

RHODOPSIN
Visual purple, photosensitive pigment, derived from vitamin A, found in the retinas of many vertebrates, including humans. Its bleaching by incident light is the basis of light-and-dark distinction in vision.

RHOMBOIDEUS
Either of two muscles that lie beneath the trapezius muscle and connect the spinous processus of various vertebrae with the medial border of the scapula.

RHOMBOID FOSSA
The floor of the fourth ventricle of the brain formed by the dorsal surfaces of the pons and medulla oblongata.

RHONCHUS
A rattling sound in the throat or bronchial tubes.

RHONCHUS RALE
An extremely course rale which originates in the larger air passages and sets up vibrations which in addition to being heard quite clearly through a stethoscope, usually can even be felt with the hand when it is laid on the chest.

RHYTHM
A regular recurrence of a function or action.
(1) A regularly recurrent quantitative change in a variable biological process as the pattern of recurrence of the heart cycle.
(2) The recurring pattern of physical and functional changes associated with the human sexual cycle.

RHYTHMICITY
The state of being rhythmic or of

responding rhythmically.

RHYTHM METHOD
A system of birth control through abstinence from sexual intercourse during the estimated monthly interval of female ovulation and fertility.

RIB
One of the 24 long, flat, curved bones forming the wall of the chest.

RIBOFLAVIN
Vitamin B_2. Deficiency of vitamin B_2 can cause many eye problems (ulceration, cataracts, corneal vascularization, burning and itching) and skin problems, as well as problems in the blood (leukocytosis or fewer than normal white blood cells) and the nervous system (neuritis). Riboflavin is found mostly in milk, meat and nuts.

RIBONUCLEIC ACID (RNA)
One of the nucleic acids found in the cell.

RIBOSOMAL RNA
A type of ribonucleic acid which lines up amino acids in the ribosomes to form proteins to a particular sequence.

RIBOSOMES
Tiny granules, of diameter about 10 nm, found in cell protoplasm. They are composed of protein and a special form of ribonucleic acid, known as ribosomal RNA. The ribosome is the site of protein synthesis.

RICCO'S LAW
A statement in physiology: when a light source of a given size and intensity is just capable of producing visual sensation, reduction of either size or intensity will make it invisible.

RICE-WATER STOOLS
A descriptive term for bowel discharges in cholera.

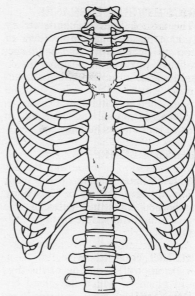

Bony thorax in anterior view. Twelve pairs of ribs make up the sides of the thoracic cavity. The ribs increase in length from the first to the seventh; then they decrease in length to the twelfth rib.

RICIN
A poisonous white powder derived from the castor bean, used in medicine to cause agglutination of red blood cells.

RICKETS
A deficiency of infancy due to lack of vitamin D, characterized by poor nutrition and changes in the bones. There is slight fever and sweating together with general symptoms.

RICKETTSIA
Organisms partway between bacteria and viruses that are obligatory intracellular organisms but have a more complex structure than viruses. They are responsible for a number of diseases (often born by ticks or lice) including typhus, scrub typhus and Rocky Mountain spotted fever; related organisms cause Q fever and psittacosis.

They are sensitive to tetracyclines and cause characteristic serological reactions.

RICKETTSIAL DISEASES
A variety of illnesses manifested by sudden onset, a course of fever of one to several weeks, headache, malaise, prostration, peripheral vasculitis and, in most cases, a characteristic rash. Most rickettsias are maintained in nature by a cycle involving an animal reservoir and an insect that infects humans.

RIDER'S BONE
An infiltration of bone into the adductor longus muscle on the inner side of the thigh. It is caused by prolonged pressure between the muscle and the saddle in horse riding.

RIEDEL'S DISEASE
A chronic inflammation of the thyroid gland in which the gland becomes hard and stony and firmly attached to the surrounding tissue.

RIGHTING REFLEX
A reflex or reflexive act which serves to return the organism to an upright position when thrown off balance or when placed on its back.

RIGIDITY
A state of strong muscular contraction. The term is also used in the sense of the inability to alter one's opinions, attitudes or actions when they are inappropriate.

RIGOR MORTIS
Stiffness of the body muscles occurring some hours after death and caused by biochemical alterations in muscle. The body is set in the position held at the onset of the changes.

RIGHTHANDEDNESS
The quality or state of being righthanded; using the right hand habitually more easily than the left.

RIGHT-TO-LIFER
Person who is opposed to abortion.

RING CHROMOSOME
A circular chromosome resulting from breakage in both arms of a chromatid followed by fusion of the broken ends to form a ring.

RINGER'S SOLUTION
Sodium chloride, potassium chloride and calcium chloride, dissolved in distilled water. It is used in cases where these chemicals and body water have been lost through vomiting or diarrhea or both.

RING PESSARY
A rubber appliance inserted into the vagina to correct the position of the uterus or to prevent it from prolapsing.

RINGWORM
Common fungus disease of the skin of humans and animals which may also affect the hair or nails. Ring-shaped raised lesions occur, often with central sparing; temporary baldness is seen on hairy skin, together with the disintegration of the nails.

Athlete's foot is ringworm of the toes, while tinea cruris is a variety affecting the groin. Various fungi may be responsible, including Trichophyton and Microspora.

Treatment includes topical ointments (e.g., benzyl benzoate or systemic antifungal antibiotics such as griseofulvin).

RINNE'S TEST
A test of hearing performed with a tuning fork to detect whether air or bone conduction of sound is the better of the two.

RISK
The probability that an event will occur, e.g, that an individual will become ill or die within a stated period of time or age. Also, a nontechnical term encompassing a variety of measures of the probability of a (generally) unfavorable outcome.

RISK FACTOR
Term used in medicine in at least three different senses.
(1) An attribute or exposure that is associated with an increased probability of a specific outcome, such as the occurrence of a disease.
(2) An attribute or exposure that increases the probability of occurrence of disease or other specific outcome.
(3) A determinant that can be modified by intervention, thereby reducing the probability of occurrence or disease or other specified outcomes.

RISUS SARDONICUS
The sardonic grin. A distortion of the face caused by muscle spasm, and seen in some cases of tetanus (lockjaw).

RITTER-LYELL SYNDROME
Another name for toxic epidermal necrolysis.

RITUAL
A system of religious or magical ceremonies or procedures, frequently with special forms of words, or a special vocabulary, and usually associated with important occasions or actions.

RIVER BLINDNESS
Another name for onchocerciasis.

RNA
Abbreviation of ribonucleic acid, an important nucleic acid. RNA is any of several nucleic acids that contain ribose and uracil as structural components and are associated with the control of cellular chemical activities.

ROCKY MOUNTAIN SPOTTED FEVER
An acute febrile disease caused by Rickettsia rickettsii and transmitted by ixodid ticks. The incubation period averages seven days.

The onset is abrupt with severe headache, chills and muscular pains. Fever may reach 40 degrees centigrade within several days and remains high for 10 to 15 days. Untreated patients may develop necrosis and circulatory failure, with such sequelae as brain and heart damage.

Starting antibiotic therapy early has significantly reduced mortality, formerly about 20 percent and much higher in localized areas and in adult over the age of 40 years. No serious sequelae result if therapy is instituted early.

RODENT ULCER
A form of malignant disease (a carcinoma) with more or less deep penetration, affecting especially the face, neck and scalp.

ROD OF CORTY
Any of the minute modified epithelial elements that rise from the basilar membrane of the organ of Corti in two spirally arranged rows so that the free ends of the members incline toward and interlock with corresponding members of the opposite row and enclose the tunnel of Corti.

ROENTGEN
The unit used internationally as a measure of radiation, named for Wilhelm Konrad Roentgen.

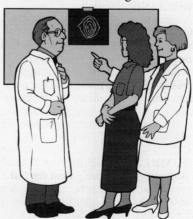

Investigation of X-ray photographs.

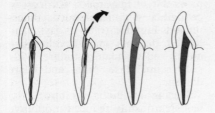

Treatment of a root canal infection.

ROENTGENOLOGY
The study of all applications of X-rays, especially those relating to medical diagnosis and therapy.

ROENTGEN THERAPY
Treatment of disease by roentgen rays (X-rays).

ROLE PLAYING
The adoption of the role of an important other in the person's life so as to come to a better understanding of the other or adoption of social roles so as to better understanding how he conceives of and functions in them.

ROLE TAKING
Ability to place oneself in the role of another; major mechanism that accounts for the way moral judgments are learned.

ROLFING
A method of systematically massaging the deep muscles that is intended to serve as both physical and emotional therapy.

ROLLOVER TEST
Test during pregnancy for susceptibility to toxemia which is a serious high blood pressure condition of unknown origin.

ROMBERG SIGN
The swaying which is evident in a person with locomotor ataxia when he tries to stand quietly with eyes closed and feet together.

ROOF
The vaulted upper boundary of the mouth supported largely by the palatine bones and limited anteriorly by the dental lamina and posteriorly by the uvula and upper part of the fauces.

ROOMING-IN
An arrangement in a hospital whereby a newborn infant is kept in a crib at the mother's bedside instead of in a nursery.

ROOT
That part of an organ (such as a tooth or hair) embedded in the tissues. The term is also applied to the part of a tooth within the socket.

ROOT CANAL
The part of the pulp cavity lying in the roof of a tooth.

ROOTING REFLEX
The head-turning and mouth-opening movements in the infant when his cheek is stroked which is involved in the reflex to turn towards the breast when being nursed.

RORSCHACH-INKBLOTS TEST
A projective test consisting of ten cards on which either black and white, black and white with color or colored symmetrical inkblots occur.

The subject is presented the cards in a prescribed sequence and requested to tell the examiner what the inkblots could be.

Responses are scored according to the various determinants used in a particular response and are indicative of the particular cognitive style and defensive mechanisms characterizing the individual's personality structure as a whole.

ROSACEA
A chronic inflammatory disorder, usually beginning in middle age or later, and characterized by telangiectasia, erythema, papules

and pustules appearing especially in the central area of the face.

Broad-spectrum antibiotics are the only regularly effective treatment.

ROSE FEVER
An allergy similar to hay fever, associated with rose pollen and usually occurring in early summer.

ROSEOLA INFANTUM
An acute disease of infants or very young children characterized by high fever, absence of localizing symptoms or signs and appearance of a rubelliform eruption simultaneously with, or following, defervescence.

The cause and mode of spread are not known, but the disease is probably communicable and caused by a virus. It occurs more often in the spring and fall. Minor local epidemics have been reported.

The treatment is symptomatic and includes measures to keep the fever down. When the temperature falls to normal and the eruption appears, the person is so nearly well that no further treatment is necessary.

ROSTRUM
A bodily part or process suggesting a bird's bill.
(1) The inferior median spine of the body of the basisphenoid bone articulating with the vomer.
(2) The reflected anterior portion of the corpus callosum below the genu.

ROTATOR CUFF
A supporting and strengthening structure of the shoulder joint that is made up of its capsule blended with tendons of the subscapularis, infraspinatus, supraspinatus, and teres minor muscles as they pass to the capsule or across it to insert on the humerus.

ROTAVIRAL ENTERITIS
A condition characterized by gastrointestinal symptoms that may be preceded by respiratory illness (cough, nasal discharge) or otitis media (red throat, inflamed tympanic membrane).

Vomiting generally starts before diarrhea, which may cause severe dehydration and rapid circulatory collapse, particularly in children aged 12-18 months (usually less below 12 months). The condition is caused by rotaviruses, the incubation period is 2 days. Control and treatment: rehydration, enteric precautions, investigation of contacts and source of infection.

ROTE LEARNING
Learning by pure repetition, regardless of meaning, and without any attempt of organization.

ROUGHAGE
Indigestible fibers of animal origin. Although they have no nutritional value, they help keep the colon functioning normally by providing bulk. The word roughage is often applied to cellulose.

ROUGHNESS
In tactual experiences, unevenness arising from a number of simultaneous or successive pressure stimuli of varying intensity.

ROUS' SARCOMA
A cancer-like growth found in some fowls and from which can be obtained a virus, which on inoculation into other fowls reproduces a similar cancer-like growth.

RUBACELL
A blood test done to determine whether a child or adult has had rubella (German measles), to screen for immunity to rubella and to determine whether a child has congenital rubella infection.

RUBEFACIENT
A substance for external application that produces redness of the skin,

not followed by blistering. A rubefacient is also known as a counterirritant, that, when applied to an area of skin, causes it to redden by increasing blood flow in vessels in that area.

RUBELLA

A contagious exanthematous disease, usually with mild constitutional symptoms that may result in abortion, stillbirth or congenital defects in infants born to mothers infected during the early months of pregnancy. The disease is caused by a virus.

The rash is similar to that of measles but is less extensive and more evanescent. It begins on the face and neck and quickly spreads to the trunk and extremities. At the onset of eruption, a flush simulating that of scarlet fever may appear, particularly on the face. The rash usually lasts about three days. On the second day, if often becomes more scarlatiniform with a reddish flush. The slight skin discoloration that remains as the rash fades, disappears in a day.

Rubella requires little or no treatment. Middle ear infection, a rare complication, requires appropriate treatment. Rubella can be prevented through immunization with the rubella vaccine, which is usually given as part of the measles-mumps-rubella (MMR) vaccine.

RUBIN TEST

One of several tests performed in cases of infertility. Specifically, it determines whether the Fallopian tubes (which carry the ovum, or egg, from the ovary to the uterus) are open or blocked. Carbon dioxide gas is forced into the uterus under pressure; if the tubes are normal (open), the gas is detected in the abdomen. occasionally the test procedure itself acts therapeutically to open blocked tubes.

RUBOR

The redness of inflammation.

RUCTUS

Intestinal rumbling. Also called borborygmi.

RUFFINI'S CORPUSCLE

Any of numerous oval sensory end organs occurring in the subcutaneous tissue of the fingers.

RUMINATION

Chewing the cud; sometimes a persistent habit in unhappy babies who regurgitate their feed and re-taste it with intense satisfaction; in psychiatry, an obsessional concentration on an idea which cannot be dislodged from the mind, seen in anxiety states.

RUMPEL-LEEDE TEST

A test in which the increased bleeding tendency characteristic of various disorders (as scarlet fever and thrombocytopenia) is indicated by the formation of multiple petechiae on the forearm following application of a tourniquet to the upper arm.

RUNNING PULSE

A very weak, frequent pulse, with no tension in the arteries, one pulse wave running into the next with no apparent intervals. It is seen after cases of extensive bleeding.

RUTIN

A yellow crystalline flavonol glycoside that occurs in various plants (as rue, tobacco, and buckwheat), that yields quercetin and rutinose on hydrolysis, and that is used chiefly for strengthening capillary blood vessels, as in cases of hypertension and radiation injury.

S

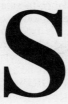

SABURRA
Dirt or filth, particularly the brown crusts which collect around the lips and teeth in persons suffering with fevers.

SACCHARIDE
Any of a large group of carbohydrates, including sugars and starches.

SACCHARIN
A sweetening agent, 550 times sweeter than sucrose, normally used as its soluble sodium salt. Not absorbed by the body, it is used by diabetics and in low-calorie diabetic foods.

SACCHAROSE
Cane sugar.

SACCHAROSURIA
The presence of saccharose in the urine.

SACRAL FORAMEN
Any of 16 openings in the sacrum of which there are four on each side of the dorsal surface giving passage to the dorsal roots of the sacral nerves and four on each side of the pelvis surface giving passage to the ventral roots of the sacral nerves.

SACRALGIA
Pain in the sacrum (rear wall of the pelvis).

SACRAL HIATUS
The opening into the spinal canal in the midline of the dorsal surface of the sacrum between the laminae of the fifth sacral vertebra.

SACRAL NERVE
Any of the spinal nerves of the sacral region of which there are five pairs and which have anterior and posterior branches passing out through the sacral foramina.

SACRAL PLEXUS
A nerve plexus that lies against the posterior and lateral walls of the pelvis, formed by the union of the lumbosacral trunk and the first, second, and third sacral nerves, and continuing into the thigh as the sciatic nerve.

SACRIFICIAL OPERATION
An operation in which some part or organ is completely removed and sacrificed because there is no alternative if the patient is to be helped.

SACROILIAC JOINT
The joint between the sacrum or lower part of the vertebral column and the iliac bones of the pelvis. Little movement occurs about the joint but it may be affected by certain types of arthritis, such as ankylosing spondylitis.

SACRODYNIA
Pain in and around the sacrum (rear wall of the pelvis).

SACROSPINAL
Relating to the sacrum (rear wall of the pelvis).

SACRUM
A curved, triangular bone composed of five united vertebrae, situated between the last lumbar vertebra above, the coccyx below and the innominate bones on each side and forming the rear wall of the pelvis. (See illustration on next page)

SADDLE BLOCK
A low spinal block to anesthetize the perineum and buttock area.

SADISM
A sexual perversion in which sexual

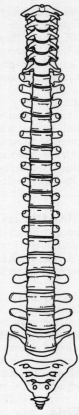

Anterior view of the vertebral column. The sacrum (below) is a triangular bone formed by the union of five sacral vertebrae. It serves as a strong foundation for the pelvic girdle.

excitement and orgasm are dependent upon the infliction of pain and humiliation of others.

SADISTIC PERSONALITY DISORDER

A pervasive pattern of cruel, demeaning, and aggressive behavior directed toward other people, beginning by early adulthood. The sadistic behavior is often evident both in social relationships (particularly with family members) and at work (with subordinates), but seldom is displayed in contacts with people in positions of authority or higher status.

Many people with this disorder use physical violence to establish dominance in interpersonal relationships. This violence is frequently resorted to or escalated when the person perceives that his or her victims are no longer willing to be intimidated or controlled.

SADNESS

An emotional mood, tending towards sorrow, characterized by relative passivity and diminished muscular tone, with sighing, and not infrequently, weeping.

SADOMASOCHISM

Sexual pleasure related to both sadism and masochism. Sadism and masochism are two kinds of kinky sex that are closely related. The essential element in both is a sexual arousal based on pain or suffering. The sadist delights in watching or making other people suffer. The masochist delights in experiencing this suffering.

SAFFLOWER OIL

An oil derived from seeds or the safflower plant; one of the richest sources of the essential fatty acids.

SAGITTAL

Arrow-shaped; the middle horizontal plane of the body from front to back.

SALAAM SPASM

Movements of the head and upper part of the body which are rhythmic and periodic; usually seen in children as part of an epileptic syndrome.

SALAAM TIC

Rhythmic head movements associated with compensatory balancing movements of the trunk in the same direction with or without extension of the upper limbs, and with nystagmus. The movements are slow and occur in oligophrenic subjects, particular in the sitting position.

SALICYLATE
Any salt of salicylic acid (prepared synthetically or obtained from wintergreen leaves of the bark of white birch).

Aspirin is one of the most common sources of salicylates as are many other drugs to minimize pain. Taking an excessive amount causes poisoning.

Salicylates are also used to relieve some symptoms caused by arthritis or rheumatism, such as swelling, stiffness, and joint pain. However, they do not cure arthritis and will help only as long as one continues to take them.

SALICYLATE POISONING
Condition usually caused by acetylsalicylic acid (aspirin) overdose. Early symptoms of toxicity are hyperventilation and vomiting, followed by lethargy, disorientation and coma.

Chronic toxicity symptoms include:
- muscle tenderness;
- muscle spasm;
- decreased auditory acuity;
- paresthesia;
- excitability;
- delirium;
- hallucinations.

SALICYLIC ACID
White crystalline solid, made from phenol and carbon dioxide; used in medicine against calluses and warts, and to make aspirin and dyes. Its sodium salt is an analgesic and is used in rheumatism. It has also proved to be of significant value in the prevention of heart and brain thrombosis.

SALINE SOLUTION
Normal, more correctly physiological, saline solution containing 0.9 percent of sodium chloride (common salt, NaCl). This fluid is in balance with the salinity of body tissues so that no osmotic pressure is exerted in either direction when it is used as a bland irrigating solution.

SALIVA
The watery secretion of the salivary glands which lubricates the mouth and food boluses. It contains mucus, some gamma globulins and ptyalin and is secreted in response to food in the mouth or by conditioned reflexes such as the smell or sight of food. Secretion is partly under the control of the parasympathetic autonomic nervous system. The various salivary glands - parotid, submandibular and sublingual - secrete slightly different types of saliva, varying in mucus and enzyme content.

SALIVARY CALCULUS
A stone in a duct or a salivary gland.

SALIVARY FISTULA
An opening between a salivary gland or its duct with the surface of the skin.

SALIVARY REFLEX
The reflex characterized by the production and flow of saliva upon perceiving food.

SALIVATION
Excessive flow of saliva.

SALMONELLA
A group of organisms which cause acute infective enteritis (food poisoning) and closely resembling the germs which cause paratyphoid (they are named after the bacteriologist who discovered them and not because they are contained in tinned salmon).

SALMONELLOSIS
Disease caused by Salmonella bacteria. Symptoms include:
- sudden abdominal pain;
- nausea;
- vomiting;
- fever;
- diarrhea.

SALPINGECTOMY
Surgical removal of a Fallopian tube (duct from ovary to the uterus).

SALPINGO-OOPHORECTOMY
Surgical excision of a Fallopian tube and its adjacent ovary.

SALPINGOTOMY
Surgical creation of an opening into a Fallopian tube (duct from ovary to uterus).

SALT
Common name for sodium chloride (NaCl), found in seawater and also as the common mineral, rock salt or halite. Some salt is obtained by solar evaporation from salt pans, shallow depressions periodically flooded with seawater; but most is obtained from underground mines.

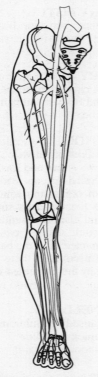

Veins of the lower extremity. The main superficial veins are great saphenous and small saphenous.

The most familiar use of salt is to flavor food. It is, however, used in much larger quantities to preserve hides in leathermaking, in soap manufacture, as a food preservative and in keeping highways ice-free in winter.

SALTATION
The dancing, skipping and jumping sometimes seen in chorea (in brain disease); in genetics, an abrupt change of sequence or variation of a species.

SALT SUBSTITUTES
Substances used by those who are on salt-free diets or who are trying to cut down on their salt intake. Two types available are potassium-chloride tablets and kelp derivatives.

SANITATION
Any measure or program, other than direct care of a diseased patient, that is directed toward the promotion and maintenance of health.

SANGUINE
Resembling blood, bloody; hopeful, optimistic.

SANGUINE PERSONALITY
Individual with rich flow of blood, causing optimism, hopefulness and warm-heartedness.

SAPHENOUS
Manifest or superficial; pertaining to the two large veins in the legs (saphena) or the nerves which accompany them.

SAPHENOUS VEIN
Either of two superficial veins of the leg, one originating in the foot and passing up to the medial side of the leg, and the other originating similarly and passing up the back of the leg.

SAPONINS
Substances found in plants which

form stable foams with water. They normally occur combined with a sugar in glucosides. The component sterols are termed sapogenins.

Many are of considerable value in medicine in spite of being highly poisonous. The heart stimulant, digitalis, is a saponin from the purple foxglove.

SAPPHISM
Sexual function and erotic practices occurring between two females.

SAPHROPHITE
An organism that lives on rotting matter.

SACROCARCINOMA
A malignant growth composed of both sarcoma and carcinoma (cancer cells).

SARCOID
Resembling flesh; the characteristic lesion in sarcoidosis; resembling a sarcoma.

SARCOIDOSIS
The cause of this disease is uncertain, some regard it as an allergy disease. It is characterized by granulomatous lesions (fibrous and inflammatory thickening) principally affecting lymph glands, skin, lungs and bones (especially in the distal parts of the extremities), but they may arise in any tissue of the body.

SARCOLEMMA
The delicate sheath which surrounds every muscle fiber.

SARCOMA
A form of tumor from connective tissue, usually of mesodermal origin in embryology. It is often distinguished from cancer as its behavior and natural history may differ, although it is still a malignant tumor. It commonly arises from bone (osteosarcoma), fibrous tissue (fibrosarcoma) or cartilage (chond-

rosarcoma). Excision is required, though radiation therapy may be helpful.

SATURATED FATS
Fats which come mainly from animal sources, and which are generally solid at room temperature. Saturated fats and cholesterol may deposit in the inner wall of arteries and thus causing damage and atherosclerosis. Foods high in saturated fats include butter, lard, fatty meats, coconut oil, palm oil, and hydrogenated fats.

SATYRIASIS
Excessive sexual desire in the male.

SCABIES
Mites; contagious skin disease, with oozing crust.
   The symptoms are:
- intensely itching;
- bumpy red rash found on finger webs;
- the same rash on wrists, elbows, buttocks, around the nipples in females and genitals in males.
Scabies is caused by the female itch mite, which tunnels into the layers of the skin and deposits her eggs. The larvae hatch within days and cluster around the hair follicles. The mites are irritating and lead to the skin inflammation and rash. Continuous scratching can lead to secondary rash and skin infections. The disease is easily transmitted by skin-to-skin contact with an infected person.

SCALA TYMPANI
The canal in the cochlea, extending from the apex to the round window.

SCALA VESTIBULI
The canal in the cochlea, from the oval window to the apex.

SCALD
A burn caused by hot fluids or vapors. If more than 30 percent of the body surface is involved severe sur-

gical shock is produced and the person must be taken to the hospital. Small scalds merely need covering with a sterile dressing, while larger ones, not amounting to emergency treatment, need antibiotic treatment under medical supervision.

SCALOTOMY
A surgical operation in which the scalenus anterior muscle is divided to remove pressure on the nerves to relieve the symptoms of the cervical rib syndrome.

SCALENUS ANTERIOR SYNDROME
Pain, numbness and weakness of the arm due to compression of the brachial plexus (a network of nerves in the neck) by the edge of the scalenus anterior muscle.

SCALES
Heaped-up particles of horny epithelium. The most common scaly rashes are:
- psoriasis;
- seborrheic dermatitis;
- superficial fungus infections;
- tinea versicolor;
- pityriasis rosea;
- chronic dermatitis of any type.

SCALP
The hair-bearing skin on the upper part of the head.

SCALPEL
A small straight thin-bladed knife used especially in surgery.

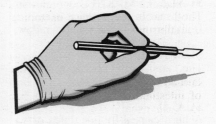

Scalpel in the hand of a surgeon.

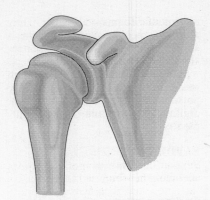

Shoulder joint; part of the scapula (right) and upper portion of the humerus (left).

SCANNING SPEECH
A peculiar, slow and measured form of speech observed in various diseases of the nervous system such as multiple sclerosis.

SCAPEGOATING
Process by which a person, group of object becomes the focus of displaced aggression.

SCAPHOID BONE
A boat-shaped bone on the thumb side of the wrist and the inner side of the instep of the foot. Also called the navicular bone.

SCAPULA
The shoulder blade.

SCAPULECTOMY
Surgical removal or part or the whole of the scapula.

SCAR
The mark resulting from the healing of a wound or disease process in a tissue, especially the skin. Also called a cicatrix. The presence of excessive scar tissue is called a keloid.

SCARLATINA
Mild scarlet fever.

SCARLET FEVER
Infectious disease caused by certain

strains of Streptococcus. It is common in children and causes sore throat with tonsillitis, a characteristic skin rash and mild systemic symptoms. Penicillin and symptomatic treatment is required. Scarlet fever occurs in epidemics; a few are followed by rheumatic fever or nephritis.

SCHEIE'S SYNDROME
A disorder of mucopolysaccharide metabolism which is transmitted as an autosomal recessive trait and is characterized by a coarse appearance, cloudy corneas, limitation of motion in the joints, normal intellect and changes in the functioning of heart and blood vessels.

SCHEUERMANN'S DISEASE
Osteochondritis (inflammation of both bone and cartilage) of the growing points of the bodies of the vertebrae.

SCHICK'S TEST
Test to measure immunity to diphtheria by injecting the germ toxin (poison) of diphtheria into the thickness of the skin.

SCHILDER'S DISEASE
Progressive disease of the nerve cells of the brain producing increasing failure of cerebral function. Often the disease starts with blindness not due to eye diseases, followed by deafness, incoordination of muscles, spastic paralysis and finally complete amentia (mental deficiency). The actual cause of the disease is unknown and there is no treatment that has any influence on its course.

SCHILLER TEST
Test for superficial cancer, especially of the cervix of the uterus. In gynecological examinations, many doctors "paint" the cervix (entrance of the uterus) with an iodine solution in order to isolate any suspected area of disease. Normal cells contain glycogen (starch), which iodine will stain.

Although the Schiller test is not a specific diagnostic tool, it does point out suspicious areas for further study. Before the cervix is stained, the cervical mucus (discharge) is also examined for threadiness. The time it takes for the thread components of the mucus to be stretched indicates the phase of the menstrual cycle.

SCHILLING TEST
A test utilizing radioactive vitamin B_{12} for gastrointestinal absorption of vitamin B_{12}. This vitamin is essential to several bodily functions (tissue growth, nervous system functioning and red blood cell production). Anemia is sometimes caused by a deficiency of B_{12} in the diet, but the more common cause is a difficulty in absorbing vitamin B_{12} through the intestine. In pernicious anemia, the "intrinsic factor" (protein in gastric secretion) does not join with the vitamin B_{12} ingested in the diet; as a result, the vitamin cannot be absorbed through the intestine into the blood.

SCHISTOSOMIASIS
A parasitic disease due to infestation with blood flukes belonging to the genus Schistosoma. Humans become infected by wading or bathing in water containing cercaria which have issued from snails.

Of all the human parasitic infections, schistosomiasis is one of the most widespread. It is second only to malaria in socioeconomic and public health importance in tropical and subtropical areas.

Intestinal schistosomiasis is caused by damage due to the eggs from adult worms living in the portal and mesenteric veins. One form of intestinal schistosomiasis is due to Schistosoma mansoni and the other to Schistosoma japonicum without geographical overlap.

The worms which cause intestinal

schistosomiasis live in the blood vessels around the intestines, and mother worms produce eggs which are found in the feces. About half of the eggs produced by the mother worms stay in the body and damage the liver (in intestinal schistosomiasis) or the bladder or kidneys (in urinary schistosomiasis).

SCHIZO-AFFECTIVE DISORDER

A subtype of schizophrenia characterized by the following symptoms:
- A disturbance during which, at some time, there is neither a major depressive or manic syndrome concurrent with symptoms that meet one of the basic criteria of schizophrenia (delusions, prominent hallucinations, incoherence or marked loosening of associations, catatonic behavior, flat or grossly inappropriate affect).
- During an episode of the disturbance, there have been delusions or hallucinations for at least two weeks, but no prominent mood symptoms.

SCHIZOID

Resembling schizophrenia.

SCHIZOID CHARACTER

An individual with a character disorder characterized by social withdrawal. Such individuals are shy, oversensitive, seclusive and often appear detached and eccentric and sometimes withdraw into autistic fantasies and daydreams though some reality contact is maintained.

SCHIZOID DEFENSES

Combined use of introjection of good objects and denial, splitting and projection of bad aspects of the self as a defense against guilt, anxiety and depression.

SCHIZOIDISM

The state of being split off, as in schizoid personality and schizophrenia, from one's social and vital environment.

SCHIZOID PERSONALITY DISORDER

A pervasive pattern of indifference to social relationships and a restricted range of emotional experience and expression, beginning by early adulthood and present in a variety of contexts. People with this disorder neither desire nor enjoy close relationships, including being part of a family. They prefer to be "loners," and have no close friends or confidants (or only one) other than first-degree relatives.

SCHIZOID POSITION

The situation occurring in early infancy in which the infant interprets rejection and frustration as evidence that his love is destructive and responds by splitting of the ego.

SCHIZOPHRENIA

Term used to describe a complex mental disorder. It describes a set of conditions which are not constant, but ever changing, a way of behaving that is not general among all sufferers, but highly personal.

In contrast to many illnesses, it is not localized in one part of the body. Rather, it affects all aspects of an individual's personality; the way he thinks, acts, and feels. No generalizations hold true for all schizophrenics. In fact, it is possible for two people to be labeled "schizophrenics" and to show entirely different symptoms. The most important criteria for establishing the diagnosis of schizophrenia are:
(1) A thought disorder characterized by:
- hallucinations or delusions in the absence of such known causes of these symptoms as encephalitis, hallucinogenic drugs, or epilepsy;
- some other form of conceptual disorganization;
(2) An early onset of symptoms,

usually in young adult life.
(3) Absence of major affective symptoms.
(4) Absence of major neurological deficits.
(5) A progressively deteriorating course of illness or an intermittent course with remissions.
(6) A history of schizophrenia in close relatives contributes but is not necessary for the diagnosis.

SCHLATTER'S DISEASE
A form of osteochondritis (inflammation of both bone and cartilage) of the tuberosity of the tibia.

SCHMORL'S NODULES
Projection of the center of an intervertebral disc into the soft, spongy substance of an adjoining vertebra. When extensive, it produces wedge-shaped vertebrae and causes severe curvature of the spine.

SCHWANN CELL
A cell that forms spiral layers around a myelinated nerve fiber between two nodes of Ranvier and forming the myelin sheath consisting of the inner spiral layers from which the protoplasm has been squeezed out.

SCHWANN'S SHEATH
The membrane covering a nerve fiber.

SCIATIC
Pertaining to the sciatic nerve or to the ischium (lowermost part of the pelvis).

SCIATICA
A characteristic pain in the distribution of the sciatic nerve in the leg caused by compression or irritation of the nerve.

The pain may resemble an electric shock and be associated with numbness and tingling in the skin area served by the nerve. One of the commonest causes is a slipped disc in the lower vertebral spine.

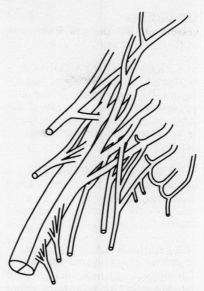

The sciatic nerve (nervus ischiadicus) originates from the lumbosacral plexus. The sciatic nerve is the source of sciatica.

SCIATIC NERVE
Largest nerve in the body, arising from the sacral plexus, leaving the pelvis through the greater sciatic foramen, running through the hip joint and down the back of the thigh.

SCINTISCAN
A map of the distribution in the body, or a part of the body, of a radioactive compound given previously; the emitted rays are printed on photographic film.

SCIRRHUS
A hard cancer, especially of the breast and sometimes of the intestine.

SCLERA
The tough, fibrous, white outer membrane of the eyeball. Also called the sclerotic coat of the eye.

SCLERECTOMY
Surgical excision of the sclera (white outer coat of the eye); surgical removal of diseased ossicles (small bones in the middle ear).

SCLEREMA
Sclerosis or hardening of tissue particularly of the skin.

SCLEREMA NEONATORUM
A disease of the newborn characterized by a hardening of the subcutaneous tissues, especially of the legs and feet, due to the presence of an abnormally dense deposit of fat.

SCLEROCONJUNCTIVITIS
Inflammation of the sclera (white outer coat of the eye) and the conjunctiva (the membrane covering the front of the eye).

SCLERODERMA
A disease characterized by induration (hardening) and thickening of the skin either in localized patches or diffuse areas and associated with pigmentation.

The skin becomes firmly adherent to the underlying tissues, sometimes causing joints to become flexed and immovable.

SCLERODERMATITIS
Inflammation and hardening of the skin.

SCLEROSIS
Hardening of a part by the overgrowth of fibrous tissue. The term is applied particularly to hardening of the nervous system from atrophy (wasting) or degeneration of the nerve elements and to a thickening of the coats of arteries by the excessive production of fibrous connective tissue.

SCOLIOSIS
A curvature of the spine to one side, with twisting. It occurs as a congenital defect or may be secondary to spinal diseases including neurofibromatosis. Severe scoliosis, often associated with kyphosis, causes hunchback deformity, loss of height and may restrict cardiac or lung function.

SCOTOMA
An area in the retina which is blind or partially blind.

SCOTOMIZATION
Psychoanalytical term for a process of depreciating or denying everything conflicting with the valuation of the ego.

SCOTOPHOBIA
A neurotic fear of darkness.

SCOTOPIA
The ability to see in the dark, dark adaptation.

SCOTOPIC VISION
Perception of shape and form without recognition of color, as occurs in dim light.

SCREAMER'S NODULUS
Another name for vocal cord nodules.

SCREEN MEMORY
Psychoanalytical term for fragmentary memory items from early childhood, represented by something trivial in processes of condensation, in the manifest dream content.

SCROFULA
Tuberculosis of the lymph nodes of the neck, usually acquired by drinking milk infected with bovine or atypical mycobacteria, and involving enlargement of the nodes with information of a cold abscess. The eradication of tuberculosis in cattle has substantially reduced the incidence. Treatment includes antituberculous chemotherapy.

SCROTOCELE
Hernia (rupture) of the scrotum (the bag containing the testicles).

SCROTUM
A pouch of skin situated below the root of the penis. It is divided internally by a septum, and this division

is marked on the surface by a ridge. The scrotal skin is dark and thin and contains numerous sebaceous glands and sparse hairs. Its subcutaneous tissue contains smooth muscle fibers. This muscle contracts in response to cold and exercises, and its contraction makes the scrotum smaller and causes its skin to be wrinkled.

SCRUB TYPHUS
A mite-borne infectious disease caused by Rickettsia tsuthsgamus and characterized by fever, a primary lesion, a macular rash, and disorder of lymph glands.

After an incubation period of six to twenty days, onset is sudden, with fever, chilliness, headache and general disorder of lymph glands. At the onset of fever, a local lesion often develops at the site of the chigger bite. In untreated patients, high fever may persists for two weeks or more, then fall by lysis over several days. With specific treatment, recovery usually begins within 36 hours and recovery is prompt and uneventful.

SCURVY
A disease caused by gross deficiency of vitamin C. It is characterized by extreme weakness, spongy gums and a tendency for hemorrhages to occur under the skin, membranes and periosteum (the membrane covering the bones).

SEASONAL DEPRESSION
Mood disorder characterized by the following symptoms:
- There has been a regular temporal relationship between the onset of an episode of bipolar disorder or recurrent major depression and a particular 60-day period of the year (e.g., regular appearance of depression between the beginning of October and the end of November).
- Full remissions (or a change from depression to mania or hypoma-

nia) also occurred within a particular 60-day period of the year (e.g., depression disappears from mid-February to mid-April).
- There have been at least three periods of mood disturbance in three separate years that demonstrated the temporal seasonal relationship defined above; at least two of the years were consecutive.
- Seasonal episodes of mood disturbance, as described above, outnumbered any nonseasonal episodes of such disturbance that may have occurred by more than three to one.

SEAWEED
Large multicellular red, brown, or green marine algae that are generally found attached to the seabed, rocks, or other solid structures. Many are commercially important as food, as fertilizers, and in pharmacological products.

SEBACEOUS CYST
A swelling formed beneath the skin by blockage of the duct of a sebaceous gland. It can occur wherever sebaceous glands are located but is peculiarly common on the scalp.

SEBACEOUS GLANDS
Small glands in the skin which secrete sebum, a fatty substance that acts as a protective and water repellant layer on the skin and allows the epidermis to retain its suppleness. Sebum secretion is fairly constant but varies from individual to individual. Obstructed sebaceous glands become blackheads which are the basis for acne.

SEBORRHEA
An excessive oily secretion from the sebaceous glands producing a greasy skin. It is an inherited characteristic and produces the condition favorable for the existence of acne (blackheads) and seborrheic dermatitis.

SEBORRHEIC DERMATITIS

An inflammatory scaling disease of the scalp, face, and occasionally, other areas of the body. despite the name, the composition and flow of sebum are normal.

SECONDARY SEX CHARACTERISTICS

Anatomical, physiological and psychological characteristics, which differentiate the sexes, but apparently play no part in reproduction.

SECRETIN

A hormone of the gastrointestinal tract secreted by cells in the duodenum epithelium in response to the presence of food and increasing the secretion of pancreas enzymes and bile.

SECRETION

The act of forming, by means of the blood, a substance which is either eliminated from the body as an excretion or carried around it to perform a special function; the substance produced by secretion.

SECTION

The act of cutting or dividing; a cut surface; a division.

SECRETORY OTITIS MEDIA

An effusion in the middle ear resulting from incomplete resolution of acute otitis media or obstruction of the Eustachian tube. The effusion is often sterile but may contain pathogenic bacteria. Secretory otitis media is common in children.

SEDATIVES

Drugs that reduce anxiety and induce relaxation without causing sleep; many are also hypnotics, drugs that in adequate doses may induce sleep. Sleeping drugs and anti-anxiety drugs have a sedative effect, and many other drugs such as antihistamines and antidepressants can produce sedation as a side effect.

SEDIMENTATION

Settling of solid material in blood or other fluid to the bottom of a container.

SEDIMENTATION RATE

Laboratory test of speed at which erythrocytes settle when an anticoagulant is added to the blood. The erythrocyte sedimentation rate (ESR) is a measure in millimeters of how far the red blood cells cling together, fall, and settle toward the bottom of a specially marked test tube in an hour's time.

SEGMENT

A part bounded by a natural or imaginary line; a natural division, resulting from segmentation; the part of a limb between two consecutive joints; a subdivision, ring, lobe, somite or metameres of any cleft or articulated body.

SEGMENTAL NEURITIS

Neuritis affecting a segment of a nerve.

SEGMENTAL REFLEX

A reflex involving only one segment of the spinal cord.

SEGREGATION

The placing apart or isolation of contacts of a serious infectious disease. In genetics, the reappearance of contrasted inherited characteristics in the young or the separation of the paired maternal and paternal genes when the egg cell splits up.

SEIZURE

A convulsion or an attack of epilepsy. A convulsive seizure is an abnormal set of movements that are caused by an abnormal electrical discharge in the brain. The seizure can be generalized, with jerking or twitching of the entire body, along with stiffening, or it can be limited to one body part. It can be associated with complete unconsciousness, or the person can appear to be awake during part of the seizure. Certain seizures involve only momentary lapses in awareness. Epilepsy is a chronic problem that is characterized by the tendency to have seizures. Seizures have a variety of causes. When a seizure occurs for the first time, it is critically important that a cause be searched for. Of greatest concern are the causes that can be corrected easily. Of additional concern is the stopping of one seizure and the prevention of any future attacks.

SELENIUM
A trace mineral, required by the body in very minute amounts and essential for heart and other muscle functions. It acts as coenzyme, necessary for certain enzyme activities. It also seems to act on, and with, vitamin E as a protective anti-oxidant in the body.

SELENIUM SULPHIDE
Preparation used for the treatment of dandruff and minor skin inflammations.

SELF
The traits and characteristics making up the individual.

SELF-ABSORPTION
A high state of abstraction for external stimuli or events, excessive or pathological egoism or narcissism.

SELF-ACCEPTANCE
A healthy attitude toward one's worth and limitations consisting of an objective recognition of each quality and an acceptance of each as being part of the self.

SELF-ACTIVITY
Changes within mental life, consciously produced by, and felt as originating in, oneself.

SELF-ACTUALIZATION
Stages of Maslow's hierarchy of needs characterized by acceptance of the world for what it actually is; autonomy, serenity and a fresh appreciation of the world.

SELF-CONCEPT
The individual's appraisal or evaluation of himself.

SELF-CONSCIOUSNESS
Awareness of one's own existence, thoughts and actions.

SELF-CONSISTENCY
A theory of personality growth which postulates that growth consists of development of a self-image and progressive harmonization of subsequent behavior consisting with that image.

SELF-DETERMINATION
Guidance, by the individual, of his own conduct.

SELF-EXPRESSION
The expression in behavior of one's own nature: usually applied to the development of an individual, through free expression of his own tastes, interests and capacities.

SELF-PRESERVATION
Group of instinctive impulses directed towards the preservation of the life of an individual.

SELF-RECOGNITION
The process by which the immune system of an organism learns to distinguish between the body's own chemicals, cells, and tissues and intruders from the outside.

SELF-SENTIMENT
A control of impulse, temperamental capacity of to integrate and strong investment of appropriate behavior integrated about the self-concept.

SELF-STIMULATION
Stimulation of oneself as a result of one's own activity or behavior.

SELF-TOLERANCE
The physiological state that exists in an organism when its immune system has learned not to attack and destroy its own bodily constituents.

SEMEN
Thick, opalescent, viscid secretion discharged from the urethra of the male at the climax of sexual excitement; it contains spermatozoa.

The semen, seminal fluid or ejaculate is the single most important test of testicle function and fertility. Besides sperm (spermatozoa), normal semen contains spermatocytes, sertoli cells, sperm nutrients, red and white blood cells, macrophages, lecithin crystals and secretions from the prostate as well as other glands (fructose, citric acid, proteins, prostaglandins and hormones).

SEMICIRCULAR CANALS
The three minute, semicircular canals in the labyrinth of the ear which occupy three planes in space and form the organ of balance for posture. Each canal contains a fluid which, when the head is moved in a particular direction, runs around the canal and by stimulating minute nerve fibers sends impulses to the brain which are interpreted as movement, so that even a blind person is able to tell whether or not he is the right way up.

SEMICIRCULAR DUCT
Any of the three loop-shaped membranous inner tubular parts of the semicircular canals that are about one-fourth the diameter of the corresponding outer bony canals, that communicate at each end with the utricle, and that have near pone end an expanded ampulla containing an area of sensory epithelium.

SEMILUNAR VALVES
Cup-shaped valves. The aortic valve at the entrance to the aorta and the pulmonary artery are semilunar valves. They consist of three cup-shaped flaps which prevent the backflow of blood.

SEMINAL VESICLES
Apparently lobulated organs, placed symmetrically on each side of the midline behind the urinary bladder and above the prostate.

Before puberty its mucous membrane shows very few folds but at puberty, under the influence of the testicular secretion, the mucosa grows very rapidly and is thrown up into folds.

SENILE DEMENTIA
Mental deterioration in old age. The dementia involves a multifaceted loss of intellectual abilities, such as memory, judgment, abstract thought, and other higher cortical functions, and changes in personality and behavior.

The onset is insidious, and the course is generally progressive and deteriorating. In the early stages, memory impairment may be the only apparent cognitive deficit. There may also be subtle personality changes, such as the development of apathy, lack of spontaneity, and a quiet withdrawal from social interactions. People usually remain neat and well-groomed, and, aside from an occasional irritable outburst, are cooperative and behave in a socially appropriate way. With progression to the middle stage of the disease, various cognitive disturbances become quite apparent, and behavior and personality are more obviously affected. By the late stage, the person may be completely mute and inattentive. At this point he or she is totally incapable of caring for himself. This stage leads inevitably to death.

SENILE GANGRENE
A type occurring in old age and due to atherosclerosis (hardening of the arteries). The condition usually affects the extremities.

SENILE PSYCHOSIS
A psychosis occurring in old age.

SENILE WARTS
Another name for seborrheic keratosis.

SENILITY
The state of old age, usually referring to the general mental and physical deterioration, often -but not always - seen in the elderly. Failure of recent memory, dwelling on the past, episodic confusion and difficulty in absorbing new information are common. The degenerative changes in skin, bone and connective tissue lead to the altered physical appearance characteristic of the elderly.

SENSATION
Immediate elementary experiences requiring no verbal, symbolic or conceptual elaboration, and related primarily to sense organ activity such as occurring in the eye or ear and in the associated nervous system leading to a particular sensory area of the brain.

SENSE FEELING
The dimension of pleasantness and unpleasantness of a sensory experience.

SENSE IMPRESSION
Condition as a result of the immediate effect of the stimulus on the sense organ; the specific contribution to sense perception of the sense organ.

SENSE PERCEPTION
The apprehension of situations or objects, determined by, or based on, stimuli affecting the sense organs at the moment.

SENSE QUALITY
The specific character of a sensation, which persists through quantitative variations, within a separate and specific sense department.

SENSES
The media through which stimuli in the environment of an organism act on it (external senses); also, the internal senses which report on the internal state of the organism (through thirst and hunger; pain, etc.). The organs of sense, the eye, ear, skin, etc., all contain specialized cells and nerve endings which communicate with centers in the nervous system. Sense organs may be stimulated by pressure (in touch, hearing and balance), chemical stimulation (smell, taste) or electromagnetic radiation (vision, heat sensors).

SENSIBILITY
The capacity to sense or to be stimulated by sense stimuli.

SENSITIVE ZONES
Regions of the skin especially susceptible to cutaneous stimulation.

SENSITIVITY
The responsiveness of an organism to stimulus energy or energy changes.

SENSITIVITY TRAINING
Training in an interacting group that is designed to increase each individual's awareness of his own feelings and the feelings of others and to enhance interpersonal relations through the exploration of the behavior, needs, and responses of the individuals making up the group.

SENSITIZATION
The process in a receptor, or receptors, of becoming or being made more excitable by sense stimuli.

SENSITIZED
Rendered sensitive, particularly to bacteria or proteins which produce an allergy.

SENSORIMOTOR
Physiological term referring to structures, processes or phenomena

involving both the sensory and the motor aspects, or parts, of the organism.

SENSORINEURAL
Physiological term referring to, or involving the aspects of sense perception mediated by nerves.

SENSORIUM
A sensory nerve center in the brain; the parts of the brain or the mind concerned with the reception and interpretation of sensory stimuli. The term is also used to designate the ability of the brain to receive and interpret sensory stimuli.

SENSORY
Pertaining to sensation; conveying nerve impulses from the sense organs to the nerve centers.

SENSORY APHASIA
A condition characterized by difficulty in understanding speech or written words, and assumed to be due to a lesion of an area below the middle part of the first temporal convolution of the brain.

SENSORY AREAS
Areas in the central nervous system especially in the cerebral cortex which receive neural stimuli from sense organs.

SENSORY CELL
A peripheral nerve cell, as an olfactory cell, located at the sensory receiving surface and being the primary receptor of a sensory impulse. The term is also used to designate a nerve cell, as a spinal ganglion cell, transmitting sensory impulses.

SENSORY CODE
The information content of a pattern of neural discharge frequencies about the nature of the stimulus impinging on a sense receptor.

SENSORY DEPRIVATION
Condition of perceptual isolation - which may result in hallucinations, thought or emotional disorders or spatiotemporal disorientation - experienced by people confined in highly unstimulating environments, a subject of such recent research.

SENSORY INTEGRATION
The postulate that the continuous stimulation of two afferent areas results in the relationship between them whereby the activity of one will cause the other to be aroused.

SENSORY INTERACTION
The interdependence of sensory processes occurring simultaneously.

SENSORY NERVE
Afferent nerve, carrying sensory signals to the spinal cord and brain.

SENSORY NEURON
A neuron that transmits nerve impulses from a sense organ towards the central nervous system (spinal cord and brain)

SENSUAL
Excessive appetite for, and indulgence in, sense pleasures, particularly those of food and drink and sex.

SENSUALISM
Being controlled by primitive passions, instincts or emotions.

SENSUOUS
Physiological and psychological term referring to the special emphasizing of the sense aspect of experience; tendency in some individuals to have affective or emotional experience from the sense aspect.

SENTIMENT
An emotional disposition, centering around the idea of an object.

SENTINEL NODES
Lymph glands situated above the left collar bone, which may be the site of spread from cancer of the

stomach, from other abdominal areas, or from within the chest.

SEPARATION ANXIETY
Anxiety caused in a child by actual separation from the mother or by a threat thereof.

SEPARATION ANXIETY DISORDER
Psychic disorder characterized by excessive anxiety, for at least two weeks, concerning separation from those to whom the child is attached. When separation occurs, the child may experience anxiety to the point of panic. The reaction is beyond that expected for the child's developmental level. Onset of the disorder is before age 18.

SEPSIS
Poisoning of body cells by infectious organisms or by the toxic substance they produce.

SEPSIS NEONATORUM
Another name for neonatal sepsis.

SEPTAL DEFECT
An abnormal opening in the wall (septum) that normally divides the right and left sides of the heart. There are both atrial and ventricular septal defects, depending on whether the upper or lower heart chambers are involved.

SEPTICEMIA
Circulation of infective bacteria and the white blood cells responding to them in the blood. Bacteria may transiently enter the blood normally but these are removed by the reticulo-endothelial system. If this system fails and bacteria continue to circulate, their products and those of the white blood cells initiate a series of reactions that lead to shock, with warm extremities, fever and hypothermia. Septic embolism may occur causing widespread abscesses. Gram's stain-negative bacteria (usually from urinary or gastrointestinal tract) and staphylococcus cause severe septicemia. Treatment includes antibiotics and resuscitative measures for shock.

SEPTUM PELLICIDUM
The thin double partition extending vertically from the lower surface of the corpus callosum to the fornix and neighboring parts, separating the lateral ventricles of the brain, and enclosing the fifth ventricle.

SERIAL BEHAVIOR
An integrated sequence of acts, as in a skilled performance, or the sequence of response in the running of a maze.

SERINE
An amino acid that can be manufactured by the body.

SEQUEL, SEQUELA
An abnormal condition produced by a disease process and directly caused by it.

SEQUESTRAL
Pertaining to a sequestrum (a detached piece of dead bone).

SEQUESTRATION
The production of a sequestrum (a detached piece of dead bone); isolation.

SEQUESTRUM
Dead piece of bone that separated from a normal healthy bone, usually the result of infection.

SERODIAGNOSIS
Diagnosis founded on the blood serum reactions of patients.

SEROLOGY
Literally, the study of serum. Refers to the determination of antibodies to infectious agents important in clinical medicine.

SEROLYSIN
A substance in blood serum which

has the ability to kill bacteria.

SEROTONIN
Chemical present in platelets, gastrointestinal mucosa, mast cells and certain groups of nerve cells in the brain. Serotonin is manufactured in the blood from tryptophan (one of the amino acids in the protein we eat) and is then metabolized into 5-hydroxyindolacetic acid (HIAA), a compound that can be tested for in the urine. Serotonin acts to transmit nerve impulses and also constricts blood vessels. An excess of serotonin seems to be implicated in both flushing and blueness of the skin, rapid heartbeat, diarrhea, precipitation of asthma and increased blood clotting.

SEROUS CAVITY
Any cavity lined by serous (moist) membrane such as the peritoneal and pleural cavities.

SERUM
The clear yellowish fluid that separates from blood, lymph and other body fluids when they clot. It contains water, proteins, fat, minerals, hormones and urea. Serum therapy involves injecting (horse or human) serum containing antibodies (globulins) which can destroy particular pathogens. Occasionally injected serum gives rise to an allergic reaction known as serum sickness; a second injection of the same serum may induce anaphylaxis.

SERUM GLOBULIN
Globulin contained in blood serum.

SERUM SICKNESS
An allergic reaction following the injection of serum, usually appearing seven to twelve days after administration, characterized by urticaria (nettle-rash), arthritis (inflammation of joints), fever and prostration. The most common cause of serum sickness is not serum, but penicillin and related drugs.

SEVER'S DISEASE
A painful condition of the heel affecting children. Heat and swelling occasionally are present. Heel pads are placed within the shoe to alleviate the pull of the achilles tendon on the heel.

SEX
Sexual behavior is an important facet of behavior; it may also be the root of aggression and territoriality in animals.

To the psychologist sex and sexual behavior are used in connection with human drives linked to reproduction and similarly fantasies, sensations, etc. To the psychoanalyst, sexual behavior has its roots in infantile sexuality as well as instinct; and the term also covers a wide range of behavior derived from or analogous to sexuality and sexual drive.

SEX CHROMATIN
A chromatin mass in the nucleus of interphase cells of females.

SEX CHROMOSOMES
The two chromosomes designated X and Y. All normal males have one Y and one X chromosome. The normal female has two X chromosomes and no Y chromosome. The other 44 chromosomes in the normal cell are known as autosomes.

SEX DETERMINATION
Genetic mechanism which determines the difference between two sexes, specifically the sex chromosomes X and Y.

SEX HORMONE
A hormone affecting the growth or function of the sexual organs or the development of secondary sex characteristics.

SEX LIMITED
Appearing in or affecting one sex only.

SEX LINKED
Applied to genes located on the X chromosome, and to the characteristics which may occur in either sex, conditioned by such genes.

SEX-LINKED INHERITANCE
Inherited characteristics carried by the X chromosomes.

SEX ROLE
Behavioral patterns expected from an individual by his social group believed to be typical of his sex. Some sex determinant behavioral patterns are biologically determined, such as, for instance, menstruation and pregnancy in females.

Certain behavioral patterns are culturally influenced, such as, for instance, ascendance-submissiveness, or occupational choices.

SEX-TYPING
The designation in a culture of certain behaviors as feminine or masculine and the training of children to adhere to these roles.

SEXUAL BEHAVIOR
The totality of normal and abnormal, conscious or unconscious, overt and covert sensations, thoughts, feelings and actions related to sexual organs and other erotogenic zones, including masturbation, heterosexual and homosexual relations, sexual deviations and techniques.

SEXUAL CYCLE
A cycle of bodily functional and structural changes associated with sex.

SEXUAL DEVIATION
Sexual behavior which does not conform with social norms of a certain culture such as sadism, masochism.

SEXUAL DISORDERS
Two groups of disorders:
(1) The paraphilias are charac-
terized by arousal in response to sexual objects or situations that are not part of normative arousal-activity patterns and that in varying degrees interfere with the capacity of reciprocal affectionate sexual activity.
(2) The sexual dysfunctions are characterized by inhibitions in sexual desire or the psychophysiologic changes that characterize the sexual response cycle.

SEXUAL DYSFUNCTION
Inhibition in the appetitive or psychophysiologic changes that characterize the complete sexual response cycle.

SEXUAL FRIGIDITY
Sexual inadequacy in females; covers a wide variety of symptoms, such as:
- lack of sexual desire;
- total inability to reach orgasm;
- inability of reaching orgasm in coitus;
- unresponsiveness to stimuli;
- complete or partial anesthesia of sexual organs;
- veganism, etc.

SEXUAL INFANTILISM
Retardation in development of sexual characters, primary or secondary, although age of puberty has been reached.

SEXUAL INSTINCT
All the impulses included under sexual, as opposed to ego instinct.

SEXUAL INTERCOURSE
(1) Heterosexual intercourse involving penetration of the vagina by the penis;
(2) Intercourse involving genital contact between individuals other than penetration of the vagina by the penis.

SEXUALLY TRANSMITTED DISEASE
Venereal disease.

SEXUAL REPRODUCTION
The process of creating a new organism through the union of male and female sex cells.

SEXUAL SADISM
The inflicting of physical or psychologic suffering on the sexual partner as a method of stimulating sexual excitement and orgasm. Generally there are insistent and persistent fantasies in which sexual excitement is produced as a result of suffering inflicted on the partner, but the fantasies alone without behavior are an insufficient basis for the diagnosis.

SEXUAL SELECTION
Selection of sexual mates which leads to natural selection. The prevalence of certain sex characteristics sought after fosters, through heredity, a prevalence of these characteristics in the forthcoming generations.

SEXUAL SYMBOLISM
The use of substitute objects to represent sexual organs or actions, such as receptacles for female organs and sharp objects for male organs.

SEXUAL SYNERGISM
Sexual excitation resulting from the combined effect of many stimuli occurring simultaneously.

SGA-INFANT
Abbreviation of small-for-gestational-age infant.

SGOT
Abbreviation for serum glutamic-oxaloacetic transaminase. Measuring the level in the blood helps demonstrate liver disorders and diagnose recent heart damage.

SGPT
Abbreviation for a laboratory study measuring the blood level of serum glutamic-pyruvic transaminase. De-viations from a normal level may indicate liver disease.

SHAFT
A long slender cylindrical body or part; the cylindrical part of a long bone between the enlarged ends. The term is also used to designate the part of a hair that is visible above the surface of the skin.

SHAKING PALSY
Another name for Parkinson's disease or parkinsonism.

SHARPEY'S FIBER
Any of the thready processes of the peritoneum that penetrate the tissue of the superficial lamellae of bones.

SHEATH
A covering structure of connective tissue, usually of an elongated part, such as the membrane covering a muscle. The term is also used for condom.

SHEEHAN'S SYNDROME
A necrosis of the pituitary gland with associated hypopituitarism resulting from postpartum hemorrhage.

SHELF LIFE
The period of time during which a material, as a food or drug, may be stored and remain suitable for use.

SHELL SHOCK
Temporary or prolonged nervous disorders, manifesting a variety of symptoms, developed through experience of war conditions in the field.

SHIATSU
A massage with the fingers applied to those specific areas of the body used in acupuncture.

SHIFT TO THE LEFT
Alteration of an Arneth index by an increase of immature leukocytes in the circulating blood.

SHIFT TO THE RIGHT
Alteration of an Arneth index by an increase in mature or overage leukocytes in the circulating blood.

SHIGELLA
A genus of nonmotile aerobic bacteria of the family Enteobacteriaceae that form acid but no gas on many carbohydrates and that cause dysentery in animals and man.

SHIGELLOSIS
An acute infection of the bowel caused by Shigella organisms. The incubation period is one to four days. In younger children, the onset is sudden, with fever, irritability or drowsiness, anorexia, nausea or vomiting, diarrhea, abdominal pain and distention. The untreated child may die in the first 12 days; if not, acute symptoms subside by the second week. Most adults do not show fever, but diarrhea and tenesmus. The disease usually resolves spontaneously in adults; mild cases in four to eight days, severe cases in three to six weeks.

SHINGLES
Another name for herpes zoster.

SHIN-SPLINTS
Painful injury to and inflammation of the tibial and toe extensor muscles or their fasciae that is caused by repeated minimal traumas, as by running on a hard surface.

SHIVER
An instance of shivering; experience of rapid involuntary muscular twitching especially in response to cold.

SHIVERING
Fine contractions of muscles, causing slight repetitive movements, employed for increasing heat production by the body; thus raising body temperature in conditions of cold or when disease induces fever. Uncontrollable shivering with gross movements of the whole body is a rigor only seen in some fevers.

SHOCK
Term used to designate a clinical syndrome with varying degrees of disturbance of oxygen supply to the tissues.

Shock signifies an emergency where swift and immediate medical intervention is necessary. Essentially, shock results when the blood supply to vital organs is decreased. The blood flow to the skin and muscles ceases first, resulting in a pale look, with moist, clammy and cold skin. The blood flow to the internal organs - intestines, kidneys, heart and brain - slows, leading to eventual collapse. Symptoms of shock are general weakness, nausea and vomiting, anxiety or panic and tiredness. Later light-headedness, difficulty breathing and eventual loss of consciousness follow. At this stage there is a risk of choking if vomiting occurs. Severe shock leads to death when the heart stops.

Shock is the body's response to injury, serious illness, overwhelming infection, blood loss or dehydration. Often if the cause receives immediate treatment, shock will be diminished, controlled or reversed.

SHOCK LUNG
A condition of severe pulmonary edema associated with shock.

SHOCK ORGAN
An organ or part that is the principal site of an allergic reaction.

SHOCK THERAPY
The treatment of psychiatric patients, by inducing coma, with or without convulsions, by means of drugs or by passing an electric current through the brain.

SHORT-TERM MEMORY
Memory that involves recall of information for a relatively short time, as a few seconds, that, for in-

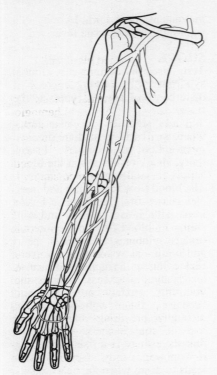

Anterior view of the arm. The shoulder, or pectoral, girdles attach the bones of the upper extremity to the axial skeleton. Structurally, each of the two shoulder girdles consists of two bones: a clavicle and a scapula.

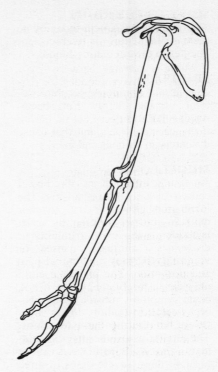

Lateral view of the arm and shoulder girdle (clavicle and scapula).

stance, is involved when a phone number if remembered just long enough to dial it.

SHORTWAVE
(1) A radio wave having a wavelength between 10 and 100 meters; (2) electromagnetic radiation having a wavelength equal or less than that of visible light.

SHORTWAVE DIATHERMY
Diathermy in which wavelengths of about 11 meters are employed; applied in physical treatment.

SHOULDER
Joint between the upper arm (humerus) and the upper trunk (scapula, collar bone and rib cage). It is an open ball-and-socket joint which is only stable by virtue of the numerous powerful muscles around it; this leads to increased maneuverability.

SHOULDER-HAND SYNDROME
Pain and stiffening of the shoulder followed by swelling and stiffening of the hand and fingers often associated with or following myocardial infarction.

SHOULDER JOINT
The ball-and-socket joint of the humerus and the scapula.

SHRAPNELL'S MEMBRANE
A triangular flaccid part of the tympanic membrane of the ear.

SHUNT
A passage between two vessels or

the two sides of the heart, as in cases where an opening exists in the wall which normally separates them. In surgery, the operation of forming a passage between blood vessels to divert blood from one part of the body to another.

SIALADENITIS
Inflammation of a salivary gland.

SIALAGOGUE
An agent which stimulates the production of saliva.

SIALECTASIS
Abnormal dilation of the ducts of a salivary gland.

SIALODOCHOPLASTY
A plastic operation performed on a duct of a salivary gland.

SIALOGRAPH
X-ray studies of the parotid and submaxillary glands after injection of contrast medium.

SIALOLITH
A stone in a salivary duct or gland.

SIALOLITHOTOMY
Surgical incision of a salivary gland for the removal of a calculus.

SIAMESE TWINS
Any twins congenitally united.

SIBLING
One of two or more individuals having one common parent.

SIBLING RIVALRY
Antagonistic interaction pattern among siblings, often resulting from children's frustration of the need to feel worthy.

SICK
In poor health; affected with nausea.

SICK-HEADACHE
Headache accompanied by nausea, irritability and vomiting.

SICKLE CELL
A sickle-shaped red blood cell.

SICKLE CELL ANEMIA
One of many hereditary blood diseases caused by abnormal hemoglobin in the red blood cells. Rather than the normal disc shape, the red cells of persons with this disease have distorted sickle or crescent shapes when their oxygen supply is low. It is from this unusual appearance of the red blood corpuscles derive their names, the hemoglobin being known as sickle hemoglobin or hemoglobin S.

The abnormal red blood cells of sickle cell anemia sufferers are considerably shorter-lived than normal red cells, which usually last about 120 days. The higher rate of red cell destruction is responsible, at least in part, for the chronic anemia seen in these persons. Also, their bone marrow may fail to produce red blood cells normally for brief anemia is superimposed on the chronic anemia.

For persons with sickle cell anemia, continuous health care is of utmost importance. Adequate nutrition, hygiene and dental care, avoidance of exposure to infections, prompt medical treatment when a crisis or other complications occur and cooperation of teachers and school authorities are all essential.

SICKLE CELL TRAIT
Carrier state of anemia. It is generally a benign condition with no clinical manifestations. The carriers have some sickle hemoglobin in their blood, but to a much lesser extend than persons with sickle cell anemia. Under special conditions, a crisis or other complication can occur.

SICKNESS
Any disease; the condition of being unwell.

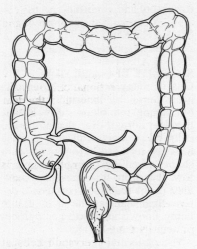

The S-shaped sigmoid connects the descending part of the colon with the rectum.

SICK SINUS SYNDROME
A variety of syndromes associated with inadequate sinus node function most commonly resulting in the cerebral manifestation of light-headedness, dizziness and near or true syncope. Coronary artery disease is the most common single cause of sinus node syndrome.

SIDE CHAIN
A branches chain of atoms attached to the principal chain or to a ring in a molecule.

SIDE EFFECT
A secondary and usually adverse effect, as of a drug. A side effect is a reaction to a drug that can be explained by the established effects of the drug itself. A side effect may be a predictable effect such as dry mouth caused by an anticholinergic drug, or an exaggeration of the normal therapeutic effect, such as bleeding caused by an anticoagulant drug.

SIDEROBLAST
An erythroblast containing cytoplasmic iron granules.

SIDEROCYTE
An atypical red blood cell containing iron not found in hemoglobin.

SIDEROPENIA
Iron deficiency in the blood serum.

SIDEROSIS
Chronic inflammation of the lungs due to prolonged inhalation of dust containing iron, occurring in those employed as iron miners and arc welders. X-rays of the chest show a characteristic nodular shadowing.

SIDS
Abbreviation of sudden infant death syndrome.

SIGH
A long indrawn breath, followed by a short breathing out or a short intake of breath followed by a long, drawn out expiratory effort.

SIGHT
(1) Something that is seen.
(2) The process, power, or function of seeing; specifically, the one of the five basic physical senses by which light stimuli received by the eye are interpreted by the brain in the construction of a representation of the position, shape, brightness, and usually color of objects in the real world.
(3) A perception of an object by the eye.

SIGMA FACTOR
A detachable polypeptide subunit of RNA polymerase that is held to determine the genetic material which undergoes transcription.

SIGMATISM
Faulty articulation of the sounds s and zh.

SIGMOID COLON
The S-shaped bend in the colon (large intestine) above the rectum. Also called the sigmoid flexure.

SIGMOIDECTOMY
Surgical removal of part or all of the sigmoid colon.

SIGMOID FLEXURE
The part of the colon between the descending colon and the rectum.

SIGMOIDITIS
Inflammation of the sigmoid colon.

SIGMOIDOPEXY
Surgical attachment of the sigmoid flexure to the wall of the abdomen for relief or a rectal prolapse.

SIGMOIDOSCOPE
An illuminating surgical instrument that is passed into the anus for the visual examination of the lower part of the bowel.

SIGMOIDOSCOPY
The process of using a sigmoidoscope for the inspection, diagnosis and treatment of the last 10 to 12 inches of the large intestine.

SIGMOIDOSTOMY
Surgical creation of an artificial anus in the sigmoid flexure.

SIGMOID SINUS
A sinus on each side of the brain that is a continuation of the transverse sinus on the same side, following an S-shaped course to the jugular foramen, and emptying into the internal jugular vein.

SIGN
Any objective evidence which the doctor is able to see, hear or feel as positive evidence of disease.

SIGNAL NODE
A supraclavicular lymph node which when tumorous is often a secondary sign of gastrointestinal cancer.

SIGNET RING
A malaria parasite in an intracellular developmental stage in which the nucleus is peripheral and the cytoplasm somewhat attenuated and annular.

SIGN LANGUAGE
A system of communicating by means of conventional chiefly manual gestures that is used by the deaf or by people speaking different languages.

SILICA GEL
Colloidal silica resembling coarse white sand in appearance but possessing many fine pores and therefore extremely adsorbent.

SILICON CARBIDE
A very hard dark crystalline compound of silicon and carbon that is used as an abrasive in dentistry.

SILICONE
Any of various polymeric organic silicon compounds which are obtained as oils, greases, or plastics and some of which have been used as surgical implants.

SILICOSIS
A form of pneumoconiosis produced by inhaling silica dust; common among sandblasters, some miners, and others who work with sand.

SILVER
A trace mineral whose function in the body and food sources has not yet been fully determined.

SILVER IODIDE
A compound AgI that darkens on exposure to light and is used in medicine as a local antiseptic.

SILVER NITRATE
A topical anti-infective agent used on wound dressings and placed in the eyes of newborns to prevent infection.

SILVESTER METHOD
A method of artificial respiration in

which the subject is laid on his back and air is expelled from his lungs by pressing his arms over his chest and fresh air drawn in by pulling them above his head.

SIMMOND'S DISEASE
A disorder due to destruction or atrophy (wasting) of the pituitary gland and manifested by extreme wasting, absence of menstrual periods and loss of appetite.

SIMULATOR
A device that enables the operator to reproduce or represent under test conditions phenomena likely to occur in actual performance.

SINGER'S NODULES
Another name for vocal cord nodules.

SINGLE-BLIND
Being an experimental procedure in which the experimenters but not the subjects know the makeup of the test and control groups during the actual course of the experiments.

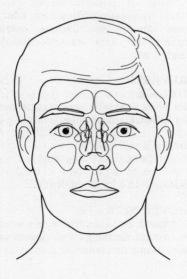

Localization of the seven sinuses in the facial skeleton.

SINISTRAL
A person exhibiting dominance of the left hand and eye; a left-handed person.

SINISTRALITY
Preference for the left hand in motor activity, or for the left one of some other double organ of the body, with respect to use.

SINISTROCULAR
Using the left eye habitually or more effectively than the right.

SINOATRIAL NODE
A small mass of specialized cells in the right upper chamber of the heart which give rise to the electrical impulses that initiate contractions of the heart.

SINOGRAM
A roentgenogram of a sinus following the injection of a radiopaque dye.

SINOGRAPHY
Roentgenography of a sinus following the injection of a radiopaque dye.

SINUS
Large air spaces connected with the nose which may become infected after obstructed upper respiratory infection and cause facial pain and fever. There are four major nasal sinuses: the maxillary, frontal, ethmoid and sphenoid. Also, a blind-ended channel which may discharge pus or other material onto the skin or other surface.

SINUS BRADYCARDIA
Abnormally slow sinus rhythm; sinus rhythm at a lower rate than 60 beats per minute.

SINUSITIS
Inflammation of a sinus. Any virus that enters the body through the nasal passages can set off a chain reaction resulting in a sinus attack.

For example, the common cold, influenza and measles all cause congestion in the nose. When this swelling involves the adjacent mucous membranes of the sinuses, air and mucus are trapped and -unless the sinuses are open enough to permit drainage - an attack of acute sinusitis occurs.

Sinusitis carries its own localized pain signals, depending upon the particular sinus affected. Headache upon awakening in the morning is characteristic of sinus involvement. A stuffy nose, though a symptom of sinusitis, occurs in other conditions and many people confuse simple nasal congestion with sinusitis. However, by physical examination and X-rays, a doctor can make a precise diagnosis and prescribe a course of treatment that will clear up the source of infection and relieve the symptoms.

SINUS RHYTHM
Normal heart rhythm as initiated by electrical impulses in the sinoatrial node or pacemaker.

SINUS TACHYCARDIA
A sinus rhythm of the heart amounting to more than 100 beats per min. in an adult.

SIRENOMELIA
A congenital malformation in which the lower limbs are fused.

SITIASIS
Another name for heat stroke.

SITOSTEROL
Any of several steroids that are widespread especially in plant products, as wheat germ or soybean oil, and are used as starting materials for the synthesis of steroid hormones.

SITUATION
(1) The way in which something is placed in relation to its surroundings;

(2) the total set of physical, social, and psychocultural factors that act upon an individual in orienting and conditioning his behavior;
(3) relative position or combination of circumstances at a particular moment.

SITZ BATH
A bath used especially in postoperative cases in which the hips and thighs are immersed in hot water for the therapeutic effect of moist heat in the perineal and anal regions.

SIXTH DISEASE
An acute infectious disease affecting small children, characterized by the sudden onset of a temperature with signs of malaise.

The temperature falls abruptly and is immediately followed by a measles-like rash that spreads from the back and shoulders to abdomen and lastly to face and limbs.

The rash fades after about two days. Since the whole complaint is over in a few days it is also called three day fever.

SIXTH NERVE
One of the cranial nerves which supplies the external rectus muscle of the eyeball. Also called the abducent nerve.

SJOEGREN-LARSSON SYNDROME
Hereditary syndrome characterized by mental retardation, spastic paralysis and ichthyosis, and occurring through the autosomal recessive type of transmission.

SJOEGREN'S SYNDROME
A chronic, systemic inflammatory disorder with unknown cause, characterized by dryness of the mouth, eyes and other mucous membranes and frequently associated with rheumatic disorders.

SKATOLE
A chemical product found in the fe-

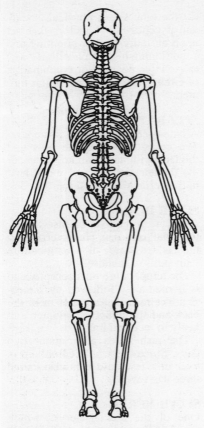

Posterior view of the human skeleton.

ces due to decomposition of protein material and causing the characteristic odor of feces.

SKATOPHAGY
The eating of feces, a behavior disorder of children.

SKELETAL
Pertaining to the skeleton.

SKELETAL MUSCLE
A muscle that is composed of striated muscle and is attached to the skeleton; striated muscle making up skeletal muscles.

SKELETAL MUSCLE RELAX-ANTS
A group of drugs prescribed to treat spasms of the skeletal muscles. The drugs are also used to relieve the pain and discomfort caused by strains, sprains, or other injury to the muscles. However, these muscles do not take the place of rest, exercise or physical therapy, or other treatment that the physician may recommend for your medical problems.

Skeletal muscle relaxants act in the central nervous system to produce their muscle relaxant effects. Their action in the central nervous system may also produce some of their side effects.

SKELETAL TRACTION
Traction exerted directly upon the long bones by transfixing them with pins, wire, and other mechanical devices to which wires and weights are attached in order to straighten fractured bones and keep them in position until the fracture is united.

SKELETON
The framework of the body, made up of 206 bones that provide structure and form for the body, protect delicate internal organs, provide for the attachment of muscles, produce red blood cells, and serve as blood reservoirs.

The skeleton is divided into two major parts: the axial skeleton, which includes the skull, vertebral column, sternum, and ribs; and the appendicular skeleton, which includes the pectoral (shoulder) girdle (clavicle and scapula) and the pelvic (hip) girdle and the upper and lower appendages (arms and legs).

SKIN
The outer covering of the body. The largest organ of the body. It protects the body from injury and invasion by microorganisms, helps (through hair follicles and sweat glands) maintain body temperature, serves as a sensory network, lubricates and waterproofs the exterior, and serves as an organ of excretion.

The skin consists of an outer layer: the epidermis, and an inner layer: the dermis, which contains nerve endings, hair follicles, glands, lymph vessels, and blood vessels.

SKIN CANCER
A neoplasm of the skin. Skin cancer is the most common and most curable malignancy. Treatment depends on the location and extent of the neoplasm; it may involve surgery, radiotherapy and/or chemotherapy.

SKIN EROTICISM
Psychoanalytic term for erotic pleasure from the experience of scratching or rubbing.

SKIN ERYTHEMA DOSE
The minimal dose of radiation required to cause perceptible reddening of the skin.

SKIN GRAFTING
The application of portions of skin, either the outer layers or the full thickness, to a raw surface to promote healing or to replace a defect.

SKINNER BOX
A laboratory apparatus in which an animal is caged for experiments in operant conditioning and which typically contains a lever that must be pressed by the animal to gain reward or avoid punishment.

SKIN REACTIVE FACTOR
A lymphokine that causes an inflammatory process in the skin, including an increase in vascular permeability.

SKIN TAGS
Common soft, small, flesh-colored or hyperpigmental pedunculated lesions, usually multiple and procuring mainly on the neck, axilla and groin.

Treatment by freezing with liquid nitrogen or cutting with a scalpel or scissors is being performed if the

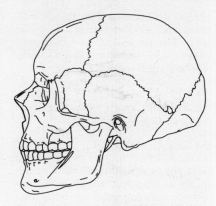
Lateral view of the human skull.

tags are irritating or for cosmetic reasons.

SKIN TEST
A test, as a scratch test, performed on the skin and used in detecting allergic hypersensitivity.

SKULL
The bony skeleton of the head, consisting of the cranium, made up of 8 bones that contain and protect the brain; and the facial skeleton, consisting of 14 bones.

SLEEP
A state of relative unconsciousness and inactivity. If deprived of sleep, humans initially experience hallucinations, acute anxiety, and become highly suggestible and eventually, coma and sometimes death result.
During sleep, the body is relaxed and most bodily activity is reduced. Cortical, or higher brain activity, as measured by the electroencephalograph, blood pressure, body temperature, rate of heart beat and breathing are decreased. However, certain activities, such as gastric and alimentary activity, are increased. Sleep tends to occur in daily cycles which exhibit up to five or six periods of orthodox sleep - characterized by its deepness - alternating with periods of paradoxical, or rapid-eye-movement (REM)

sleep - characterized by its restlessness and jerky movements of the eyes. Paradoxical sleep occurs only when one is dreaming and occupies about 20 percent of total sleep time.

SLEEP APNEA
Intermittent apnea occurring as a sleep disorder.

SLEEP DISORDER
Common symptom of many mental and physical disorders, such as depressive disorders and physical conditions causing pain or other discomfort, and can be associated with the taking of certain medications. Sleep disorders are divided into two major subgroups: the dyssomnias and the parasomnias. In the dyssomnias, the predominant disturbance is in the amount, quality, or timing of sleep. In the parasomnias, the predominant disturbance is an abnormal event occurring during sleep.

SLEEP INDUCERS
Night-time sedatives to aid in falling asleep.

SLEEPING PILLS
Drugs that induce sleep; properly called hypnotics.

SLEEPING SICKNESS
Infectious disease caused by trypanosomes occurring in Africa and carried by tsetse flies. It initially causes fever, headache, often a sense of oppression and a rash; later the characteristic somnolence follows and the disease enters a chronic, often fatal stage. Treatment is most effective if started before the late stage of brain involvement.

SLEEP PARALYSIS
A complete temporary paralysis occurring in connection with sleep and especially upon waking.

SLEEP TERROR DISORDER
Sleep disorder characterized by repeated episodes of abrupt awakening from sleep, usually beginning with a panicky scream. The episode usually occurs during the first third of the major sleep period and lasts one to ten minutes. This condition has also been called pavor nocturnus.

SLEEPWALKING DISORDER
Sleep disorder characterized by repeated episodes of a sequence of complex behaviors that progress to leaving the bed and walking about, without the person's being conscious of the episode or later remembering it. The episode usually occurs during the first third of the major sleep period (the interval of NREM sleep that typically contains EEG delta activity, sleep stages 3 and 4) and lasts from a few minutes to about a half-hour.

SLIME MOLD
Any of about 500 species of primitive organisms resembling both protozoa and fungi.

SLIPPED DISC(K)
A common condition in which the intervertebral discs of the spinal column degenerate with extrusion of the central soft portion through the outer fibrous ring. The protruding material may cause back pain, or may press upon the spinal cord or on nerves as they leave the spinal cord (causing sciatica). Prolonged bed rest is an effective treatment in many cases, but traction, manipulation or surgery may also be required particularly if there is paralysis or nerve involvement.

SLIPPING RIB
Excessive mobility of a lower intercostal joint (the cartilaginous joints at the rib tips).

SLIT LAMP
An apparatus used by an eye specialist to study optical sections of the front portion of the eye.

SLOW VIRUS
A virus that produces disease with a greatly delayed onset and protracted course.

SLUDGED BLOOD
Blood in which the red blood cells become massed along the walls of the blood vessels and reduce the lumen of the vessels and the rate of blood flow.

SMALL-FOR-GESTATIONAL -AGE-INFANT
Any infant whose weight is below the 10th percentile for gestational age, whether premature, full-term or postmature. Despite his size, a full-term 1.4 kg (3 lb) small-for-gestational-age infant does not have the problems related to organ system immaturity that the premature infant has.

SMALL INTESTINE
The part of the intestine that lies between the stomach and colon, consisting of duodenum, jejunum, and ileum, secreting digestive enzymes, and that is the chief site of the absorption of digested nutrients.

SMALL MUSCLE SKILLS
Ability to perform movements - such as picking up and manipulating small objects - that require precise coordination of the small muscles. Also called fine motor skills.

SMALLPOX
An acute, highly contagious viral disease, initiated by sudden severe constitutional symptoms and characterized by a progressive cutaneous eruption often resulting in permanent pits and scars.

This disease is of historical interest only. The WHO (World Health Organization) declared the world free of smallpox in 1980, and smallpox vaccination is only indicated for laboratory workers directly involved with the virus or related agents.

SMEAR
A thin layer of tissue of fluid spread on a glass slide for microscopic examination.

SMEGMA
A thick, cheesy secretion found under the foreskin and around the lips of the vagina.

SMELL
The property of a thing that affects the olfactory organs. The term is also used to designate the perception of odor or scent of through affecting the olfactory nerves. The nose is the organ of smell. Respiratory air is drawn into the nostrils and passes across a specialized receptor surface - the olfactory epithelium. Receptor cells detect the tiny concentrations of odors in the air stream and stimulate nerve impulses that pass to olfactory centers in the brain for coding and reception.

Certain animals depend mainly on the sense of smell, while humans are predominantly visual animals. But with training, they can achieve sensitive detection and discrimination of odors.

SMELL FUNCTION
Olfactory perception that refers to the ability to distinguish different odors. Before smell function can be determined, nasal airway resistance must be measured. Once nasal resistance is eliminated, specific familiar odors are introduced directly into one side of the nose and then the other.

SMITH FRACTURE
A fracture of the lower end of the radius with forward displacement of the lower fragment.

SMITH-PETERSEN NAIL
A triflanged nail which is driven into the upper end of the femur (thighbone) in order to fix the head of the femur in cases of fractures of the neck of the femur.

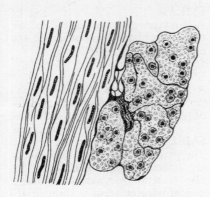

Microscopic structure of smooth muscle.

SMOKER'S PATCH
An area of chronic inflammation on the tongue, seen in pipe smokers.

SMOKER'S SORE THROAT
A chronic catarrhal condition of the throat, common in heavy smokers.

SMOOTH MUSCLE
Muscle tissue that lacks cross striation, made up of elongated spindle-shaped cells having a central nucleus, and that is found in visceral structures, as the stomach and bladder, as thin sheets performing functions not subject to conscious control by the mind.

SNELLEN CHART
The chart used in the Snellen test with black letters of various size against a white background.

SNELLEN TEST
A test for visual acuity presenting letters of graduated size to determine the smallest size that can be read at a standard distance.

SNORE
The sound made during sleep when breathing causes the soft palate to vibrate.

SNOW BLINDNESS
Irritation of the eyes caused by continuous exposure to the reflection of light from vast expanses of snow.

SNUFFLES
A common condition of nasal catarrh in babies causing them to make the characteristic snufling sound. In some cases it is due to inherited syphilis.

SOCIAL BEHAVIOR
Behavior of an individual dependent on the presence of other people.

SOCIAL CHARACTER
General term to mean the character matrix shared by members of a social group. It develops in the process of active adaptation to the economic, social and cultural conditions common to the group.

SOCIAL CONSCIOUSNESS
Awareness of one's relations to the social group or community, and other individuals in the community.

SOCIAL DISEASE
A disease, as tuberculosis, whose incidence is directly related to social and economic factors.

SOCIAL ELIMINATION
The social steps taken - functioning as a type of selection - to destroy or remove from active social participation individuals who are inferior, or seriously maladjusted.

SOCIAL FACILITATION
The increase in the efficiency of responses as a result of the social stimuli from others engaged in the same operations.

SOCIAL INTELLIGENCE
The types of intelligence involved in an individual's dealing with other people, and with social relationships.

SOCIALIZED MEDICINE
Term comprising the various systems of free health care supported by the state from tax revenue.

SOCIAL MATURITY
An index of the level of social development including the acquisition of social behavior and standards expected at a particular age.

SOCIAL MEDICINE
Field of medicine covering the study of factors affecting the welfare or health of society, so far as these can be considered as coming under the head of preventive medicine in a wide sense.

SOCIAL PSYCHIATRY
A branch of psychiatry that deals in collaboration with related specialties, as sociology and anthropology, with the influence of social and cultural factors on the causation, course, and outcome of mental illness. The term is also applied to designate the application of psychodynamic principles to the solution of social problems.

SOCIAL PSYCHOLOGY
The branch of psychology which studies the psychological conditions underlying the development of social groups, the mental life, so far as it manifests itself in their social organization, and their institutions and culture.

SOCIODRAMA
A dramatic play in which several individuals set out assigned roles for the purpose of studying and remedying problems in group or collective relationship.

SOCIOGENESIS
The process by which other persons affect the self, either the body or the mind.

SODIUM
One of the blood electrolytes. It is essential to maintaining the body's normal water metabolism and acid-base balance, and to keep the proper amounts of fluids in the bloodstream and in the tissues around the cells (potassium holds the water in each cell).

SODIUM CHLORIDE
Common salt.

SOLAR PLEXUS
The ganglion of nerve cells and fibers situated at the back of the abdomen which subserve the autonomic nervous system function for much of the gastrointestinal tract. A sharp blow on the abdomen over the plexus causes visceral pain and "winding".

SOLEUS
SOLITARY PLAY
Characterized by a child pursuing his own activity alone, without reference to what other children are doing.

SOLVENT

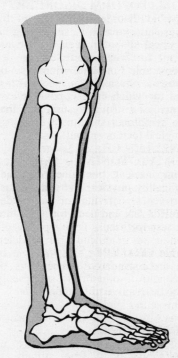

The soleus and the gastrocnemius occupy the dorsal part of the leg between the knee joint and ankle joint.

SOLVENT
A liquid capable of dissolving a substance to form a solution.

SOMA
The body as distinguished from the mind; the whole body, excluding the germ cells; the main part of the body without the limbs.

SOMATIZATION
The conversion of mental experiences or states into bodily symptoms.

SOMATIZATION DISORDER
A neurotic illness characterized by the presence of multiple somatic symptoms, including those seen in classical conversion hysteria.

The cause is not known, although the disorder often runs in families.

SOMATOFORM DISORDER
Psychic disorder characterized by physical symptoms suggesting a physical disorder (hence, somatoform) for which there are no demonstrable organic findings or known physiologic mechanisms, and for which there is positive evidence, or a strong presumption, that the symptoms are linked to physiological factors or conflicts.

SOMATOTONIA
Temperament component characterized by physical and personal assertiveness, striving for power, desire for risk and need for adventure and competition.

SOMATOTYPE
In anthropometry, descriptions of physique, sometimes supposedly also descriptive of temperament.

SOMESTHESIA
Indefinite sensory experience of one's own body, from stimuli affecting mainly touch and temperature receptors on the surface of the body, but not excluding internal stimuli.

SOMNAMBULISM
State in which the body is able to walk and perform automatic tasks while consciousness is diminished. Often seen in anxious children, it is said to be unwise to awaken them as intense fear may be felt.

SOMNOLENTIA
To be drunk with sleep, a condition of incomplete sleep in which some of the faculties are excitable whilst the others are in repose.

SOOT-CANCER
A form of cancer of the scrotum (the bag containing the testicles) occurring in chimney sweeps.

The constant presence of soot in that region acts as a surface irritant and starts skin cancer between the legs.

SORE
Painful or tender; an ulcer or wound.

SORE THROAT
Mostly caused by virus infection which antibiotics cannot cure.

With simple treatment one normally gets better in four to five days.

SOUFFLE
A soft, auscultatory sound. A cardiac souffle is any heart or vascular murmur of a blowing quality.

SOUND
The sensation produced by stimulation of the organ of hearing; an instrument for insertion into a cavity to detect a foreign body or structure; a noise, normal or abnormal, heard within the body.

SPACE
An enclosed or partly circumscribed area in or about the body. There are about 70 such areas of the body and

each has a special name, for example the axillary space (armpit).

SPACE MEDICINE
The specialized branch of medicine concerned with the special physical and psychological problems arising from the space flight. In particular, the effects of prolonged weightlessness and isolation are studied, simulated space flight forming the basis for much of this work.

SPACE ORIENTATION
Awareness of one's position in space and adjustment accordingly, both mental and physical.

SPACE PERCEPTION
Perception of spatial order and spatial relationships of bodies, i.e. of position, direction, distance, form and magnitude.

SPASM
A sudden muscular contraction.

SPASMODIC TORTICOLLIS
Tonic or intermittent spasm of the neck muscles, causing rotation and tilting of the head. The cause varies and often cannot be defined, but underlying psychologic disturbances, disease of the basal parts of the brain, neuronal infections or tumors in the bones may occasionally be implicated.

SPASMODISM
A spasmodic condition produced by an excitable state of the brain.

SPASMOPHILIA
A morbid tendency to convulsions and tonic spasms (prolonged contractions before relaxation), such as those observed in tetany.

SPASTIC
Relating to or characterized by spasm. The term is also applied to one who suffers from congenital spastic paralysis.

SPASTIC COLON
Another name for irritable bowel syndrome.

SPASTICITY
The condition of being spastic. Form of paralysis due to disease of the brain (for example, stroke) or spinal cord (for instance, multiple sclerosis), in which the evolved muscles are in a state of constantly increased tone (or resting contraction). Spasticity is a segmental motor phenomenon where muscle contractions occur without voluntary control.

SPECULUM
A surgical instrument, sometimes fitted with reflectors and sometimes with electric lights, used for examining the interior of body cavities.

SPEECH
The expression of thoughts and ideas by vocal sounds.

SPEECH THERAPY
Treatment of speech disorders, such as lisping, stuttering, and speech difficulties associated psychiatric disorder, mental retardation, defects in learning, and aftereffects of stroke.

SPERM
The male gamete or sex cell in animals. Sperm cells are usually motile, having a single flagellum.

SPERMATIC CORD
Duct or canal for passage of semen. This cord extends from the internal ring to the back part of the testicle.

Where it emerges from the inguinal canal it lies immediately under the skin and superficial fascia and is easy to palpate.

It then passes in front of the pubis to reach the scrotum.

The spermatic cord contains the vas deferens, arteries for the testicles, veins, lymph vessels and nerves, all bound together by loose connective tissue.

SPERMATOCELE
Mass in the scrotum caused by a cyst on the spermatic cord. A symptom is a painless enlargement of the scrotum, usually in adolescent or adult males. The swelling may be high, above or at the top of one testicle. The condition is caused by the formation of a cyst (fluid-filled pocket) in or near the spermatic cord, which carries sperm from the epididymis to the prostate gland. There may have been mild injury that led to the cyst formation. The cyst usually contains sperm.

SPERMATOGENESIS
The production of spermatozoa.

SPERMATOPHOBIA
Neurotic dread of the emission of semen.

SPERMATOZOON
The male germ cell manufactured in the testicles. It has an oval-shaped head and a long tail, which it uses to propel its way over the most internal surface of the uterus (womb) to gain entry into the Fallopian tube (the duct from ovary to uterus), where it meets the ovum (female egg cell).

SPHENOID
Shaped like a wedge; the wedge-shaped bone at the base of the skull.

SPHENOIDITIS
Inflammation of the sphenoid sinus (a cavity in the skull).

SPHENOPALATINE GANGLION
An autonomic ganglion of the maxillary nerve that is situated in the pterygopalatine fossa, that receives preganglionic parasympathetic fibers from the facial nerve by way of the greater petrosal nerve and sends postganglionic fibers to the nasal mucosa, palate, pharynx, and orbit, and that gives passage without synapses to sympathetic fibers comprising the deep petrosal nerve.

SPHINCTER
Muscle, group of muscles or aggregation of smooth (visceral) muscle fibers, that can temporarily prevent movement of the contents of hollow viscera under autonomic or voluntary control.

SPHINCTERALGIA
Severe pain in or around a sphincter muscle.

SPHYNGOGRAPH
An instrument used to make recording of the pulse.

SPHYNGOMANOMETER
An instrument for measuring arterial blood pressure.

SPINA BIFIDA
A congenital deformity in which there is a fissure in the lower part of the spine, allowing the spinal membranes to protrude. The condition is leading to a variable degree of leg paralysis and loss of urine and feces sphincter control; it may be associated with other malformation - particularly hydrocephalus.

It is an embryological disorder due to failure of fusion of the neural tube. Surgery has made it possible to treat mild cases by closure of the defect and orthopedic procedures can be applied to balance muscle power.

SPINA BIFIDA OCCULTA
A congenital cleft of the spinal column without hernial protrusion of the meninges.

SPINAL
Relating to a spine, the spinal cord, or spinal column.

SPINAL ANESTHESIA
Injection of anesthetic solutions into the spinal canal to freeze the whole

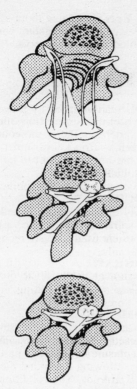

Various types of spina bifida. From top to bottom: open, semi-open and closed spina bifida.

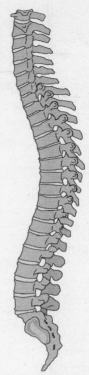

Lateral view of the spine or vertebral column. From top to bottom: cervical, thoracic, lumbar, sacral and coccygeal vertebrae.

area below the level of injection.

SPINAL ANALGESIA
The injection into the spinal canal of local anesthetics, which paralyse the body below the level of injection.

SPINAL CANAL
A canal that contains the spinal cord and is delimited by the neural arches on the dorsal side of the vertebrae.

SPINAL COLUMN
The vertebral column, consisting of the vertebrae, the intervertebral discs and associated ligaments.

SPINAL CORD
That part of the central nervous system contained within the spinal column and extending from the skull to the level of the first or second lumbar vertebra; the nerve structures and nerve pathways within the vertebral canal, extending from the skull opening to the second lumbar vertebra.

SPINAL MENINGITIS
Inflammation of the meninges of the spinal cord.

SPINAL NERVE
Any of 31 pairs of nerves connected to the spinal cord. Each spinal nerve divides into branches, some serving the voluntary nervous system, others the autonomic nervous system.

SPINAL SEGMENT

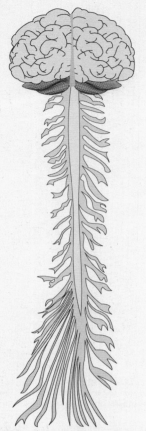

Spinal nerves emerge at regular intervals from the spinal cord.

A segment of the spinal cord including a single pair of spinal nerves and presenting the spinal innervation of a single primitive metamere.

SPINAL SHOCK
A temporary condition following transection of the spinal cord that is characterized by muscular flaccidity and loss of motor reflexes in all parts of the body below the point of transection.

SPINAL TAP
Removal of fluid from the spinal canal by means of a needle and syringe for examination.

SPINA VENTOSA
Enlargement of a bone due to destruction or malignant growth.

SPINE
Vertebral column.

SPINOUS PROCESS
A bony backward projection from a spinal vertebra. These projections can be felt as firm knobs under the skin of the fingers when run up the spinal column.

SPIROCHETE
A variety of germ distinguished by slender spiral filaments. One variety is responsible for syphilis.

SPIROGRAPH
An instrument used for recording respiration.

SPIROMETER
An instrument used for measuring the capacity of the lungs. Also called a pneumonometer.

SPLANCHA
The intestines or viscera (internal organs).

SPLANCHNIC
Pertaining to the viscera (internal organs).

SPLANCHNIC NERVE
Any of three important nerves situated on each side of the body and formed by the union of branches from the six or seven lower thoracic and first lumbar ganglia of the sympathetic system. The greater splanchnic nerve is the superior one ending in the celiac ganglion. The lesser splanchnic nerve is the middle one ending in a detached ganglionic mass of the celiac ganglion at the origin of the renal artery. The least splanchnic nerve as the inferior one ending in the renal plexus.

SPLANCHNICOTOMY
Surgical division of a splanchnic

nerve (the nerves of internal organs).

SPLANCHNOLOGY
The branch of medicine which deals with the viscera.

SPLAY-FOOT
Flat-foot; also called pes planus.

SPLEEN
Large, dark-red, oval organ situated on the left side of the body between the diaphragm and stomach. It is part of the lymphatic and reticulo-endothelial systems, functioning to destroy worn out erythrocytes and platelets, to produce leukocytes, lymphocytes, and other cells involved in immune responses; it also stores blood and produces red blood cells before birth.

SPLENECTOMY
Surgical removal of the spleen.

SPLENOMEGALY
Enlargement of the spleen.

SPLENOTOMY
Surgical incision into the spleen.

SPLINT
Material or a device used to protect and immobilize a body part, such as a plaster for a fractured leg or arm.

SPLIT-BRAIN
Relating to, concerned with or having undergone separation of the two cerebral hemispheres by surgical division of the optic chiasm and corpus callosum.

SPONDYLITIS
A form of arthritis affecting the spine. Ankylosing spondylitis, the commonest form, most prevalent among men between the ages of twenty and forty.

In severe cases, complete fixation of the spine may occur.

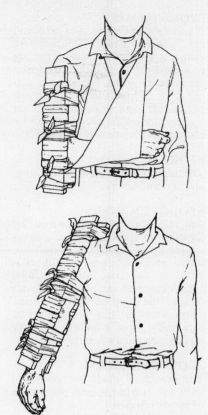

Splinting a fractured humerus. Top: elbow bending easily; bottom: elbow not bending easily.

SPONDYLITIS DEFORMANS
Spondylitis, alleged to be caused by a rheumatic affection of the joints of the spine which become fixed causing forward spinal deformity. The individual may be so bent forwards that he has to look through his eyebrows to see where he is going. Also called ankylosing spondylitis.

SPONDYLOLISTHESIS
Deformity of the spinal column produced by the sliding forwards of a lumbar (loin) vertebra on the sacrum (rear wall of the pelvis), thus obstructing the inlet of the pelvis.

SPONDYLOSIS
A painful disease complex affecting the spinal column. Degenerative changes similar to those occurring in osteoarthritis not only affecting the vertebral joints but also the spinal discs and the surrounding tissues, so that pain is produced either by pressure on the nerve roots or by changes in the joints themselves.

SPORE
The reproductive element of fungi and certain bacteria.

SPOROTRICHOSIS
An infectious disease caused by Saprophyte sporothrix, and characterized by the formation of nodules, ulcers and abscesses, usually confined to the skin and superficial lymph channels but occasionally affecting the lung or other tissues. Farm laborers and horticulturists, especially those handling barberry bushes, are most often infected.

SPORTS MEDICINE
The branch of medicine concerned with the treatment and prevention of sports injuries.

SPOTTED FEVER
Another name for Rocky Mountain spotted fever.

SPRAIN
Injury to a ligament (which connects bone to bone in a joint). The symptoms are: rapid swelling and inflammation and some initial pain and stiffness around a joint. Swelling and pain seem worse 24 to 48 hours after injury occurs. Discoloration and limitation in motion and function may also take place. The treatment is with cold compresses after the injury occurs and elevation of the injured joint, if possible. The joint should be immobilized and a compression wrap used.

SPRUE
A non-febrile, chronic disease common in white people in South East Asia and the East and West Indies. It is due to an inability of the intestines to adequately absorb fat, glucose, calcium and certain vitamins, and is characterized by the passage of large, soft, frothy stools, weakness, wasting, changes in the tongue and anemia.

SPUTUM
The mucous secretion (phlegm) from the lower respiratory system (the lungs, the bronchi, the trachea and the larynx).

SQUAMA
A scale or scale-like substance; the curved platelike posterior portion of the occipital bone. The term is also used to designate the vertical portion of the frontal bone that formes the forehead.

SQUAMOUS CELL CARCINOMA
A carcinoma made up of or arising from squamous cells.

SQUINT
Strabismus; an instance or habit of squinting.

STAB CELL
A young blood granulocyte with a densely staining unsegmented nucleus.

STAB WOUND
A small surgical incision, as for drainage, made by a thrust with a sharp instrument.

STADER SPLINT
A splinting device consisting of two stainless steel pins inserted in the bone above and below a fracture and a bar joining the pins for drawing and holding the broken ends together.

STAGE
The definite period of a disease characterized by certain symptoms.

STAGGERS
A term applied to various diseases which are characterized by lack of coordination in movement and a staggering gait, examples are:
- encephalomyelitis of horses;
- botulism;
- grass tetany;
- brain diseases such as Parkinson's disease;
- tabes dorsalis.

STAGNATION
A cessation of motion; in pathology, a cessation of motion in any fluid, stasis. In dentistry, the accumulation of debris on a tooth because its antagonist in the other jaw has been removed.

STAIN
A dye used to color bacteria or tissues to make them visible for examination under the microscope.

STAIRCASE ILLUSION
A visual illusion of reversible or ambiguous perspective, in which a set of steps can be seen as from above or from below, and the two views keep alternating.

STAIRCASE SIGN
A difficulty in walking downstairs, an early symptom of locomotor ataxia (syphilis of the brain).

STAMINA
The strength or vigor of bodily constitution; capacity for standing fatigue or resisting disease.

STAMMERING
Hesitant or interrupted speech. This is a frequent speech defect in emotional children and persists only when the child loses confidence in his ability to speak and when his difficulty becomes an obsession.

STANFORD ACHIEVEMENT TEST
A test designed for use in measuring a pupil's progress in paragraph meaning, word meaning and grammatical usage.

STANFORD-BINET TEST
Intelligence test that measures general ability to deal with abstractions. The intelligence test was prepared at Stanford University as a revision of the Binet-Simon scale and commonly employed with children.

STAPEDECTOMY
Surgical removal of the stapes (a bone in the middle ear).

STAPEDIUS
A small muscle of the middle ear that arises from the wall of the tympanum, inserted into the neck of the stapes by a tendon that sometimes contains a slender spine of bone, and serves to check and dampen vibration of the stapes.

STAPES
The innermost of the three ossicles (small bones) of the ear. It is shaped like a stirrup.

STAPHYLO-ANGINA
An inflammation of the throat, producing a pseudomembrane, caused by staphylococci (a type of germ).

STAPHYLOCOCCAL FOOD POISONING
An acute syndrome of vomiting and diarrhea caused by the ingestion of food contaminated by Staphylococcus enterotoxin. The potential for outbreaks is high when food handlers with skin infections contaminate foods left at room temperature.

Custards, cream-filled pastry, milk, processed meat and fish provide media where staphylococci grow and produce enterotoxin.

The treatment is supportive. Rapid replacement of fluid and electrolyte losses by intravenous infusion often brings dramatic relief.

STAPHYLOCOCCUS
A genus of bacteria so called be-

cause when cultured on nutrient media they form into clusters resembling a bunch of grapes. There are many different types of staphylococci, only a few of which are harmful to humans.

STAPHYLODERMATITIS
Inflammation or disease of the skin caused by staphylococci.

STARCH
A carbohydrate consisting of chains of glucose arranged on one or two forms to give the polysaccharides amylose and amylopectin. Amylose consists of an unbranched chain of 200-500 glucose units, whereas amylopectin consists of chains of 20 glucose units joined by cross links of chains of 20 glucose units links to give a highly branched structure. Most natural starches are mixtures of amylose and amylopectin; for instance, potato and cereal starches are 20 to 30 percent amylase and 70 to 80 percent amylopectin. Starch is found in plants, occurring in grains scattered throughout the cytoplasm.

STARLING'S LAW OF THE HEART
A statement in physiology: the strength of the heart's systolic contraction is directly proportional to its diastolic expansion with the result that under normal physiological conditions the heart pumps out of the right atrium all the blood returned to it without letting any back up in the veins.

STARTLE REFLEX
Reflex, observed in the newborn child, and elicited, according to the result of investigation, with very young children, by loud sounds, withdrawal of support, pain or experience of shaking.

STARVATION
Structural and functional changes due to inadequate intake of nutrients and energy sources. Primary starvation may result from inadequate intake of all nutrients, which may be involuntary as in famine, imprisonment, shipwreck and other circumstances of deprivation, and severe anorectal disease, or voluntary as in fasting and anorexia nervosa.

Secondary starvation may be caused by impaired absorption, in malabsorption syndromes, metabolic disorders, severe infections, injuries, burns, draining wounds or severe kidney disorders.

STASIS
Cessation of flow of any body fluid, particularly the blood.

STASIS DERMATITIS
Persistent inflammation of the skin of the lower legs with a tendency toward brown pigmentation, commonly associated with venous incompetence.

STATIC REFLEX
A postural reflex which maintains the balanced posture of the body or restores it.

STATIC SENSE
The sense of equilibrium or posture. The receptors of the static sense are located in the semicircular canals in the inner ear.

STATOKINETIC REFLEX
Postural reflex which adjusts the balance posture while the body is in motion.

STATOLITHS
Minute stones or concretions found in the labyrinth of the ear.

STATUS
A state or condition, often a severe or intractable condition.

STATUS ASTHMATICUS
Rapidly recurring attacks of asthma or a prolonged asthmatic attack

which refuses to respond to treatment and in which the person's general condition is deteriorating.

STATUS EPILEPTICUS
Condition in which one epileptic fit follows another in rapid succession without periods of consciousness between them.

STATUS LYMPHATICUS
Condition in which the lymphoid (lymph-containing) tissues are very prominent in the body, especially the thymus gland and spleen. It is alleged to cause sudden death, especially if the patient has to undergo anesthesia.

STEADY STARING
An apparently passive state during which a baby or toddler actually is taking in a substantial amount of environmental stimuli through the eyes.

STEADY STATE
A state or condition of a system or process that does not change in time. The term is also used to designate a state of physiological equilibrium especially in connection with a specified metabolic relation or activity.

STEATOMA
A fatty tumor; a sebaceous (sebum-containing) cyst.

STEATORRHEA
An increased flow of the secretion (sebum) of the sebaceous glands (grease glands) in the skin; fatty stools.

STEINMANN PIN
A stainless steel spike used in the internal fixation of fractures of long bones.

STELLATE GANGLION
A composite ganglion of the autonomic nervous system formed by fusion of the inferior cervical and first thoracic ganglion of the sympathetic chain.

STENOSIS
Constriction or narrowing, especially of a channel or aperture.

STENSEN'S DUCT
The tube carrying the saliva from the parotid gland into the mouth and opening on the inside of the cheek.

STEPPING-GAIT
The peculiar high-stepping gait seen in tabes dorsalis (brain syphilis) and

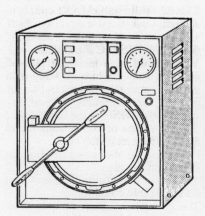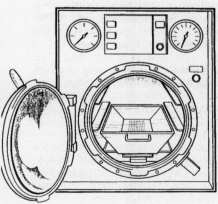

Apparatus for sterilization of surgical instruments. Left: closed autoclave; Right: open autoclave.

some forms of multiple neuritis.

STERCOBILIN
The chief constituent of the brown coloring found in feces. Derived from bilirubin, which originates in the gallbladder, and reduced by the action of bacteria in the intestine.

STEREO-AGNOSIA
Failure to recognize an object by touching.

STEREOGNOSIS
The faculty of recognizing the nature of an object by touch.

STEREOTAXIC
Relating to, or being a technique or apparatus used in neurological research or surgery for directing the tip of a delicate instrument, as a needle or an electrode, in three planes in attempting to reach a specific locus in the brain.

STEREOTYPE
Something conforming to a fixed or general pattern; a standardized mental picture that is held in common by members of a group and that represents an oversimplified opinion.

STEREOTYPY
Frequent almost mechanical repetition of the same posture, movement, or form of speech, as in schizophrenia.

STERILITY
The condition of being incapable of producing offspring; freedom from germs.

STERILIZATION
(1) A surgical procedure in which a woman or man is rendered incapable of reproducing; in males the procedure is a vasectomy; in females, a form of tubal ligation.
(2) A means of rendering objects free of microorganisms (germs) that may produce disease by boiling,

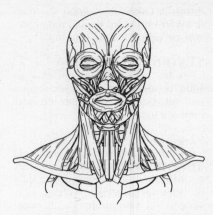

The sternocleidomastoid muscle connects the breastbone, clavicle and mastoid process of the skull. The muscle plays an important role in movements of the head.

subjecting to steam in an autoclave, or by use of disinfectants and antiseptics.

STERILIZER
An apparatus for destroying germs by heat.

STERNALGIA
Pain in the sternum (breastbone).

STERNOCLAVICULAR
Pertaining to the sternum (breastbone) and the clavicle (collarbone).

STERNOCLEIDOMASTOID
A thick superficial muscle on each side that arises by one head from the first segment of the sternum and by a second from the inner part of the clavicle, that inserts into the mastoid process and occipital bone, and that acts especially to bend, rotate, flex, and extend the head.

STERNOCOSTAL
Pertaining to the sternum (breastbone) and the ribs.

STERNUM
The breastbone. It is composed of three parts; the top part is called the manubrium, and articulates with the clavicles (collarbones); the center

portion is called the gladiolus; and the lower end is known as the ensiform, or xiphoid cartilages.

STEROID
A group name for compounds which resemble cholesterol (a fatlike substance) chemically. The group includes sex hormones, bile acids, sterols and some cancer-producing hydrocarbons.

STEROID HORMONE
Any of numerous hormones, as the sex hormones, cortisone, and adrenalcortical hormones, having the characteristic ring structure of steroids.

STEROLS
Naturally occurring secondary alcohols with a fused ring structure of three six-membered carbon rings and one five-membered carbon ring, all of which are hydrogenated and contain in total one or more double bonds.
   Sterols are generally colorless crystalline non-saponifiable compounds. Important sterols include cholesterol, the major sterol found in most animals, and sitosterol, found in plants.

STETHOGRAPH
An instrument for registering the respiratory movements of the chest.

STETHOSCOPE
Instrument devised by Rene Laennec (1781-1826) for listening to sounds within the body, especially those from the heart, lungs, abdomen and blood vessels.

STEVENS-JOHNSON SYNDROME
A severe and sometimes fatal form of erythema multiforma that is characterized especially by purulent conjunctivitis, Vincent's angina, and ulceration of the genitals and anus and that often results in blindness.

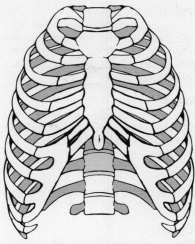

Anterior view of the ribcage. The sternum, or breastbone, is a flat, narrow bone measuring about 6 inches (15 cm) in length. It is located in the median line of the anterior thoracic wall. The sternum, consists of three basic portions: from top to bottom: manubrium, body, and xiphoid process.

STIFFNESS-MAN SYNDROME
Chronic progressive disorder of uncertain etiology that is characterized by painful spasms and increasing stiffness of the muscles.

STIGMA
A small spot or mark, especially a hemorrhage spot in the palm or sole, sometimes found in hysterical people; any mark or sign characteristic of a disease or condition; an opening between cells, a stoma.

STILLBIRTH
The birth of a dead child after the 28th week of pregnancy. Prior to the 28th week of pregnancy it would be called a miscarriage or an abortion.

STILL'S DISEASE
Chronic polyarthritis (inflammation of many joints) which affects children and is marked by enlargement of lymph (tissue fluid) glands and spleen and by irregular fever.

STIMULANT

An agent, such as a drug, that activates or increases the activity of a body part or system. Amphetamines and caffeine are central nervous system stimulants.

STIMULUS

Any energy change which excites a receptor; employed in the sense of any object or event which has such an effect.

STING

A sharp prick with an acute burning sensation.

STIRRUP

The stapes; one of the three small bones in the middle ear.

STITCH

A sudden sharp pain occurring in a muscle, usually the diaphragm, after unaccustomed exercise.

STOKES-ADAMS SYNDROME

Fainting and convulsions induced by complete heart block with a pulse rate of 40 beats per minute or less.

STOMACH

An expendable, sac-like organ that forms part of the digestive tract between the esophagus and duodenum. It is located below the diaphragm in the right upper part of the abdomen, partly under the liver. The stomach receives partly digested food from the esophagus through the cardiac sphincter. In the stomach the food is churned by muscular layers of the stomach and mixed with the secretions of the gastric glands, chiefly hydrochloric acid and the enzyme pepsin. The semiliquid mass then passes through the pyloric sphincter to the duodenum.

STOMACHACHE

Pain in or in the region of the stomach.

STOMACH PUMP

A pump for removing the contents of, or to wash out, the stomach.

STOMACH TUBE

A rubber tube for irrigation or evacuation of the stomach contents.

STOMATITIS

An inflammation of the mouth, occurring as a primary disease or as a symptom of a systemic disease.

STOMATOLOGY

A branch of medical science dealing with the mouth and its disorders.

STOOL

Waste material discharged from the bowels. Iron and bismuth turn the stool black, and certain vegetables and berries darken it or produce a distinct color. Pathological stools are usual grayish or have a whitish glistening color and tarry in hemorrhage, or show fresh blood.

Fatty stools are observed in obstructive jaundice, cancer of the pancreas and in indigestion or overfeeding in infants. Frothy, poorly formed stools may indicate a spastic colon, the presence of gas or inflammatory processes in the intestines. Mucous stools exist in catarrhal or inflamed conditions of the intestines or rectum.

STOOL CULTURE

Incubation of a sample of feces in nutrient material to determine growth and types of infection-causing microorganisms.

STRABISMUS

A condition in which the two eyes do not see the identical images simultaneously; usually one eye is directed in a slightly different direction from the other. Most often this condition is the result of an eye muscle weakness (eye movement is controlled by six different muscles); it can also come from brain and nerve involvement.

STRAIGHT SINUS
A venous sinus of the brain that is located along the line of junction of the falx cerebri and tentorium cerebelli, formed by the junction of the great cerebral vein and the inferior sagittal sinus, and passing posteriorly to terminate in the confluence of sinuses.

STRAIN
An act of straining or the condition of being strained. The term is used in two senses:
(1) excessive physical or mental tension;
(2) bodily injury from excessive tension, effort or use.

STRAIT JACKET
A cover or overgarment of strong material (as canvas) used to bind the body and especially the arms closely in restraining a violent prisoner or patient.

STRANGER ANXIETY
A temporary phenomenon, common during the second half of the first year of life, in which a baby expresses extreme discomfort about being in the company of unfamiliar adults.

STRANGLE
To choke or throttle by compression of the trachea (windpipe); the closing of any opening by constriction.

STRANGULATED HERNIA
Hernia in which the blood supply of the herniated viscus is so constricted by swelling and congestion as to arrest its circulation.

STRAPPING
The application of adhesive plaster in overlapping strips upon or around a part, as a sprained ankle or dislocated shoulder joint or the chest in pleurisy, to serve as a splint to reduce motion or hold surgical dressings in place upon a surgical wound.

STRATEGY
An adaptation or complex of adaptations, as of behavior, metabolism, or structure, that serves or appears to serve an important function in achieving evolutionary success.

STRATUM
A layer of tissue.

STRAWBERRY MARK
A nevus, a red mark visible on the skin of a baby shortly after birth.

STRAWBERRY TONGUE
The description of the tongue in cases of scarlet fever.

STREAM OF CONSCIOUSNESS
The belief that consciousness is a stream of thought, a changing continuum, a unity in diversity rather than a series of discrete separate elements.

STREPTOCOCCUS
Bacteria responsible for many common infections including:
- sore throat;
- tonsillitis;
- scarlet fever;
- impetigo;
- cellulitis;
- erysipelas;
- puerperal fever.

A related organism is a common cause of pneumonia and one type may cause endocarditis on damaged heart valves. Penicillin is the antibiotic of choice. Rheumatic fever is a late immune response to streptococcus.

STRESS
Any factor - physical, emotional or other - that requires a change in response or affects health in any way, especially having an adverse effect on the functioning of the body or any of its parts.

Continual stress brings about widespread neurological and endocrine responses that over a period of time lead to changes in the functioning of many body organs, often leading to disease (for instance, hypertension and allergic responses).

STRESS BREAKER
A flexible dental device used to lessen the occlusal forces exerted on teeth to which a partial denture is attached.

STRESS ELECTROCARDIOGRAM
An electrocardiogram tracing that is made while the patient exercises on a treadmill or stationary bicycle, to evaluate heart muscle function.

STRESS FRACTURE
A usually hairline fracture of a bone that has been subjected to repeated stress. Stress fractures occur especially among joggers.

STRESS INCONTINENCE
Involuntary leakage of urine during activity that raises the pressure in the abdomen. The symptoms are: sudden, unexpected loss of urine control during lifting, sneezing, coughing or other activity that puts pressure on the bladder.

The cause may be inability of the urinary sphincter (closure muscle) to remain closed under pressure. In women, it happens with loss of muscle tone due to aging or having children. In men, the condition may follow surgical removal of the prostate gland.

Stress incontinence is not a health problem, but one of potential embarrassment. Some mild cases may be corrected by exercises of the pelvic muscles. Where the problem is severe, correction by surgery is recommended.

STRESS TEST
A diagnostic method used to determine the body's responses to physical exertion (stress). Usually involves taking an electrocardiogram and other physiological measurements (such as breathing rate and blood pressure) while the person is exercising - usually jogging in a treadmill, walking up and down a short set of stairs or pedaling in a stationary bicycle.

STRETCH REFLEX
Contraction of a muscle in response to sudden brisk stretching.

STRIAE ATROPHICAE
Whitish wrinkles or lines on the skin of the abdomen or breast following stretching by obesity, pregnancy or other cause.

STRIAE GRAVIDARUM
The white lines seen on the skin of the abdomen in women who have borne children or who have been pregnant.

STRIATAL SYNDROME
Disease of the striatum (basal ganglia of the hemispheres of the brain) characterized by:
- rigidity;
- tremor;
- hypokinesis;
- impairment of associated movements;
- absence of sensory disturbances or true paralysis.

STRIATE BODY
A part of the base of both cerebral hemispheres which is striated by nerve fibers and consists of several nuclei. This part of the brain is considered to be important in maintaining muscle tone and posture.

STRICTURE
Abnormal narrowing of a canal or hollow organ. The results of inflammation or other changes in the wall of an organ and occasionally occurs through external pressure.

STRIDOR
A harsh, vibrating sound produced during expiration in certain conditions.

STROKE

A sudden and severe attack. Commonly the term stroke is used for apoplexy. A stroke occurs when the blood supply to a part or the brain tissue is cut off, and as a result, the nerve cells in that part of the brain cannot function.

The effects of a stroke may be very slight or they may be severe. They may be temporary or they may be permanent. It depends in part on which brain cells have been damaged, how widespread the damage is, and how effectively the body can repair its system of supplying blood to the brain, or how rapidly other areas of brain tissue can take over the work of the damaged nerve cells.

STROKE IN EVOLUTION

The clinical condition manifested by neurologic defects that increase over a 24-48 hour period, reflecting enlarging infarction or progressive edema, usually in the territory of the middle cerebral artery.

STROKE VOLUME

The quantity of blood ejected by the left ventricle (lower heart chamber) during a single heartbeat.

STROMA

The supporting framework of an organ.

STRONGYLOIDIASIS

An infection caused by Strongyloides stercoralis and characterized by epigastric pain and blood disorders.

The larvae generally molt in the soil and develop into the infective filariform stage. Heavy intestinal infection may cause epigastric pain and tenderness, vomiting and diarrhea.

STROPHULUS

A popular name for a skin condition of infants and young children called lichen urticatus, probably caused by a mild gastrointestinal disturbance. The skin eruption consists of spotty papules (raised, solid spots) which may be pale or pink and are usually more numerous on the limbs but may occur on the loins and about the waist.

STRUCTURAL DEVELOPMENT

Refers to physical growth, such as changes in cells, tissues, organs and systems; the emergence of psychological structures.

STRUCTURAL SCOLIOSIS

One in which a series of vertebrae remain constantly out of position and accompanied by some degree of rotation. Organic and congenital forms of scoliosis are structural and the functional type may become so.

STRUMA

A goiter (enlargement of the thyroid gland).

STRYCHNINE

Poisonous alkaloid from Nux vomica seeds causing excessive spinal cord stimulation. Death results from spinal convulsions and asphyxia.

STUPOR

A condition of greatly dulled or completely suspended sense of sensibility. The term is also used for a chiefly mental condition marked by absence of spontaneous movement, greatly diminished responsiveness to stimulation, and usually impaired consciousness.

STUTTERING

A type of hesitating speech characterized by repeated attempts to pronounce a syllable or word.

Various other types of speech dysfluencies may also be involved, including blocking of sounds or interjections of words or sounds. The extent of the disturbance varies from situation to situation and is more severe when there is special pressure to communicate, as during a job interview.

ST. VITUS' DANCE
Another name for chorea minor.

STYLET
A small probe; a wire passed into a hollow such as a hypodermic needle, in order to keep the channel clear.

SUBARACHNOID
Located beneath the arachnoid (the central of the three membranes covering the brain and spinal cord).

SUBARACHNOID HEMORRHAGE
Bleeding into the subarachnoid space, that is between the two innermost of the three membranes covering the brain and spinal cord.

SUBARACHNOID SPACE
The space between the arachnoid and the pia mater through which the cerebrospinal fluid circulates and across which extend delicate trabeculae of connective tissue.

SUBCALLOSAL AREA
A small area of cortex in each cerebral hemisphere below the genu of the corpus callosum.

SUBCLAVIAN STEAL SYNDROME
An uncommon cerebrovascular symptom complex in which an obstruction in the subclavian artery proximal to the origin of the vertebral artery is envisaged as causing reversed flow down the latter.

SUBCLINICAL
Applied to a disease in which signs and symptoms are so slight as to be unnoticeable and even not demonstrable.

A condition which is inferred rather than diagnosed.

SUBCOMMISURAL ORGAN
An aggregation of columnar cells situated between the posterior commissure and the third ventricle of the brain.

SUBCONJUNCTIVAL
Lying beneath the conjunctiva (the membrane lining the eyelids and covering the front of the eye).

SUBCONSCIOUS
A psychologic term used in two senses:
(1) existing in the mind but not immediately available to consciousness;
(2) imperfectly conscious; partially but not fully aware.

The term is also used for the mental activities just below the threshold of consciousness.

SUBCONSCIOUS PROCESS
A process of which the personality is unaware and thus it is outside personal consciousness but which is a factor in determination of conscious and bodily phenomena.

SUBCORTICAL
Referring to neural structures lying below the cerebral cortex which mediate functions that are not controlled by the cortex.

SUBCUTANEOUS
Beneath the skin.

SUBCUTANEOUS EMPHYSEMA
Air of gas beneath the skin due to injury or infection by a gas forming organism.

SUBCUTANEOUS INJECTION
A method of administering a drug by which the drug is injected just beneath the skin.

The drug is then slowly absorbed over a few hours into the surrounding blood vessels. Insulin is given in this way.

SUBCUTANEOUS SENSIBILITY

Sensitivity to pressure stimuli, residing in the deeper layers of the skin and the underlying tissues, as well as in the fasciae and capsules of the joints.

SUBDURAL

Beneath the dura (outermost of the three membranes covering the brain).

SUBDURAL HEMATOMA

A hematoma that occurs between the dura mater and arachnoid in the subdural space and that may apply neurologically significant pressure to the cerebral cortex.

SUBGLOTTIC

Below the glottis (a structure in the throat).

SUBJECTIVE

Relating only to the individual concerned; a term used to indicate that the symptoms of which the person complains are probably imaginary and for which there is no supporting evidence. On some occasions it is a polite way of indicating that the person is malingering.

SUBLIMATION

The act of vaporizing and condensing a solid. In psychiatry, a psychic device whereby undesirable primitive cravings gain outward expression by converting their energies into socially acceptable activities. Sigmund Freud used the term to indicate the deviation of sexual feelings to aims and objects of non-sexual character.

SUBLIMINAL

Below the threshold of consciousness or awareness.

SUBLIMINAL SELF

The portion of an individual's personality that lies below the threshold of consciousness.

SUBLINGUAL

Beneath the tongue. Some drugs are administered sublingually in tablet form. The drug is then very rapidly absorbed through the lining of the mouth into the bloodstream within a few seconds. Nitrate drugs may be given this way to provide rapid relief of an angina attack.

SUBLINGUAL GLAND

A small salivary gland on each side of the mouth lying beneath the mucous membrane in a fossa in the mandible near the symphysis.

SUBMANDIBULAR GANGLION

An autonomic ganglion that is situated on the lingual nerve about the deep part of the submandibular gland, receiving preganglionic fibers from the facial nerve by way of the chorda tympani, and sending postganglionic fibers to the submandibular and sublingual glands.

SUBMUCOSA

The space or area beneath a mucous membrane.

SUBOCCIPITAL NERVE

The first cervical nerve that supplies muscles around the suboccipital triangle including the rectus capitis posterior major, obliquus capitis superior, and obliquus capitis inferior and that sends branches to the rectus capitis posterior minor and semispinalis capitis.

SUBORDINATION

The condition of being under subjection; the condition of organs that depend upon or are controlled by other organs.

SUBPHRENIC

Beneath the diaphragm (the muscular partition between chest and abdominal cavities).

SUBPUBIC

Beneath the pubic arc or symphysis pubis of the pelvis.

SUBSTITUTION
The replacement of one thing by another. In chemistry, the replacing of one or more elements or radicals in a compound by other elements or radicals.

SUBSTITUTION THERAPY
Providing one with a substance which his body should normally be able to manufacture for itself. For instance, the provision of insulin in cases of diabetes and treatment by cortisone and hormones.

SUCROSE
Cane sugar, disaccharide carbohydrate, commercially obtained from sugar beet, sugar cane and sweet sorghum. It comprises a glucose unit joined to a fructose unit.

SUCTION LIPECTOMY
Vacuuming of fat tissue. Through a small incision, a surgeon inserts a hollow tube that is attached to a suction pump. He repeatedly thrusts the tube into the fat so that small amounts are sucked out section by section, leaving the fat tissue as full of holes as cheese. The tissue is then compressed and the treated area tightly wrapped to prevent fluid accumulation.

SUDDEN CARDIAC DEATH
Death due to a primary cardiac cause or mechanism occurring within 24 hours of the onset of acute illness in a person thought to be free of heart disease or with symptomatically mild heart disease. In adults more than 90 percent of sudden cardiac deaths are due to coronary heart disease.

SUDDEN INFANT DEATH SYNDROME (SIDS)
The unexpected and unexplained death of an apparently well, or virtually well, infant. It is the most common cause of death between the age of two weeks and one year, accounting for one-third of all deaths in this age group. The cause is uncertain. In 10 to 15 percent of the cases, autopsies show an unsuspected disorder of the heart or blood vessels or anomaly of the central nervous system, or evidence of an overwhelming infection.

SUGAR
One of the group of foods called carbohydrates. In a way, the term sugar is misleading because there are really several different kinds of sugar, the most common being sucrose, glucose, fructose and lactose. These sugars may occur naturally, for example in fruit, vegetables and milk.

SUGGESTIBILITY
Readiness to accept suggestion, as a temporary or permanent characteristic of the individual, whether due to the temporary condition, or as a congenital characteristic.

SUGGESTION
Process whereby an individual loses his critical faculties and thus accepts ideas and beliefs that may be contrary to his own. People under hypnosis are particularly suggestible.

SUICIDE
Act or instance or taking one's own life voluntarily. Taking one's life appears to be a conscious decision that only human beings can make.

SULFA DRUGS
Synthetic compounds that inhibit the multiplication of invading bacteria, thus allowing the body's cellular defense mechanisms to suppress infection. Sulfa drugs are effective against streptococci, certain venereal diseases and meningitis.

SULFATE
Any of numerous chemical compounds related to sulfuric acid.

SULFIDE
Any of three classes of chemical compounds containing the element sulfur.

SULPHEMOGLOBIN
A substance not normally present in the blood, but found in persons who have taken certain drugs in excess, or in cases of hydrogen sulphide poisoning.

SULPHUR
A mineral needed for conditioning the blood and for keeping fingernails, hair and skin healthy. It is available mainly in protein foods, such as meat, eggs, legumes, nuts and fish.

SULPHONAMIDES
Sulfa drugs.

SUMMER DIARRHEA
A form of infectious gastroenteritis of children, seen usually during the summer and often initiated by food contamination from flies.

SUNBURN
An inflammation of the skin caused by excessive exposure to the sun's rays. In addition to the acute effects of sunburn, exposure to the sun's ultraviolet rays can cause chronic damage, permanently destroying the elastic fibers that keep the skin tight and young-looking.

Ultraviolet radiation also damages the DNA, or genetic material, in skin cells. Eventually, accumulated DNA damage can result in the formation of cancerous cells.

SUNSTROKE
Rise in body temperature and failure of sweating in hot climates, often following exertion. Delirium, coma and convulsions may develop suddenly and rapid cooling should be effected.

SUPERCILIARY RIDGE
A prominence of the frontal bone above the eye caused by the projection of the frontal sinuses.

SUPEREGO
A term coined by Sigmund Freud meaning the intrapsychic, mostly unconscious structure of personality which represents societal and cultural standards. The superego develops as a result of an introjection and identification of the child with the parents.

SUPERFICIAL
Related to a surface. In referring to several layers, the top one may be called superficial as opposed to the lowest one, which is called deep. The superficial fascia and deep fascia beneath the skin, for instance.

SUPERINFECTION
A second or subsequent infection caused by the same germ, as seen in tuberculosis for instance.

SUPERIORITY COMPLEX
Overvaluation by an individual of his abilities, usually a defense mechanism countering an inferiority complex.

SUPERIORITY FEELING
Exaggerated self-evaluation; not in-

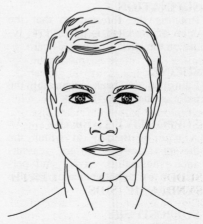

The superciliary ridge is a bony ridge just above the orbit.

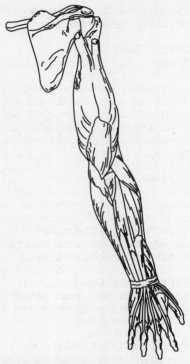

The supinator muscle (located just below the elbow) turns the palm downward or posteriorly.

frequently appearing as a reaction or defense against an inferiority feeling or inferiority complex.

SUPINATION
Rotating the forearm so that the palm of the hand is uppermost; lying on the back.

SUPINE
Lying on the back or turning the palm upwards.

SUPPORTIVE THERAPY
A type of therapy in which the therapist actively offers reassurance, suggestion, advice and persuasion to help the person resolve problems.

SUPPOSITORY
Medical substance incorporated into a gelatin or greasy base and in-

tended for introduction into the rectum. A suppository is usually a bullet-shaped pellet containing a drug for insertion into the rectum.

SUPPRESSION
A sudden cessation of secretion such as the urine or menstruation during pregnancy; in psychiatry, a mode of adjustment to urges and desires considered to be unacceptable or unworthy, through attempting to control or prevent their occurrence or expression in consciousness.

SUPPURATION
The formation of pus.

SUPRAOPTIC NUCLEUS
A small nucleus of closely packed neurons that overlies the optic chiasm and is intimately connected with the neurohypophysis (posterior part of the pituitary gland).

SURFACE
The outer surface of the body; a term frequently used in anatomy to describe bones.

SURFACTANT
An agent that lowers surface tension.

SURFER'S KNOT
A knobby lump just below a surfer's knee or on the upper surface of his foot caused by friction and pressure between surfboard and skin.

SURGERY
The branch of medicine which treats diseases and deformities by manual or operative methods.

SURGICAL EMPHYSEMA
Distention of the subcutaneous tissues by air communicating with the lungs.

SURGICAL SHOCK
A very serious condition of complete collapse of bodily functions

resulting from severe bleeding, extensive burns or scales, or severe crush injuries.

SUSPENSION
Temporary cessation in the function of an organ; hanging or fixing in a higher position, a method or treatment such as suspension of the womb; the dispersion of solid particles throughout the body of a liquid.

SUSPENSORY
Serving to suspend; a muscle, ligament or a bandage or sling for suspending a part.

SUTURE
In anatomy, a line of junction or closure between bones, such as those in the cranium; to close a wound by sewing; fine cord-like structures, such as gut, silk, wire or nylon, used to sew up a wound.

SWAN-GANZ CATHETER
A soft catheter with an expandable balloon tip that is used for measuring blood pressure in the pulmonary artery.

SWEAT GLAND
A simple tubular gland of the skin that secretes perspiration, widely distributed in nearly all parts of the skin, and consisting typically of an epithelial tube extending spirally from a minute pore on the surface of the skin into the dermis or subcutaneous tissues where it ends in a convoluted tuft.

SWEAT TEST
A test for cystic fibrosis that involves measuring the subject's sweat for abnormally high sodium chloride content.

SWELLING
A symptom that can have many causes. It can be localized to a small area of the body as a response to inflammation, with redness and swelling as a part of the body's defense mechanism against infection.

SWING SICKNESS
Another name for motion sickness.

SYCOSIS
An inflammatory disease affecting the hair follicles of the skin, particularly of the beard area (when it is called sycosis barbae, popularly known as barber's rash) and characterized by papules (small swellings) and pustules (pus-containing swellings) together with crusting of the skin surface.

SYDENHAM'S CHOREA
A disease of the central nervous system, often of insidious onset but of finite duration, characterized by involuntary, purposeless, nonrepetitive movements, and subsiding without neurologic residue.

SYLVIAN FOSSA
A depression that forms in the lateral surface of each embryonic cerebral hemisphere during the third month of development and contains the insula at its bottom which is later covered by the operculum whose edges form the border of the fissure of Sylvius.

SYMBIOSIS
The relationship between two organisms of different species in which mutual benefit is derived by both participants.

SYMBOL
An object or activity representing and standing as a substitute for something else. In the psychoanalytical terminology symbol stands for a representation by something not directly connected with it, of unconscious, usually repressed sexual, material.

SYMBOLIC PLAY
Characterized by games that imply both representation of an absent ob-

ject and make-believe representation.

SYMBOLISM
The art or practice of using symbols
especially by investing things with
a symbolic meaning or by expressing the invisible or intangible by
means of visible or sensuous representation.

SYMBOLIZATION
The process of employing symbols
in dreams, myths and the like; characteristically present also in neurotic symptoms.

SYMPATHETIC
Pertaining to sympathy or to the
sympathetic nervous system.

SYMPATHETIC NERVOUS SYSTEM
That part of the autonomic nervous
system which consists of centrally
located nerves in the thoracic and
lumbar part of the spinal cord, the
ganglionic chain, lying outside and
parallel to the spinal cord, with its
nerves.

The sympathetic nervous system
is concerned especially with preparing the body to react to situations of stress or emergency, that
contains chiefly adrenergic fibers
and tends to suppress secretion,
decrease the tone and contractility
of smooth muscle, and cause the
contraction of blood vessels, and
that comprises essentially of preganglionic fibers arising in the thoracic and upper lumbar parts of the
spinal cord.

SYMPATHETIC OPHTHALMIA
A severe bilateral granulomatous
uveitis that occurs as a hypersensitivity reaction to uveal pigment following trauma to one eye.

SYMPATHICOMIMETICS
A large group of drugs that mimic
the effects of stimulation of the
sympathetic part of the autonomic
nervous system.

SYMPATHICUS
Abbreviation for sympathetic nervous system.

SYMPATHOLYTIC
A term meaning blocking the effect
of the sympathetic part of the autonomic nervous system.

Sympatholytic drugs work by reducing the release of the stimulatory neurotransmitter noradrenalin
from nerve endings, or by occupying the receptors that the neurotransmitters adrenalin and noradrenalin normally bind to, thereby
preventing their normal actions.
Beta-blockers are examples of sympatholytic drugs.

SYMPATHOMIMETIC
Imitating the action of the sympathetic nervous system; having the
same effect as stimulation of the
sympathetic part of the autonomic
nervous system, for example, an increase in the heart rate and widening of the airways.

A drug with a sympathomimetic
action may work either by causing
the release of the stimulatory neurotransmitter noradrenalin from nerve
endings or by mimicking the action
of neurotransmitters.

Sympathomimetic drugs include
certain bronchodilators and decongestants.

SYMPATHY
The mutual relationship between
two parts or more or less distant,
whereby a change in one has an effect upon the other.

SYMPHYSECTOMY
Surgical excision of the symphysis
pubis (the junction of the pubic
bones at the front lower part of the
pelvis).

SYMPHYSIOTOMY
Surgical division of the symphysis

pubis (junction of the pubic bones at the front lower part of the pelvis) in order to increase the diameter of the pelvis and thus facilitate delivery in a difficult labor.

SYMPHYSIS
The junction line of two meeting bones.

SYMPHYSIS PUBIS
The joint between the two pubic bones at the front lower part of the pelvis.

SYMPTOM
The complaint described by the patient as indicating some disease or disorder as opposed to a sign, which is that the doctor observes himself.

SYMPTOMATIC REACTION
One following therapeutic injection of an allergen and characterized by the reproduction of the original symptoms under investigation or treatment.

SYMPTOMATOLOGY
The study of symptoms; all the symptoms of a disease considered as a whole.

SYMPTOM-SUBSTITUTION THEORY
An expression of the contention that simple removal of a symptom through behavior modification, hypnosis or suggestion will result in the appearance of another symptom.

SYNAPSE
The point of connection between two nerves or between nerve and muscle fiber. An electrical nerve impulse releases a chemical transmitter which crosses a small gap and initiates electrical excitation (or inhibition) of the succeeding nerve or muscle.

SYNAPTIC CLEFT
The space between neurons at a nerve synapse across which a nerve

impulse is transmitted by a neurotransmitter.

SYNCOPE
Swooning or fainting, temporary loss of consciousness from anemia of the brain.

SYNCYTIUM
A mass of protoplasm with numerous nuclei; the exterior covering of the chorionic villi, associated with the fetal membrane within the womb.

SYNDESMOSIS
A form of joint in which the bones are connected by ligaments.

SYNDROME
A group of symptoms and signs which together characterize a disease.

SYNECHIA
A morbid union of parts, especially adhesion of the iris (colored portion surrounding the pupil) to the lens capsule or cornea (transparent front portion of the eye).

SYNERGISM
The working together of two or more agencies (e.g. synergistic muscles, or a chemical with a mechanical phenomenon, or even a chemist with a physicist) to greater effect than both would have working independently.

SYNERGIST
(1) an agent that increases the effectiveness of another agent when combined with it; especially a drug that acts in synergism with another.
(2) An organ, as a muscle, that acts in concert with another to enhance its effect.

SYNESTHESIS
Phenomena in which sensations in one sense department carry with them sensory impressions belonging to another sense department.

SYNOVIAL FLUID

Clear lubricating fluid secreted by the synovial membrane of a joint. All body joints contain a small amount of straw-colored syrupy liquid called synovial fluid that helps lubricate the bone or cartilage surfaces.

SYNOVIAL MEMBRANE

The dense connective-tissue membrane that secretes synovia and that lines the ligamentous surfaces of articular capsules, tendon sheaths where free movement is necessary, and bursae.

SYNOVITIS

Inflammation of a synovial membrane (the membrane lining joints). It usually leads to a vast output of fluid, causing the joint to swell.

SYNTACTICS

A branch of semiotic that deals with the formal relations between signs or expressions in abstraction from their significance and their interpreters.

SYPHILIS

A highly contagious venereal disease, caused by a spirochete, the treponema pallidum, and characterized by a variety of lesions, the chancre, the mucous patch and the gumma being the most distinctive.

The microbe that causes syphilis is transmitted from person to person by direct sexual contact, such as: sexual intercourse, oral-genital contact, anal-genital contact.

SYPHILITIC NODE

Localized swelling on bones due to syphilis.

SYRINGE

A simple pump for drawing and ejecting liquids. The ear syringe is merely a tapering tube with a rubber bulb at one end. The hypodermic syringe, used to give injections, has a cylindrical barrel containing a piston and with an attached hollow needle.

SYRINGOBULBIA

A fluid-filled neuroglial cavity of the brain stem. It is a congenital lesion, but for unknown reasons often expands during the teens or young adult years.

SYRINGOMYELIA

A slow progressive disease of the nervous system which affects adults.

A cavity forms in the spinal cord, causing loss of sensation of heat, cold and pain.

The sense of touch is not affected. As the disease progresses, the legs may become spastic and extensive deformity and paralysis develop.

In some cases, the disease spontaneously stops worsening and the person affected is left with a moderate to severe physical disability. Mental faculties are not affected.

SYRINGOMYELOCELE

A defect of the spine with protrusion of a sac containing a portion of the spinal cord whose central canal is greatly distended with cerebrospinal fluid.

SYSTEM

A methodical arrangement; a combination of parts into a whole, such as the digestive, nervous, circulatory and respiratory systems; the body as a whole.

SYSTEMIC

Medical term used in the sense of or concerning the whole body, not confined to a particular part, such as a systemic infection caused by a virus.

A systemic agent usually causes a generalized effect, such as physical or chemical changes throughout the body.

For a drug to have a systemic effect it must be absorbed into the bloodstream, usually via the digestive tract, by injection or by rectal suppository.

SYSTEMIC CIRCULATION
Circulation of blood in the body, with the exception of the pulmonary circulation.

SYSTEMIC LUPUS ERYTHE-MATOSUS
An inflammatory connective tissue disorder of unknown cause occurring predominantly in young women, but also in children and older adults. The characteristic molar butterfly erythema is one of several cutaneous lesions that may oc-cur. Recurrent pleurisy is frequent. Kidneys, joints and lungs may be involved. The prognosis varies widely, depending on the organs involved and the intensity of the inflammatory reaction.

SYSTOLE
The period of the heart's contraction; the contraction itself.

SYSTOLIC PRESSURE
The highest arterial blood pressure of a cardiac cycle occurring immediately after systole of the left ventricle of the heart.

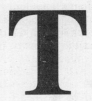

TABES
Any progressive wasting of the body or part of it; the short term for tabes dorsalis.

TABES DORSALIS
Form of tertiary syphilis in which certain tracts in the spinal cord - particularly those concerned with position sense - degenerate, leading to a characteristic high-stepping gait, sensory abnormalities and sometimes disorganization of joints. Attacks of abdominal pain and abnormal pupil reactions are typical.

TABLE
In medicine, the external or internal layer of compact bone of the skull separated by cancellous diploe.

TABLET
Solid dosage form containing medicine.

TABLET TRITURATE
A small tablet made by molding fine moistened powder containing a medicinal and a diluent.

TABOO
Polynesian word meaning that which is forbidden. Negative taboos arise from fear of possible ill effects (for instance, incest); positive taboos from awe or reverence (for instance, approaching a god). The term is also used to designate a prohibition imposed by social custom or as a protective measure.

TABOPARESIS
Paresis occurring with tabes and especially with tabes dorsalis.

TACHYCARDIA
Abnormally fast heart rate. Generally, anything over 100 beats per minute is considered tachycardia.

TACHYPHYLAXIS
Diminished response to increments in a sequence of applications of a physiologically active substance, as the diminished response that follows repeated injections of renin.

TACHYPNEA
Rapid breathing; increased rate of respiration.

TACHYSTEROL
An oily liquid alcohol isomeric with ergosterol that is formed by ultraviolet irradiation of ergosterol or lumisterol and that on further irradiation yields vitamin D_2.

TACTILE CELL
One of the oval nucleated cells, as in a Meissner's corpuscle, that are in close contact with the expanded ends of nerve fibers in the deeper layers of the epidermis and dermis of some parts of the body and probably serve a tactile function.

TACTILE CIRCLE
An area of the cutaneous surface within which two points of simultaneous pressure are sensed as a single point.

TACTILE CORPUSCLE
One of the numerous minute bodies, as a Meissner's corpuscle, in the skin and some mucous membranes that usually consist of a group of cells enclosed in a capsule, containing nerve terminations, and that are held to be end organs of touch.

TACTILE RECEPTOR
An end organ, as a Meissner's corpuscle or a Pacinian corpuscle, that responds to light touch.

TACTUAL
Involving, or referring to, the sense

of touch. Used to describe a specific type of cutaneous sensation.

TAEDIUM VITAE
A morbid weariness of life, a form of depression which sometimes leads to suicide.

TAENIA
Tapeworms, ribbon-like parasitic flatworms of the class cestoda.

TAENIA COLI
Any of three external longitudinal muscle bands of the large intestine.

TAENIA SAGINATA INFECTION
Another name for beef worm infection.

TAG
A small abnormal projecting piece of tissue especially when potentially or actually neoplastic in character.

TAIL BUD
A knob of embryonic tissue not divided into germ layers that arises at the primitive knot and contributes to the formation of the posterior part of the vertebrate body.

TAKAYASU'S DISEASE
Progressive obliteration of the arteries branching from the arch of the aorta and comprising the innominate artery, left common carotid artery, and left subclavian artery that is marked by diminution or loss of the pulse in and symptoms of ischemia in the head, neck, and arms.

TALALGIA
Pain in the heel or ankle.

TALC
A native hydrous magnesium silicate, sometimes with a small amount of aluminum silicate, used as a dusting powder.

TALENT
Natural aptitude in some special direction, e.g., a talent for mathematics or music.

TALIPES EQUINOVARUS
A congenital deformity of the foot in which both equinus and talipes varus occur so that walking is done on the toes and outer side of the sole.

TALIPES EQUINUS
A congenital deformity of the foot in which the sole is permanently flexed so that walking is done on the toes without touching the heel to the ground.

TALIPES VARUS
A congenital deformity of the foot in which it is rotated outward so that walking is done on the outer side of the sole.

TALISMAN
An object believed to possess magical protective power in favor of the individual possessing it or carrying it.

TALOCRURAL
Pertaining both to the talus (anklebone) and the legbones.

TALOTIBIAL
Pertaining both to the talus (anklebone) and the tibia (shinbone).

TALUS
The astralagus or anklebone; the bone bears the weight of the body and forms with the tibia and the fibula the ankle joint. (See illustration on next page)

TAMPON
A plug of soft material inserted into a cavity; to plug a cavity with a tampon.

TAMPONADE
The closure or blockage, as of a wound or body cavity, by or as if by a tampon especially to stop bleeding as in case of a wound.

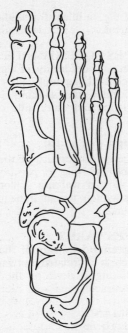

Dorsal aspect of the foot. The tarsus is a collective designation for the seven bones of the ankle. The talus, the uppermost tarsal bone, is the only bone of the foot that articulates with the fibula and tibia.

TANGIERS DISEASE
A familial disorder characterized by recurrent polyneuropathy, disorder of the lymph glands, orange-yellow tonsillar hyperplasia and enlargement of the spleen and liver, associated with a marked decrease in high-density lipoproteins. There is no treatment.

TANNATE
Any of the salts of tannic acid, all of which are astringent.

TANNIN
Any of various soluble astringent complex phenolic substances of plant origin used in tanning, dyeing, the making of ink, and in medicine as astringents and formerly in the treatment of burns.

T-ANTIGENS
Tumor antigens, probably protein products of the viral genome present only on infected neoplastic cells.

TANTRUM
A violent display of bad temper, usually employed by children as a means of obtaining or avoiding something. In severe cases tantrums are part of a psychopathic behavior.

TAPETUM
Any of the various membranous layers or areas especially of the choroid and retina of the eye. The term is also used to designate a layer of nerve fibers derived from the corpus callosum and forming part of the roof of each lateral ventricle of the brain.

TAPETUM LUCIDUM
A layer in the choroid chiefly of nocturnal mammals that reflects light causing the eyes to glow when light strikes them at night and that is made up of several layers of flattened cells covered by a zone of doubly refracting crystals.

TAPEWORMS
Intestinal parasites, so named because they are long and flat, forming the class cestoda of the flatworm phylum platyhelminthes.

TAPHEPHOBIA
Morbid dread of being buried alive. In some cases a severe neurosis exists that should be treated by psychotherapy.

TAPOTEMENT
Tapping movements used in massage.

TARDIVE DYSKINESIA
Involuntary movements of the jaw, lips and tongue caused by an unpredictable drug action. It is a central nervous system disorder characterized by twitching of the face and tongue and involuntary motor movements of the trunk and limbs

and occurring especially as a side effect of prolonged use of antipsychotic drugs, as phenothiazines. This condition is distinct from parkinsonism that may also be caused by such drugs.

TARGET CELL
A cell that is acted on preferentially by a specific agent, as a virus, drug, or hormone.

TARGET GLAND
An endocrine organ of which the functional activity is controlled by tropic hormones secreted by the pituitary gland.

TARSAL
Relating to the tarsus (instep) of the foot; relating to the tarsal plate (tissue framework) of the upper eyelid.

TARSAL PLATE
The plate of strong dense fibrous connective tissue that forms the supporting structure of the eyelid.

TARSECTOMY
Surgical removal of part of the tarsus (instep) of the foot or of the tarsal plate (tissue framework) in the upper eyelid.

TARSOGRAPHY
The operation of suturing the eyelids together entirely or in part.

TARSUS
The bones forming the instep of the foot; the tissues forming the upper eyelid.

TARTAR
An incrustation on the teeth consisting of salivary secretion, food residue, and various salts, as calcium carbonate.

TARTRAZINE DYE
A dye used in foods and medicine preparations that may cause an allergic reaction in some people.

TASK
The performance that is required of the subject in a psychological experiment or test and that is usually communicated to a human being by verbal instruction.

TASTE
Special sense concerned with the differentiation of basic modalities of food or other substances in the mouth; receptors are distributed over the surface of the tongue and are able to distinguish salt, sweet, sour, bitter and possibly water as primary tastes. Much of what is colloquially termed taste is actually smell perception of odors reaching the olfactory epithelium via the naso-pharynx. Receptors for sweet are concentrated at the tip of the tongue, for salt and sour along the sides, with bitter mainly at the back. Taste nerve impulses pass via the brain stem to the cortex.

TASTE BLINDNESS
Inability to taste certain substances.

TASTE BUD
A structure, containing the receptor cells (sensors) for taste, in the fungiform, circumvallate and foliate papillae of the tongue.

TASTE CELL
A neuroepithelial cell that is located in a taste bud and is the actual receptor of the sensation of taste.

TASTE FUNCTION
The ability to taste four distinctive flavors on both sides of the tongue equally is important to the diagnosis of certain brain lesions. Nerves of taste located on the front of the tongue come from a different part of the brain than nerves of taste located on the back of the tongue.

TASTE HAIR
The hairlike free end of a neuroepithelial cell in a taste bud.

TAT
Abbreviation of thematic apperception test.

TATTOO
An inedible mark or figure fixed upon the body by insertion of pigment under the skin or by production of scars.

TATTOOING
The introduction of vegetable and mineral substances into the skin in order to color it. Many practicing this trade are less than careful with their antisepsis (AIDS), and apart from adding their design, which most young men love to respect, there is a risk of introducing infections into the skin.

TAU EFFECT
An illusion, affecting the perception of spatial intervals, due to the influence of temporal factors.

TAXIS
Manipulation of a misplaced organ into its normal position, as, for instance, the reduction of a rupture, or the replacing of a misplaced womb; the involuntary response of an organism involving change of place, either towards (positive taxis) or away from (negative taxis) a stimulus.

TAY'S DISEASE
Inflammation of the choroid (vascular coat of the eye), occurring in old age and probably due to hardening of the arteries.

TAY-SACHS DISEASE
An inherited disorder that seems to occur primarily in Jewish people from Eastern Europe. Its occurrence in those of non-Jewish origin is rare. Children born with the disease have little or no active hexosaminidase enzyme, the lack of which causes fat to accumulate in the brain's ganglions.

The consequences are mental retardation, paralysis, blindness and cherry-red spots on the retina of the eye. The disorder is usually fatal before the child reaches the age of four.

T-CELL
A thymus-derived cell which participates in a variety of cell-mediated immune reactions. The T-cell is characterized by specific surface antigens, and specialized to function in cell-mediated immunity especially by killing foreign cells or virus-infected cells, by helping other T-cells or B-cells respond to antigens, or by suppressing the activity of specific populations of B-cells or T-cells.

T-CELL GROWTH FACTOR
A glycoprotein that is released by T-lymphocytes on stimulation with antigens and which functions as a T-cell growth factor by inducing proliferation of activated T-cells.

TEACHER'S NODULES
Another name for vocal cord nodules.

TEACHING NURSING HOME
A nursing home affiliated with a university medical school or medical center. In addition to the "teaching" function of the teaching nursing school, another of its purposes is to conduct research on the chronic health problems that often lead older persons to be institutionalized (problems such as dementia, incontinence, loss of mobility, depression, and sleep disorders).

TEARS
Watery secretions of the lacrimal glands situated over the eyes which provide continuous lubrication and protection of cornea and sclera. A constant flow runs across the surface of the eye to the nasolacrimal duct at the inner corner, where tears drain into the nose. Excess tears produced in states of high emotion

and conjunctival or corneal irritation overflow over the lower eyelid.

TECTORIAL MEMBRANE
A membrane having the consistency of jelly that covers the surface of the organ of Corti.

TECTUM
(1) A bodily structure resembling or serving as a roof.
(2) The dorsal part of the midbrain including the corpora quadrigemina.

TEETHING
The entire process resulting in eruption of the teeth; also called dentition.

TEGMENTUM
The part of the ventral midbrain above the substantia nigra formed of longitudinal, white fibers with arched transverse fibers and gray matter.

TEGMENTUM TYMPANI
A thin plate of bone that covers the middle ear and
separates it from the cranial cavity.

TEGUMENT
The skin covering the body.

TELA CHOROIDEA
A fold of pia mater roofing a ventricle of the brain.

TELANGIECTASIA
Dilation of small blood vessels in the skin. One form is the web-like network of veins seen on the skin of the legs of middle-aged women.

TELEDIAGNOSIS
The diagnosis of physical or mental ailments based on data received from a patient by means of telemetry and closed-circuit television.

TELEKINESIS
Term employed in psychical research (parapsychology) for movement of objects in the presence of a medium, apparently without contact or direct communication, as a result of occult forces.

TELEMEDICINE
The practice of medicine when the doctor and patient are widely separated using two-way voice and visual communication especially satellite, telemetry, closed-circuit television and teleconferencing by way of computer systems.

TELENCEPHALON
The anterior subdivision of the forebrain comprising the cerebral hemispheres and associated structures.

TELEOLOGY
Doctrine emphasizing the character of vital, including mental, phenomena, as directed toward and determined by a goal or purpose.

TELEONOMY
The quality of apparent purposefulness in living organisms that derives from their evolutionary adaptation.

TELEPATHY
Parapsychological term for alleged communication, by other than known physical means, or thoughts, experiences, feelings, etc., from one mind to another.

TELEPLASM
Hypothetical substances emanating from the body of a medium, and taking ultimately the form of a person.

TELERGY
The supposed or alleged action of the mind of one person on the mind of another. The term is part of the terminology of psychical research or parapsychology.

TEMPER
The degree of strength of individual instinctive impulses, particularly the aggressive.

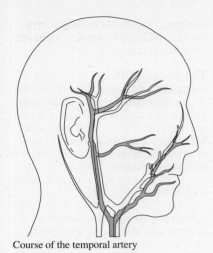

Course of the temporal artery

TEMPERANCE
Habitual moderation in the indulgence of the appetites or passions.

TEMPERAMENT
General nature of an individual, especially on the character side.

TEMPERATURE
The normal mouth temperature usually lies between 97 and 99 degrees Fahrenheit (36-37.2 degrees Celsius), the average being about 98.6° F (37.0°C). It fluctuates daily and in women monthly. The temperature setting is higher than normal in fever. When the body is too hot, the blood vessels near the skin expand to carry more blood and to lose heat by radiation and convection, and the sweat glands produce perspiration which cools by evaporation.

When the body is too cold, the blood vessels near the skin contract, the metabolic rate increases and shivering occurs to produce more heat.

TEMPERATURE SPOT
Cutaneous area sensitive to either cold or heat.

TEMPLE
The flat portion of the head behind the eye and above the ear.

TEMPORAL
Relating to the temple; relating to time.

TEMPORAL ARTERITIS
A chronic generalized inflammatory disease of the branches of the aorta arch; found principally in the temporal and occipital arteries, but may develop in almost any large artery.

The onset may be acute or gradual and may simulate an infection such as an influenza-like syndrome, with low-grade fever, malaise, anorexia, severe weakness and weight loss.

The disorder is characterized by aching and stiffness involving mainly the trunk. Treatment should start as soon as the diagnosis is suspected.

TEMPORAL ARTERY
Either of two branches of the maxillary artery that supply the temporalis muscle and anastomose with the middle temporal artery.

TEMPORAL FOSSA
A broad fossa on the side of the skull behind the orbit that contains the muscles for raising the lower jaw and that is occupied by the temporalis muscle, separated from the orbit by the zygomatic bone, bounded laterally by the zygomatic arch, and lying above the infratemporal crest of the greater wing of the sphenoid bone.

TEMPORAL GYRUS
Any of three major convolutions of the external surface of the temporal lobe of a cerebral hemisphere that are arranged approximately horizontally with one above the other. The superior temporal gyrus is the one that is uppermost and borders the fissure of Sylvius.

The middle temporal gyrus is the one lying in the middle between the other two. The inferior temporal gyrus is the inferiormost of the three.

TEMPORAL LOBE
The section of the cerebral hemisphere lying below the lateral fissure and in front of the occipital lobe, that is the cortical area for the reception of auditory stimuli.

TEMPORAL SIGN
A characteristic of a memory mechanism of which it is located in time.

TEMPOROMANDIBULAR JOINT DISEASE
Problem in which there are symptoms related to opening and closing the mouth. There can be many causes.

Pain or discomfort and limitation of motion of the jaw are the most common complaints. There may be a sensation of cracking in the jaw with movement or a feeling that the jaw is stuck and unable to move or open. Inflammation or degenerative changes in the jaw joint most often result from injury or aging, although the jaw can be involved with many forms of arthritis.

Pain in the jaw without arthritis can be caused by muscle tension and strain due to continual or repeated jaw-clenching or tooth-grinding, as a result of anxiety or habit. Malocclusion of the teeth or dentures that fit badly can contribute to any jaw pain.

TENDENCY
A definite direction of progression of movement, or of thought, towards a goal.

TENDINOUS
Pertaining to a tendon.

TENDO ACHILLES
The powerful tendon which joins the calf muscles to the back of the heel.

TENDON
An inelastic cord of a fibrous connective tissue by means of which a muscle is attached to a bone. Sometimes tendons are located between muscle parts.

TENDON REFLEX
A reflex act, as a knee jerk, in which a muscle is made to contract by a blow upon its tendon.

TENDON SENSATION
A sensation depending on receptors situated within the tendon. Tendon sense organs are sensitive to stretch stimuli.

TENDON SHEATH
A synovial sheath covering a tendon, as in the hand or foot.

TENDOVAGINITIS
Inflammation of a tendon and its sheath.

TENESMUS
A painful straining, particularly a painful straining effort to empty the bladder, or bowel, usually without success.

TENNIS ELBOW
A name commonly applied to almost every disorder in which there is pain at the side of the elbow caused by energetic use of the arm. Only in few persons is the playing of tennis the original cause, for any occupation requiring a tight grip and rotatory movement of the forearm may be responsible.

TENON'S CAPSULE
A thin connective membrane ensheathing the eyeball behind the conjunctiva.

TENON'S SPACE
A space between Tenon's capsule and the sclerotic coat of the eye that is traversed by strands of reticular tissue and by the optic nerve and ocular muscles.

TENOSYNOVITIS
Inflammation of a tendon sheath;

also called tendovaginitis or teno-vaginitis.

TENSION
Strain which results from muscular contractions and through which muscles, tendons, etc. are stretched and maintained in that position.

TENSION HEADACHE
Headache due primarily to contraction of the muscles of the neck and scalp.

TENSION PNEUMOTHORAX
Pneumothorax resulting from a wound in the chest wall which acts as a valve that permits air to enter the pleural cavity but prevents its escape.

TENSOR FASCIAE LATAE
A muscle that arises especially from the anterior part of the iliac crest and from the anterior superior iliac spine, inserting into the iliotibial band of the fascia late about one third of the way down the thigh, and acting to flex and abduct the thigh.

TERATOLOGY
The study of birth monstrosities.

TERATOMA
A tumor containing teeth, hair or other material, not found in the part wherein it grows and resulting from the misplacement of tissue during the growth of the fetus.

TERES MAJOR
A thick somewhat flattened muscle that arises chiefly from the lower third of the axillary border of the scapula, passes in front of the long head of the triceps to insert on the medial border of the bicipital groove of the humerus, and functions in opposition to the muscles comprising the rotator cuff by extending the arm when it is in the flexed position and by rotating it medially.

TERES MINOR
A long cylindrical muscle that arises from the upper two-thirds of the axillary border of the scapula, passes behind the long head of the triceps to insert chiefly on the greater tubercle of the humerus, contributes to the formation of the rotator cuff of the shoulder, and acts to rotate the arm laterally and draw the humerus toward the glenoid fossa.

TERMINAL
Pertaining to the end, being at the end, forming the end.

TERMINAL DISINFECTION
A method of removing disease-causing organisms and their toxins from a room previously occupied by a person who has an infectious disease.

TERMINAL SENSITIVITY
The highest intensity of sensation, in any sense modality, which an organism is capable of experiencing.

TEST
A standardized type of examination, given to a group of individuals to determine the presence or absence of a particular capacity, knowledge or skill, or determine the degree in which such is present. In the broadest sense the term test is also used for the determination of chemical, physical, etc. characteristics of cells, tissues and organs, for instance, blood test.

TEST CHART
A chart or card containing rows, graded as to size of the letters, characters or pictures displayed, for testing visual acuity.

TESTICULAR
Pertaining to the testicles.

TESTICULAR ARTERY
Either of a pair of arteries which supply blood to the testes of which

one arises on each side from the front of the aorta a little below the corresponding renal artery and passes downward to the spermatic cord of the same side and along it to the testis.

TESTICULAR FEMINIZATION
A genetic defect characterized by the presence of a phenotypically female individual of the normal X and Y chromosomes of a male, undeveloped and undescended testes, and functional sterility.

TESTIS
Either of a pair of male gonads, or sex glands, that produces sperm and secretes androgens. The adult testes, each about 4 cm long and oval-shaped, are suspended in the scrotum below the abdomen.

Each testis consists of many hundred seminiferous tubules where sperm develop. The sperm pass from there through efferent ducts to the epididymis, after which they pass into the vas deferens for movement toward the penis.

TESTOSTERONE
Androgen steroid produced by the interstitial cells of the testes, and to a lesser extent by the adrenal gland cortex, under the control of luteinizing hormone. It is responsible for most male sexual characteristics - voice change, hair distribution and sex-organ development.

TEST PROFILE
An instrument that yields several separate measures of different variables resulting in a picture, or profile of the individual's characteristics across several areas.

TEST SCORE
The value of the performance in a test, expressed usually in numerical terms.

TEST TUBE FERTILIZATION
Popular term for in vitro fertiliza-

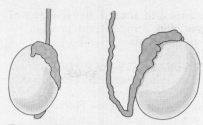

Testes, epididymis and ductus deferens.

tion; a process by which an egg is fertilized by sperm in a test tube or dish. Briefly, the technique is as follows: exploratory surgery is performed to determine the ovulatory capacity of the woman's reproductive organs; following a period of close observation of her menstrual cycle, some eggs are harvested. Sperm are also collected and placed in a special solution to allow survival. After fertilization the egg is transplanted back into the womb.

TETANUS
Lockjaw, bacterial disease in which a toxin produced by anaerobic tetanus bacilli growing in contaminated wounds causes muscle spasm due to nerve toxicity. Minor cuts may be infected with the bacteria which are common in soil.

The first symptoms may often be painful contraction of jaw and neck muscles; trunk muscles including those or respiration and muscles close to the site of injury are also frequently involved.

Untreated, many cases are fatal, but artificial respiration, antiserum and penicillin have improved the outlook. Regular vaccination and adequate wound cleansing are important in prevention.

TETRACYCLINES
Broad-spectrum antibiotics (including aureomycin and terramycin) which may be given by mouth. While useful in bronchitis and other minor infections, they are especially valuable in disease due to rickettsia and related organisms; they can also

be used in acne. Tetracyclines will not work for colds, flu, or other virus infections.

TETRALOGY OF FALLOT
A form of congenital heart disease characterized by:
(1) narrowing of the pulmonary artery (main artery of the lungs);
(2) a hole in the septum (dividing wall) between the ventricles (lower chambers of the heart);
(3) dextroposition of the aorta (main artery from the heart);
(4) enlargement of the right ventricle.

TETRAPLEGIA
Paralysis of both arms and both legs.

THALAMIC RADIATION
Any of several large bundles of nerve fibers connecting the thalamus and the cerebral cortex.

THALAMUS
A mass of gray matter at the base of the brain, developed from and forming part of the wall of the third ventricle (a brain cavity). Practically all the sensory nerve impulses must pass through this area to reach the sensory area in the cortex (outer layer) of the brain, and the primary centers for vision are situated in the rear portion of it.

THALASSEMIA
A disease in the Mediterranean region, characterized by enlargement of the spleen, anemia and changes in the bones, with pigmentation of the skin.

THALASSOTHERAPY
Treatment by means of sea bathing, sea voyages, sea air, seaside holidays.

THALLIUM POISONING
Condition characterized by neurological symptoms including myoclonic jerking and rigidity. Chronic ingestion often results in residual cerebral difficulties including intellectual, motor and personality changes.

THANATOLOGY
The description or study of the phenomena of death and of psychological mechanisms for coping with them.

THANATOPHOBIA
Morbid fear of death. In severe cases a neurosis may develop that should be treated by psychotherapy.

THEMATIC APPERCEPTION TEST (TAT)
Projective technique in which the subject projects or reads into a series of pictures his own feelings and interpretations. The test is widely used in clinical psychology to make personality, psychodynamic, and diagnostic assessments based on the subject's verbal responses to a series of black and white pictures.

THENAR
The palm of the hand or sole of the foot, but especially the palm of the hand; the fleshy mass of muscle at the base of the thumb, which is also called the thenar eminence.

THERAPEUTIC BARGAIN CONCEPT
In psychiatric therapy, the patient must have a choice of something better, before a symptom or trait can be modified or surrendered.

THERAPEUTIC WINDOW
The range of plasma concentrations with the greatest probability of therapeutic success.

THERAPY
The treatment of disability or disease, as by some remedial or curative processes.

THERMALGESIA
State of an organism when a warm

stimulus produces a pain sensation.

THERMOANESTHESIA
Insensibility to temperature stimuli.

THERMO-ANESTHESIA
Loss of normal powers of detecting temperature changes.

THERMOCAUTERY
An instrument consisting of a loop of platinum which is usually heated by an electric current to a dull red. It is used for cutting through tissues and by its burning action seals off bleeding points.

THERMOGENESIS
The production of heat, especially within the body.

THERMOGRAPH
An instrument for recording temperature variations.

THERMOGRAPHY
Method to measure the slightest variations in temperature of soft tissue in the body using infrared heat sensors. The technique is often used in mammography (breast examination) to detect any growth in the breast (the mass will have a different temperature from other breast tissue).

THERMOMETER
An instrument for measuring temperatures.

THERMORECEPTOR
Sense organ or sensor responding to changes in the environmental temperature.

THIAMINE
Vitamin B_1 used as a supplement for a number of medical conditions: (1) Dietary supplement to promote normal growth, development and health. (2) Treatment for beri-beri (a thiamine-deficiency diseases). (3) Dietary supplement for alcohol-

ism, cirrhosis, overactive thyroid, infection, breast-feeding, absorption diseases, pregnancy, prolonged diarrhea, burns.
   Thiamine combines with an enzyme to metabolize carbohydrates.

THIAZIDES
A group of chemicals that cause diuresis (loss of water through the kidney. These medicines are frequently used to treat high blood pressure and congestive heart failure.

THIOGUANINE
Generic name of an anticancer drug prescribed for the treatment of some forms of leukemia. The drug interferes with the growth of cancer cells.

THOMAS' SPLINT
A splint consisting of a leather-padded ring which surrounds the top of the thigh and from which metal bars extend on either side of the limb. Slings are tied to the metal bars and the limb lies on these slings. It is used primarily as a first-aid treatment for fractures of the femur (thighbone).

THORACENTESIS
The removal of fluid from the space around the lungs.

THORACIC
Pertaining to the chest.

THORACIC CAVITY
Space containing the heart and lungs.

THORACIC GANGLION
Any of the ganglia of the sympathetic chain in the thoracic region that occur in 12 or fewer pairs.

THORACIC NERVE
Any of the spinal nerves of the thoracic region that consists of 12 pairs of which one pair emerges just below each thoracic vertebra.

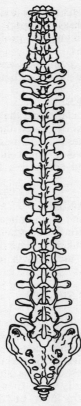

Dorsal or posterior view of the spine. The thoracic vertebrae (12) are located between the cervical and lumbar parts of the spine.

THORACIC VERTEBRA
Any of the 12 vertebrae dorsal to the thoracic region and characterized by articulation with the ribs.

THORACO-ABDOMINAL
Pertaining to both the chest and abdomen.

THORACODORSAL NERVE
Branch of the posterior cord of the brachial plexus that supplies the latissimus dorsi muscle.

THORACOPLASTY
Surgical removal of parts of all the ribs on one side to allow both the chest wall and the underlying lung to collapse and close cavities in the lung.

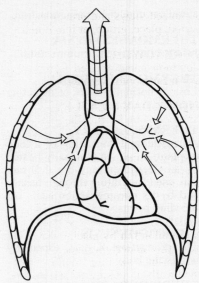

The thorax in exhalation of air.

THORACOTOMY
Surgical incision into the chest wall.

THORAX
The chest, that part of the body between neck and abdomen.

THORNWALDT'S CYST
A frequently infected cyst found in the midline of the nasopharynx. The cyst lies superficial to the superior constrictor muscle of the pharynx and is covered by mucous membrane. If infected, it may cause persistent purulent drainage with a foul taste and odor, obstruction of the Eustachian tube and sore throat.

THOUGHT
Psychological and neurophysiological term used in several meanings.
(1) The action or process of thinking.
(2) A reasoning power or the power to imagine.
(3) Something that is thought as an individual act or product of thinking. The term is also used to designate something as an opinion of belief in the mind.
(4) The intellectual product or the

organized views and principles of a period, place, group, or individual.

THREADWORM
Common name applied to the pinworm Enterobius vermicularis.

THREE-DAY MEASLES
Another name for rubella.

THRESHOLD
The lower limit of stimulus capable of producing an impression upon consciousness or evoking a response; the entrance of a canal.

THRILL
A vibration felt by placing the hand over the underlying aneurysm (a balloon-like swelling of the weakened walls of a blood vessel), over a heart with valvular disease, and over hydatid cysts.

THROAT
The pharynx; the fauces; the front part of the neck.

THROAT CULTURE
Incubation of a sample of throat secretions in nutrient material, to determine the presence and type of infection-causing micro-organisms.

THROMBECTOMY
An operation to remove a blood clot from a blood vessel.

THROMBIN
The enzyme that causes clotting of shed blood.

THROMBINOGEN
A substance which is the precursor of thrombin (a clotting factor present in blood plasma). Also called prothrombin, thrombogen and proserozyme.

THROMBOANGIITIS OBLITERANS
A disease of the blood vessels of the extremities, primarily the legs, which occurs most commonly in men and is associated with tobacco use. It is characterized by inflammation of the veins, arteries and nerves and by thrombosis in the vessels (blood clot formation). This leads to poor circulation and gangrene.

THROMBO-ARTERITIS
Clotting accompanied by inflammation of an artery.

THROMBOCYTE
A blood platelet.

THROMBO-EMBOLISM
Lodgment of a blood clot in a pulmonary artery with subsequent obstruction of blood supply to the lung tissue. The most common type of pulmonary embolus is a thrombus which usually has formed in the leg or pelvic veins.

THROMBOKINASE
A substance capable of transforming thrombinogen to thrombin, part of the mechanism of the formation of a clot.

THROMBOLYTIC AGENTS
Substances which dissolve blood clots. Two examples are streptokinase and urokinase.

THROMBOPHLEBITIS
Inflammation and blood clotting in a vein.

THROMBOSIS
The formation of a clot (thrombus) in the heart or blood vessels. It commonly occurs in the legs and is associated with varicose veins but is more serious if it occurs in the heart or in the brain arteries. Detachments from a thrombus in the legs may be carried to the lungs as an embolus; this may have a fatal outcome if large vessels are occluded. The treatment includes anticoagulants.

THROMBUS
A clot of blood formed within the

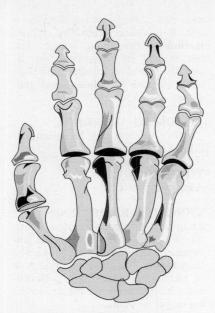

The skeleton of the thumb consists of a metacarpal bone and two phalanges.

heart or blood vessels, usually due to a slowing of the circulation or to alteration of the blood or walls of the blood vessels.

THRUSH
An infection due to the fungus Candida albicans. It occurs usually in children and is characterized by small, whitish spots on the tip and sides of the tongue and the lining membrane of the mouth.

THUMB
The short and thick first or preaxial digit of the human hand that difers from the other fingers in having only two phalanges, in having greater freedom of movement, and in being opposable to the other fingers.

THYMECTOMY
Surgical removal of the thymus gland.

THYMITIS
Inflammation of the thymus gland.

THYMOPATHY
Any disorder of the thymus gland.

THYMUS
A lymphoid organ situated in the superior and front part of the mediastinum, which reaches its maximum weight at about puberty and then undergoes involution. It is necessary in early life for development and maturation of cell-mediated immunological responses.

At birth, when it is largest in relation to the body weight, it weighs 10-15 g and at the age of eight to ten years it reaches its maximum absolute weight of 35-50 g. Although a lymphoid organ, it is not concerned with the handling of lymph, and unlike a lymph node it has no lymphatic channels of sinusoidal type in its parenchyme.

The functions of the thymus gland may be summarized as follows:
(1) In the newborn the thymus is necessary for the development of the peripheral lymphoid tissues. In its absence, lymphoid aplasia, lymphopenia and a failure of cellular immunity lead to wasting and death from infection. By adolescence the lymphoid system is fully developed and then the thymus involutes.
(2) In the adult the function of the involuted thymus is one of maintenance. It ensures the supply of fresh, immunologically uncommitted lymphocytes able to react to new antigens.
(3) The thymus stimulates both its own and peripheral lymphopoiesis by a humoral factor produced by its medullary epithelial cells. The production of thymic lymphocytes is autonomous; the thymus governs its own lymphopoietic rate, its ultimate population of lymphocytes and the onset of its involution.
(4) The bone marrow supplies the stem cells from which lymphocytes develop in the thymus, under the influence of the humoral factor.
(5) The thymus is responsible for the gradual restoration of cellular

immune competence in animals rendered experimentally tolerant to antigens.

(6) In auto-immune diseases the thymus often shows germinal follicle formation and in some of these diseases may play an initiating part. The thymus gives some protection against experimentally induced carcinoma.

THYROID ANTIBODIES
Antibodies present in various diseases, such as thyroid disorder, allergic disorders and pernicious anemia.

THYROID GLAND
A large endocrine gland situated at the base of the neck. It consists of two lobes, one on each side of the trachea, connected by an isthmus. Under the influence of thyroid-stimulating hormone (TSH) released from the anterior pituitary gland, the thyroid secretes the hormone thyroxin into the bloodstream; it is essential for normal growth and development in children and normal metabolic rates in adults.

THYROIDISM
The condition resulting from overuse of thyroid gland preparations; the disturbances due to overactivity of the thyroid gland; the after-effects caused by surgical removal of part or the whole of the thyroid gland.

THYROIDITIS
Inflammation of the thyroid gland.

THYROID SCAN
An organ imaging procedure done after injecting a radioactive substance into a vein, to determine the thyroid's size, shape, loca-tion and function, or any abnormality such as cancer.

THYROXINE
The active hormone of the thyroid gland. It can now be prepared by

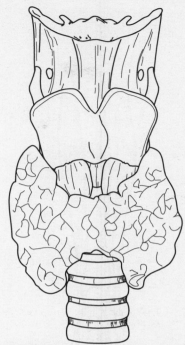

Localization of the thyroid in relation to the trachea and larynx.

synthesis, and is used to treat underactivity of the thyroid gland.

TIA
Abbreviation of transient ischemic attack.

TIBIA
The larger of the two bones in the lower part of the leg. Also called shinbone. (See illustration on next page)

TIBIAL
Relating to, or located near a tibia.

TIBIALGIA
Pain in the tibia (shinbone).

TIBIAL NERVE
The large nerve in the back of the leg that is a continuation of the sciatic nerve and terminates at the medial malleolus in the lateral and medial plantar nerves.

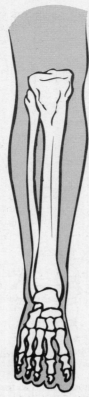

The skeleton of the leg consists of the tibia (right) and fibula (left). Anterior view.

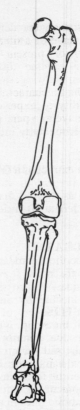

Posterior view of the right leg. The tibia is on the left.

TIC
An involuntary, sudden, rapid, recurrent, nonrhythmic, stereotype, motor movement or vocalization. It is experienced as irresistible, but can be suppressed for varying lengths of time. All forms of tics are often exacerbated by stress and usually are markedly diminished during sleep. They may become attenuated during some absorbing activities, such as reading or sewing. Both motor and vocal tics may be classified as either simple or complex, although the boundaries are not well defined.

TIC CONVULSIVE
A muscular spasm occurring in the face, in the area supplied by the seventh cranial nerve.

TIC DOULOUREUX
A form of intense neuralgia, occurring in the area at the side of the face supplied by the fifth cranial nerve (the trigeminal nerve). The pain is very severe and can be precipitated by a causal movement such as brushing the hair.

TICK
The popular name for a number of blood-sucking parasites.

TICK FEVER
Any infectious disease transmitted by the bite of a tick such as African relapsing fever, Rocky Mountain spotted fever or Texas fever.

TIME SENSE
The direct experience of the lapse

of time, based on the definite impression we have of a time interval within the sensory present.

TIMIDITY
An individual characteristic of marked liability to experience fear in which the average person experiences no such emotion.

TINCTURE
An alcoholic extract of a drug.

TINEA
Ringworm; a fungus infection of the skin.

TINEA BARBAE
Ringworm of the beard area. Also called barber's itch, barber's rash and tinea sycosis.

TINEA CAPITIS
Ringworm of the scalp. In its earliest stage, it appears as a small scaly spot, about the size of a dime, with a few broken hairs present on the patch. May occur in epidemic form amongst children through wearing each other's cap.

TINEA VERSICOLOR
An infection characterized by multiple, usually asymptomatic, patches of lesions varying in color from white to brown, and caused by Pityrosporon orbiculare.

TINNITUS
Purely subjective sensation of sounds, such as ringing, roars or banging in the inner ear.

Hearing sounds, such as buzzing, roaring, banging, hissing or ringing, that do not actually exist in the nearby environment. It is a common symptom of most ear disorders, including otosclerosis, tumor, presence of foreign body in the ear, organic ear obstruction and inner ear infection.

Tinnitus itself is not a severe or disabling problem, although it can be irritating or frustrating. However, a medical diagnosis is important in determining whether an underlying cause requires treatment.

TISSUE
Group or layer of similarly specialized cells which together perform certain special functions.

TISSUE TYPING
The determination of the degree of compatibility of tissues or organs from different individuals based on the similarity of histocompatibility antigens especially on lymphocytes and used especially as a measure of potential rejection in an organ transplant procedure.

TITER
The strength, or concentration, of a substance in fluid, such as the lowest dilution of serum at which antibody is still present.

TOBACCO
Dried leaves of varieties of the tobacco plant (Nicotiana tabacum), used for smoking, chewing and as snuff. Consumption is increasing despite the health hazards of smoking.

TOBACCO AMBLYOPIA
Loss of vision due to excessive tobacco smoking. It is caused by nicotine poisoning which prevents the body from absorbing and using vitamin B. It is now possible to correct this form of blindness with injections of vitamin B.

TOBACCO HEART
An irritable condition of the heart caused by excessive use of tobacco.

TOE
One of the terminal members of man's foot.

TOILET TRAINING
The process of training a child to control bladder and bowel movements and to use the toilet.

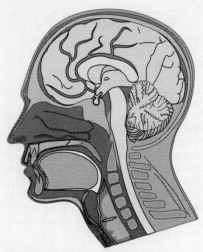

Median section of the head. The tongue occupies a large part of the oral cavity.

TOLERANCE
The capacity to endure the influence of a drug, particularly when it is being administered for a long time. Tolerance is also defined as a decreasing response to repeated constant doses of a drug or a need to increase doses to produce the same physical or mental response.

TOMOGRAPHY
A special X-ray technique that visualizes layers of tissue.

TONE
The normal state of tension of a part; a particular quality of sound or of the voice.

TONGUE
Freely movable muscular organ lying partly in the floor of the mouth and partly in the pharynx. Its function is manipulation of food in mastication and deglutition; speech production and taste. Its surface is covered with mucous membrane, with papillae and taste buds.
It is the main organ of taste. There are four basic tastes (in different papillae): sour (sides of the tongue), bitter (back of the tongue), sweet and salty (front of the tongue).

TONIC IMMOBILITY
State of total stillness, usually due to the stimulation of specific brain centers upon a set of sensory stimuli.

TONIC NECK REFLEX
A natural response in the newborn that results in the "fencer's pose.' When the newborn is in a faceup position and the head is turned to one side, the arm on that side will extend while the arm on the opposite side will bend.

TONICITY
The state of normal tone of the body.

TONICS
A diverse group of remedies prescribed or bought over the counter for relieving vague symptoms such as malaise, lethargy, and loss of appetite, for which no obvious cause can be found. Tonics sometimes contain vitamins and minerals, but there is no scientific evidence that such ingredients have anything other than a placebo effect. Nevertheless, many individuals feel better after taking a tonic for a few weeks.

TONOMETER
An instrument for measuring tension, especially that within the eyeball, to test for glaucoma.

TONOMETRY
The specific measurement of the intraocular pressure. It is used primarily to test for glaucoma, although there are rare instances of intra-ocular hypertension without glaucoma.

TONSIL
One of the two small oval-shaped, fleshy bodies, situated on each side of the back of the throat.

TONSILLECTOMY
Surgical removal of a tonsil.

TONSILLITIS
Inflammation and infection of the tonsils (lymph tissues located in the throat). The symptoms are: soreness of the throat, with aching pain much of the time and more severe pain with swallowing. The tonsils in the throat are usually very red and swollen, with pus on the tonsils. Usually fever, generalized aching, headache and nausea.

The cause is usually a bacterial or viral infection. Strep throat - tonsillitis caused by group A beta-hemolytic streptococcus - is one of the more serious infections.

TONSILLOTOME
A surgical instrument used in removing a tonsil.

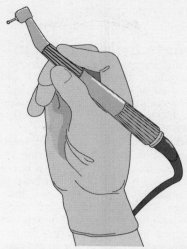

Cleaning teeth with a special drill helps in preventing dental decay.

TONSILLOTOMY
Surgical cutting away of the whole or a part of a tonsil.

TONUS
Slight degree of contraction normally occurring in muscles not in active movement.

TOOTH
One of the small bone-like structures of the jaws for the biting and mastication of food.

TOOTH DECAY
A gradual pathologic disintegration and dissolution of tooth enamel and dentin, with eventual involvement of the pulp.

Except for the common cold, this is the most prevalent human disorder.

TOPHUS
A mineral concretion in the body, especially about the joints; deposits of sodium urate in the skin about a joint, in the ear or in a bone, a characteristic of gout.

TOPICAL
Applied locally or to a particular area of the skin. Topical medica-

tions normally affect only the area to which they are applied, although some topical medications (such as estrogen creams) may be absorbed into the bloodstream. Disorders of the skin, eye, outer ear, nasal passages, anus, and vagina are often treated with drugs applied topically.

TOPICAL STEROID
Corticosteroid drug applied to the skin.

TORPOR
Sluggishness, lack of reaction to normal stimuli.

TORSION
Twisting; the rotation of the eye about its visual axis; the tilting of the vertical meridian of the eye.

TORSION DYSTONIA
A progressive disorder characterized by twisting movements causing dystonic, often bizarre, postures of the extremities and trunk. No pathologic changes have been identified in the brain, but the symptoms suggest an extrapyramidal origin. Some psycho-pharmacological drugs have been partially effective in some persons.

TORSION SPASM
Another name for torsion dystonia.

TORTICOLLIS (WRY NECK)
Temporary or permanent deformity in which the head is tilted and twisted in its position on the neck. The symptoms are: unusual position of the head noticed during the first few weeks after birth.

Treatment involves the tightened neck muscles regularly during infancy. In addition, the baby is encouraged to turn his or her head to stretch the muscle. Heat and massage of the lump in the neck might be helpful. If the condition is not helped by these measures, surgery to release the scar tissue in the muscles might be necessary but not until one year of age.

TORULUS
A small prominence or elevation.

TOUCH
The sensory system concerned with surface sensation, found in all external body surfaces including the skin and some mucous membranes. Touch sensation is crucial in the detection and recognition of objects at the body surface, including those explored by the limbs, and also in the protection of these surfaces from injury.

TOUCH SPOT
A point on the skin especially sensitive to light pressure, as by a stiff hair.

TOURETTE'S SYNDROME
Neuropsychiatric disorder characterized by multiple motor and one or more vocal tics. These may appear simultaneously, or at different periods during the illness. The tics occur many times a day, nearly every day or intermittently throughout a period of more than one year. The anatomic location, frequency, complexity, and severity of the tics change over time.

The tics typically involve the head and, frequently, other parts of the body, such as the torso and upper and lower limbs. The vocal tics include various sounds such as clicks, grunts, yelps, barks, and coughs, or words. Coprolalia, a complex vocal tic involving touching, squatting, deep knee bends, retracing steps, and twirling when walking are often present.

The cause is unknown. The disorder is usually lifelong, though periods of remission lasting from weeks to years may occur. In some cases, the severity and frequency of the symptoms diminish during adolescence (the median age at onset is 7 years), and adulthood, and the symptoms do not vary in severity over time as much as before. In other cases, the symptoms of the disorder disappear entirely, usually by early adulthood.

TOURNIQUET
Any apparatus for controlling bleeding from any part of the body where direct pressure can be brought upon the blood vessels by means of straps, cords, rubber bands or pads.

TOXEMIA
A general infection of blood poisoning in which the blood contains germ poisons but not the actual germs. It may also be caused by poisonous products of body cells.

TOXEMIA OF PREGNANCY
General term that refers to the hypertensive diseases of pregnancy. The symptoms depend on severity, but rapid weight gain, swelling, headaches and dizziness; in late stages convulsions may occur.

Elevated blood pressure, along with edema, protein in the urine and excessive weight gain are symptoms found by the doctor.

The condition is potentially very serious if not detected and controlled. For the baby, there is risk of growth retardation, stillbirth and placental abruption; for the mother, convulsions (eclampsia) plus all the risks of hypertension The treatment depends on the cause and severity and requires close medical supervision.

TOXICITY
Poisonous reaction to a drug that impairs body functions or damages cells.

TOXICODERMATITIS
Inflammatory skin disease caused by poisons.

TOXICOLOGY
The study of poisons.

TOXICOMANIA
A neurotic desire for poisonous substances.

TOXIC PSYCHOSIS
A psychic disorder caused by poisons or poisonous agents, such as opium or alcohol.

TOXIC REACTION
Unpleasant and possibly dangerous symptoms caused by a drug, the result either of an overdose or an adverse reaction.

TOXIC SHOCK SYNDROME
Very serious illness most commonly seen in (but not limited to) women who have used tampons.
The symptoms are:
– sudden high fever;
– generalized aches and pains;
– vomiting and diarrhea;
– collapse and shock may follow in hours or days.
There is often a rash on the body that peels at the end of the illness. Palms of hands and soles of feet may also peel, even though rash may not have visible signs. The cause is a toxic substance caused by staphylococcus organisms. The disease requires immediate medical treatment.

TOXIN
Substance produced by a cell or group of cells, or by bacteria during their growth, that produces a poisonous effect. Drugs that are usually safe in normal doses may produce toxic effects when taken in overdose. An adverse reaction may be produced by a toxin.

TOXOID
A non-poisonous product similar to a toxin but with the ability to provoke the body into producing antibodies after it has been injected.

TOXOPHOBIA
Morbid dread of phobia of being poisoned. In some cases a severe neurosis may develop, which should be treated by psychotherapy.

TOXOPLASMOSIS
An infection caused by a parasite. For unexplained reasons the domestic cat is the primary source of the microorganism, and infected cats, while showing no symptoms of the condition, will still excrete the parasite in their feces. Symptoms and signs include nerve and muscle damage, lymph gland swelling, eye problems and heart muscle damage.
The most serious complication comes when a pregnant woman contracts the disease, shows no symptoms and passes it on to her fetus. The consequences include spontaneous abortion, stillbirth or a child with the disease and all its complications, including encephalitis or physical birth defects.

TRACE ELEMENTS
Those elements that occur in not more than one part in 20,000 in the tissues of the body. Some of these elements are essential dietary constituents; others are probably not required, but are incorporated from the soil into crops used for human and animal food.
Examples are: iodine, fluoride,

copper, cobalt, zinc, manganese, selenium.

TRACHEA
Windpipe; a cylindrical cartilaginous tube (11-12 cm) long in the adult, from the larynx to the bronchial tubes. It extends from the sixth cervical to the first thoracic vertebra. Here it divides into two bronchi, one for each lung.

TRACHEITIS
Inflammation of the trachea (windpipe). This is the "raw chest" experienced during a cold or early attack of bronchitis.

TRACHEOBRONCHITIS
An inflammation involving both the trachea (windpipe) and the bronchi (main air passages of the lungs).

TRACHEOSCOPY
Examination of the interior of the trachea (windpipe) by means of an instrument fitted with an electric light and a mirror.

TRACHEOSTOMY
Surgical creation of an opening into the trachea through the neck.

TRACHEOTOMY
Surgical incision into the trachea (windpipe).

TRACHEOTOMY TUBE
A metal tube which is placed in the aperture made from the outside of the neck into the trachea (windpipe) to enable the patient to breathe when he or she is in danger of asphyxiation due to obstruction in the normal breathing channels.

TRACHOMA
A chronic conjunctivitis caused by Chlamydia trachomatis and characterized by progressive exacerbations and remissions, with follicular subconjunctival hyperplasia, corneal vascularization and cicatrization of the conjunctiva, cornea and lids. Tetracycline eye ointments are usually effective.

TRACT
A pathway or course; a bundle of nerve fibers; any of the nervous pathways of the spinal cord or brain; a group of parts of organs serving some special purpose, such as the intestinal respiratory or genito-urinary tract.

TRACTION
The act of drawing or dragging.

TRAIT
Any distinguishable, relatively enduring way one individual varies from another.

TRANCE
Condition of mental dissociation, characterized by lack of voluntary movement, and frequently by automatisms in act and thought. A trance is usually illustrated by hypnotic and mediumistic conditions.

TRANQUILLIZER
Agent which induces a state of quietude in anxious or disturbed persons. Minor tranquillizers are valuable in the anxious patient. In psychosis, especially schizophrenia and mania, major tranquillizers are required to suppress abnormal mental activity as well as to sedate.

TRANSACTION ANALYSIS
A system of psychotherapy involving analysis of individual episodes of social interaction for insight that will aid communication, as by the substitution of constructive verbal exchanges for destructive immature ones.

TRANSCENDENTAL MEDITATION
A technique of meditation that involves the repetition of a mantra.

TRANSDERMAL PATCHES
Medications that work via patches

on the skin. There are more and more medications in such a form. If you are using this form, follow these instructions.

Choose an area of skin without cuts, scars or hair, such as the upper arm, chest, or behind the ear. Thoroughly clean the area where patch is to be applied. If patch gets wet and loose, cover with an additional piece of plastic. Apply a fresh patch if the first one falls off. Apply each dose to a different area of skin if possible.

Drugs administered by way of transdermal patches include nitrates (for the treatment of angina attacks), remedies for travel sickness, and estrogens.

TRANSFERENCE
One of the basic principles in psychoanalytic treatment. The patient transfers his past emotional attachments to the psychoanalyst in accordance with the repetition compulsion principle. The analyst is a substitute for the parental figure.

TRANSFER FACTOR
A dialyzable extract of immune lymphocytes that is capable in transferring cell mediated immunity in humans and possibly in other animal species.

TRANSFERRIN
An iron binding protein in the blood; levels are increased in iron deficiency and decreased in inflammatory conditions and liver disease.

TRANSFUSION
A transfer of blood into the veins; the introduction of blood, saline solution or other liquids directly into the bloodstream; the pouring of liquid from one vessel to another.

TRANSIENT ISCHEMIC ATTACKS (TIAs)
Focal neurologic abnormalities of sudden onset and brief duration (usually minutes, never more than a few hours) that reflect dysfunction in the distribution of either the internal carotid-middle cerebral or the vertebral-basilar arterial system.

The attacks are often recurrent and at times presage a stroke. Most attacks are due to cerebral emboli arising from atherosclerotic vessels.

In addition to treating the atherosclerosis, high blood pressure or other underlying disorder, vascular surgery or anticoagulants may be indicated.

TRANSIENT TIC DISORDER
Single or multiple motor and/or vocal tics that occur many times a day, nearly every day for at least two weeks, but for no longer than twelve consecutive months. The most common tic is eye-blinking or another facial tic. However, the whole head, torso, or limbs may be involved.

In addition, there may be vocal tics. A person may have only one or a number of tics; if the latter, the tics may be performed simultaneously, sequentially, or randomly.

The age of onset is always during childhood or early adolescence, and may be as early as two years of age. The tics may disappear permanently, or recur, especially during periods of stress. The cause is unknown.

TRANSITIONAL OBJECT
A toy, blanket, or other such item that provides a feeling of security as a baby moves from complete helplessness to early independence.

TRANSLOCATION
The transfer of a piece of one chromosome to a different chromosome.

TRANSLOCATION MONGOLISM
A form of mongolism which may be hereditary and which results from a piece of a chromosome in pair 21 breaking off and attaching itself to another chromosome.

TRANSMISSION
The communication or transfer of anything, especially disease, from one person to another, or from one place to another.

TRANSMUTATION
The act of changing; the turning of one substance into another.

TRANSPLANTATION
Transfer of living tissues or cells from one individual to another, with the objective of maintaining the functional integrity of the transplanted tissue in the recipient. Rejection of the transplanted organ is the most serious problem in transplantation. Rejection is in this respect defined as the destruction of transplanted material at the cellular level by the host's immune mechanisms. The principal mechanism of rejection is the acute lymphocyte-mediated immune reaction against transplantation antigens, a so-called host-versus-graft reaction. Careful typing of tissues and the use of specific immunosuppressive drugs have minimized the problems of rejection nowadays.

TRANSPLANTATION ANTIGEN
The genetically determined antigens that stimulate the immunologic response occurring when blood cells or tissues are transplanted from a donor into a recipient.

TRANSPOSITION
Usually refers to a change in the position of internal organs, such as finding an organ situated on the opposite side of the body to normal. Occasionally the heart is found on the opposite side (a condition called dextrocardia), and sometimes also the appendix is found on the left side of the body instead of on the right.

TRANSSEXUALISM
A gender identity disorder whereby the transsexual believes that he is the victim of a biologic accident, cruelly imprisoned within a body incompatible with his real sexual identity. Most are men who consider themselves to have feminine gender identity and regard their genital organs and masculine features with repugnance.

TRANSUDATE
Any substance which has passed through a membrane.

TRANSUDATION
The passing of fluids through a membrane, especially of blood serum through the walls of the capillaries (minute blood vessels).

TRANSURETHRAL
Refers to any operation performed by passing an instrument down the urethra (the canal through which the urine is discharged from the bladder).

TRANSVERSE PRESENTATION
That in which the child lies with its long axis across the womb so that the presenting part to the mouth of the womb may be the shoulder, back or abdomen.

TRANSVESTIC FETISHISM
Recurrent, intense, sexual urges, and sexually arousing fantasies, of at least six months' duration, involving cross-dressing. The person has acted on these urges, or is markedly distressed by them. Usually the person keeps a collection of women's clothes that he intermittently uses to cross-dress when alone. While cross-dressed, he usually masturbates and imagines other males being attracted to him as a woman in his female attire.

Transvestic phenomena range from occasional solitary wearing of female clothes to extensive involvement in a transvestic subculture. Some men wear a single item of women's apparel under their masculine attire. When more that one article of women's clothing are involved, the man may wear makeup and dress entirely as a woman. An associated feature may be the presence of sexual masochism.

TRANSVESTISM
Dressing by men in the clothes of the opposite sex. Usually the transvestite achieves a certain amount of sexual excitement, and public display gives much satisfaction. Despite their deviation, many transvestites manage to have reasonably happy marriages.

TRAPEZIUM
The first bone on the thumb side of the second row of carpal bones of the wrist and hand. Also applied to a band of fibers in the brain.

TRAUMA
Any injury, wound or shock, most frequently physical or structural, but also mental or psychological, in the form of an emotional shock, producing a disturbance, more or less enduring, of mental functions.

TRAUMATIC NEUROSIS
A neurotic disorder precipitated by a trauma such as an incident.

TRAVELLER'S DIARRHEA
Diarrhea that occurs with a change in dietary habits and food during travel to other countries. The symptoms are:
- diarrhea, mild to severe;
- cramping of the abdomen;
- nausea;
- weakness and,
- occasionally, vomiting;
- fever is rare.

The diarrhea is loose to watery, but there is no blood or mucus present. The condition lasts from one to five days usually, although a few people have difficulties for several weeks. The cause is not completely known but believed to be caused by exposure to different intestinal bacteria than people are accustomed to.

Treatment consists of rest and adequate liquids to prevent dehydration. There is no specific cure.

TREMOR
Involuntary movements in one or more parts of the body produced by successive fast contractions of muscles, due to metabolic, neurological or psychiatric disturbances.

TRENCH FEVER
A disease caused by rickettsia (Rochalimacea quintana) and characterized by:
- sudden or slow onset;
- fever;
- headache;
- muscular pains;
- enlargement of the spleen;
- short episode (five-day fever) or relapses;
- sometimes macular rash, typhoid like.

The following transmission mechanisms are known: feces of body louse through skin breaks, man and louse are the only reservoirs. Treatment by antibiotics.

TRENDELENBURG'S OPERATION
An operation in which the long saphenous vein in the thigh is tied as part of the treatment of varicose veins in the leg.

TRENDELENBURG'S POSITION
The patient lies on his back with the operating table tilted so that the head is low. This position enables the surgeon to operate in the lower part of the abdomen.

TREPHINE
A saw-like surgical instrument for removing a disc of bone or other tissue; to remove with such an instrument either a circular segment of bone from the skull or part of the sclera (the white outer coat of the

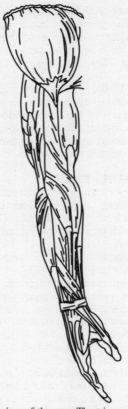

Lateral view of the arm. The triceps muscle occupies the dorsal part of the upper arm. Action of the muscle causes extension in the elbow joint.

eye) to relieve excessive pressure within these structures.

TREPONEMA
A class of germs which cause such diseases as syphilis and yaws.

TREPONEMATOSIS
Infestation with Treponema; a genus of spirochetes, parasitic in humans, with undulating or rigid bodies.

TRIAL AND ERROR
A type of learning marked by the successive trial of various responses to a situation, ostensibly at random, until one is successful and attains the goal.

TRICEPS
The major arm muscle concerned with straightening the elbow. It has three heads or bellies at its upper end that have separate insertions.

TRICEPS REFLEX
Extension of the forearm in response to a brisk tap against the triceps tendon behind the elbow joint.

TRICHINOSIS
Infestation with the larva of a worm (Trichinella), contracted from eating uncooked pork, etc., causing a feverish illness. Edema around the eyes, muscle pains and diarrhea occur early; later the lungs, heart and brain may be involved.

The disease is avoided by the adequate cooking of pork. Chemotherapy may be helpful in severe cases.

TRICHINA   AGGLUTININ TEST
A test performed to detect the presence of trichinosis, a disease contracted by persons who eat undercooked, infected pork or beef.

TRICHIURASIS
An infection caused by Trichiuris trichiura and characterized by abdominal pain and diarrhea. Infection results from ingestion of eggs that have incubated in soil for two or three weeks. The larva hatches in the small intestine, migrates to the colon, and embeds its anterior head in the mucosa. Prevention depends upon adequate toilet facilities and good personal hygiene. Mebendazole 100 mg taken by mouth for three days have been highly effective and is the drug of choice.

TRICHOGLOSSIA
A thickening of the tongue papillae (nipple-like elevations) producing an appearance as if the tongue were covered with hair.

TRICHOMONAS
A variety of ciliate (possessing

lash-like appendages) protozoa, a low form of life.

TRICHOMONAS INTESTINALIS

A variety which attacks the intestines, producing diarrhea and enteritis.

TRICHOMONAS VAGINALIS

A variety of Trichomonas found in the vagina. It produces a form of white discharge called leukorrhea.

TRICHOPHOBIA

A morbid fear of hair.

TRICHOPHYTOSIS

A contagious disease of the skin and hair, occurring mostly in children and due to the invasion of the skin by the trichophyton fungus. It is characterized by circular scaly patches and partial loss of hair.

TRICHOTILLOMANIA

Recurrent failure to resist impulses to pull out one's own hair. The person with this disorder experiences an increasing sense of tension immediately before engaging in the behavior and achieves a sense of release or gratification from pulling out the hair. The avulsion of hairs results in patchy areas of incomplete alopecia in easily accessible regions, principally the scalp. Other areas commonly involved are the eyebrows, eye-lashes, and beard. Less commonly the trunk, armpits, and pubic area may be involved. Hair loss often is characterized by short, broken strands appearing together with long, normal hairs in the affected area. The disorder usually begins in childhood, but cases have been reported with onset as late as 60. Some suggest that adult onset is strongly linked to the presence of a psychotic disorder.

TRICROTIC

Having three waves to one pulse beat.

TRICROTIC PULSE

A pulse in which the three waves normally present are abnormally distinct.

TRICUSPID

Having three cups; acting upon the tricuspid valve, a heart valve situated in the opening between the right atrium (upper chamber) and the right ventricle (lower chamber).

TRICYCLIC ANTIDEPRESSANTS

Group of psychoactive drugs that affect part of the brain that controls messages between nerve cells. The drug is prescribed for a number of medical conditions:
(1) gradually relief of symptoms of depression;
(2) treatment of bedwetting;
(3) pain relief;
(4) treatment of narcolepsy, ulcers, bulimia, panic attacks, cocaine withdrawal, attention deficit disorder.

TRIGEMINAL NERVE

The fifth cranial nerve, which divides into three main branches and supplies the face. The trigeminal nerve arises by a small motor and a large sensory root which both emerge from the side of the pons with the sensory root bearing the Gasserian ganglion and dividing into ophthalmic, maxillary, and

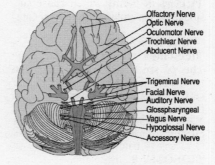

Olfactory Nerve
Optic Nerve
Oculomotor Nerve
Trochlear Nerve
Abducent Nerve

Trigeminal Nerve
Facial Nerve
Auditory Nerve
Glosspharyngeal
Vagus Nerve
Hypoglossal Nerve
Accessory Nerve

The trigeminal nerve is the largest of the cranial nerves.

mandibular nerves and the motor root supplying the fibers to the mandibular nerve and through this to the muscles of mastication.

TRIGEMINAL NEURALGIA

Bouts of severe brief lancinating pain in the distribution of one or more divisions of the fifth cranial nerve. The cause is unknown, and no pathological changes can be found. Older persons are usually affected.

The pain is often set off by touching a trigger point or by activity such as chewing or brushing the teeth. Pain is intense, and although each bout is brief; successive bouts may incapacitate the person.

Carbamazepine is generally the effective treatment.

TRIGGER ZONE

A sensitive area of the body which when stimulated gives rise to reaction elsewhere in the body; especially a hypersensitive area that evokes referred pain elsewhere when stimulated.

TRIGLYCERIDE

The main type of lipid (fatty substance) found in adipose (fat) tissue of the body and also the main dietary lipid. High levels of triglycerides in the blood may be associated with a great risk of coronary heart disease (atherosclerosis).

TRISMUS

Lockjaw, an early symptom of tetanus.

TRISOMY

The presence of three, rather that two, chromosomes in a particular set; for instance, individuals with three sex chromosomes, XXX, XXY or XYY, are trisomic for sex chromosomes.

TRISOMY 9

An autosomal hereditary anomaly caused by three instead of two chromosomes number 9. Common features are:
- mental retardation;
- microcephaly;
- small palpebral fissures;
- prominent nose;
- high-arched palate;
- low-set ears;
- small penis;
- undescended testes;
- long flexed fingers;
- dislocation of hips;
- congenital heart disease.

The latter condition may be fatal.

TRISOMY 13

Autosomal hereditary anomaly caused by three instead of two chromosomes number 13. Infants tend to be small at birth. Apneic spells in early infancy are frequent, and mental retardation is severe.

Most children are so severely affected that they die before the age of six months.

TRISOMY 18

An autosomal hereditary aberration characterized by severe mental retardation. Survival for more than a few months is rare, and mental retardation is severe in those who survive.

TRISOMY 21

The presence of three chromosomes rather than the normal pair designated 21. This genetic defect is the chromosomal abnormality most frequently observed with Down's syndrome (mongolism). Trisomy 21 is sometimes used as an alternative name for this syndrome.

TRITANOPIA

Partial color blindness, affecting the blue and yellow colors; rare as a congenital condition, but occurring fairly frequently as an acquired condition.

TROCAR

A surgical instrument consisting of a perforator enclosed within a metal tube (a cannula) and used for puncturing in a cavity. The perforator is then removed leaving the cannula within the cavity to drain out fluid.

TROCHANTER
One of two bony knobs at the upper end of the femur (thighbone). The major trochanter is on the outer side and the minor trochanter is on the inner side of the bone.

TROCHLEAR NERVE
Either of the fourth pair of cranial nerves that arise from the dorsal aspect of the brain stem just below the inferior colliculus and supply the superior oblique muscle of the eye with motor fibers.

TROPHIC
Pertaining to the functions concerned in nutrition, digestion and assimilation of food.

TROPHIC CENTERS
The nerves governing the nutrition of organs.

TROPHIC ULCER
One due to a disturbance of the nutrition of a part, for instance a varicose ulcer.

TROPHOBLASTIC DISEASE
The occurrence of tumors of trophoblastic origin.

TROPICAL MEDICINE
Branch of medicine concerned with the particular diseases encountered in and sometimes imported from the tropics. These largely comprise infectious diseases due to viruses (for instance, yellow fever, smallpox, lassa fever), bacteria (for instance, cholera), protozoa (for instance, malaria, trypanosome diseases) and worms (for instance, filariasis) which are generally restricted to tropical zones.

TROPICAL SORE
Another name for oriental sore.

TROPICAL SPRUE
A disease of unknown etiology characterized by malabsorption, multiple deficiencies and abnormalities in the small bowel mucosa. Tropical sprue is an acquired disease related in some way to environmental and nutritional conditions. The best treatment is folic acid and tetracycline.

TRUE-FALSE TEST
A mental or psychological test, usually intended to test for mental consistency. The subject is faced with a series of statements to be checked as true or false.

TRUE RIBS
The seven upper ribs on each side that are attached in front to the sternum (breastbone).

TRYPANOSOMA
A type of parasite which infests the blood plasma of both animals and humans, producing disease and transmitted by insects. The protozoa are responsible for trypanosomiasis of the African (sleeping sickness) and South American (Chagas' disease) varieties, carried by the tsetse fly and certain bugs respectively.

TRUNCUS ARTERIOSUS
An arterial trunk arising from the fetal heart which develops into the aorta and pulmonary artery. It is a congenital defect if it persists past the birth of the infant.

TRUNK
The central part of the body, situated between the shoulder and pelvis. Topographically, we can distinguish three groups of organs: the chest organs in the thoracic cavity; the abdominal organs in the abdominal cavity and the pelvic organs in the pelvic cavity.

The skeleton of the trunk is formed by part of the vertebral column, the ribs and the sternum. (See illustration on next page)

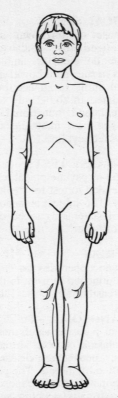

Outline of the body of a child. The trunk occupies a relative large part of the body.

TRYPSIN
Enzyme catalyzing the breakdown of proteins in the vertebrate digestive system; produced by the pancreas.

TRYPTOPHAN
One of the eight essential amino acids. It is believed that tryptophan is needed for the reproductive system and for the skin.

TSETSE FLY
An insect almost wholly restricted to Africa. This fly carries trypanosomes, the causative agents of sleeping sickness in humans and a similar disease, nagana, in cattle.

TSS
Another name for toxic shock syndrome.

TUBAL MOLE
Remains of a fetus which has grown in a Fallopian tube, died and become infiltrated with blood.

TUBAL PREGNANCY
A form of ectopic pregnancy which takes place in the Fallopian tube (the duct from the ovary to uterus) and not in the uterus.

TUBE
A hollow cylindrical structure, especially the uterine tube or the auditory tube.

TUBECTOMY
Surgical excision of a tube. Usually refers to the removal of the Fallopian tube, when the operation is called salpingectomy.

TUBERCLE
A small nodule; a rounded prominence on a bone; the specific lesion produced by the germ of tuberculosis, consisting of a collection of round cells and sometimes including giant cells.

TUBERCULIN
Protein derivative of the mycobacteria responsible for tuberculosis. This may be used in tests of cell-mediated immunity to tuberculosis, providing evidence of previous disease (often subclinical) or immunization (BCG).

TUBERCULIN REACTION
Localized inflammation of the skin following injection of a small quantity of tuberculin, indicating that the body has been sensitized by tubercle bacilli.

TUBERCULOSIS
An infectious disease caused by the tubercle bacillus Mycobacterium tuberculosis, and characterized pathologically by:
- inflammatory infiltrations;
- formation of tubercles;
- caseation;

- necrosis;
- abscesses;
- fibrosis;
- calcifications.

It most commonly affects the respiratory system but other parts of the body such as gastrointestinal and genito-urinary tracts, bones, joints, nervous system, lymph nodes and skin may become infected. Infection occurs primarily by inhalation. Infectious droplets, which are aerolized by coughing and dry when suspended in air, may contaminate the air in closed spaces for long periods. Many cases occur nowadays in older individuals, and in persons known to have had clinical tuberculosis in the past who were never adequately treated with specific drugs.

TUBEROUS SCLEROSIS
A condition characterized by multiple tumors on the skin of the cheeks and face, mental deficiency and epileptic fits.

TUBULAR
Shaped like a tube; relating to a tubule; occurring in a tube.

TULAREMIA
Infectious disease caused by a bacterium and characterized by:
- sudden onset;
- fever;
- chills;
- swollen and tender lymph nodes.
The incubation period amounts to 2-10 days. Transmission by contact with blood or tissue of infected wild animals. Treatment by antibiotics.

TUMOR
A growth of tissue, characterized by uncontrollable cell proliferation. A tumor may be benign or malignant (cancer).

TUNING FORK TEST
Test for hearing function. Tuning forks are metal instruments that vibrate when struck, giving off a pure tone of a predetermined number of cycles per second. They are used primarily to measure the ability to hear sounds by both air and bone conduction.

TUNNEL ANEMIA
The popular name for hookworm disease or ankylostomiasis. A disease due to the infestation of the intestines with a worm. Characterized by anemia, digestive upsets and mental inertia.

TUNNEL VISION
The extremely contracted visual field characteristic of hysteria.

TURNER'S SYNDROME
A congenital abnormality characterized by shortness of stature, webbing (a filling out of the skin from the top of the neck to the shoulder area) of the neck, swelling of the tissues, defective nails and short fingers, and cubitus valgus (the forearms being carried outwards instead of forwards).

TYMPANIC CAVITY
Cavity behind the eardrum containing three vibrating ear bones which transmit sounds to the internal ear. It communicates with the post-nasal space by means of the Eustachian tube.

TYMPANIC MEMBRANE
A thin membrane that separates the middle ear from the inner part of the external auditory meatus and functions in the mechanical reception of sound waves and in their transmission to the site of sensory reception.

TYMPANIC NERVE
A branch of the glossopharyngeal nerve arising from the petrosal ganglion and entering the middle ear where it takes part in forming the tympanic plexus.

TYMPANIC PLATE
A curved platelike bone that is part

of the temporal bone and forms the floor and anterior wall of the external auditory meatus.

TYMPANOMETRY
Test to measure the functioning of the eardrum.

TYPE
A class of individuals, having a characteristic or a pattern of characteristics in common, such as direction of interest, temperament, etc. on the mental side, or on the physical.

TYPE A PERSONALITY
Personality that is marked by impatience, aggressiveness, and competitiveness and that is held to be associated with an increased risk of cardiovascular disease.

TYPE B PERSONALITY
Personality that is marked by a lack of excessive aggressiveness and tension and that is held to be associated with reduced risk of cardiovascular disease.

TYPHOID FEVER
Infectious disease due to a salmonella species causing the following symptoms:
- fever;
- a characteristic rash;
- lymph node enlargement;
- increase in size of the spleen;
- gastrointestinal tract disturbance with bleeding and ulceration;
- malaise or prostration.

It is contracted from other cases or from disease carriers, the latter often harboring asymptomatic infection in the gallbladder or urine. Treatment is by antibiotics.

TYPHUS FEVER
An acute, infectious louse-borne disease, characterized by a sustained high temperature, a skin rash, nervous irritability and profound prostration which continues for some two weeks. It is a disease that occurs in crowded, insanitary and unhygienic conditions. Also known as epidemic typhus, fleck typhus, jail fever, and camp fever.

TYPING
Classifying blood, tissues, and other material so they can be compared to standards.

TYRAMINE
Normal chemical compound of the body that helps sustain blood pressure. The blood level of tyramine can rise to fatal levels in combination with some drugs.

TYROSINE
An amino acid that the body can manufacture.

U

UBIQUINONE
A quinone that contains a long iso-prenoid side chain and that functions in the part of cellular respiration comprising oxidative phosphorylation as an electron-carrying coenzyme in the transport of electrons from organic substrates to oxygen.

ULCER
- Pathological defect in skin or other epithelium, caused by:
- inflammation secondary to infection;
- loss of blood supply;
- failure of venous return;
- cancer.

Various skin lesions can cause ulcer, including:
- infection;
- arterial disease;
- varicose veins;
- skin cancer.

Peptic ulcers include gastric and duodenal ulcers, although the two have different causes: they may cause characteristic pain, acute hemorrhage or lead to perforation and peritonitis.

ULCERATIVE
Relating to ulceration or characterized by the presence of ulcers.

ULCERATIVE COLITIS
A chronic, nonspecific inflammatory and ulcerative disease of the colon, characterized most often by bloody diarrhea. Any age may be affected, but the disease frequently begins between ages 15 and 40. Although there is a familial tendency, the etiology is unknown.

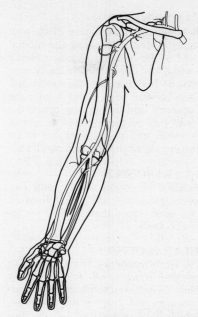

Anterior view of the right arm. The ulna is on the right.

ULEGYRIA
A condition in which the convolutions of the cerebral cortex are abnormally narrow and misshapen due to scarring following the production of lesions in fetal or postnatal life.

ULNA
The larger of the two bones of the forearm.

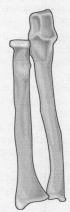

Skeleton of the forearm; radius (left) and ulna (right).

ULNAR NERVE
A large superficial nerve of the arm that is a continuation of the medial cord of the brachial plexus, passing around the elbow superficially in a groove between the olecranon and the medial epicondyle of the humerus, and continuing down the inner side of the forearm to supply the skin and muscles of the little-finger side of the forearm and hand.

ULTRASONICS
Science of sound waves with frequencies above those that humans can hear (more than 20,000 cycles per second).

ULTRASOUND
(1) High-frequency sound waves to project images of various body parts. A transducer produces the ultrasound and catches the response, which is displayed on an oscilloscope.
(2) The diagnostic or therapeutic use of ultrasound and especially a technique involving the formation of a two-dimensional image used for the examination and measurement of internal body structures and the detection of bodily abnormalities.

ULTRAVIOLET RADIATION
Electromagnetic radiation of wavelengths between 0.1 nm and 300 nm, produced using gas discharge tubes. Although it constitutes 5 percent of the energy radiated by the sun, most falling on the earth is filtered out by atmospheric oxygen and ozone, thus protecting life on the surface from destruction by the solar ultraviolet light.

The principal use is in fluorescent tubes but important medical applications include germicidal lamps, the treatment of rickets and some skin diseases and the vitamin D enrichment of milk and eggs.

ULTRAVIOLET RAYS
Light waves beyond the violet rays of the spectrum. They cannot be seen by the eye. They are capable of destroying bacteria, are used for their tonic effect, as in ultra-violet baths, and also for provoking a violent inflammatory reaction in the skin to dry it in such cases as acne (blackheads).

UMBILICAL
Pertaining to the umbilicus (navel), its cord or vessels.

UMBILICAL ARTERY
Either of a pair of arteries that arise from the hypogastric arteries of the fetus and pass through the umbilical cord to the placenta to which they carry the oxygenated blood from the fetus.

UMBILICAL CORD
Long structure linking the developing embryo or fetus to the placenta through most of pregnancy. It consists of blood vessels taking blood to and from the placenta, and a gelatinous matrix. At birth the cord is clamped to prevent blood loss and is used to assist delivery of the placenta. It undergoes atrophy (wasting) and becomes the navel.

UMBILICAL GRANULOMA
A gray mass of tissue that develops where the umbilical cord separates. Treatment may require cauterization.

UMBILICAL VEIN
A vein that passes through the umbilical cord to the fetus and returns the oxygenated blood from the placenta to the fetus.

UMBILICUS
The round depressed scar in the middle of the abdomen marking the point of entry of the umbilical cord. Also called the navel.

UNCINATE PROCESS
An irregular downwardly and backwardly directed process of each lat-

eral mass of the ethmoid bone that articulated with the inferior nasal concha.

UNCONDITIONED RESPONSE
Involuntary reflexes that are automatically elicited by chemical and/or physical stimulation.

UNCONDITIONED STIMULI
Events that elicit unconditioned responses.

UNCONSCIOUS
That part of the mind in which take place events of which the individual is unaware; i.e., the part of the mind that is not conscious. Unconscious processes can, however, alter the behavior of the individual. Freud renamed the unconscious the ID.

UNCONSCIOUSNESS
Lack of awareness, the commonest example of which is sleep; or the lack of self-awareness displayed by most, if not all, animals.

UNCONSCIOUS STATE
The aggregate of the dynamic elements constituting the personality, of some of which the individual may be aware as part of his makeup, of others entirely unaware, all being structural, rather than process.

UNCTION
(1) The application of a soothing or lubricating oil or ointment;
(2) something that is used for anointing.

UNCUS
(1) A hooked anatomical part or process;
(2) the anterior curved end of the hippocampus.

UNDERDOSAGE
The administration or taking of an insufficient dose.

UNDERNUTRITION
A deficient bodily nutrition due to inadequate food intake or faulty assimilation.

UNGUINAL
Pertaining to a fingernail or toenail.

UNIDEXTRALITY
The use of one hand or one side of the body rather than the other.

UNILATERAL
Relating to one side.

UNIQUE TRAITS
Traits that apply only to a given person and are not found in other people in exactly the same form.

UNIT CHARACTER
A character which is transmitted as a whole, or as a unit, when inherited. The term is used to designate a character that is dependent on the presence or absence of a single gene.

UNITARY TYPE
The type of individual whose afterimages, memory images and eidetic images are closely similar in type.

UNIVERSAL ANTIDOTE
An antidote for ingested poisons having activated charcoal as its principal ingredient.

UNIVERSAL DONOR
(1) The blood group O characterized by a serum that does not agglutinate the cells of any other ABO blood group.
(2) A person with blood group O.

UNIVERSAL RECIPIENT
(1) The blood group AB characterized by a serum that is not agglutinated by any other ABO blood group.
(2) A person with blood group AB blood.

UNIVERSAL SEROLOGIC RE-ACTION
The Kahn test used to detect sero-

logical changes characteristic of various diseases, as tuberculosis, malaria, and leprosy.

UNNA'S BOOT
A compression dressing for varicose veins or ulcers consisting of a paste made of zinc oxide, gelatin, glycerin, and water that is applied to the outside of the bandage.

UNPHYSIOLOGICAL
Not characteristic or of appropriate to an organism's normal functioning.

UNREALITY FEELING
The feeling that an experience, including the experience of oneself, lacks objectivity or reality. The feeling is usually pathologic in nature.

UNSATURATED FAT
Fat whose molecules have one or more double bonds, so that it is capable of absorbing more hydrogen. Mono-unsaturated fats, such as olive oil, have only one double bond (the rest are single) and seem to have little effect on blood cholesterol.

Poly-unsaturated fats, such as corn oil and safflower oil, have two or more double bonds per molecule and tend to lower blood cholesterol.

UPPER RESPIRATORY TRACT
The part of the respiratory system including the nose, nasal passage, and nasopharynx.

UPTAKE
An act or instance of absorbing and incorporating something especially into a living organism.

URACHUS
A cord of fibrous tissue extending from the bladder to the umbilicus and constituting the functionless remnant of a part of a duct of the allantois to the embryo.

URACIL
A pyrimidine base that is one of the four bases coding genetic information in the polynucleotide chain of RNA.

UREA
A soluble weakly basic nitrogenous compound that is the chief solid component of urine and an end product of protein decomposition and that is administered intravenously as a diuretic drug.

UREA CLEARANCE
The amount of urea filtered and removed from the blood by the kidneys within a given period of time.

UREA CONCENTRATION TEST
Performed to test the efficiency of the kidney. The person drinks 100 ml of water containing 15 g of urea. The concentration of the urea in the urine is then measured at the end of one hour and again at the end of two hours.

UREMIA
The retention in the blood of constituents more normally found in the urine due to failure of the kidneys to excrete them. It is characterized by headache, giddiness, vomiting, blindness, convulsions and coma.
The condition can result from several factors including:
– structural abnormalities of the kidneys;
– chronic kidney infection;
– severe hypertension;
– diabetes.

URETER
The tube that conveys the urine from the kidney to the bladder.

URETERAL INFECTION
Blockage of an ureter (the tube conveying urine from the kidney to the bladder) by a calculus (a stone), preventing the passage of urine and

causing back pressure on the kidney.

URETERECTOMY
Surgical removal of the ureter.

URETERITIS
Inflammation of the ureter.

URETEROCELE
A dilation of the lower end of the ureter, forming a cyst.

URETEROLITHIASIS
The presence of stones in the ureter.

URETHRA
The canal through which the urine is discharged, extending from the neck of the bladder to the urethral (external) opening.

URETHRAL PHASE
The developmental stage, according to Sigmund Freud, between anal and phallic stage. Urethral eroticism is basically auto-erotic; it may, however, be directed toward others with fantasies about urinating on them or being urinated on.

URETHRAL EROTICISM
Sexual feelings in connection with the urethral region. The term was first coined by Sigmund Freud and is part of a specific developmental theory.

URETHRITIS
Inflammation of the urethra. One cause of urethritis is the venereal disease gonorrhea, which produces a copious discharge of yellow pus from the urethra.
Urethritis has many different names and any of the following terms may be used by doctors:
- NSU: non-specific urethritis;
- NGU: non-gonococcal urethritis;
- PGU: post-gonococcal urethritis.
All three terms are used to describe urethritis when the germ causing the infection has not been discovered by laboratory tests.

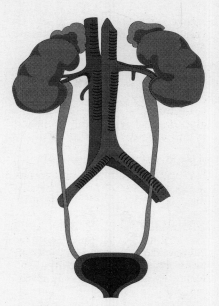

Urinary apparatus. From top to bottom: kidneys, ureters, bladder, beginning of the urethra.

URETHROCYSTITIS
Inflammation of the urethra and the bladder.

URETHROSCOPE
An endoscopic instrument containing a light and lenses for examining the interior of the urethra.

URGENCY
A compelling desire to urinate or defecate due to some abnormal stress, as inflammation or infection.

URIC
Relating to the urine.

URIC ACID
The end-product of protein metabolism in birds, invertebrates and snakes, and of purine metabolism in many insects, reptiles, birds, primates (including humans). Sufferers from gout have a high blood level of uric acid.

URICEMIA
An excess of uric acid in the blood.

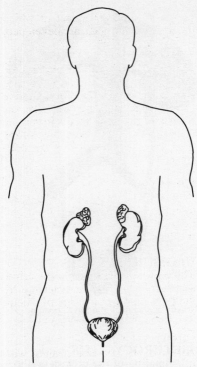

Location of the urinary tract in the aldominal and pelvic cavity.

URICOSURICS
A group of drugs that promotes excretion of uric acid in the urine. These drugs include probenecid and sulfinpyrazone.

URIDINE
A crystalline compound that consists of uracil · attached to ribose, that is derived by hydrolysis from nucleic acids, and that in the form of phosphate derivatives plays an important role in carbohydrate metabolism.

URINAL
Relating to urine.

URINARY BLADDER
A distensible membranous sac that serves for the temporary retention of the urine, situated in the pelvis in front of the rectum, receiving the urine from the two ureters and discharging it at intervals into the urethra through an orifice closed by a sphincter, and that is lined with transitional hypoblastic epithelium, and develops from the proximal part of the allantois of the embryo.

URINARY CALCULUS
A calculus occurring in any portion of the urinary tract and especially in the pelvis of the kidney.

URINARY INCONTINENCE
The involuntary loss of urine during the day or night.

URINARY INFECTION
Usually an infection in the bladder or kidneys. If left untreated, permanent damage may occur. Usually, symptoms are burning during urination, pressure on the bladder, fever and backache.

When the clinical symptoms present the characteristic portrait of a urinary tract infection, treatment is initiated immediately with one of the sulpha drugs or antibiotics.

URINARY ORGANS
Those organs concerned with the production and discharge of urine, that is the kidneys, the ureters (the canals conveying urine from kidneys to bladder), the urinary bladder and the urethra (the canal which discharges urine from the bladder).

URINARY REFLEX
The desire to pass urine in response to its accumulation within the bladder.

URINARY SYSTEM
The organs of the urinary tract comprising the kidneys, ureters, urinary bladder, and urethra.

URINARY TRACT
The tract through which urine passes and which consists of the renal tubules and pelvis of the kidney, the ureters, the bladder, and the urethra.

URINE
Fluid secreted by the kidneys, transported through the ureters to the bladder, where it is stored until excreted from the body through the urethra. Normal urine is straw-colored and slightly acid. Changes in the color, acidity and other characteristics of urine are important clues to many diseases.

UROBILIN
A bile pigment produced by the putrefaction of bilirubin in the gut and excreted by the kidney into the urine. The principal pigment that colors the urine yellow.

UROBILINEMIA
The presence of urobilin in the blood, jaundice.

UROBILINOGEN
A bilirubin metabolism product found in urine or feces; increased in certain types of blood diseases and decreased in certain liver, gallbladder and related diseases.

UROBILINURIA
An excess of urobilin in the urine.

UROCHROME
A yellow pigment to which the color of normal urine is principally due.

URODYNIA
Pain that arises with the passage of urine.

UROGENITAL MEMBRANE
A double layer of pelvic fascia with its included muscle that is situated between the ischial and pubic rami, supporting the prostate in the male, and that is traversed by the vagina in the female, giving passage to the membranous part of the urethra, and enclosing the sphincter muscle of the urethra.

UROGENITAL RIDGE
A pair of dorsolateral mesodermal ridges in the embryo out of which the urogenital organs are developed.

UROGENITAL STATUS
The ventral part of the embryonic mammalian cloaca that is formed by the growth of a fold dividing the cloaca where the gut and allantois meet and that eventually forms the neck of the bladder and some of the more distal portions of the genitourinary tract.

UROKINASE
An enzyme that is similar to streptokinase, found in human urine, and used to dissolve blood clots, as in the heart.

UROLITHIASIS
The presence of stones in the urine; a condition that is characterized by the formation or presence of calculi in the urinary tract.

UROLOGY
A branch of medicine dealing with the urinary or urogenital organs.

UROMETER
An instrument for measuring the specific gravity of the urine.

UROSCOPY
Examination or analysis of the urine, as for the purpose of medical diagnosis.

URTICARIA
A skin condition characterized by intensely itching weals with elevated, usually white, centers and a surrounding area of red skin. The term urticaria is usually thought of as a pathological process confined to the skin and lips in which there is a rapidly reversible increase in vascular permeability.

UTERINE
Pertaining to the uterus (womb).

UTERINE ARTERY
An artery that arises from the inter-

nal iliac artery and after following a course between the layers of the broad ligament reaches the uterus at the cervix and supplies the uterus and adjacent parts and during pregnancy the placenta.

UTERINE GLAND
Any of the branches of tubular glands in the mucous membrane of the uterus.

UTERINE MILK
A nutritive secretion that is produced by uterine glands especially during the early phases of mammalian gestation and that nourishes the young mammalian embryo prior to implantation.

UTERINE PLEXUS
A plexus of veins tributary to the internal iliac vein by which blood is returned from the uterus.

UTERINE TUBE
The Fallopian tube.

UTERITIS
Inflammation of the uterus (womb).

UTEROSACRAL LIGAMENT
A fibrous fascial band on each side of the uterus that passes along the lateral wall of the pelvis from the uterine cervix to the sacrum and that serves to support the uterus and hold it in place.

UTEROVAGINAL
Pertaining to the uterus (womb) and the vagina.

UTEROVESICAL POUCH
A pouch formed by the peritoneum between the uterus and the bladder.

UTERUS
That part of the female reproductive system specialized to allow the implantation, growth and nourishment of a fetus during pregnancy.
The non-pregnant uterus is a hollow, pear-shaped organ, about 7.5 cm (3 inches) long suspended in the pelvic cavity by ligaments. Its upper end is connected to the Fallopian tubes, its lower end narrows into a neck, or cervix, that opens into the vagina. The uterus has three layers:
- an inner mucous layer, the endometrium, which undergoes the menstrual cyclic changes during the menstrual cycle and helps form the placenta in pregnancy;
- a muscular layer, the myometrium, contractions of which expel a child during labor and childbirth;
- an outer connective tissue parametrium that extends into the broad ligament.

UTERUS BICORNIS
One divided into two compartments, due to a developmental defect.

UTERUS DIDELPHIS
A double uterus. It is possible for a pregnancy to occur in each part.

UTRICLE
A delicate membranous sac communicating with the semicircular canals (organs of balance) of the ear.

UVEA
The pigmented part of the eye, including the iris, ciliary body and the choroid.

UVEITIS
Inflammation of the uveal tract (iris, ciliary body, choroid).

UVULA
A small, conical, fleshy projection suspended from the soft palate over the root of the tongue.

UVULECTOMY
Surgical excision of the uvula.

U WAVE
A positive wave following the T wave on an electrocardiogram.

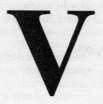

V

VACCINAL FEVER
A feverish reaction that follows vaccination.

VACCINATION
Method of inducing immunity to infectious disease due to bacteria or viruses. Vaccination leads to the formation of antibodies and the ability to produce large quantities rapidly at a later date; this gives protection equivalent to that induced by an attack of the disease. It is occasionally followed by a reaction resembling a mild form of the disease, but rarely by the serious manifestations. Persons on corticosteroids, with immunity disorders or eczema may suffer severe reactions and should not generally receive vaccinations.

VACCINE
A preparation of attenuated (weakened) or killed microorganisms (germs) administered for the prevention or treatment of infectious disease. When introduced in the body the vaccine stimulates the production of antibodies, creating immunity to the disease.

VACCINIA
Cowpox, a contagious disease of cows, characterized by blisters and ulcers of the skin, which usually appear around the teats and the udders and is transmissible to humans by handling infected cows and by vaccination

VACUOLAR
Pertaining to, or like a vacuole.

VACUOLATION
The development or formation of vacuoles, such as neuronal vacuoles in certain neurological diseases.

VACUOLE
A small cavity or space in the tissues of an organism containing air or fluid. The term is also used to designate a cavity or vesicle in the protoplasm of a cell containing fluid.

VACUOLIZATION
The formation of vacuoles; appearance or formation of drops of clear fluid in growing or aging cells.

VACUUM EXTRACTOR
Device, using a suction cup attached to the fetal head, for applying traction to the fetus during delivery. Its use may be hazardous except in the hands of experts.

VACUUM TREATMENT
Insertion of a limb in a partial vacuum.

VAGAL
Relating to, mediated by, or being the vagus nerve.

VAGAL TONE
Impulses from the vagus nerve producing inhibition of the heartbeat.

VAGINA
A muscular tube belonging to the female genital organs, measuring about 8 cm (3 inches) in length. When a woman stands erect, the vagina does not descend vertically but is directed downward and forward from the uterus at an angle of about 70 degrees.

It receives the penis during coitus, ejaculation of semen usually occurring in the upper vagina, from where the sperm move upward to fertilize the ovum.

The vagina is normally sufficiently elastic to allow the passage of a child.

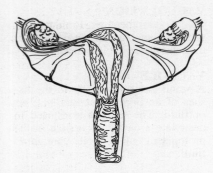

Schematic anterior section of the female genital organs. The vagina connects the uterus with the outside world.

VAGINAL DISCHARGE

A common gynecological disorder characterized by distressing, often whitish, non-bloody discharge from the genital tract.

A complaint regarding vaginal discharge may represent merely the woman's perception of normal secretions or the presence of disease, and the source of the discharge may be anywhere in the genital tract.

VAGINAL HYSTERECTOMY

A hysterectomy (surgical removal of the uterus) performed through the vagina.

VAGINAL SMEAR

A smear taken from the vaginal mucosa for cytologic diagnosis.

VAGINAL THRUSH

Candidiasis of the vagina or vulva.

VAGINISMUS

Spasm of the vagina as a conditioned contraction of the lower vaginal muscles resulting from a woman's unconscious desire to prevent penetration. Since intromission is often impossible, vaginismus is frequently seen in cases of unconsumated marriage. Some women with vaginismus enjoy clitoral orgasms.

VAGINITIS

Any type of vaginal infection. It is usually characterized by an abnormal vaginal discharge and symptoms such as vaginal pain, itching, painful intercourse and painful urination.

One out of every two women consulting a gynecologist is suffering from vaginitis.

There are many possible causes. Infections that cause it include:
- candidiasis (yeast infection), often seen after antibiotic treatment, during pregnancy or in people with diabetes;
- sexually transmitted infections such as trichomoniasis, herpes infections, chlamydia infection and gonorrhea.

Atrophic vaginitis, caused by lack of estrogen hormone, is seen after menopause.

Use of vaginal creams, douches and sprays can cause a contact dermatitis or allergic reaction. The treatment depends on the cause.

VAGINODYNIA

Neuralgic pain in the vagina.

VAGINOSCOPE

An instrument and especially a speculum used to examine the interior of the vagina; *vaginoscopy*: visual examination of the vagina with a special inspection instrument. This may be a speculum or an optical instrument.

VAGOTOMY

Surgical division of the vagus nerve, sometimes performed in the treatment of peptic ulcer.

VAGOTONIA

Hyperirritability of the parasympathetic part of the autonomic nervous system.

VAGOTROPIC

Drug or substance acting selectively upon the vagus nerve.

VAGOVAGAL

Relating to or arising from both afferent and efferent impulses of the vagus nerve.

VAGUS
The tenth cranial nerve, a mixed nerve containing both sensory tracts and motor tracts. It supplies the soft palate, back of the throat and voice box and also the non-striped muscles of the respiratory and alimentary tracts.

VAGUS PULSE
A slow pulse due to the inhibitory action of the vagus nerve on the heart.

VALENCY
The combining power of an element or radical, which may be defined as the number of atoms of hydrogen (or its equivalent) that one atom of the element or one radical will combine with or displace.

VALERIAN
(*Valeriana officinalis*) Fragrant valerian, a perennial plant, about 2 to 4 feet high, which has escaped from cultivation to inhabit roadsides and thickets.
   A sedative tonic can be prepared from the rootstock.

VALGUS
A term used to denote position, a turning outwards.
   The term is used specifically to denote a deformity in which an anatomical part is turned outward away from the midline of the body to an abnormal degree, as a deformity of the ankle.

VALINE
One of the eight essential amino acids. It affects the nervous system and body coordination.

VALLATE
A brim surrounding a depression; papillae with taste buds on the back part of the tongue.

VALSALVA'S MANEUVER
Attempts to forcibly exhale with the glottis, nose and mouth closed. It the eustachian tubes are not obstructed the pressure on the tympanic membranes will be increased. The maneuver can also be done with just the glottis closed, but only intrathoracic pressure will be increased. This causes increased intrathoracic pressure, slowing of the pulse, decreased return of blood to the heart and increased venous pressure.

VALUE
The measure of how strongly something is desired for its physical or moral beauty, usefulness, rarity, etc., especially expressed in terms of the effort one is willing to expend in acquiring, retaining possession of, or preserving it.

VALVE
A flap of tissue which prevents backflow of blood to keep it moving through the heart and circulatory system in the right direction. There are tiny valves along the inside of the veins and four large valves at the entrances and exist of the ventricles in the heart.

VALVE OF THEBESIUS
Valve of the coronary sinus in the right atrium of the heart.

VALVOTOMY
Surgical cutting of a heart valve to overcome an obstruction (stenosis) to the flow of blood.

VALVULA
A small valve or fold, as the valvula coli.

VALVULAR INSUFFICIENCY
Valves which close improperly and permit a backflow of blood in the wrong direction.

VALVULOTOME
An instrument for incising a valve.

VALVULOTOMY
Process of cutting through a valve, as a rectal fold which is too rigid or a heart valve which is constricted by connective tissue.

VANILLA
A commercially important extract of the vanilla bean that is prepared by soaking comminuted vanilla beans in water and ethyl alcohol and that is used especially as a flavoring in pharmaceutical preparations.

VANILLIC ACID
An odorless crystalline phenolic acid found in some varieties of vanilla, formed by the oxidation of vanilla, and used chiefly in the form of esters as food preservatives.

VANILLISM
Irritation of the skin, mucous membranes and conjunctivae sometimes experienced by workers handling vanilla. It is caused by a mite.

VANILLYLMANDELIC ACID
Approximately 90 percent of the catechol-amines adrenalin and noradrenalin are metabolized to vanillylmandelic acid and are secreted in the urine. Persons with pheochromocytoma produce excess amounts of catecholamines; this vanillylmandelic acid is present in urine in an increased amount.

VAPOR
A substance in gaseous state but below its critical temperature, and so liquefiable by pressure alone; a liquid, especially water, dispersed and suspended in the air in the form of very small drops.

VAPOR DENSITY
The density of a vapor or gas by comparison with that of some standard.

VAPORIUM
Apparatus for applying hot, cold or medicated vapors for bronchitis.

VAPORIZATION
Therapeutic use of a vapor.

VAPORIZER
Device for converting liquids into a vapor spray.

VARIANT
An individual or species deviating in some character or characters from type.

VARIATION
Change in an organism or species due either to environmental conditions, or to herediry, or to mutation.

VARICELLA
Another name for chicken pox.

VARICELLA-ZOSTER
A herpesvirus that causes chicken pox and herpes zoster.

VARICOCELE
Dilation of the veins running down each side of the scrotum, forming a soft elastic swelling that feels like a collection of worms under the skin, and more prominent on the left side than on the right.

VARICOCELECTOMY
Excision of a portion of the scrotal sac with ligation of the dilated veins to relieve varicocele.

VARICOSE
Resembling or having the characteristics of a varix.

VARICOSE ULCER
A chronic ulcer of the skin due largely to malnutrition of the skin resulting from stagnant venous congestion by varicose veins. Popularly called a leg ulcer.

VARICOSE VEINS
Enlarged, swollen and knotted condition of the veins, usually observed

in the legs. Early symptoms include feelings of heaviness and fatigue in the legs, especially during the evening or menstruation. Swelling and pain occur later.

VARICOTOMY
Surgical removal of a varicose vein.

VARIOLA
Any of several virus diseases, as smallpox or cow pox, marked by a pustular eruption.

VARUS
Relating to, or being a deformity of a bodily part characterized by bending or turning inward toward the midline of the body to an abnormal degree.

VAS
Original latin term for a vessel, either a lymph vessel of a blood vessel. Vasa is the plural form of vas.

VASCULAR
Pertaining to the blood vessels.

VASCULAR AREAS
Scattered areas developed between endoderm and mesoderm of the yolk sac, beginning of primitive blood vessels.

VASCULAR BED
An intricate network of minute blood vessels that ramifies through the tissues of the body or of one of its parts.

VASCULAR HEADACHE PREVENTATIVES
Medicines prescribed to prevent the occurrence of or reduce the frequency and severity of vascular headache such as migraine.

VASCULARITY
The quality of being vascular.

VASCULARIZATION
Development of new blood vessels

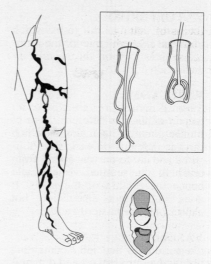

The occurrence of varicose veins in the lower extremity.

in a structure or organ in the body. The term is also used to denote the process of becoming vascular. Sometimes the term is used for the abnormal or excessive formation of blood vessels, as in the retina or the cornea.

VASCULAR SENSATION
A sensory complex, attending abrupt changes in cutaneous circulation, and circulation changes in the underlying tissues as in blushing.

VASCULAR SYSTEM
The total of arteries, veins and capillaries.

VASCULATURE
The arrangement of arteries and veins in the body or any part of it, including their relationship and functions.

VASCULITIS
Inflammation of blood vessels, which is often segmental and may be generalized or localized, constituting the basic mechanism of the production of lesions in a variety of rheumatic diseases and syndromes.

VAS DEFERENS
Excretory duct of the testis which joins the excretory duct of the seminal vesicle to form the ejaculatory duct.

VASECTOMY
Surgical division or resection of all or part of the vas deferens; form of family planning in males in which the vas deferens on each side is ligated and cut to prevent sperm from reaching the seminal vesicles and hence the urethra of the penis. It does not affect ejaculation but causes permanent sterilization.

VASELINE
Cream, lotion and jelly containing petrolatum, mineral oil and dimethicone as active ingredients. This preparation is clinically proven to help healing clapping, scaling, raw cracked skin, redness, soreness and itching caused by severely dry skin.

VASOCONSTRICTION
Narrowing of blood vessels, facilitating control of blood pressure and body temperature.

VASOCONSTRICTOR
A drug that narrows blood vessels often prescribed to reduce nasal congestion. Vasoconstrictors are also frequently given with injected local anesthetics. Ephedrine is a commonly-prescribed vasoconstrictor.

VASODEPRESSSOR
An agent that depresses circulation; also: having a depressing influence on the circulation, lowering blood pressure by dilatation of blood vessels.

VASODILANTIN
Product of protein disintegration corresponding in properties with histamine.

VASODILATION
Widening of blood vessels, facilitating control of blood pressure and body temperature.

VASODILATOR
Causing the dilatation of blood vessels; an agent that causes dilatation of the blood vessels.

VASOGRAPHY
X-ray photography of the blood vessels.

VASOMOTOR
Nerves supplying muscles in the wall of blood vessels and regulating the caliber (diameter) of blood vessels, through containing both vasoconstrictor and vasodilator fibers.

VASOMOTOR CENTER
Center in the brain stem which is supposed to control muscle tone in blood vessels.

VASOMOTOR RHINITIS
A chronic rhinitis characterized by intermittent vascular engorgement of the mucous membrane of the nose, sneezing and watery discharge from the nose.

The treatment is empirical and not always satisfactory.

Persons benefit from humidified air, e.g., from a humidified heating system or vaporizer in the workroom and bedroom. Drugs such as ephedrine give symptomatic relief but are not recommended for regular long-term use.

VASOPRESSIN
Antidiuretic hormone (ADH), hormone produced by the hypothalamus and posterior pituitary gland, which is a mild vasoconstrictor, but primarily inhibits diuresis or loss of water in urine. It is a vital link in the system for preserving the homeostasis or constancy of body fluids.

VASOSPASM
Spasm of any vessel, especially of a blood vessel.

VASOVAGAL SYNCOPE
A usually transitory condition that is marked by anxiety, nausea, respiratory distress and fainting and that is believed to be due to joint vasomotor and vagal disturbances.

VASOVASOSTOMY
Surgical anastomosis of a divided vas deferens to reverse a previous vasectomy.

VASOVESICULITIS
Inflammation of the vas deferens and the seminal vesicles.

VAS SPIRALE
A large blood vessel beneath the tunnel of Corti in the basilar membrane.

VASTUS
One of three muscles of the thigh; part of the quadriceps muscle.

VASTUS INTERMEDIUS
The division of the quadriceps muscle that arises from and covers the front of the shaft of the femur.

VASTUS LATERALIS
A division of the quadriceps muscle that covers the outer anterior aspect of the femur, arising chiefly from the femur, and inserting into the outer border of the patella by a flat tendon which blends with that of the other divisions of the muscle and sends an expansion to the capsule of the knee.

VASTUS MEDIALIS
A division of the quadriceps muscle that covers the inner anterior aspect of the femur, arising chiefly from the femur and the adjacent intermuscular septum, inserting into the inner border of the patella and into the tendon of the other divisions of the muscle, sending also a tendinous expansion to the capsule of the knee joint, and that is closely and in the upper part often inseparably united with the vastus intermedius.

VATER'S AMPULLA
Dilation of the united common bile duct and pancreatic duct.

VD
Abbreviation for venereal disease.

VECTOR
(1) An agent that transmits a pathogen from one organism to another either mechanically or as a carrier (for instance, the housefly for typhoid) or biologically, with a role in a life cycle (for instance, the mosquito for the malaria parasite); (2) a quantity that is specified by magnitude, direction and sense, that may be represented in some reference system by an orientated arrowed line segment whose length is a simple function of the magnitude.

VECTORCARDIOGRAM
Electrocardiogram represented by vectors. At any moment the electrical activity of the heart can be represented as an electrical vector with a specific direction and magnitude. These vectors may be established for the entire heart cycle.

VEGETARIAN
A person who abstains from eating meat, either keeping strictly to a vegetable, grains, nuts and fruits diet, or also eating eggs, milk, butter and cheese.

VEGETARISM
The restriction of one's food to substances of vegetable origin. A vegetarian who abstains from eating eggs, milk, butter and cheese is called an ovo-lacto-vegetarian.

VEGETATION
A morbid luxurious outgrowth on any part, especially wartlike projections made up of collections of fibrin in which are enmeshed white and red blood cells, sometimes seen on denuded areas of the endocardium covering the valves of the heart.

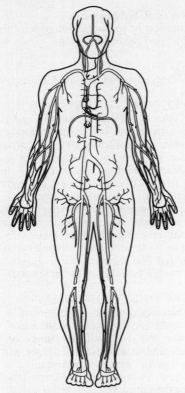

Schema of the venous system of the body.

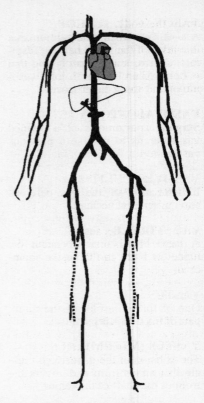

The major veins of the human body.

VEHICLE
A fluid used as a medium for a suspension of a pigment; a substance with which the active agent of a medicine is compounded.

VEIN
(Latin: vena) Vessel carrying dark red (unsaturated) blood to the heart, except for the pulmonary vein, which carries oxygenated blood. Like arteries, veins have three coats in their walls. There is, however, very much less muscle and elastic tissue and the wall is much thinner in proportion to the diameter of the vessel.

VEIN SCAN
Scanning procedure performed after intravenous injection of a radiopharmaceutical, to detect blood clots or inflammation.

VELUM
A membrane or structure similar to a veil.

VENA CAVA
Either of two large veins by which the blood is returned to the right atrium of the heart.

VENA CAVA INFERIOR
A vein that is the largest vein in the body, is formed by the union of the two common iliac veins at the level of the fifth lumbar vertebra, and returns blood to the right atrium of the heart from bodily parts below the diaphragm.

VENA CAVA SUPERIOR
A vein that is the second largest

vein in the body, is formed by the union of the two innominate veins at the level of the space between the two first ribs, and returns blood to the right atrium of the heart from bodily parts above the diaphragm.

VENEREAL
Pertaining to or produced by sexual intercourse. The word originates from the Latin for Venus, goddess of love.

VENEREAL DISEASES
Those infectious diseases transmitted mainly or exclusively by sexual contact, usually because the organism responsible is unable to survive outside the body and the close contact of genital organs provide the only means for transmitting viable organisms.

VENEREAL WARTS
Warts caused by sexually transmitted viruses. Women with monilia seem to have a higher incidence of contracting them, probably because the Ph changes make the vagina more susceptible.

VENEREOLOGIST
A doctor who specializes in the treatment of venereal or sexually transmitted diseases.

VENEREOLOGY
The scientific study and treatment of venereal or sexually transmitted diseases.

VENEREOPHOBIA
Neurotic dread of sexual intercourse; fear of being infected with venereal disease.

VENESECTION
The taking of blood from a vein.

VENIPUNCTURE
A surgical puncture of a vein especially for the withdrawal of blood or for intravenous medication.

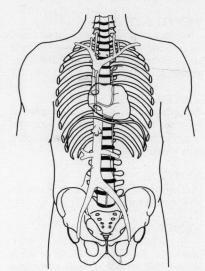

Upper (vena cava superior) and lower (vena cava inferior) caval veins. Both transport venous blood to the right atrium.

VENOGRAPHY
A radiographic procedure that shows the internal structures of veins after the patient receives an injection of contrast medium.

VENOM
Poison, particularly that secreted by certain snakes, reptiles and insects.

VENOUS BLOOD
The dark type of blood found in the veins.

VENOUS HUM
The murmur heard on listening over a vein.

VENOUS PRESSURE
The pressure of blood within the veins.

VENOUS SINUS
A large vein or passage, as the canal of schlemm, for venous blood.

VENTER
A belly-shaped part; the cavity of the abdomen; a wide swelling part or belly of a muscle.

VENTILATION
Circulation of air or amount of fresh air in a room and withdrawal of foul air. The term is also used for oxygenation of blood.

VENTILATION SCAN
Procedure in which the person breathes in radioactive gas and the lungs are scanned for areas that don't receive air.

VENTRAL
Pertaining to or situated on lower or abdominal surface.

VENTRAL HORN
A longitudinal subdivision of gray matter in the anterior party of each lateral half of the spinal cord that contains neurons giving rise to motor fibers of the ventral roots of the spinal nerves.

VENTRAL ROOT
The one of the two roots of a spinal nerve that passes anteriorly from the spinal cord separating the anterior and lateral funiculi and that consists of motor fibers.

VENTRICLE
One of the cavities within the heart or the brain. In the heart there are two ventricles (left and right); in the brain there are four ventricles filled with cerebrospinal fluid.

VENTRICULAR FIBRILLATION
An irregular and chaotic ventricular arrhythmia with a rapid rate and disorganized spread of impulses throughout the ventricular heart muscle.

Acute myocardial infarction is the most common cause.

VENTRICULAR TACHYCARDIA
A regular ventricular rhythm with broad QRS complexes in the electrocardiogram and a rate between 100 and 200 beats per minute.

VENTRICULO-ATRIOSTOMY
The surgical establishment of a shunt to drain cerebrospinal fluid, as in hydrocephalus, from a ventricle of the brain to the right atrium.

VENULE
Small vein of vessel conducting venous blood from the capillaries to a vein.

VERBALISM
The use of words which sound well but have little content in reality, or an instance of this.

VERDOHEMOGLOBIN
A greenish pigment occurring as an intermediate product in the formation of bilirubin from hemoglobin.

VERMICIDE
A chemical compound for destroying intestinal worms.

VERMICULAR
Resembling a worm in appearance or movement.

VERMIFORM APPENDIX
A long, worm-shaped tube connected to the cecum. It varies in length from 2 to 20 cm with an average of 8 cm. Its distal end is closed. It is lined with mucosa similar to that of the large intestine. Inflammation of it is called appendicitis.

VERMIS
Either of two annulated median portions of the cerebellum:
(1) one slightly prominent on the upper surface, called superior vermis;
(2) one of the lower surface sunk in the vallecula, called also inferior vermis.

VERNIX CASEOSA
A hand-cream-like sebaceous substance which protects the fetal skin in the uterus and may be seen at birth.

VERRUCA

Tumor of the epidermis of the skin; it produces a circumscribed elevated area of hypertrophy of the papillae.

VERRUCA ACUMINATA

A pointed reddish wart about the genitals and the anus. It develops near mucocutaneous junctures, forming pointed, tufted or pedunculated, pinkish or purplish projections of varying lengths and consistency.

VERRUCA DIGITATA

Form seen on the face and the scalp, possibly serving as starting point of cutaneous horns, forming several filiform projections with horny caps closely grouped on a comparatively narrow base which in turn may be separated from the skin surface by slightly contracted neck.

VERRUCA FILIFORMIS

Small thread-like growth on the neck or the eyelids, covered with smooth and apparently normal dermis.

VERRUCA PLANTARIS

Warts on the soles of the feet.

VERRUCA VULGARIS

Common warts, usually on the back of the hand and fingers but may occur anywhere on the skin.

VERSION

Altering the position of the fetus in the uterus. This is done in order to facilitate delivery.

VERTEBRA

Any of the 33 bones forming the spinal column or spine. They comprise seven cervical (neck) vertebrae, twelve thoracic or dorsal (chest) vertebrae, five lumbar (in the small of the back), five sacral, which are fused together to form the sacrum (the rear wall of the pelvis), and four coccygeal vertebrae, which

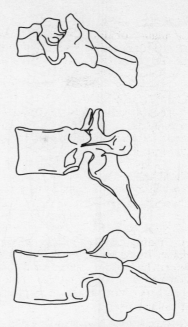

Lateral view of three characteristic vertebrae. From top to bottom: cervical, thoracic, and lumbar vertebra.

are fused together to form the coccyx (the vestige of a tail in the human).

VERTEBRAL

Relating to a vertebra.

VERTEBRAL ARTERY

A large branch of the subclavian artery that ascends through the foramina in the transverse processes of each of the cervical vertebrae except the last one or two, entering the cranium through the foramen magnum, and uniting with the corre-

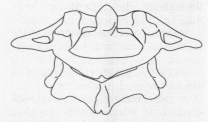

Atlas and axis. The vertebral artery runs through a hole in the transverse process.

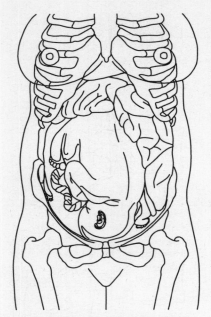

Vertex presentation of a fetus in the uterus.

sponding artery of the opposite side to form the basilar artery.

VERTEBRAL COLUMN
Spine, spinal column.

VERTEBRAL FORAMEN
The opening formed by a neural arch through which the spinal cord passes.

VERTEBRAL GANGLION
Any of a group of sympathetic ganglia which form two chains extending from the base of the skull to the coccyx along the sides of the spinal column.

VERTEBRAL NOTCH
Either of two concave constrictions of which one occurs on the inferior surface and one on the superior surface of the pedicle on each side of a vertebra and which are arranged so that the superior notches of one vertebra and the corresponding inferior notches of a contiguous vertebra combine to form an invertebral foramen on each side.

VERTEBRA PROMINENCE
The seventh cervical vertebra characterized by a prominent spinous process which can be felt at the base of the neck.

VERTEBRATION
Division into segments or parts resembling vertebrae.

VERTEX
The crown of the head.

VERTEX PRESENTATION
The normal presentation with the back part of the skull presenting at the mouth of the womb.

VERTIGO
A disturbance in which the individual has a subjective impression of movement in space or of objects moving around him, usually with a loss of equilibrium.

The vertigo, as distinguished from faintness, lightheadedness or other form of dizziness, results from a disturbance somewhere in the equilibrium or balance system in the ear. Treatment depends on determining and eliminating the cause.

VESICA
The bladder.

VESICA FELLEA
The gallbladder.

VESICAL PLEXUS
A plexus of nerves that comprises preganglionic fibers derived chiefly from the hypogastric plexus and postganglionic neurons whose fibers are distributed to the bladder and adjacent parts.

VESICLE
Dermatologic condition characterized by a circumscribed, elevated lesion less than 5 mm in diameter, containing serous fluid. Vesicles are commonly caused by primary irritants, allergic contact dermatitis,

physical trauma, sunburn, insect bites or viral infections.

VESICO-URETERAL REFLUX
Reflux of urine from the bladder into the ureter. The disorder predisposes to damage of the upper urinary tract by bacteria, infection and by increased hydrostatic pressure. The condition is most often due to congenital malimplantation of the ureter into the bladder.

VESICULA
A vesicle (blister or small bladder).

VESICULAR
Relating to or composed of vesicles.

VESICULAR BREATHING
The sound produced by air entering and leaving healthy lungs, the normal sound of breathing heard through the stethoscope.

VESICULAR DERMATITIS
A severe dermatitis characterized by vesicle formation.

VESICULASE
An enzyme from secretion of prostate gland, capable of coagulating contents of seminal vesicles.

VESICULITIS
Inflammation of a vesicle (small bladder), especially of a seminal vesicle (the storage sac for semen).

VESTIBULAR
Of or relating to the vestibule of the inner ear, the vestibular apparatus.

VESTIBULAR APPARATUS
The vestibule of the inner ear together with the end organ and nerve fibers that function in mediating the labyrinthine sense.

VESTIBULAR GANGLION
A sensory ganglion in the trunk of the vestibular nerve in the internal auditory meatus that contains cell bodies supplying nerve fibers comprising the vestibular nerve.

VESTIBULAR GLAND
Any of the glands (as the Bartholin's glands) that open into the vestibule of the vagina.

VESTIBULAR LIGAMENT
The narrow band of fibrous tissue contained in each of the false vocal cords and stretching between the thyroid and arytenoid cartilages.

VESTIBULAR MEMBRANE
A thin cellular membrane separating the scala media and scale vestibuli.

VESTIBULAR NERVE
A branch of the auditory nerve that consists of bipolar neurons with cell bodies collected in the vestibular ganglion, with peripheral processes passing to the semicircular canals, utricle, and saccule, and with central processes passing to the vestibular nuclei of the medulla oblongata.

VESTIBULAR NUCLEUS
Any of four nuclei in the medulla oblongata on each side of the floor of the fourth ventricle of the brain in which fibers of the vestibular nerve terminate.

VESTIBULE
A cavity leading into another cavity or passage, as the cavity of the ear labyrinth; the space between the labia minora containing the opening of the urethra; the portion of the ventricle of the heart directly below the opening of the aortic arch.

VESTIBULUM
Any vestibule, but frequently the vestibule of the ear.

VESTIGE
A small degenerate or imperfectly developed organ or part which may have been complete and functional in some ancestor.

VESTIGIAL
Small and imperfectly developed.

VESTIGIAL ORGAN
An anatomical structure which is non-functional and frequently underdeveloped in a modern species but which represents the remnant of an organ which in the remote past was fully functional in an ancestor species; for instance, the vermiform appendix in humans.

VIABILITY
Ability to live after birth. Refers principally either to premature labor or Cesarean operations performed before them.

VIBRATOR
Device for causing artificial vibration of the body or its parts.

VIBRATORY
Having a vibrating or oscillatory movement. The vibratory sense is defined as the ability to perceive vibrations transmitted through the skin to deep structures. Usually tested by placing a vibrating tuning fork over bony prominences.

VIBRISSAE
The hairs that grow from inside the nostrils. Also refers to the whiskers of animals such as the cat.

VICARIOUS
Taking the place of something else; a habitual discharge occurring in an abnormal situation.

VICIOUS CIRCLE
A course of action in which the result achieved defeats the purpose of the act; a combination of problems or disorders which aggravate one another; often said of inflammation that cannot be controlled by antibiotics.

VILLUS
A minute, elongated projection from the surface of a mucous or other membrane. Whilst villi occur in several parts of the body, those most commonly referred to are the intestinal villi which project into the lumen of the small intestine.

VIOLENCE
The use of force or physical compulsion. It may be expected in acute delirious mania. After epileptic furor, patients have no memory of their violent attacks. Many attacks of violence may be averted by recognizing warning signs and by knowing the person.

VIOLINIST'S CRAMP
A nervous disorder affecting violin players and marked by spasms of the fingers.

VIRAL DISEASES
Generally infectious diseases due to viruses. The common cold, influenza, chickenpox, measles and German measles are common in childhood, while yellow fever is an important tropical virus disease. AIDS is an important sexually transmitted viral disease.

Viruses may also cause specific organ disease such as:
- hepatitis;
- encephalitis;
- meningitis;
- myocarditis;
- pericarditis.

Most virus diseases are self-limited and mild, but there are few specific drugs effective in cases of severe illness. Prevention by vaccination is therefore crucial.

VIRGIN
A person who has not had sexual intercourse, especially a girl or a woman.

VIRILE
Having characteristics of a mature male.

VIRILE REFLEX
Sudden downward movement of the

penis when the prepuce or glans of a completely relaxed penis is pulled upward.

The term is also used for the contraction of the bulbocavernosus muscle on percussing the dorsum of the penis.

VIRILESCENCE
The acquisition of masculine characteristics in the female.

VIRION
A virus particle, consisting of a protein coat, called a capsid, and a nucleic acid core.

VIROID
Ultramicroscopic entity or symbiont theoretically existing in living organisms, and able to give rise to viruses by mutation. A viroid is regarded as the smaller known agent of infectious disease: short strands of RNA.

They cause several plant diseases and possibly are implicated in enigmatic diseases of man.

VIROLOGY
The study of viruses, their growth, development, and relationships to disease.

VIRULENCE
The capacity of a given organism or group of organisms to introduce disease of various degrees of severity.

VIRUS
A small particle that is not living and does not exhibit signs of life but which can reproduce itself within a living cell. A virus reproduces by infecting a host cell, and taking over the nucleic acid of that host cell, making more virus nucleic acid and protein. As new virus particles develop, the host cell bursts, releasing the new virus particles.

VISCERA
The plural of viscus, any one of the organs situated in the chest or abdomen.

The term applies particularly to the organs of the abdominal cavity, such as the liver, spleen, kidneys, pancreas, gallbladder, urinary bladder, stomach and intestines.

VISCERAL
Pertaining to a viscus or viscera.

VISCERALGIA
Neuralgia (pain in the course of a nerve) of any of the viscera.

VISCOSITY
The condition of being viscous. It normally refers to the flow rate of a fluid, that is, its ability to flow fast or slow.

VISIBLE SPECTRUM
The part of the electromagnetic spectrum to which the human eye is sensitive extending from a wavelength of about 400 nm for violet light to about 700 nm for red light.

VISION
The special sense concerned with reception and interpretation of light stimuli reaching the eye; the principle sense in humans.

VISUAL
Relating to vision.

VISUAL ACUITY
The degree of discrimination, as of separation of points of apprehension of form, of which the eye is capable.

VISUAL AIDS
Devices to assist understanding or memory by displaying what is to be understood or memorized in a visible form.

VISUAL ANGLE
The angle subtended at the eye by any visual object, upon which the magnitude of the retinal image depends.

VISUAL APPERCEPTION TEST

A projective technique for use with subjects 12 years of age and older. The subject is presented with 12 plates consisting of lines randomly drawn under controlled conditions and is asked to color in whatever object or pattern he sees in the doodles and title the finishing drawing.

VISUAL FIELD

The area within which objects may be seen when the eye is fixed.

VISUAL ORGANIZATION

The complex relationships existing among the various elements of the visual field, reflecting the fact that the phenomenal visual field always appears patterned and meaningful.

VISUAL PROCESS

Activity of the organism contributing to seeing; operations of the eye, nerve tract and brain centers involving seeing.

VISUAL PROJECTION

The process involving the attribution of objective location to a visually perceived object.

VISUAL PURPLE

An organic pigment of the retina (visual coat of the eye) which is bleached to yellow by light. It is a protein closely related to vitamin A and is called erythropsin or rhodopsin.

VISUAL WHITE

The product of visual yellow irradiated by ultraviolet light.

VITAL CAPACITY

The volume of air that can be breathed out from the lungs after a complete respiration.

VITAL FORCE

Form of bodily energy manifested in living phenomena when considered distinct from chemical, physical, and mechanical forces.

VITALISM

The theory, dating from Aristotle, that there is a distinguishing vital principle ("life force") in living organisms that is absent from non-living objects.

VITAL STATISTICS

Statistics of births, deaths, marriages and diseases.

VITAMER

Compound having a chemical structure and physiological effect similar to that of a natural vitamin.

VITAMIN

(from the Latin vita = life, + amine). Any of a group of organic substances other than proteins, carbohydrates, fats, minerals, and organic salts which are essential for normal metabolism, growth and development of the body. Vitamins are not sources of energy nor do they contribute significantly to the substance of the body, but they are indispensable for normal functions and the maintenance of health.

VITILIGO

Piebald skin, a skin disorder marked by a loss of the natural pigment in patches, leaving white areas.

VITREOUS CHAMBER

The part of the eyeball situated behind the lens.

VITREOUS HUMOR

The transparent jelly-like substance which fills the vitreous chamber of the eye.

VITREOUS MEMBRANE

The innermost layer of the connective tissue sheath surrounding a hair follicle. The term is also used for the inner membrane of the choroid.

VITREOUS TABLE

The inner layer of the compact tissue characteristic of most of the bones of the skull.

VITRIFICATION
Condition of cells or organisms instantaneously frozen but able to resume all vital activities on being thawed out.

VITUS' DANCE, ST
A functional nervous disorder causing muscular spasms.

VIVISECTION
Strictly, the dissection of living animals, usually, in the source of physiological of pathological research; however, the use of the term is often extended to cover all animal experimentation. Although the practice remains the subject of considerable popular controversy, it is doubtful whether research, particularly medical research, can be effectively carried on without a measure of vivisection.

VOCABULARY TEST
A type of mental test which aims at the determination of an individual's store of understood words; usually given by presenting the subject with a standard list of words, which he is required to define, or indicate which of a number of words given is nearest in meaning.

VOCAL CORD NODULES
Nodules caused by chronic voice abuse, such as screaming or shouting, or using an unnaturally low fundamental frequency. The nodules are condensations of hyaline connective tissue. Hoarseness and a breathy voice quality result.

Treatment involves surgical removal of the nodules and correction of the underlying voice abuse. Vocal nodules in children usually regress with voice therapy alone.

VOCAL CORDS
Two cords situated within the larynx (voice box), controlled by muscles, which open and close to produce alterations in sound.

VOCAL FREMITUS
The vibration which the doctor feels when he places his hand on the patient's chest and asks him to say "ninety-nine."

VOCAL IMMATURITY
Voice disorder due to the inhibition of laryngeal growth, usually caused by dysfunctioning of the sex glands, and characterized by a voice of higher than normal frequency.

VOCAL LIGAMENT
A strong band of elastic tissue lying within the vocal folds.

VOCAL MUSCLE
The inner portion of the thyreoarytenoid muscle which lies in the vocal lip lateral to and in contact with the vocal ligament.

VOICE
The sound emitted in speech, the method of communication exclusive to Homo sapiens. It is dependent for its generation upon the passage of air from the lungs through the trachea, larynx, pharynx and mouth and its quality in each individual is largely determined by the shape and size of these structures and the resonance of the nose and nasal sinuses.

VOLAR
Pertaining to the palm or sole.

VOLITION
The conscious adoption by the individual of a line of action; self-conscious activity towards a determined end, manifested primarily as decision and intention.

VOLKMANN'S CANALS
Simple canals piercing circumferential or periosteal lamellae of bone, for blood vessels, and joining the haversian canal.

VOLKMANN'S CONTRACTURE
Degeneration, contracture, fibrosis and atrophy of a muscle resulting from injury to its blood supply, usually seen in the hand.

VOLUNTARY
Controlled by the will.

VOLVULUS
A twisting of the bowel upon itself so as to cause obstruction, occurring most frequently in the sigmoid flexure (that part of the colon above the rectum).

VOMER
The thin plate of bone forming the back part of the nasal septum (the partition between the nostrils).

VOMITING
The forceful expulsion of gastric contents produced by involuntary contraction of the abdominal musculature when the gastric fundus and lower esophageal sphincter are relaxed.

VON WILLEBRAND'S DISEASE
A hereditary bleeding disorder with a prolonged bleeding time and a mild to severe factor VIII deficiency, inherited as an autosomal dominant treat. It is one of the commonest hemorrhagic diatheses. Mild bleeding into the skin and mucosa, characteristic of a vascular or platelet disorder, is common. Treatment is provided by commercially produced factor VIII.

VORTEX
Spiral arrangement of muscle fibers at the apex of the heart; spiral arrangement of hairs.

VOYEURISM
The condition of becoming sexually aroused by looking at unsuspecting women who are naked, in the act of disrobing or engaging in sexual activity. The essential feature of this condition is a repetitive seeking-out of these situations. Orgasm usually produced by masturbation may occur during the voyeuristic activity. The voyeur does not initiate further sexual contact.

VULNERABILITY
Susceptible to injury or infection.

VULVA
The external genital organs at the opening of the vagina consisting of the labia minora and the labia majora (the fleshy lips on each side of the vagina). Usually a part of the vulva are the anus (rectal opening) and the pubic hair.

VULVITIS
Inflammation of the vulva, caused by trauma, mechanical and chemical irritations, neglect of hygiene, urinary, vaginal or fecal contamination or local allergic reactions to clothing, detergents or drugs. Parasitic infections are common.

VULVOVAGINITIS
Inflammation of both the vulva and the vagina at the same time, or of the vulvo-vaginal glands.

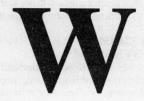

W

WAARDENBURG'S SYNDROME
Genetic disorder characterized by white forelock, deafness, hypertelorism and heterochromia of the iris. Less than 20 percent of cases have significant hearing loss. Some, with none of the features except white forelock, have had children with serious congenital deafness.

WACHENDORF'S MEMBRANE
A thin membrane occluding the pupil of the embryo.

WAGSTAFF'S FRACTURE
Fracture with separation of the internal malleolus of the ankle.

WAIST
Narrow part of the human body between ribs and hips.

WAISTLINE
The waist of the human body, considered with respect to position or size.

WAKEFUL
Unable to sleep, marked by lack of sleep.

WALCHER'S POSITION
Position in which the patient assumes dorsal recumbent position with the hips at the edge of the bed and the legs hanging down.

WALDEYER'S RING
The ring of tonsillar (lymphatic) tissue which encircles the nasopharynx and the oropharynx. The ring consists of the two palatine tonsils, lingual and pharyngeal tonsils.

WALKING CASTE
A cast that is worn on a patient's leg and has a stirrup with a heel or other supporting device embedded in the plaster to facilitate walking.

WALLENBERG'S SYNDROME
A complex of symptoms resulting from occlusion of the posterior inferior cerebellar artery or one of its branches supplying the lower portion of the brain stem. The following symptoms may result:
- dysphagia;
- muscular weakness or paralysis;
- impairment of pain and temperature senses;
- cerebellar dysfunction.

WALLERIAN DEGENERATION
The fatty degeneration of the process of a nerve cell cut off from the cell body, which results in a condition that takes on certain stains, so that its course can be traced in a series of microscopic sections.

WALLEYE
Eye in which the iris is light-colored or white. The term is also used to denote leukoma or dense opacity of the cornea.

WANGENSTEEN'S METHOD
Technique for relieving postoperative abdominal distention, nausea, vomiting and certain cases of mechanical bowel obstruction. It involves the use of an intranasal catheter in combination with a suction siphonage apparatus.

WARDROP'S OPERATION
Ligation of an artery for aneurysm at a distance beyond the sac.

WARM SPOT
A small area of cutaneous surface,

peculiarly sensitive to punctuate stimulation by objects above body temperature.

WARM-UP
The act or an instance of warming up; a procedure, as a set of exercises, used in warming up. A warm-up usually consists of a set of stretching exercises.

WAR NEUROSIS
Neurosis caused by an experience connected with warfare in an emotionally unstable person so disposed to react in such a way.

WARTS
Common, contagious benign epithelial tumors caused by papovaviruses. Viral warts may occur at any age, but are most frequent in older children and uncommon in the aged.

WASSERMAN REACTION
The complement-fixing reaction that occurs in a positive complement-fixation test for syphilis using the serum of an infected individual.

WASSERMANN TEST
A test of a sample of blood or cerebrospinal fluid for the presence of syphilitic infection.

WASTE PRODUCTS
Material, for instance, feces, excreted from a living human or animal body.

WASTING
Undergoing or causing decay or loss of strength; tuberculosis is a wasting disease.

WATER BALANCE
The ratio between the water assimilated into the body and that lost from the body. The term is also used to designate the condition of the body when this ratio approximates unity.

WATER BLISTER
A blister with a clear watery content that is not purulent or sanguineous.

WATERHOUSE-FRIDERICH–SEN SYNDROME
Blood vessel collapse and shock accompanying meningitis. A prodromal respiratory illness or sore throat often precedes the fever, headache, stiff neck and vomiting that characterizes acute meningitis.

Adults become desperately ill within 24 hours; the course can be even shorter in children. In older children and adults, changes in consciousness progress through irritability, confusion, drowsiness, stupor and coma.

WAVELENGTH
The distance, measured parallel to the path of propagation of a wave, between any point and the next successive points of maximum of minimum amplitude on the wave form.

WEAKNESS
A feeling of lack of strength; common to many problems but especially prominent in certain of the more serious illnesses.

While certain diseases are characterized by weakness of only some of the muscles, others are accompanied by generalized weakness as well as by a feeling of fatigue or tiredness.

WEANING
Psychological term for breaking up of a fixation or transference situation.

WEANLING
A young child or infant recently changed from breast to formula feeding.

WEANLING DIARRHEA
Severe gastroenteritis which sometimes occurs in infants who recently have been weaned.

WEB

A tissue or membrane, resembling a piece of cloth in the process of being woven on a loom or just taken off the loom.

WEBER-CHRISTIAN DISEASE

Relapsing, febrile, nodular, non-suppurative panniculitis; a generalized disorder of fat metabolism characterized by recurring episodes of fever and development of crops of subcutaneous fatty nodules.

WEBER-FECHNER LAW

An approximately accurate generalization in psychology: the intensity of a sensation is proportional to the logarithm of the intensity of the stimulus causing it.

WEBER'S TEST

Test to determine the nature of the unilateral hearing loss in which a vibrating tuning form is held against the forehead at the midline and conduction deafness is indicated if the sound is heard more loudly in the affected ear and nerve deafness is indicated if it is heard more loudly in the normal ear.

WECHSLER ADULT INTELLI-GENCE SCALE

An updated version of the Wechsler-Bellevue test having the same structure but standardized against a different population to more accurately reflect the general population.

WECHSLER-BELLEVUE TEST

A test of general intelligence and coordination in adults that involves both verbal and performance tests and is now superseded by the Wechsler Adult Intelligence test.

WEDGE RESECTION

Any of several surgical procedures for removal of a wedge-shaped mass of tissue, as from the ovary or a lung.

WEIGHTLESSNESS

The condition of a body arising when there is no apparent gravitational pull upon it.

WEIGHT TRACTION

That exerted by means of a weight connected to a limb to maintain a fractured bone in position during recovery.

WEIL-FELIX TEST

A test to determine the presence of typhus and other rickettsial diseases. It is an agglutination test for various rickettsial infections as typhus and scrub typhus, using particular strains of bacteria of the genus proteus that have antigens in common with rickettsias to be identified.

WEIL'S DISEASE

An inclusive term for all infections due to an organism of the genus Leptospira. The disease is a zoonosis, occurring in several domestic and wild animal hosts and varies from inapparent illness to fatal disease.

A carrier state exists in which animals shed leptospiras in their urine for months. Human infections occur by direct contact with an infected animal's urine or tissue, or indirectly by contact with contaminated water or soil.

Abrased skin and exposed mucous membranes (conjunctival, nasal or oral) are the usual portals of entry in humans.

The main symptoms are:
- jaundice;
- hemorrhages;
- anemia;
- disturbances in consciousness;
- continued fever.

Antibiotics are effective in experimental infections, but their value in humans is uncertain.

WELT

An elevation on the skin produced by a lash, blow or an allergic stimulus. The skin is unbroken and the mark is reversible.

WELTSCHMERZ
A conviction of sadness of things, dissatisfaction with the world as it is mingled with yearning for an ideal world.

WEN
A slowly growing benign cystic tumor of the skin containing follicular, keratinous and sebaceous material and frequently found on the scalp, ears, face, back or scrotum. On palpation, the cyst is firm, globular, movable and non-tender. It seldom causes discomfort unless infected.

The treatment may consist of a small surgical procedure by which the contents are evacuated; then the cyst wall is removed through the incision with a curette or hemostat.

WENCKEBACH PERIODICITY
Deviation in the normal electrocardiogram by which the P-R interval progressively lengthens until finally one P wave fails to result in a QRS complex. The cycle then repeats.

WERNER'S SYNDROME
A hereditary disorder characterized by premature aging with associated abnormalities as dwarfism, cataracts, osteoporosis, and hypogonadism.

WERDNIG-HOFFMANN DISEASE
Another name for infantile spinal muscular atrophy.

WERLHOF'S DISEASE
A blood disorder characterized by thrombocytopenia without a readily apparent exogenous cause or underlying disease and marked by increased destruction of platelets.

WERNICKE AREA
The area in the first and second convolutions of the temporal lobe of the left hemisphere (in right-handed persons), identified as the cerebral center for hearing and understanding of spoken language.

WERNICKE'S APHASIA
Loss or impairment of the capacity to use words correctly. Sometimes the words are uttered fluently but inappropriately, as a form of jargon.

WERNICKE'S SIGN
An eye sign which occurs in cases where there is blindness in one half of the visual field. If a light is shone on the blind half there is no pupil reaction, but if shone on the good half the pupil contracts, indicating that the disease process is situated in front of the geniculate bodies of the brain.

WERNICKE'S SYNDROME
Loss of memory and other symptoms associated with senility. Also called presbyophrenia.

WESTERGREN METHOD
A method for estimating the sedimentation rate of red blood cells in fluid blood by observing the level to which the cells fall in one hour in a tube of 2 to 2.5 mm bore that is 300 mm long and is graduated downward in mm from 0 to 200 when 4.4 ml of venous blood is mixed with 0.3 ml of 3.8 percent aqueous solution of sodium citrate.

WET LUNG
Respiratory failure with life-threatening respiratory distress and hypoxemia, associated with various acute lung injuries. The condition is part of the acute respiratory distress syndrome.

WET NURSE
A woman who cares for and suckles young not her own.

WET PLEURISY
Pleurisy with effusion of exudate into the pleural cavity.

WHARTON'S DUCT
The duct of the submaxillary gland in the mouth.

WHARTON'S JELLY
A gelatinous intercellular substance consisting of primitive connective tissue of the umbilical cord. It is rich in hyaluronic acid.

WHEAL
Dermatologic condition characterized by a transient, elevated lesion caused by local edema. Wheals are a common allergic reaction; for instance, from drug eruptions, insect stings or bites or sensitivity to cold, heat, pressure or sunlight.

WHEEZE
A whistling or sighing sound resulting from narrowing of the lumen of a respiratory passageway. Often only noted by the use of a stethoscope. A wheeze may occur in asthma, croup, hay fever, mitral stenosis and pleural effusion. It may also result from a tumor, foreign obstructions, bronchial spasms, obstructive emphysema or edema.

WHIPLASH
A form of neck injury resulting when the head is rapidly shaken back and forth. The symptoms are the following:
- pain and stiffness in the neck;
- inability to bend the neck forward, backward or to the side without pain;
- sometimes headache

The cause is a rapid shaking of the head back and forth that causes stretching of the ligaments and muscles of the neck. The severity of the problem is variable and can be worsened if there is already degenerative joint disease in the cervical spine. Treatment consists of rest, prevention of movement at the neck.

WHIPPLE'S DISEASE
An illness occurring predominantly in males aged 30 to 60, characterized clinically by;
- anemia;
- skin pigmentation;
- joint symptoms (arthralgia and arthritis);
- weight loss;
- diarrhea;
- severe malabsorption.

The typical presentation is malabsorption in an adult male with additional features of polyarthritis, disorders of the lymphatic apparatus and abnormal pigmentation. Untreated the disease is progressive and fatal. Many different types of antibiotics are curative.

WHIPWORM INFECTION
Another name for trichuriasis.

WHITE BLOOD CELLS
One of the three kinds of formed elements found in the blood. There are various types of white blood cells. Their best-known function is defense: they destroy foreign bodies, such as bacteria, in areas of infection. Also called leukocytes.

WHITE COMMISSURE
Anterior commissure, a transverse band of white matter forming the floor of the median ventral fissure of the spinal cord.

WHITE MATTER
Parts of the central nervous system (brain and spinal cord) consisting mainly of myelinated nerve fibers, giving a characteristic white appearance.

WHO
Abbreviation of World Health Organization.

WHOOPING COUGH (PERTUSSIS)
Long, contagious preventable respiratory infection with characteristic cough. It usually affects infants and children who are not immunized against it, but it can affect adults

who are no longer immune. The disease can be prevented by immunization with the diphtheria-tetanus-pertussis (DTP) vaccine.

WIDAL REACTION
A blood test used in typhoid fever. It is a specific reaction consisting in agglutination of typhoid bacilli or other salmonellas when mixed with serum from a patient having typhoid fever or other salmonella infection and constituting a test for the disease.

WILLIS' CIRCLE
A circle of arteries situated at the base of the brain at the back of the skull.

WILM'S TUMOR
A malignant tumor of the kidney observed in early childhood.

WILSON'S DISEASE
There are two diseases known by this name. One is a rare progressive disease of the nervous system named after the neurologist S.A.K. Wilson.

The other disease, named after the dermatologist W.J.E. Wilson, is an inflammatory reaction of the skin characterized by shedding of its surface.

This condition sometimes follows the administration of certain drugs, such as the sulphonamides, and poisoning by such substances as arsenic. It is also known as exfoliative dermatitis.

WINTER DEPRESSION
Depression occurring solely in the winter period. Although the cause of the condition is not clear, it is suspected that it is tied to disturbances in circadian rhythms, the internal rhythms that orient a person to cycles in the environment, such as the day-night cycle, the phases of the moon or the seasons. Most sufferers are in their twenties and thirties and did not experience the con-

dition when they were children. Specific dosages of light during certain times of the day may alleviate the condition.

WINTER ITCH
Itching occurring only in cold weather. Probably due to drying of the skin which is deficient in natural lubrication.

WINTON DISEASE
Cirrhosis of the liver resulting from the chronic poisoning by toxic constituents of ragwort and other noxious plants.

WISDOM TOOTH
Four molar teeth which complete the permanent set in humans, erupting later.

WISH FULFILLMENT
The realization of the aim of a Freudian wish or impulse, whether that is an acknowledged wish or impulse or not.

WISHFUL THINKING
Acceptance of the thought that conditions are as an individual would wish them to be, and rejection of the thought that they are otherwise.

WISKOTT-ALDRICH SYNDROME
A sex-linked recessive disorder with a defect of lymphocytic cell function, characterized by eczema and blood disorders.

WITCH'S MILK
Milk that sometimes appears in the breasts of newborn babies.

WITHDRAWAL DELIRIUM
A alcohol delirium that develops after recent cessation of or reduction in an alcohol consumption, usually within one week.

Marked autonomic hyperactivity, often indicated by tachycardia and sweating, is present. Vivid hallucinations, which may be visual, auditory, or tactile, are common. Delusions and agitated behavior are also frequently present. There may be a course, irregular tremor.

WITHDRAWAL SYNDROME

The development of a substance-specific syndrome that follows the cessation or reduction in, intake of a psychoactive substance that the person previously used regularly. The syndrome that follows varies according to the psychoactive substance that person was using. Common symptoms include:
- anxiety;
- restlessness;
- irritability;
- insomnia;
- impaired attention.

The nature of the psychoactive substance determines the associated features, which may range from physiologic symptoms, such as nausea and vomiting following cessation of heavy alcohol intake, to diffuse malaise, such as that following chronic use of certain sedatives, or a compelling desire to resume taking the substance. There may be changes in sleep patterns and mood, as can be seen after withdrawal from amphetamines, or convulsions after sedative withdrawal.

WOLFF-PARKINSON-WHITE SYNDROME

A form of premature excitation of the ventricles (lower chambers) of the heart which may be permanent, transient or paroxysmal.

WOLMAN'S DISEASE

A familial condition characterized by enlargement of the liver and spleen, fatty stools and adrenal calcification. Large amounts of neural lipids accumulate in the body tissues. There is no specific therapy, and death usually occurs by six months of age.

WOMB

Uterus, female reproductive organ which is specialized for implantation of the egg and development of the embryo and fetus during pregnancy.

The regular turnover of its lining under the influence of estrogen and progesterone is responsible for menstruation.

WORD-ASSOCIATION TEST

A test of personality and mental function in which the subject is required to respond to each of a series of words with the first one that comes to mind or with one of a specified class of words.

WORD BLINDNESS

Inability to understand written or printed words.

WORD DEAFNESS

Inability to understand the spoken word.

WORD SALAD

A jumble of meaningless words, used by some persons suffering from a psychosis, especially schizophrenia.

WORK-LOSS DAY

A day on which a person did not work at his or her job or business for at least half of his or her normal workday because of a specific illness or injury.

WORLD HEALTH ORGANIZATION (WHO)

Specialized agency of the United Nations founded in 1948; based in Geneva. Its services are available to all nations and territories.

WHO advises countries on how to develop health services, combat epidemics and promote health education and standards of nutrition and sanitation. It also coordinates the standardization of drugs and health statistics, and studies pollution.

WORM

Any disruption by physical means

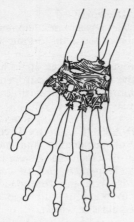

Posterior view of the wrist with its numerous ligaments.

of the continuity of the body's external or internal surfaces.

WOUND

An injury to the body constituting of a laceration or breaking of the skin or mucous membrane usually by a hard or sharp instrument forcefully driven or applied. The term is also to an opening made in the skin or a membrane of the body incidental to a surgical operation or procedure.

WOUND CULTURE

A culture done on a sample of wound drainage to determine the presence of disease-causing organisms.

WRENCH

A sharp twist or sudden jerk straining muscles or ligaments.

WRIGHT'S STAIN

A stain that is a modification of the Romanowsky stain and is used in staining blood and parasites living in blood.

WRISBERG'S GANGLION

A small ganglion that sometimes occurs in the superficial part of the cardiac plexus at the right side of the ligamentum arteriosum.

WRIST

The part connecting the forearm and the hand, consisting of eight carpal bones and their ligaments. Also called the carpus.

WRISTBONE

The styloid process of the radius in man that forms a prominence on the outer side of the wrist above the thumb.

WRISTDROP

Inability to bend the hand backwards due to paralysis of the extensor muscles. It is characteristic of lead poisoning but may occur in other ailments.

WRITER'S BLOCK

A psychological inhibition preventing a writer from proceeding with a piece of writing.

WRITING TREMOR

Shaky movements in writing, arising from a variety of causes, such as senility, intoxication, writer's cramp, disorders of the brain, etc.

WRYNECK

Another name for spasmodic torticollis.

X

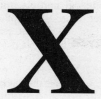

XANTHEMIA
The presence of yellow pigments in the blood.

XANTHELASMA
Flat or slightly raised yellowish tumor occurring in elderly persons, found most frequently on the upper and lower eyelids, especially near the inner canthus.

XANTHELASMOIDEA
Chronic disease of childhood marked by wheals and followed by brownish-yellow patches.

XANTHINE
A nitrogenous extractive contained in muscle tissue, liver, spleen, pancreas and other organs and in the urine, formed during the metabolism of nucleotides.

XANTHINE-DERIVATIVE BRONCHODILATORS
Medicines used to treat the symptoms of bronchial asthma, chronic bronchitis, and emphysema. These medicines relieve cough, wheezing, shortness of breath, and troubled breathing. They work by opening up the bronchial tubes or air passages of the lungs and increasing the flow of air through them.

XANTHINE OXIDASE
A crystallizable flavoprotein enzyme containing iron and molybdenum that promotes the oxidation of hypoxanthine and xanthine to uric acid and of many cellular aldehydes to acids.

XANTHINES
Substances that stimulate muscle tissue, especially that of the heart. Types of xanthines include aminophylline, caffeine, diphylline, oxtriphylline, theophylline.

XANTHOCHROMIA
Yellow discoloration of the skin in patches or of the cerebrospinal fluid, resembling jaundice.

XANTHOCYTE
A cell containing yellow pigment.

XANTHODERMA
A yellow color of the skin.

XANTHOGRANULOMA
A tumor having characteristics of both an infectious granuloma and a xanthoma.

XANTHOMA
A disorder characterized by the presence of yellow nodules on the skin, and due to disturbance of lipoid (fat) metabolism.

XANTHOMATOSIS
A disorder of lipoid (fat) metabolism characterized by excessive deposits of lipoids in the body.

XANTHURENIC ACID
A yellow crystalline acid, closely related to kynurenic acid and excreted in the urine when tryptophan is added to the diet of experimental animals deficient in pyridoxine.

X-CHROMOSOME
A chromosome associated with sex-determination. It occurs simply in males, in duplicate in the normal female.

X-DISEASE
Any of various usually virus diseases of obscure etiology and relationships, as a viral encephalitis and meningitis of man first detected in Australia.

XENODIAGNOSIS
The detection of a parasite (as of man) by feeding a suitable intermediate host (as an insect) on supposedly infected material (as blood) and later examining it for the parasite.

XENOGENESIS
The supposed production of offspring completely unlike either parent.

XENOGENOUS
Originating outside the organism; caused by external stimuli.

XENOGRAFT
A tissue or organ graft between members of two distinct or different species.

XENOMENIA
Menstruation from a part of the body other than the normal one.

XENON
A heavy, colorless, and relatively inert gaseous element that occurs in air as about one part in 20 million by volume.

XENOPHOBIA
A neurotic dread of strangers or foreigners or people of foreign origin.

XENOPHONIA
Alteration in accent and intonation of a person's voice due to a defect of speech.

XENOPHTHALMIA
Traumatic conjunctivitis (inflammation caused by injury to the conjunctiva, the membrane lining the eyelids).

XENOPLASTIC
Graft established in a different host.

XENOREXIA
An abnormality of appetite marked by persistent swallowing of foreign subjects.

XENOTROPIC
Replicating or reproducing only in cells other than those of the host species. One speaks of xenotropic viruses.

XERODERMA
Dry skin; a disease characterized by dry, harsh, scaly, discolored skin, which rubs off as a dust. Also called ichthyosis.

XERODERMA PIGMENTOSA
A rare disease of the skin starting in childhood marked by disseminated pigment discolorations, ulcers, cutaneous and muscular atrophy and death.

XEROGRAPHY
X-ray method of soft tissues. The method is mainly used for diagnostic procedures of the breast. A fine calcified stippling in the area of the lesion is suspicious of cancer and may occasionally be seen even without a palpable mass. However, a negative mammogram made with xerographical methods does not rule out malignancy.

XEROPHTHALMIA
Eye condition caused by retinol deficiency. Primary deficiency is usually caused by prolonged dietary deprivation. Secondary deficiency may be due to inadequate conversion of carotene, or to interference with absorption, storage or transport in celiac disease, sprue, cystic fibrosis, operations on the pancreas, duodenal bypass, obstruction of the bile ducts and cirrhosis of the liver.

The eye disorders may be irreversible and lead to blindness. The earliest, rod dysfunction, can be detected by various specialized methods. Prevention is by vitamin A preparations.

XEROSIS
Excessive dryness of the skin or conjunctival membrane (lining of the eyelids).

XEROSTOMIA
Dryness of the mouth caused by the arresting of normal salivary secretion. It occurs in diabetes, hysteria, paralysis of facial nerve involving chorda tympani, acute infections, some types of neuroses and is induced by certain drugs as nicotine and atropine.

XIPHODYNIA
Pain in the xiphoid cartilage at the lower end of the sternum.

XIPHOIDITIS
Inflammation of the xiphoid (or ensiform) cartilage at the lower end of the sternum (breastbone).

XIPHOID PROCESS
The lowest portion of the breastbone or sternum, a sword-shaped cartilaginous process supported by bone. It has no ribs attached to it, but some of the abdominal muscles are attached to it. It ossifies in the aged.

X-LINKAGE
Transmission of a trait by a gene on the X-chromosome.

X-RAYS
Electromagnetic radiations produced by passing a high-voltage electric current through a vacuum tube with a cathode consisting of a spiral filament of incandescent tungsten and an anode of massive tungsten. The rays so produced being similar to the gamma rays emitted by radio-active substances. X-rays can penetrate tissues and are used both for taking photographs of the internal structures of the body and for the treatment of some skin conditions and deeplying growths.

X-RAY THERAPY
Medical treatment, as of cancer, by controlled application of X-rays.

XX-MALE
Genetic syndrome closely resem-

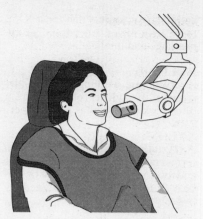

Apparatus for X-raying the teeth and temporomandibular joint.

bling Klinefelter's syndrome. It is rare and probably not associated with mental retardation.

XXX-SYNDROME
Genetic syndrome characterized by the presence of three X-chromosomes. These individuals have three X-chromosomes and two Barr bodies or sex chromatin masses. Though sterility sometimes occurs, several XXX normal females have had offspring who have been both chromosomally and phenotypically normal.

XXXX-SYNDROME
Genetic syndrome characterized by the presence of four X-chromosomes in somatic cells. Although rare, these females show no consistent phenotype, though the risk of mental retardation and congenital abnormalities increase markedly with an increase in the number of X-chromosomes, especially when there are more than 3.

XXY-SYNDROME
Relatively common genetic disorder occurring in about 1:700 live male births. The typical affected individual is tall and eunuchoid, with small, firm testes and gynecomastia. However, clinical variation is great,

and it is now known that most XXY (47,XXX) males are normal in appearance and intellect.

XYLITOL
A crystalline alcohol that is a derivative of xylose, obtained from birch bark, and used as a sweetener.

XYLOSE
A crystalline aldose sugar that is not fermentable with ordinary yeasts and occurs as a constituent of xylans from which it is obtained by hydrolysis.

XYLULOSE
A ketone sugar of the pentose class that plays a role in carbohydrate metabolism and is found in the urine in cases of pentosuria.

XYROSPASM
Occupational neural disorder of the fingers seen in barbers.

XYY-SYNDROME
Genetic disorder characterized by the presence of one X- and two Y-chromosomes in males.

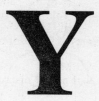

YAGE
A powerful hallucinogenic beverage prepared from any of several tropical plants of the genus Banisteriopsis of the family Malphighiaceae.

YANG
Masculine principle; the masculine and positive principle (as of activity, height, light, heat, or dryness) in nature that according to traditional Chinese cosmology combines and interacts with its opposite yin to produce all that comes to be.

YAWNING
An involuntary gaping open of the mouth, often accompanied by involuntary stretching of the muscles and accompanied by a deep inspiration. It usually occurs during the drowsy state produced by a fatigue or boredom and is a prelude to sleep.

YAWS
Disease caused by Treponema pertenue. It produces lesions in the skin, bone and cartilage, but not in deeper tissues or organs. Like other pathogenic treponema, it is easily killed by drying, exposure to oxygen and elevated temperature.

Yaws is transmitted by direct (person-to-person) non-sexual contact with the exudate or serum from infectious yaws lesions.

Y-CARTILAGE
Cartilage joining ilium, ischium and pubes in the acetabulum.

Y-CHROMOSOME
A sex chromosome that occurs singly in the normal male, but is absent in the normal female.

YEAST
A substance found on the surface of fermenting sugary liquids containing actinomycetes, that multiply by budding and cause the fermentation of sugars, with the production of alcohol and carbon dioxide. The term is also used for any of various fungi that produce alcohol and carbon dioxide from sugar.

YELLOW BILE
The one of the four humors of ancient and medieval physiology that was believed to be secreted by the liver and cause irascibility.

YELLOW CARTILAGE
A cartilage with matrix invaded by yellow or elastic connective tissue fibers.

YELLOW ENZYME
A combination of riboflavine, a protein and phosphoric acid, essential in the respiratory mechanisms of cells. The name is also applied to any of several flavoprotein respiratory enzymes widely distributed in nature.

YELLOW FEVER
An acute arbovirus infection of variable severity, characterized by:
- sudden onset;
- fever;
- relatively slow pulse;
- headache;
- albuminuria;
- jaundice;
- hemorrhage, especially hematemesis.

The virus of urban yellow fever is transmitted by the bite of Aedes aegyptii mosquito infected two weeks previously by feeding on a person with a high concentration of virus in the blood.

Active immunization with live attenuated yellow fever vaccine effectively prevents outbreaks and spo-

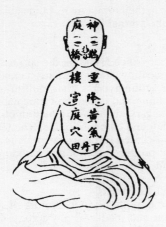 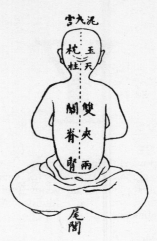

Old Chinese pictures explaining the principles of Yin and Yang.

radic cases. Management is supportive and direct toward alleviating major symptoms. Complete bedrest and nursing care is important. Hemorrhagic tendencies will be combatted with calcium gluconate. Transfusion with heparin will be considered if there is evidence of disseminated intravascular coagulation.

YELLOW-FEVER MOSQUITO
A small dark-colored mosquito of the warmer parts of the world that is the usual agent in the transmission of yellow fever.

YELLOW SPOT
(1) Yellowish nodule of the anterior end of the vocal cord.
(2) Center of the retina, the point of clearest vision.

YERSINIA
A genus of gram-negative bacteria of the Enterobacteriaceae that includes several important pathogens, as the plaque bacterium Yersinia pestis.

YIN
The feminine and negative principle (as of passivity, depth, darkness, cold, wetness) in nature that according to traditional Chinese cosmol-

ogy combines with its opposite yang to produce all that comes to be.

YIN AND YANG
Two forces through whose essences, according to Taoist cosmology, the universe was produced and cosmic harmony is maintained. Yin is dark, female and negative, and Yang is light, male and positive.

YOGA
(1) Union of the individual self with the universal spirit;
(2) a major orthodox system of Hindu philosophy based on Sankhya but differing from it in being theistic and method of liberating the self;
(3) the suppression through progressive discipline of all activity of the body, mind, and individual will in order that the self may realize its distinction from them and attain liberation from all pain and suffering;
(4) a system of exercising for attaining bodily or mental control and well-being;
(5) a discipline by which the individual prepares himself for liberation of the self and union with the universal spirit.

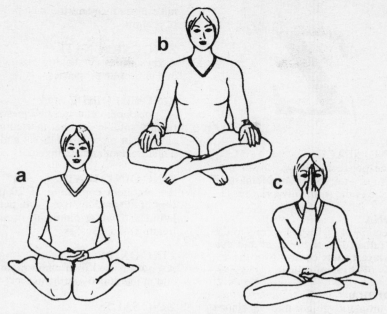

Yoga-postures. Breathing exercises: a: deep breathing; b. inhalation and exhalation; c: breathing through the nose.

YOGHURT
A fermented slightly acid often flavored semisolid food made of whole or skimmed cow's milk and milk solids to which cultures of bacteria of the genus Lactobacillus (Lactobacillus bulgarius) and Streptococcus (Streptococcus thermophilus) have been added.

YOGI
A person who practices yoga; in particular, an ascetic seeking self liberation through bodily and mental disciplines, as of posture, breathing, or concentration, and sometimes credited with supernormal powers.

YOHIMBINE
An alkaloid that is a weak blocker of alpha-adrenergic receptors and has been used as an aphrodisiac.

YOLK
Material stored in an ovum that supplies food to the developing embryo and consists chiefly of proteins, lecithin, and cholesterol.

YOLK SAC
Membranous sac attached to the embryo and containing yolk which passes to the intestine through the vitelline duct and acts as food for the developing embryo.

YOUNG-HELMHOLTZ THEORY
A theory in color vision: the eye has three different and separate elements each of which is stimulated by a different primary color.

Y-SHAPED LIGAMENT
The iliofemoral ligament.

ZANG' SPACE
Space between the two lower tendons of the sternocleidomastoid muscle in the supraclavicular fossa.

Z-DNA
A section of DNA that spirals to the left rather than to the right and that may exert some control over the activity of adjacent genes.

ZEDORA
An aromatic ginger-like substance made from the rootstock of East Indian plants of the genus Curcuma and used in medicine and perfumery.

ZELOTYPIA
Morbid or monomaniacal zeal in the interest of any project or cause.

ZEN
A form of Mhayana Buddhism emphasizing the value of meditation and intuition.

ZENKER'S DEGENERATION
A glassy or waxy, hyaline degeneration of skeletal muscle in acute infectious diseases, especially typhoid.

ZEOLITE
Any of various hydrous silicates that can act as ion-exchangers; any of various natural or synthesized silicates of similar structure used in water softening and as adsorbents.

ZINC
A mineral needed for the utilization of carbohydrates, production of

male hormones and the metabolism of protein.

ZINC CARBONATE
A crystalline salt having astringent and antiseptic properties.

ZINC CHLORIDE
A poisonous caustic deliquescent readily soluble salt that is used as a catalyst in organic synthesis and as a disinfectant and astringent.

ZINC OINTMENT
An ointment consisting of 20 percent of zinc oxide mixed with petrolatum and white ointment, used in treating skin diseases.

ZINC OXIDE
A powder used as a white pigment and in medicinal ointments.

ZINC SALTS
A bluish-white metal used to make various containers and also to galvanize iron to prevent rust. The most commonly used compounds are zinc oxide as a pigment for paints, in ointments and in chloride and sulphate which resemble Epsom salts.

ZINC SULPHATE TURBIDITY TEST
A test done to determine the gamma globulin
concentration in blood increased in infection, allergy and auto-immune illnesses, and decreased in some leukemias, cancers and hypo-immune conditions.

ZINC SUPPLEMENTS
Preparations containing zinc as nutritional supplement such as egozinc, orazinc, verazinc, zinc gluconate, zinc sulfate, zincate.
  Zinc supplements are used to:
(1) treatment of zinc deficiency that may lead to growth retardation, appetite loss, changes in taste or smell, skin eruptions, slow wound healing, decreased immune func-

tion, diarrhea or impaired night vision.

(2) In absence of a deficiency, the preparations are used to treat burns, eating disorders, liver disorders, prematurity in infants, intestinal diseases, parasitism, kidney disorders, skin disorders and stress.

(3) Zinc supplements may be useful as a supplement for those who are breast-feeding or pregnant (under a doctor's supervision).

ZOLLINGER-ELLISON SYNDROME

A syndrome characterized by marked hypergastrinemia, gastric hypersecretion and peptic ulceration. Usually there is a specific tumor in the pancreas.

ZOMBIE

A dull or apathetic person. The term is also used to designate a corpse said to be revived by witchcraft.

ZONA

Another name for herpes zoster.

ZONA ARCUATA

The inner part of the basilar membrane, supporting the spiral organ of Corti.

ZONA GLOMERULOSA

The outermost of the three layers of the adrenal cortex that consists of round masses of granular epithelial cells that stain deeply.

ZONA GRANULOSA

Granular zone around the ovum in the Graafian follicle in the ovary, formed by cells of the membrana granulosa.

ZONA ORBICULARIS

Circular fibers of the capsule of the hip joint, around the neck of the femur.

ZONA PECTINATA

Outer division of the basilar membrane of the cochlea.

ZONA PELLUCIDA

Thick transparent membrane surrounding the ovum in the ovary.

ZONA RADIATA

Radially striated inner egg envelope.

ZONA RETICULARIS

The innermost of the three layers of the adrenal cortex that consists of irregularly arranged cylindrical masses of epithelial cells.

ZONE THERAPY

Therapy called reflexology.

ZONESTHESIA

A sensation like that produced by a tight girdle encircling the waist. Also called a girdle pain.

ZONULA CILIARIS

The hyaloid membrane forming the suspensory ligament of the lens of the eye.

ZONULE OF ZINN

The suspensory ligament of the crystalline lens of the eye; also called ciliary zonule.

ZOOLAGNIA

Sexual interest and attraction to animals.

ZOONOSES

Diseases common to humans and animals. They include the following:
Bacterial diseases
– anthrax;
– brucellosis;
– leptospirosis;
– pasteurellosis;
– salmonella;
– staphylococcal and streptococcal infections;
– tuberculosis
Fungal infections
– ringworm
Protozoal infections
– toxoplasmosis
Parasitic infections

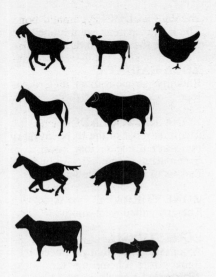

Many animals act as vectors for human diseases. Helminths are common in mammals; birds may cause various kinds of viral diseases.

- worms;
- hydatid diseases;
- fleas;
- lice;
- scabies.

ZOOGENOUS
Produced or caused by animals.

ZOOPHILIA
Sexual excitement produced by the act or phantasy of engaging in sexual activity with animals as the preferred or exclusive method. The animal is preferred even when other forms of sexual outlet are available.

Shame, guilt and social isolation with depression, anxiety and loneliness may result from the intense and persistent desire to engage in this extremely rare form of sexual activity.

ZOOPHOBIA
Morbid fear of animals.

ZOOPLASTY
Transplantation of animal tissue to humans.

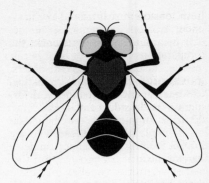

Flies may be vectors for various infectious diseases.

ZOOPSIA
Hallucinations of vision taking the form of animals.

ZOOTOXINS
Those produced by animals. They include snake venom and the poisons of spiders.

ZOSTER AURICULARIS
Herpes zoster of the ear.

ZOSTER OPHTHALMICUS
Herpes affecting the ophthalmic nerve, a major branch of the trigeminal nerve.

Z-PLASTY
A technique with a Z-shaped incision used in plastic surgery to re-

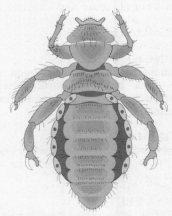

Lice may be carriers of plague.

lieve tension in scar tissue. The area under tension is lengthened at the expense of the surrounding elastic tissue.

ZUCKERKANDL'S BODIES
Chromaffin tissue of paraganglia lying on each side of the fetal abdominal aorta.

ZYGAPOPHYSIS
Any of the articular processes of the neural arch of a vertebra of which there are usually two anterior and two posterior.

ZYGOCITY
The number of ova from which a pair of twins are derived; the condition of monozygotic or dizygotic.

ZYGODACTYLY
Fusion of two or more fingers or toes.

ZYGOMA
The bony arch of the cheek formed by connection of the zygomatic and temporal bones.

ZYGOMATIC BONE
A bone of the side of the face below the eye that forms part of the zygomatic arch and part of the orbit and articulates with the temporal, sphenoid, and frontal bones and with the maxilla of the upper jaw.

ZYGOMATIC NERVE
A branch of the maxillary nerve that divides into a facial branch supplying the skin of the prominent part of the cheek and a temporal branch supplying the skin of the anterior temporal region.

ZYGOMATIC PROCESS
Any of several bony processes that articulate with the zygomatic bone as:
(1) a long slender process of the temporal bone helping to form the zygomatic arch;
(2) a narrow process of the frontal bone articulating with the zygomatic bone;
(3) a rough triangular eminence of the maxilla of the upper jaw articulating with the zygomatic bone.

ZYGOTE
Cell produced by the fusion of two gametes and which contains the diploid chromosome number. The offspring is produced by mitotic division of the zygote to give 2, 4, 8, 16, 32 etc, cells.

ZYMASE
Enzyme complex found in yeast which catalyzes the alcoholic fermentation of carbohydrates.

ZYMOGEN
A substance capable of being transformed into a ferment; for instance precursor of an enzyme.

ZYMOGENESIS
The production of an enzyme by a zymogen activated by a kinase.

ZYMOPROTEIN
Any of the proteins having catalytic capacity.

ZYMOSIS
Reactions induced by an enzyme or enzymes.

ZYMOSTHENIC
Enhancing the activity of an enzyme.